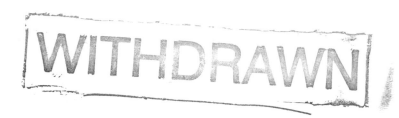

PHARMACEUTICAL DOSAGE FORMS

PHARMACEUTICAL DOSAGE FORMS

Disperse Systems

In Three Volumes
VOLUME 1
Second Edition, Revised and Expanded

EDITED BY

Herbert A. Lieberman

H. H. Lieberman Associates, Inc.
Livingston, New Jersey

Martin M. Rieger

M. & A. Rieger Associates
Morris Plains, New Jersey

Gilbert S. Banker

University of Iowa
Iowa City, Iowa

Marcel Dekker, Inc.   **New York•Basel•Hong Kong**

Library of Congress Cataloging-in-Publication Data

Pharmaceutical dosage forms—disperse systems / edited by Herbert A. Lieberman,
    Martin M. Rieger, Gilbert S. Banker. — 2nd ed.
        p. cm.
    Includes bibliographical references and index.
    ISBN 0-8247-9387-0 (v. 1 : hardcover : alk. paper)
    1. Drugs—Dosage forms. 2. Dispersing agents. I. Lieberman, Herbert A.
II. Rieger, Martin M. III. Banker, Gilbert S.   [DNLM: 1. Dosage Forms.
2. Chemistry, Pharmaceutical. 3. Emulsions. 4. Suspensions. QV 785 P5349
1996]
RS200.P42   1996
615'.19—dc20
DNLM/DLC
for Library of Congress   96-15604
                                                                                       CIP

The publisher offers discounts on this book when ordered in bulk quantities. For more
information, write to Special Sales/Professional Marketing at the address below.

This book is printed on acid-free paper.

Marcel Dekker, Inc.
270 Madison Avenue, New York, New York 10016

Current printing (last digit):
10 9 8 7 6 5 4 3 2 1

PRINTED IN THE UNITED STATES OF AMERICA

Preface to the Second Edition

This second edition, which appears about eight years after the first, includes significant changes that further enhance the value of this series. The chapters contain about 25% new material, the references have been updated, and several new chapters have been added. As a result, the second edition now comprises three volumes rather than two.

Volume 1 of *Disperse Systems* covers the theoretical aspects involved in the formulation of many different types of disperse system drug products. In such products, an array of substances, the disperse phase, is distributed within another blend of chemical materials, identified as the continuous phase, or vehicle. Pharmaceutical disperse system products include: suspensions, emulsions, creams, aerosols, ointments, pastes, and suppositories. These dosage forms are administered by different routes, for example, oral, topical, ophthalmic, parenteral, respiratory, and rectal. The challenge in formulating disperse system products is the need to overcome their nonequilibrium state. A formula must be developed that provides the required energy barriers to delay the drug's rate of attaining thermodynamic equilibrium. To achieve the desired shelf life of the product, as well as to make the product as independent of processing variables as possible, the formulator must overcome some formidable obstacles. The concepts of equilibrium and surface and/or interfacial free energy form the basic framework necessary to formulate marketable disperse system products.

The chapter on the theory of suspensions describes several parameters involved in characterizing suspension-type products, particularly their classification, methods of preparation, and ways of achieving stable products. As in the first edition, the emphasis is on particle size and shape; there is also a new section on light-scattering techniques and improvements in microscopy. Different techniques for measuring particle size are compared. Methods used to study particles in other industries are described with the intent of encouraging the reader to apply them to the study and development of pharmaceutical products.

In this edition, the important topic of emulsification has been expanded. The fundamental relationships between droplet size and energy input per volume and time are emphasized. In practice, emulsification with only part of the continuous phase present, followed by addition of the remaining part after emulsification, has proven to be an excellent procedure for obtaining small internal phase droplets.

Colloids are a subject of growing importance in the field of disperse systems, in general, and in the design of colloidal drug delivery systems, in particular. The chapter on colloids has been updated with many new references relating to colloid theory and a discussion of the growing number of applications of colloids and pseudolatex polymer dispersions in drug product design and controlled-release medication.

The measurement of viscoelastic moduli and of mechanical properties of disperse system dosage forms has evolved considerably over the past two decades. Modern instrumentation now provides data to the formulator that previously were rarely measured. Mathematical models are included to illustrate how much rheological techniques have advanced to help pharmaceutical scientists to formulate and evaluate disperse dosage forms.

The interfacial effects of surfactants are required in diverse industrial processes and in the compounding of many health care and cosmetic products. The description of micelle structure has been de-emphasized, but a section on changes of micellar shape as a function of concentration has been added. The concept of the critical packing parameter in surfactant self-assembly and liposome formation is explored.

Polymers are employed in suspensions and emulsions to minimize or control sedimentation through an increase in viscosity. The viscosity-controlling agents may be either water-soluble or -insoluble, and only small amounts of the many different polymers discussed here are required to bring the viscosity of a liquid to almost any desired value.

A drug's efficacy critically depends on its bioavailability in any pharmaceutical dosage form. The chapter on bioavailability of disperse dosage forms has been extensively rewritten, reorganized, and enlarged to describe the physicochemical and the formulation factors that influence drug release from topical, oral, parenteral, ophthalmic, and rectal products. Drug delivery from some of the more recently developed microparticulate carriers is described.

Disperse system drugs must be adequately preserved, and awareness of the chemistry and microbiology of preservatives and their combinations is required. Information on the ever-changing regulatory and compendial concepts of preservative efficacy and safety are updated in the chapter on preservation. The inactivation (neutralization) of preservatives, both in the formulas and during efficacy testing, is again highlighted, and a procedure for validating preservative efficacy is now included.

The revised and updated chapter on experimental design, modeling, and optimization strategies provides an overview of current mathematical and statistical techniques and strategies useful for the development of pharmaceutical products. The techniques include statistically designed experiments, regression analyses, and optimization algorithms.

The chapter authors were chosen because of their expertise in their respective topics. We are particularly grateful for their cooperation in modifying and adding material to their chapters based on our suggestions. The editorial staff of Marcel Dekker, Inc., is due recognition for its help in bringing this volume to publication.

We hope that this volume, as well as others in the series, will prove invaluable in teaching and providing information to a broad range of industrial pharmacists and to others in related industries, academia, and government.

Herbert A. Lieberman
Martin M. Rieger
Gilbert S. Banker

Preface to the First Edition

Pharmaceutical Dosage Forms is the title of a series of books describing the theory and practice of product development associated with specific types of pharmaceutical products. The first three volumes describe tablets, and the two that follow are devoted to parenteral medications. This book is the first of two volumes that covers disperse system products, namely various types of liquid and semisolid emulsions, liquid and paste-like suspensions, and colloidal dispersions. A more specific product description of this type of pharmaceutical preparation would include: injectables, suppositories, aerosols, ingested and topically applied emulsions, abrasive pastes, such as toothpastes, and ingestable types of suspensions, such as liquid antacids.

Despite the diversity of disperse systems, there are unifying theoretical concepts that are applicable to all of them. Thus, the principles of rheology, of surface activity, and of the potential energy barriers to coalescence offer a systematic approach to an understanding of disperse systems. As a result, chapters with an emphasis on theory are included in the first volume of this two-volume treatise. From an understanding of these scientific fundamentals, product development formulators can develop their own approaches to the compounding of specific products. In addition, an understanding of theory and basic concepts may lead the development scientist to new ideas and technology necessary for novel drug delivery advances.

The pharmaceutical chemists, in developing a particular dosage form, must pursue many objectives. The integrity of the drug substance must be maintained; the pharmacological activity should be optimized; a uniform and consistent amount of drug must be dispensed throughout the lifetime of the product; the product must be physically and chemically stable as well as provide good user acceptance throughout its intended shelf and usage life. Successful completion of these objectives requires information on the practical aspects of formulation. Experienced practitioners have acquired this type of knowledge during many years of painstaking trials and errors. Therefore, for the second volume of this treatise, on formulation aspects, we chose as chapter contributors specialists in developing particular types of products.

A comprehensive book on disperse systems must teach two things: underlying principles and practical approaches. The novice requires detailed guidance, and the experienced formulator seeks information on new technologies and theories. Our task was to help select subject matter for this two-volume text to achieve these objectives. Thus, the book will teach the novice product development scientist the theoretical principles and practical aspects necessary for developing a disperse system product. In addition, the information is sufficiently comprehensive and extensive in order to offer knowledgeable formulators specific information that will enable them to achieve their goals.

Any multiauthor book includes redundancies. We deliberately did not strive to completely eliminate this type of duplication because authors may cover subjects from different points of view, which can help to clarify a particular subject matter. In fact, the background, experience, and bias of the various authors, in our opinion, help to contribute materially to learning and to broaden the comprehension of the subject matter for the reader.

We acknowledge the diligence with which the authors worked on their contributions. We also recognize gratefully the authors' forbearance in conforming with our numerous requests for modifications and additions. The real credit for this book belongs to each contributing author. On the other hand, the editors must assume the major responsibility for any criticism of the choice of subject matter in the text.

We sincerely hope that this book will be of help to students in the pharmaceutical sciences. In addition, we look for this book in the dosage form series to be a useful source of information for the product development specialists in the pharmaceutical industry, as well as others in related industries, academia, and government who have a need for this knowledge.

Herbert A. Lieberman
Martin M. Rieger
Gilbert S. Banker

Contents

Contributors

Daniel A. Alderman   Manager of Technical Services and Development, The Dow Chemical Company, Midland, Michigan

Claude B. Anger, M.S.   Director, R and D Microbiology/Cytotoxicology, Allergan, Inc., Irvine, California

Joseph J. Berry   Manager, International Formulation and Process Technology, World-wide Pharmaceutical Technology, Bristol-Myers Squibb Company, New Brunswick, New Jersey

Jeffrey E. Browne, Ph.D.   Director, Health Care Research and Development, R. P. Scherer North America, St. Petersburg, Florida

David C. Cooper   Senior Systems Manager, Department of Statistics, Glaxo-Wellcome Inc., Research Triangle Park, North Carolina

Maureen D. Donovan, Ph.D.   Associate Professor, College of Pharmacy, University of Iowa, Iowa City, Iowa

Michael J. Falkiewicz, Ph.D.   Research Associate, Phosphorus Chemicals Division, FMC Corporation, Princeton, New Jersey

Douglas R. Flanagan, Ph.D.   Professor, College of Pharmacy, University of Iowa, Iowa City, Iowa

Robert M. Franz, Ph.D.   Director, Process Science and Technology, Glaxo-Wellcome Inc., Research Triangle Park, North Carolina

Stig E. Friberg   Professor, Department of Chemistry, Clarkson University, Potsdam, New York

Martha L. Hilton   Research Associate, Department of Chemistry, University of Missouri—Rolla, Rolla, Missouri

Allen R. Lewis, M.S. Manager, Information Technology, The Upjohn Company, Kalamazoo, Michigan

Priscilla Lo Allergan, Inc., Irvine, California

Lisa Goldsmith Quencer Project Leader, The Dow Chemical Company, Midland, Michigan

Galen W. Radebaugh, Ph.D. Senior Director, Department of Product Development, Parke-Davis Pharmaceutical Research, Warner-Lambert Company, Morris Plains, New Jersey

Martin M. Rieger, Ph.D. President, M. & A. Rieger Associates, Morris Plains, New Jersey

David Rupp Allergan, Inc., Irvine, California

Harun Takruri, Ph.D. Director, Pharmaceutical Development, IOLAB Corporation, Claremont, California

John W. Vanderhoff Professor, Department of Chemistry, Lehigh University, Bethlehem, Pennsylvania

Norman Weiner, Ph.D. Professor of Pharmaceutics, College of Pharmacy, University of Michigan, Ann Arbor, Michigan

Joel L. Zatz Department of Pharmaceutics, Rutgers—The State University of New Jersey, Piscataway, New Jersey

Contents of Pharmaceutical Dosage Forms: Disperse Systems, Second Edition, Revised and Expanded, Volumes 2 and 3

edited by Herbert A. Lieberman, Martin M. Rieger, and Gilbert S. Banker

VOLUME 2

VOLUME 3

Contents of Pharmaceutical Dosage Forms: Tablets, Second Edition, Revised and Expanded, Volumes 1–3

edited by Herbert A. Lieberman, Leon Lachman, and Joseph B. Schwartz

VOLUME 1

VOLUME 2

Contents of Pharmaceutical Dosage Forms: Parenteral Medications, Second Edition, Revised and Expanded, Volumes 1–3

edited by Kenneth E. Avis, Herbert A. Lieberman, and Leon Lachman

VOLUME 1

VOLUME 2

VOLUME 3

1

Introduction

Norman Weiner

University of Michigan, Ann Arbor, Michigan

I. OVERVIEW

A *dispersion* can be defined as a heterogeneous system in which one phase is dispersed (with some degree of uniformity) in a second phase. The state of the dispersed phase (gas, solid, or liquid) in the dispersion medium defines the system as a *foam, suspension,* or *emulsion*. Likewise, the particle size of the dispersed phase provides further classification (*colloidal dispersion* vs. *suspension* and *microemulsion* vs. *macroemulsion*). These definitions, particularly the latter set, are somewhat arbitrary, since there is no specific particle size at which one type of system begins and the other ends. Furthermore, almost without exception, disperse systems are heterogeneous in particle size. To complicate matters even further, many commercial disperse systems cannot (and should not) be categorized easily and must be classified as complex systems. Examples include multiple emulsions (water-in-oil-in-water emulsions, in which small water drops are dispersed in larger oil drops that are dispersed in a continuous water phase), and suspensions, in which the solid particles are dispersed in an emulsion base. If the difficulty in defning these complex systems were merely a matter of semantics, the issue would be trivial, but these complexities influence the physicochemical properties of the system which, in turn, determine most of the properties with which formulators are concerned. Figure 1 illustrates the more common types of disperse systems.

Of the various pharmaceutical dosage forms, liquid disperse systems are the most complex. Method of manufacture, formulation approach, component materials selection, and the effect of environmental factors, such as temperature and holding-time, profoundly affect the variability in the product's bioavailability, stability characteristics, and a host of other variables (to be discussed under specific headings in future chapters). For this reason, there is a general reluctance on the part of the pharmaceutical industry to develop traditional disperse systems (emulsions and suspensions) when other alternatives are available (solid dosage forms or solutions). Also, there exist very few commercial successes of novel disperse systems, such as microemulsions, despite the substantial amount of experimentation in these areas.

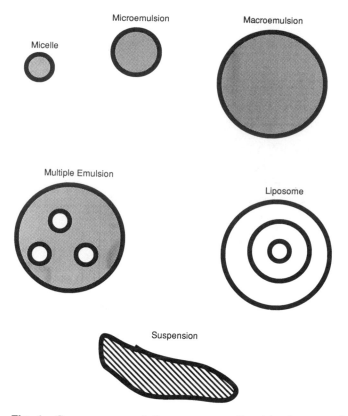

Fig. 1 Common types of disperse systems found in pharmaceutical formulations. Note that in many instances more than one of these forms will be encountered in a given formulation: white, water; shaded, oil; striped, solid; black, barrier.

Liposomes, however, have shown great potential as a drug delivery system. An assortment of molecules, including peptides and proteins, have been incorporated in liposomes, which can then be administered by different routes. Various amphipatic molecules have been used to form the liposomes, and the method of preparation can be tailored to control their size and morphology. Drug molecules can either be encapsulated in the aqueous space, or intercalated into the lipid bilayer; the exact location of a drug in the liposome depends on its physicochemical characteristics and the composition of the lipids. Because of their high degree of biocompatibility, liposomes were initially conceived of as delivery systems for intravenous delivery. It has since become apparent that liposomes can also be useful for delivery of drugs by other routes of administration. The formulator can use strategies to design liposomes for specific purposes, thereby improving the therapeutic index of a drug by increasing the fraction of the administered drug that reaches the target tissue, or alternatively, decreasing the percentage of drug molecules that reach sites of toxicity. Clinical trials now underway use liposomes to achieve a variety of therapeutic objectives, including enhancing the activity and reducing the toxicity of a widely used antineoplastic drug (doxorubicin) and an antifungal drug (amphotericin B) delivered intravenously. Other clinical trials are evaluating the ability of liposomes to deliver intravenously immunomodulators (MTP-PE) to macrophages and imaging agents (indium 111) to tumors. Recent studies in animals have reported the delivery of water-insoluble drugs into the eye, and the prolonged release of an immunomodulator (interferon) and a peptide hormone (calcitonin) from an intramuscular depot. These trials and animal studies provide evidence of the versatility of liposomes [1–5].

There are hundreds of books, chapters of books, and review articles written about various aspects of disperse systems, from both a theoretical and a practical point of view. Although disperse systems are associated with the pharmaceutical, cosmetic, food, and paint industries, liquid dispersions are prevalent in almost all industrial settings when a liquid product is involved. Industries as varied as oil refining, explosives, and printing share the problems associated with disperse systems. In most cases, therefore, it seems somewhat surprising that such products are formulated on a trial and error basis, with little or no theoretical input. Admittedly, many theories dealing with disperse systems have little apparent practical value, but there is a large body of available knowledge that, when used properly, enables the formulator to prepare better products more efficiently and evaluate them in a more systematic and realistic manner.

The problems or challenges (depending on perspective) in working with disperse systems are mostly related to their nonequilibrium state. Since an almost infinite number of nonequilibrium states are possible, each slight variation in product design or processing can lead to a different nonequilibrium product. Although these differences may not seem apparent initially, long-term stability may be affected. Of equal importance, the product is continuously seeking to reach thermodynamic equilibrium. In practical terms, thermodynamic equilibrium is synonymous with a completely coalesced emulsion or a settled, nonredispersible suspension. Thermodynamics tells us that this final state is inevitable, and the task of the formulator is to merely delay its occurrence (a stable emulsion is a thermodynamic anomaly, with the possible exception of microemulsions [6]). Basically, the formulator must seek, in a thermodynamic sense, to formulate the system such that the product is as independent of processing variables as possible and that the necessary energy barriers are introduced to delay thermodynamics equilibrium for the desired shelf life of the product. The concept of equilibrium, coupled with an understanding of free energy—particularly surface or interfacial free energy— is the basic framework that links all of the disperse systems of interest. An *interface* is defined as a boundary between two phases. [If one of the boundaries associated with the interface is a gas phase (e.g., air), the interface is referred to as a *surface*.] With suspensions, the solid–liquid interface is of primary interest, and with emulsions, the liquid–liquid interface is of primary concern. Other interfaces, such as the liquid–gas (foams) or solid–gas (wetting problems) interfaces may also come into play.

II. FREE ENERGY CONSIDERATIONS

The most important and fundamental property of any interface is that it possesses a positive free energy. Essentially, this means that the molecules at the interface are in a higher energy state than if they were located in the bulk phase (Fig. 2).

The greater the preference of the molecule of interest for the bulk, as compared with the interface, the higher the interfacial free energy [7]. Although interfacial free energies cannot be measured directly, interfacial tension values (which can be obtained experimentally) give reasonably good approximations. As a rule, accurate interfacial and

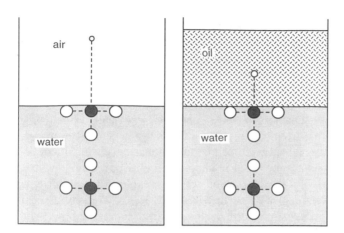

Fig. 2 Diagrammatic representation of the derivation of positive free energy of interfaces. Note that the molecule of interest (shaded) at the interface is in a higher energy state than the molecule of interest in the bulk phase because the former is being pulled down by its neighbor and there is only a weak upward force tending to equalize it.

surface tension measurements are very difficult to obtain, since impurities in the system and instrument-wetting problems introduce large errors [8]. Since most of the surfactant systems used in industry are either mixtures of surfactants, or contain significant amounts of impurities, surface or interfacial tension values associated with these systems have little meaning. Most often, these measurements are carried out without purpose, for there is usually no apparent relation between surface or interfacial tension and the formulation parameter of concern (e.g., emulsifier or solubilizer efficiency [9]). Whenever there is a real need to determine surface or interfacial tension, the Wilhelmy plate apparatus is the instrument of choice for rapid and accurate determinations. No correction factors are necessary, and wetting problems are usually absent.

In any event, surface or interfacial tension should simply be looked on as a mathematical approximation of surface or interfacial free energy. The principal problem for formulators is nature's continuous attempt to reduce this positive interfacial free energy value to zero (true equilibrium) by various means. One approach is simply to reduce the amount of interface; that is, a twofold reduction of the amount of interface results in a similar reduction in the interfacial free energy of the product. For example, when emulsion droplets collide, they can either bounce away or coalesce into larger droplets, ultimately leading to the destruction of the emulsion. The latter event will result in a reduction of interfacial free energy and, unless barriers are placed in the way, will occur with each collision. Thus, in the absence of an emulsifying agent, oil and water will separate almost instantaneously. Most often, compounders are not changing the ultimate thermodynamic fate of the product by altering the formulation (or even the processing), but are merely changing the thermodynamic path which, in practical terms, means increasing the shelf life of the product.

Another important method that nature uses to reduce interfacial free energy is to vary the composition of the interface to make it rich in surface active material, and poor in highly polar compounds (e.g., water; a surface active agent or surfactant contains at least one prominent polar group and one prominent nonpolar group). This mechanism is advantageously used by introducing materials (emulsifiers) into the formulation that concentrate at the oil–water droplet interface [10] and present barriers to droplet coalescence. The principal mechanism by which emulsifiers stabilize emulsions is not a reduction of the interfacial free energy of the system, but involves the introduction of a mechanical barrier to delay the ultimate destruction of the system. Although the concentration of surface active emulsifier is greater at the oil–water interface than in either of the bulk phases, most of the emulsifier molecules are in the water phase (hydrophilic emulsifier), or in the oil phase (hydrophobic emulsifier), and not at the emulsion droplet interface. A reduction of the interfacial free energy probably does help somewhat in the ease of preparing the emulsion (since energy needs to be added to the system to prepare the product), but it is not a major factor for long-term stability.

Finally, proper orientation of the molecules at the interface (polar groups directed toward the water phase and nonpolar groups directed toward the oil phase) further reduces interfacial free energy. It is extremely important for the formulator to keep in mind that, throughout the processing of the formulation (whether by simple mixing with a stirring rod or the use of high-energy shear equipment), the emulsifier molecules are continuously partitioning between the bulk phases and the interface, and are continually changing their orientation at the interface. Moreover, when a combination of emulsifiers is used (as usually happens), the ratio of the hydrophilic and hydrophobic emulsifier at the interface continuously changes during the preparation of the emulsion. Since equilibrium is never established, the final configuration is very much a function of processing. Thus, choosing the correct emulsifying blend (and other components as well) and processing the emulsion in such a manner that small changes in processing and storage variables do not result in large changes in the properties of the emulsion, are extremely important considerations.

Whereas emulsions have been used as an example of the importance of interfacial free energy, these concepts are applicable to all disperse systems. The importance of interfacial properties in determining the overall characteristics of the formulation, to a great extent, depends on the interface/bulk ratio of molecules in the disperse phase. In other words, the greater the percentage of molecules at the interface (e.g., the smaller the particle size), the more important are the surface properties for describing the system. For example, surface properties are much more important for colloidal dispersion than for coarse suspensions. Likewise, surface properties are much more important for microemulsions than for macroemulsions. Even though the properties of products can be altered by formulation factors affecting primarily the bulk phase (e.g., addition of hydrophilic polymers to increase viscosity), interfacial properties are much more important as a determine of the preparation's overall appearance, performance, and stability. A strategy that fails to utilize surface behavior to stabilize thermodynamically unstable formulations is unlikely to be productive. For example, if one attempts to stabilize a suspension by relying entirely on minimizing the rate of settling (Stokes' law approach; i.e., use of a small particle size and very high viscosity), the particles will ultimately settle and form a dense cake that is likely to be difficult to resuspend [11].

On the other hand, a strategy based on an appreciation of the surface properties of the system is much more likely to succeed. In the previous example, an understanding of the surface charge characteristics of the suspended particles allows formulation of the suspension so that a porous flocculated particle network is intentionally formed that can be easily redispersed (controlled flocculation approach [12]). The use of electrolytes to stabilize suspensions by this approach is based on classic electrical double-layer theory.

Thus, an understanding of this concept (to be discussed in detail in Chapters 2 and 6), facilitates the experimental determination of the amount of electrolyte necessary to produce the surface charge resulting in the most stable suspension [13]. Similarly, an understanding of this concept permits the experimental determination of the pH at which a particle containing a pH-dependent surface charge is most stable [14]. In both of the foregoing cases, the intuitive approach (greatest surface charge = greatest degree of repulsion = greatest stability) will most likely lead to a product that will settle slowly, but will not be resuspendable.

A knowledge of the surface properties of the system also helps identify the various available options and the most successful strategies for preparing the best formulation. For suspensions, surface properties of the system, other than surface charge, can be employed. Adsorption of small hydrophilic colloids or nonionic polymers provides alternative pathways to stabilize suspensions. The former increases the particle's interaction with water, and the latter sterically hinders adjacent particles from entering the primary energy minimum, where they will interact in such a way that a nonsuspendable cake will form. Whereas none of these strategies will provide permanent stability to the formulation, they can create a strong enough energy barrier, that, for practical purposes, the formulation can be considered *stable*. Similar arguments and strategies can be used for formulating emulsions and other disperse systems.

Since interfacial free energy always has a positive value, energy has to be put into the system to prepare a disperse system. Theoretically (and to a great extent, practically), enough energy can always be put into the system to overcome the thermodynamic obstacles necessary to prepare the product. The source of energy must eventually be removed (when the plug is pulled), and thermodynamics of a closed system comes back into play. The crux of the matter is that there are often two approaches at hand to formulate products: (a) the use of mechanical energy and (b) the use of the inherent energy of the system. The first relies on processing, and the second relies on formulation factors; as a practical matter, a combination of the two is used.

As instability and other problems begin to appear with products under development, modifications in processing may be employed as one approach to solve these problems. Generally, these modifications involve the introduction of more mechanical energy into the system. Whereas this strategy may appear to alleviate the situation initially, it results in an increase in the interfacial free energy of the system and invites future stability problems. If the inherent energy of the system is not sufficient to meet the increased thermodynamic demands that processing imposes, shelf life will likely be shortened. Modifications of the manufacturing procedure can be used to increase stability, but these modifications should result in improvements in energy barriers, rather than increases in interfacial free energy. In other words, a processing change that results in reorientation of the emulsifier film at the emulsion droplet interface so that a better barrier to coalescence is attained, or a processing change that allows a more uniform (not necessarily smaller) droplet size to develop will likely result in an increased shelf life.

Even under the most optimized manufacturing procedure, a disperse system will not be at thermodynamic equilibrium, but will possess a positive interfacial free energy value. Each modification of the procedure will change this value, thereby potentially resulting in different product characteristics, including stability. Since small variations in large-scale manufacture of products must be expected (e.g., holding time or temperature), processes must be avoided in which these small unavoidable variations result in major changes in the surface properties of the system. This situation is much more likely to occur with high-energy processing. If instead, reliance is placed on lower-energy processing and optimization of the system by controlling such factors as method of preparation (e.g., oil/water or water/oil ratio, for emulsions), rate of addition, and initial location of the emulsifiers, chances of improving the stability of the product will increase [15].

The reason that the latter approach has been so successful can be explained by the examination of Fig. 3, which represents hypothetical interfacial free energy pathway plots.

Point A represents the interfacial free energy of the product (e.g., smaller particle size will increase this value), and point C represents the lowest free energy state attainable (complete coalescence of the emulsion or a *cementing* of the suspension). Although thermodynamics teaches that point C will eventually be reached, it does not each how long it will take, or along what pathway the system will travel. The curves for products 1 and 2 represent different pathways that can be imposed on the system as a function of processing or formulation. Each pathway has a different energy barrier (e.g., it can be a function of how efficiently the emulsifier film prevents coalescence when emulsion drops collide, point B). Product stability could be enhanced by lowering the interfacial free energy of the product (point A), but the most efficient mechanism for stabilization involves increasing the value of the interfacial free energy barrier (point B). Actually, the stability of the system is a function of the difference in energy values between point B and point A for each product.

The curve for product 1 might result from a strategy of attempting to improve stability by primary reliance on increasing the energy output. Note that the energy values of both products (point A) are nearly the same, since, as a practical matter, changes in formulation or processing affect point B to a much greater extent than their effect on

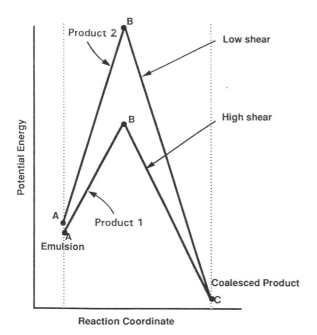

Fig. 3 Hypothetical potential energy diagram demonstrating how the energy barrier affects emulsion or suspension stability. See text for explanation.

point A. However, there is a lack of a high-energy barrier for this product (the emulsifier molecules did not have the opportunity to align properly), and there are very few thermodynamic impediments in the way for the system to reach its desired free energy (point C); thus, this product will show poor shelf life. The curve for product 2 would result from a strategy of attempting to improve stability by optimizing the process, as discussed previously. Since ample opportunity is allowed for the molecules to align in a favorable orientation, the energy barrier (point B) is strengthened, leading to a formidable barrier against product instability. Another advantage to this approach is that minor changes in manufacturing procedure are less likely to change the curve. The energy barrier can be further increased by simply changing the components in the formulation (e.g., changing the emulsifier blend or increasing its concentration). In fact, formulation changes, rather than processing changes, should be the preferred strategy of product improvement.

An intuitive understanding of free energy concepts has enormous practical value in developing formulation strategies for disperse systems. Since microemulsions are essentially at equilibrium (interfacial tension = zero), their surface properties have been completely defined by quantitative thermodynamic parameters. Importantly, many of the concepts developed by microemulsions are applicable to macroemulsions, if one remembers that the single most important difference between the two systems is that for microemulsions, nature is supplying the needed energy for emulsification (spontaneous emulsification), whereas for macroemulsions, equipment is needed in the form of mechanical energy (Fig. 4). This is perhaps the most intuitive explanation of why low-energy processing generally equates with excellent shelf life.

III. STABILITY CONSIDERATIONS

The chemical stability of individual components within the emulsion system may be very different from their stability after incorporation into other formulation types. For example, many unsaturated oils are prone to oxidation, and their degree of exposure to

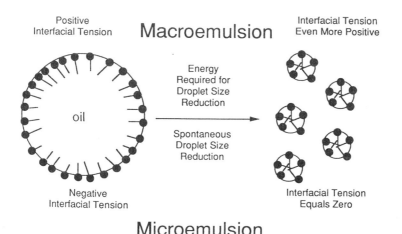

Fig. 4 Diagrammatic representation of differences between microemulsions and macroemulsions, based on free energy concepts.

oxygen may be influenced by factors that affect the extent of molecular dispersion (e.g., droplet size).

The determination of the amount of antimicrobial agent needed to achieve a minimum effective concentration is very difficult, particularly if the agent is a weak acid. Usually, the aqueous phase is most prone to microbial attack, but a large portion of the antimicrobial agent is quite likely to partition into the oil phase and the interface. Also, the ionized fraction of the antimicrobial agent in the aqueous phase is not effective (Fig. 5).

Most products generally are quite complex in the number of the *formulation's* components. For example, emulsions usually contain at least two emulsifiers (further complicated by their heterogeneous nature), more than one oil, and other components that tend to accumulate at interfaces and affect the film. Therefore, it is not surprising that small changes or alterations in temperature, in the method of manufacture, or int the source of supply of raw materials can result in altered nonequilibrium states, which equate to altered product performance. The formulator has the responsibility to anticipate, as far as possible, which parameters are likely to affect the product and which parameters can be controlled. Generally, the more complex the formulation, the less control the formulator has.

Many formulators give little thought to scale-up problems, particularly at the early stages of product development. In fact, expensive laboratory-processing equipment is sometimes used in the formulation stage of product development that has no resemblance to the production-scale equipment available. There is little practical value in preparing 100 ml of a product when a completely different procedure must be used to produce larger batches. When scale-up problems are not scrutinized early, and when a given laboratory formulation becomes final, high-energy processing often is necessary to solve the problem. Such a solution rarely works satisfactorily.

Of the many pharmaceutical dosage forms that are encountered, disperse systems are the most difficult to deal with from a stability standpoint. Homogeneous dosage forms, such as solutions, are already at thermodynamic equilibrium, and chemical de-

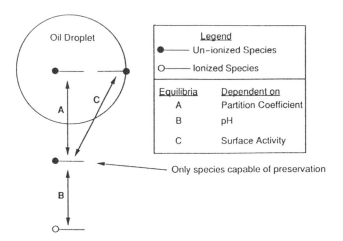

Fig. 5 Diagrammatic representation of partitioning of preservative in the various phases of an emulsion.

composition is usually the only concern. Accelerated stability testing is reasonably straightforward, and quantitative estimates of the rate of chemical decomposition can be obtained with a fair degree of certainty. Solid dosage forms usually have fewer stability problems than liquid disperse systems, even though the solid systems (e.g., capsules and tablets) are not at thermodynamic equilibrium, since the molecules have little opportunity to reorient themselves. Furthermore, solid dosage forms generally are quite chemically stable because of the absence of an aqueous environment.

Stability testing of liquid disperse systems is one of the most difficult problems faced by pharmaceutical scientists [16]. The scientist is often asked to predict the shelf life of a product or choose between experimental formulations from estimates of how well they will hold up over time. There are no standardized tests available to determine stability and, quite often, there is no certainty of what type of stability is being investigated. Once again, a conceptual understanding of the thermodynamics of these systems, particularly their interfacial properties, can provide some insight into the expected types of instability and, equally important, into the most sensible tests for predicting shelf life.

The first order of priority for solving stability problems of disperse systems is to define clearly the type or types of stability of concern. Categorizing stability as either physical or chemical is not sufficient. The various groups that are concerned with the product (product development, production, analytical, marking, and such) must have a clear and precise reference frame of stability. For example, with emulsions, various types of stability problems can occur. Creaming (a reversible separation of the emulsion into dilute and concentrated regions) may be tolerable under certain circumstances. The rate of creaming—if not complicated by other factors—is predictable, and since the various factors that influence creaming (droplet size, density differences between phases, and viscosity) are known, there are many strategies available to alleviate creaming problems successfully. Coalescence (an irreversible destruction of the emulsion) is intolerable to all groups concerned and is a function of the strength of the emulsifier film at the droplet interface (i.e., the interfacial free energy barrier shown in Fig. 2). The factors affecting coalescence and the factors affecting creaming are very difference [17], and accelerated stability testing for coalescence is, at best, difficult and risky. Various other types of stability problems can also occur, such as phase inversion, changes in rheological characteristics (as a result of creaming, coalescence, or other factors), various changes in physical properties owing to water evaporation, flocculation of the droplets, microbial contamination, and chemical decomposition, to name a few. The various types of emulsion instabilities require different testing procedures and have different degrees of reliability for making shelf life predictions. Figure 6 diagrammatically depicts the various types of emulsion instability. Similar analogies can be made for other disperse systems, such as suspensions.

An understanding of the factors that lead to stability problems can help determine which methods of testing are most likely to yield information applicable to the estimation of the product's shelf life. Stability tests commonly stress the system to limits beyond those that the product will ever encounter. Typical examples of stress tests include exposure of the product to high temperatures [18] and large gravitational forces [19]. It is important to understand whether these tests are being performed because the product is expected to encounter these conditions, or because, even though these conditions will never be approached, the results may help predict shelf life at more moderate conditions.

For example, accelerated stability testing to determine rates of creaming by the use of centrifugation can be performed if it is assumed that the factors that control cream-

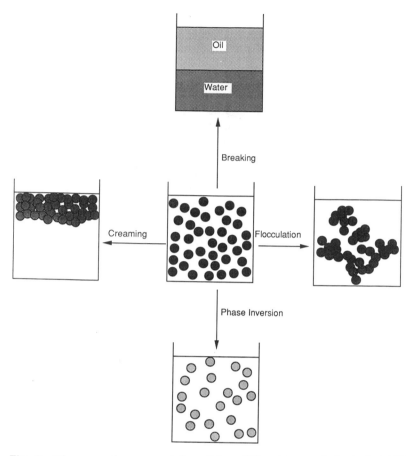

Fig. 6 Diagrammatic representation of four different types of physical stability problems seen with emulsion formulations.

ing (droplet size and viscosity) remain constant during the life of the product. More importantly, the testing procedure itself should not produce changes in the emulsion that affect the creaming rate (e.g., high-speed centrifugation may result in a weakening of the emulsifier film, leading to coalescence [20]). For predictive testing for coalescence of an emulsion or nonreversible settling of a suspension, there is little evidence that pushing the system far beyond what it will encounter in the marketplace yields any reliable information useful for shelf life predictions. Moreover, overstressing the system creates the risk of throwing away formulations that would be perfectly acceptable under realistic conditions.

High-temperature testing ($>25°C$) is almost universally used for both emulsions and suspensions. Various laboratories store this products at temperatures ranging from $4°C$ (refrigerator temperature) to $50°C$ (or perhaps even higher). The temperatures used in heat–cool cycling are also quite varied, often without considering the nature fo the product. What will the increase in temperature likely do to the properties of the systems under study?

For emulsions, higher temperatures will dramatically alter the nature of the interfacial film, especially if nonionic emulsifiers are used. The principal mechanism for stability in these systems is the hydration of the polyoxyethylene groups of the emulsifier molecules [21]. The choice of the emulsifier blend to be used (whether determined by the hydrophilic–lipophilic balance [HLB] or other methods) is based on their interfacial properties at room temperature. At higher temperatures, at which the stability tests are being run, the emulsifiers are much less hydrated, their HLB values are completely different, and, in fact, they can be considered as different molecules. Thus, if one expects the product to be exposed to a temperature of 45°C for an extended period, or for short durations (shipping and warehouse storage), studies at 45–50°C (long-term and heat–cool cycling) are quite justified. A study of a product at these temperatures determines (a) how the emulsion is holding up at this higher temperature, and (b) whether the damage is reversible or irreversible when the product is brought back to room temperature. If temperatures higher than the system will ever encounter are used, even in short-term, heat–cool cycling, there is a risk of irreversibly damaging the product so that when it is brought back to room temperature, the emulsion cannot heal. This is particularly true if higher temperatures cause large changes in the physical properties of the product, such as viscosity. These changes can be irreversible if the changes result from the precipitation of depolymerization of polymers in the dispersion.

An understanding of the mechanism by which a given blend of emulsifiers stabilize an emulsion is not merely an academic exercise. Such an understanding allows one to predict variables that will be most likely to diminish shelf life or lead to incompatibilities. For example, if one relies on a nonionic emulsifier blend, the interfacial film is tight, but changes in temperature are likely to lead to instability, since hydrogen-bonding, the major stabilizing force, is temperature-sensitive. On the other hand, if one relies on an anionic emulsifier, the interfacial film is much more diffuse, and addition of electrolytes, especially divalent cations, will influence stability, since the major stabilizing force is now electronic repulsion. A diagrammatic representation of this effect is shown in Fig. 7.

With suspensions, higher temperatures may dramatically alter the solubility of the suspended drug. During the heat–cool cycling, the saturated layer around the suspended particles will change, resulitng in a greater tendency for aggregation of particles, particularly in suspensions in which particle size is not uniform. Higher temperatures will also affect various other parameters, such as the stabilizing efficiency of polymer additives, which depends on hydration, a very temperature-dependent phenomenon. Once again, questions arise: What factors are temperature-dependent in the formulation? Which are reversible when the temperature is lowered? Is this study realistic enough to help predict shelf-life? One should keep in mind that a product that appears to be the best one at room temperature may perform poorly over the range of temperatures and other conditions it will encounter. Perhaps the use of dual emulsifiers and preservations commonly found in emulsion systems allows the system the needed flexibility to perform well over the range of conditions encountered during its lifetime.

Studies on the effect of time on particle size distribution is perhaps the single most important test to evaluate emulsion (and to some extent suspension) stability. Deterioration of the rheological properties of an emulsion on aging is largely due to changes in particle size distribution. However, since most emulsions contain a heterogeneous distribution of particles, one must be extremely careful in analyzing the droplet size distribution of an emulsion. These systems change their size distributions with time to

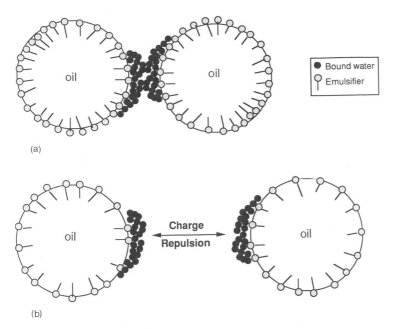

Fig. 7 Diagrammatic representation of interfacial stabilizing factors for ionic and nonionic emulsifiers: (a) nonionic emulsifier; (b) ionic emulsifier.

produce a more diffuse distribution, and the average droplet diameter will shift to higher values. Additionally, emulsions produced by high-energy processing will have a greater tendency to yield bimodal droplet size distributions. If one takes a simple example of an emulsion that comprises 97% droplets, with a radius of 1 μm, and 3% droplets with a radius three times greater (3 μm), one finds that the 3% of the larger drops will contain almost half the oil volume.

Finally, one must pay very close attention to exactness required for predictive physical stability testing. For example, determination and analysis of particle size profiles are complex.

IV. PROTOCOLS

Protocols stability testing should have flexibility that takes into consideration special properties of the product that may prove troublesome as well as special conditions the product may encounter. For example, if controlled flocculation is the strategy that is used to stabilize a suspension, one must make certain that the energy barrier that is responsible for stabilizing the product is deep enough to protect the product from destabilizing factors, such as the vibration caused by shipping. Thus, testing of this type of product should include use of a reciprocating shaker. Sunscreen emulsions that may be left in the glove compartment of a car and attain temperatures of 70–80°C, or agricultural suspensions that will be diluted in the field with ditch water, are other examples of products that require special testing.

Another example of the need for flexible testing protocols is in the rheological examination of products. The rheology (flow characteristics) of emulsions, suspensions, and other disperse systems is often the single most important characteristic that identifies the product to the consumer. Changes in the viscosity of the product while still in the container, its properties on handling, its flow properties from the container, and its properties on application to the skin are easily identifiable to the consumer. Product consistency is not only critical to product acceptance, but it may be related to therapeutic effectiveness and product stability. The product formulator has the responsibility to achieve the desired flow characteristics of the product; the responsibility of the manufacturing pharmacist is to retain these properties under large-scale manufacture; and the responsibility of all concerned is to test for and ensure rheological consistency between batches and throughout the shelf life of the product. Unfortunately, the common practice is to base rheological testing on the instrumentation available and on the protocol used with previous products. Instead, the protocol to test the rheology of the product must be based on a conceptual understanding of its physical properties and how these properties relate to the instrumentation to be used.

For example, the shearing stress associated with the spreading of a thin film of cream on the skin and the shearing stress associated with the settling of particles in the container are different by orders of magnitude. A one-point rheological determination, or even a multiple-point rheogram, may not even include the shearing stress of interest. In fact, if one is studying the spreading of a cream or its tackiness, the product's yield value may be of more interest than its absolute viscosity. Since the primary purpose for rheological testing is that of a quality control tool, rather than that of an instrument to gather theoretical insight, one should be more concerned with instrumental appropriateness, as opposed to absolute viscosity values. Thus, Wood et al. [22] modified an extrusion rheometer so that collapsible tubes containing thixotropic material could be used. Green [23] designed an instrument to analyze the rheological factors that contribute to tack (stickiness), and Havemeyer [24] described an apparatus for measuring a product's spreadability.

In conclusion, formulators spend much time and energy developing product formulations and exhaustively testing these products. Formulation chemists are not (and probably never will be) in a position to sit at their desk and, based on theoretical concepts, design a product that is certain to meet all of the desired specifications. However, as formulators, they are in a position to use a combination of theoretical concepts, experience, and practical thinking to avoid the formulation of unstable products and the evaluation of products with tests that have no validity.

REFERENCES

1. G. Gregoriadis, ed., *Liposome Technology*. CRC Press, Boca Raton, FL, 1993. (a very useful three-volume series).
2. N. Weiner, F. Martin, and M. Riaz, *Drug. Dev. Ind. Pharm.*, 15:1523 (1989).
3. M. Riaz, N. Weiner, and F. Martin, Liposomes, in *Pharmaceutical Dosage Forms: Disperse Systems, Vol. 2* (H. A. Lieberman and G. S. Banker, eds.). Marcel Dekker, New York, 1989, pp. 567–603.
4. G. Poste, *Biol. Cell*, 47:19 (1983).
5. M. Ostro, ed., *Liposomes*. Marcel Dekker, New York, 1983.
6. L. J. Osipow, *J. Soc. Cosmet. Chem.*, 14:277 (1963).
7. A. W. Adamson, *Physical Chemistry of Surfaces*, 2nd ed. Interscience, New York, 1960, p. 1.
8. N. D. Weiner and G. L. Flynn, *Chem. Pharm. Bull.*, 22:2480 (1974).

9. P. Becher, *Emulsions Theory and Practice*, 2nd ed., Reinhold, Washington, DC, 1965, p. 105.
10. T. J. Lin, *J. Soc. Cosmet. Chem.,* 30:167 (1979).
11. E. N. Hiestand, *J. Pharm. Sci.,* 53:1 (1964).
12. A. N. Martin, *J. Pharm. Sci.,* 50:513 (1961).
13. W. Schneider, S. Stravchansky, and A. Martin, *Am. J. Pharm. Ed.,* 42:280 (1978).
14. D. N. Shah, R. Feldkamp, J. L. White, and S. L. Hem, *J. Pharm. Sci.,* 71:266 (1981).
15. T. J. Lin, H. Kurihara, and H. Ohta, *J. Soc. Cosmet. Chem.,* 26:121 (1975).
16. G. Zografi, *J. Soc. Cosmet. Chem.,* 33:345 (1982).
17. S. R. Reddy and H. S. Fogler, *J. Colloid Interface Sci.,* 82:128 (1981).
18. P. Sherman, *Soap Perfum. Cosmet.,* 44:693 (1971).
19. L. Lachman, H. A. Lieberman, and J. L. Kanig, *Theory and Practice of Industrial Pharmacy*, 3rd ed., Lea & Febiger, Philadelphia, 1985.
20. P. Sherman, *Emulsion Science.* Academic Press, New York, 1968, Chap. 2.
21. R. G. Laughlin, *J. Soc. Cosmet. Chem.,* 32:371 (1981).
22. J. H. Wood, G. Catacalos, and S. V. Lieberman, *J. Pharm. Sci.,* 52:296 (1963).
23. H. Green, *Ind. Eng. Chem. (Anal.),* 13:632 (1941).
24. R. N. Havemeyer, *J. Pharm. Sci.,* 45:121 (1956).

2

Theory of Suspensions

Michael J. Falkiewicz

FMC Corporation, Princeton, New Jersey

I. INTRODUCTION

Suspensions are defined operationally as a class of materials in which one phase, a solid, is dispersed in a second phase, generally a liquid. This represents the most common system that is of importance to the pharmaceutical or formulation scientist.

While suspensions find applications in many everyday consumer products, such as drugs, cosmetics, and foods, industrial applications also exist in which a suspension may play an important role in processing or may be the final form of some household or industrial product.

This chapter discusses the principles that are at work in the field of suspensions, their classification, methods of preparation, and routes to stabilization. The focus will be on theoretical factors that impinge on these areas. Recent work that has attempted to better define the theoretical concepts of suspensions and dispersions will be emphasized. In addition, a discussion of the rheological aspects of suspensions and the effect of additives on the stability of suspensions will provide the background knowledge needed for raw material selection and use.

II. CLASSIFICATION OF DISPERSED SYSTEMS

Solutions are generally described as homogeneous mixtures of two or more substances forming a single phase. One is unable to visualize the particles of any component of a solution. Precipitates are generally easily recognized by eye. However, in the field of food, pharmaceutical, and cosmetic products, many materials are neither soluble or precipitated. The science of suspensions and dispersions provides the fundamental description of these preparations and of various industrial products as well.

Many of the terms that are used to describe dispersions can also be extended to suspensions. Most simply, the difference is one of size; however, there are no sharp boundaries. Dispersions, often called colloidal dispersions, span the gap between true solutions and suspensions. In a suspension, one can usually see the particles or the suspended phase either with the naked eye or with the microscope.

The transition from colloidal to coarse suspensions is gradual. Thus, the theoretical concepts that govern colloidal dispersions can also be applied to the larger particles found in suspensions.

A suspension or dispersion is a system that generally consists of two phases of matter, although the number of components can be higher. Depending on the state of each phase, one can have a wide series of possibilities. Table 1 depicts the various combinations that might exist [1]. Similar to the terminology of solute and solvent, the key terms in dispersions are *dispersed phase* and *dispersing medium*. The former refers to the suspended particles, and the latter to the vehicle or liquid in which the particles are suspended. From the examples in Table 1, it is apparent that dispersions are a common part of life. Notwithstanding the important area of health and medical services for which the necessity of a properly formulated product is so important relative to the delivery of an active ingredient, it is apparent that dispersions are important from morning to night in many aspects of our everyday life.

This discussion is focused mainly on solid aerosols, emulsions, or sols. The term *sol* is used for systems in which the dispersing medium is a liquid. Since this chapter deals with suspensions, the dispersion medium is a liquid, and the emphasis will be on solids that are dispersed in liquids. Again, the boundaries between sols (colloidal) and macroscopic suspensions are gradual.

Other materials can function as suspension aids and actually be in solution. For example, cellulose-based polymers can be water-soluble, as in sodium carboxymethylcellulose; other cellulose materials are suitable for solubilization in organic liquids. These materials provide a thickening of the suspension medium, but they may not be visible under the microscope.

In addition to carboxymethylcellulose, there are other water-soluble polysaccharides that also can sustain a suspension of heavy particles. These hydrocolloids achieve this primarily through their effect on the rheology of the total composition.

III. PARTICLE PROPERTIES

Both the number of particles dispersed and the size and shape of the particles can influence the overall properties, physical and chemical, of pharmaceutical suspensions of interest.

Table 1 Types of Dispersion

Dispersed phase	Medium	Dispersion	Example
Liquid	Gas	Liquid aerosol	Liquid spray, fog
Solid	Gas	Solid aerosol	Smoke, dust
Gas	Liquid	Foam	
Liquid	Liquid	Emulsion	Milk
Solid	Liquid	Sol, paste	Toothpaste, paint, drugs, suspensions
Gas	Solid	Solid foam	
Liquid	Solid	Solid emulsion	Pearl
Solid	Solid	Solid suspension	Plastics

Source: Ref. 1.

A. Particle Morphology

Particles can have various shapes or morphologies, ranging from simple geometries, to irregular boundaries. The most common shapes are spheres, cylinders, rods, needles, and various crystalline shapes. Other terms to describe more irregular types of shapes have been listed by Allen [2] (Table 2).

Although most of these shapes can be easily visualized, the actual measurement and characterization of the shapes can be difficult to express in a mathematical formula. For these reasons, workers try to provide only a general classification of the shape of the particle(s) of importance to their suspension. There have been many improvements in equipment for viewing particle morphology and size. The use of video equipment for displaying microscope fields is now a fairly common aid. These types of instrumentation and equipment serve to ease the job of the industrial microscopist. They provide a screen or monitor with which to observe particles, rather than looking through the conventional eyepiece.

Many suspended materials, especially those in liquids, might have spherical particles, as in emulsions and latices; others can have irregular shapes. Solids that are used to promote the stabilization of suspensions are termed *suspending agents*. These solids consist of materials of small particle size. Many solid suspending agents have rod-shaped or platelike structures.

Deviation from sphericity is often used to characterize particle morphology, as in the ellipsoids. With ellipsoids, the ratio of the two radii describing the particle is a measure of the deviation from a true spherical shape.

The relation between particle sizing and the shape of particles becomes more difficult when one deviates from an established geometric form (such as a sphere), which can be characterized by one or more dimension; for example, a radius or diameter, or length. Heywood [3] has introduced shape coefficients, which led to an expression with coefficients developed from a large number of experimental measurements.

Heywood, using grains of sand as a model system, derived the following relationship [2,4], incorporating such terms as elongation ratio, flatness ratio, and a coefficient relating to geometric form:

$$f = 1.57 + c\left(\frac{k}{m}\right)^{4/3}\frac{n+1}{n} \tag{1}$$

Table 2 Definitions of Particle Shape

Shape	Definition
Acicular	Needle-shaped
Angular	Sharp-edged or roughly polyhedral
Crystalline	Freely developed in a field medium of geometric shape
Dendritic	Having a branched crystalline shape
Fibrous	Regularly or irregularly threadlike
Flaky	Platelike
Granular	Having approximately an equidimensional irregular shape
Irregular	Lacking any symmetry
Modular	Having rounded, irregular shape
Spherical	Global

Source: Ref. 2.

where

    f = surface coefficient
    k = volume coefficient
    n = elongation ratio (length/breadth)
    m = flatness ratio (breadth/thickness)
    c = coefficient depending on geometric form

The surface and the volume are important properties, the ratio of which helps define the shape of the particle. Some typical shape coefficients are $c = 4.36$ for a tetrahedron, $c = 2.55$ for a cube, and $c = 1.86$ for a sphere.

For additional details, the reader should review the references.

Information on the shapes of particles is important in postulating mechanisms for the behavior of suspensions. Shape can also be a factor in understanding the packing of sediment and settling characteristics. The settling and resuspendability of suspensions is related to the packing environment into which suspended particles may be placed. The shape of particles, as well as their size, can have an influence on the prospects for reversible change. For example, one can imagine the situation in which an opportunity for attraction between two dispersed particles will be affected by the surface characteristics of the particles. Particles that have the ability to exert attractive forces across large surface will most likely result in greater attraction and adhesion. This results in heavier, larger particles which are less likely to be suspended.

B. Particle Size Analysis

The particle size of the suspended or dispersed phase is a very important part of the knowledge required for a thorough understanding of a suspension. In addition, the environment encountered by a suspended or dispersed particle has an effect on the physical properties of the particle.

Knowledge of the average size or, preferably, the particle size distribution of the suspended particles can provide direction to a formulator. For example, observation of the settling characteristics of a suspension quickly tells one something about the size of the particles, be they dispersed or flocculated.

The capability of measuring the particle size distribution is of definite value to the formulator, since it is one additional parameter over which he or she may have some control by milling or sieving.

Various instruments can be used to gain knowledge about the size of particles. The microscope provides direct observation of the sample, whereas other techniques generally rely on the measurement of some other physical or electrical property. Microscopy can also provide information on both the shape and the degree of aggregation of powder particles. Usually, one estimates size by the use of an eyepiece graticule or scale. A graticule is a scale that is used for the location and measurement of objects, using an optical instrument. A slide with known scale spacings is brought into focus and calibrated versus another scale, which is part of the eyepiece. By using this technique at a known magnification, one then knows that each ocular scale division represents a known length.

These graticules or scales are well suited to measuring the linear dimensions of particles (Fig. 1). Use of Feret's diameter, or an end-to-end measurement, provides a fairly quick estimation for particles of irregular shapes [5]. *Feret's diameter* is defined

SLIDE WITH KNOWN SPACINGS

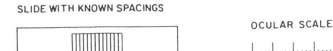

Fig. 1 Sizing with a calibrated scale.

as the mean value of the distance between two parallel tangents, on opposite sides of the particle profile. With any technique, a sufficient number of particles should be examined to ensure that a representative sample has been taken. New optical equipment has made this task much easier. Monitors accompany many new microscopic systems. In addition, the material for examination should be prepared to ensure that a truly unbiased, representative sample is obtained. This is best accomplished by using a sampling procedure, such as quartering, or a device that riffles the samples.

Another technique for the determination of particle size is sieve analysis, which can be either vibratory or by suction. A typical procedure to follow in a vibratory sieve analysis involves several steps. First, one decides on the number and size of each sieve to be included in the test. Generally, four or five sieves are stacked one upon the other, with the largest openings, inversely related to mesh per inch, being at the top of the stack. At the bottom of the stack is placed the sieve with the smallest opening, or largest mesh size, and beneath that a pan to collect all the particles that are finer than the smallest sieve. Each sieve has uniform openings of a certain size. The powder to be analyzed is placed on the top sieve and the set of sieves is vibrated in a mechanical device. In this way the powder is separated into discrete fractions. The results are usually obtained by weighing the amount of material retained on each sieve as well as the amount collected in the pan. Since the initial weight of the sample placed on the top sieve was known, one can determine the "cumulative percent finer" obtained for each succeeding sieve. An alternative suction method uses one sieve at a time and examines the amount retained on the single screen. In both these methods (vibratory and suction), one can obtain a histogram or a cumulative type of plot.

The histogram is essentially a bar graph that shows the quantities of material that fall into various size ranges. A cumulative type of plot generally indicates the amount of particulate material that is less than a certain particle size. A typical curve appears in Fig. 2. Cumulative plots often use a logarithmic scale on the *x*-axis for equivalent spherical diameter. The *y*-axis is generally a linear description of the cumulative percent finer.

The sieve analysis is a fairly rapid procedure that provides sizing information on the solids that are to be suspended. The assumption is that there is a dispersity, or nonuniformity, in the particle size distribution. Some systems, such as lattices, are characterized as *monodisperse*, meaning that just about every discrete particle is the same size. These types of systems, if unstable kinetically, can lead to finely suspended particles that might settle in the form of a hard cake.

Another method of determining the particle size distribution of a powder is based on sedimentation. The most common procedure is based on Stokes' law [2] for the

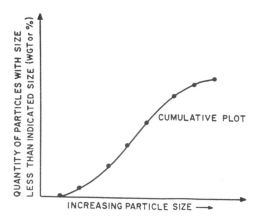

Fig. 2 Cumulative type of graph of particle size.

settling velocity of a particle in a particular fluid. The general equation for this is as follows:

$$V = d^2 \frac{(\rho_s - \rho_l)g}{18\eta} \tag{2}$$

where

    V = settling velocity
    d = Stokes' diameter
    ρ_s = density of solid
    ρ_l = density of liquid
    g = acceleration due to gravity
    η = viscosity of liquid

Practical techniques include simple sedimentation methods, such as the Andreason pipette and the Cahn sedimentation balance. The Andreason pipette method involves measuring the percentage solids that settle with time in a graduated sedimentation vessel. Samples are withdrawn over time from the bottom of the vessel through a pipette. The concentration of solids can be determined by drying and weighing. The quantities determined as settling are related to the largest possible size present, according to the Stokes equation.

The Cahn sedimentation balance electronically records the amount of dispersed powder settling out, as a function of time. From this, one finds the percentage weight of particles greater than a certain diameter. One of the advantages of this method is that the mass of particles is continuously recorded.

Both the Andreason and Cahn techniques allow one to measure the amount of solids settling from a homogeneous dispersion during a reasonable time. Under the influence of a gravitational field, these methods are appropriate when the particle size diameter is broad and when the smallest particles are 5 μm or larger. Many of these details are best found in texts dealing with particle size analysis or in the respective vendor's literature. Appendix I lists some firms that offer particle-sizing equipment.

When one wishes to measure particles smaller than 5 μm, generally some type of centrifugal method is employed to speed up the data collection. This involves use of a centrifuge to overcome the effects of convection and diffusion of small particles. Some of the more common methods involve photosedimentation devices in which the transmittance of light is measured through a cell filled with a dispersion of the material of interest. As the material settles with time, according to Stokes' law, the light intensity increases, enabling one to calculate a particle size distribution.

A recent study on the use of a sedimentation balance for the evaluation of a pharmaceutical suspension indicated mixed results, depending on the dispersed species. Although reasonable reproducibility was obtained with barium sulfate, more complex sulfur drug suspensions were not in agreement with microscopic analysis [6]. Therefore, the method is not suitable for all pharmaceutical suspensions. One must work with several methods to prove the reliability of the data.

One of the disadvantages of sedimentation devices, such as the Andreason pipette, is the length of time to do an analysis. It is not uncommon for this procedure to last for 12 h or more. An improvement to this technique is claimed by the use of multiple-sensing devices along the length of the path of the settling particles. Good agreement is claimed with both a Sedigraph and typical sedimentation balance for an inorganic powder suspended in water [7].

In a typical particle size analysis, three factors require calculation: the sedimentation time, the centrifugation time, and the cumulative percent finer. The *sedimentation time* is the time required for a particle of a certain size to settle in a liquid. This calculation uses Stokes' law to calculate the time of settling for a particular-sized particle. One can calculate a theoretical time of settling for each particular size and, thus, construct a *t-x* chart (time of sedimentation vs. particle diameter).

All the calculations are based on a spherical shape. If the particles are spherical, as in a typical latex or emulsion, the assumption is valid. However, when there is a deviation from sphericity, measurements are corrected to an equivalent spherical diameter. In such instances, one is generally more concerned about relative shifts in a particle size distribution than about absolute measurements of particle size.

The time of centrifugation must be calculated if the sample contains particles smaller than 4–5 μm. To calculate, one must take into account a centrifugal force factor, the cell height, and the revolutions per minute (rpm) chosen for centrifugation. The details can be found by referring to the literature of the vendors listed in Appendix I.

Finally, the cumulative percent finer must be calculated. The easiest way is to develop a table, showing the amount of material in a particular size range. Starting with the smallest range, a running cumulative total is taken. For each succeeding size the specific total is divided by the running cumulative total to give the cumulative percent finer. This indicates what percentage of particles is under a certain size. After this calculation has been completed, a graph of cumulative percent finer versus equivalent spherical diameter is plotted, generally on semilogarithmic paper. A typical graph is shown in Fig. 3. Recent studies on the theory of sedimentation in colloidal suspensions deal with the interactions of particles. A recent paper by Barker and Grimson considers the interactions between particles while settling [8].

To obtain meaningful data, it is imperative that the sample be dispersed in a liquid that has no effect on the shape or size of the particles under examination. In some cases, prior confirmation of the absence of such an effect can be gained by microscopic techniques. In sedimentation analysis, one must keep the concentration of the particles

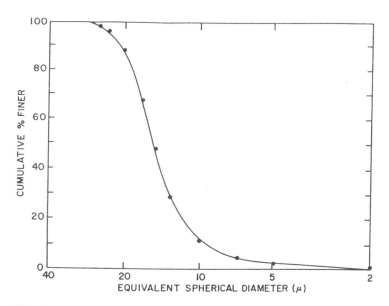

Fig. 3 Typical particle size curve depicting cumulative percent finer.

in the liquid medium low enough to minimize interaction among particles, which could change the velocity of sedimentation. In addition, depending on the technique involved, Brownian motion and thermal effects could place limitations on the accuracy of the settling times of the fine particles. In sedimentation techniques better resolution is obtained by the use of what is known as a "line start" technique in centrifugal methods. An example of this is given in a recent reference in which a range of different particle sizes were examined [9].

Another instrument uses an x-ray beam and follows the change in beam intensity as a function of time. The limitation is the type of materials that can be effectively examined, since the atomic number must be high enough to interact with the x-ray radiation. This technique is generally reserved for minerals or substances with an atomic number greater than 12. For additional information on the theory of sedimentation in suspensions, the reader is referred to a work on sedimentation in suspensions, wherein an attempt is made to develop equations describing the velocity of the particles to the forces acting on the particles in suspension [10].

Another commonly used device takes advantage of the change in an electrical sensing zone that occurs when a particle passes through a orifice positioned between two electrodes. The device counts the number of particles and their volume by changing the value of the resistance in an electrolyte by displacement of a volume of liquid proportional to the size of the particle passing through the orifice. The signal is then amplified, sized, and counted. Generally, several cells are needed to cover a broad particle size distribution range. This technique must be calibrated by well-known particle size data obtained by another method. Examples of such instruments are the Coulter Counter and the Electrozone Counter [2].

Most of the available particle size instrumentation assumes that the particles being examined are spherical. Light scattering has also made great advances in the last decade as a tool for particle size evaluation. Equipment provided by several companies incorporates different light sources, some of which are based on tungsten–halogen and some of which are based on helium neon lasers. These newer pieces of equipment rely upon light scattering as the principle of measurement and can now cover some fairly wide ranges. In some cases, various detectors need to be employed. To elaborate on these methods is really beyond the scope of this chapter. The reader is referred to several references that provide an update on the advances that have been made. An excellent review article deals with the issues that are generally encountered in trying to establish the particle sizes of particulate pharmaceutical systems [11]. A theoretical review of optical methods using laser light scattering, giving consideration to the interaction between laser beams and small particles, is also suggested [12].

Quasielastic light scattering has been used as a method for assessing the particle size distribution of suspensions. This procedure can look at very small particles. The sample is preferably dilute. A review article on this subject has been written covering the fundamentals of the method and some of the corrections necessary for light-scattering measurements [13].

Relative to the measurement of particle size distribution, a large number of new pieces of equipment that are based on laser light scattering have found application in various types of suspensions. Basically these instruments are of two main types, one employing primarily forward angle light scattering and the other using wide angles and back scattering.

In the Fraunhofer, forward angle or angular-scattering technique, corrections need to be applied for sizes smaller than dimensions of several microns to correct for the transmission of light through the particles. Equipment that features wider angles and back scattering is capable of working with more concentrated dispersions [14].

Most scientists using these techniques are looking primarily for differences among a set of samples that will confirm that a change in a process or raw material has led to a reduction or change in particle size. This is a more practical concern, rather than knowledge of the absolute particle size.

The importance of understanding the particle size distribution of material used in suspensions has been mentioned. In suspensions, one generally wants to minimize settling of the suspended particles. Since this is not always possible, the next most reliable procedure is to assure that, when settling does occur, it is of a reversible type, requiring only minimal to moderate agitation to achieve resuspension. This situation is particularly important in pharmaceutical suspensions and will be addressed in detail later in this chapter. The term *hindered settling*, which is encountered in particle size analysis by sedimentation, refers to conditions other than free settling of isolated particles. It can result from flocculation or from a colloidal structure. These flocs, if formed by electrolyte or pH changes, will respond to shear in a way different from flocs formed with polymers.

In looking for the best method to apply to a particular system, one should consider work done outside the field of pharmaceuticals. For other types of materials, one can find a technique that can help in the approach to assessing a particular size distribution. For example, in the field of ceramics, a comparative study was conducted on a variety of particle size determination techniques as applied to ceramic materials. The techniques evaluated were sedimentation using an x-ray source and laser light diffraction [15].

Another field of interest is that of water. With the ever-increasing emphasis on the quality of both wastewater and potable water, the application of particle technology has played an important role in the detection of contaminants. A review article on the subject of particle size determination in wastewater compares different treatment processes and their effect on the particle size distribution [16]. Similarly in potable water, flocculation and sedimentation of suspended particulates is an important step before the filtration of potable water supplies. In-line particle size measurement is appropriate in this case.

Again, comparing analyses conducted on different types of particles, a study on aluminum oxide revealed the effect of particle shape on the size distribution obtained by an image analyzer. As the shape of particles become less spherical, variability in measurements seems to increase [17].

In pharmaceuticals, polymer lattices are used to provide taste-masking or drug delivery control. In looking at methods used in other industries, one can use a method developed for measuring agglomerated and dispersed particles from electron micrographs. The technique was verified on controlled latex samples [18].

For the present, knowledge of the average size, and preferably the range of sizes of a suspended particle, will be of value to a formulator of pharmaceutical products. With this information, one can anticipate settling trends and perhaps employ alternative-processing methods, such as milling or homogenizing, to modify the particle size distribution and, thereby, improve overall product quality, effectiveness, and stability. Some of the new particle-sizing equipment features automated sampling systems for measuring the particulates in liquid suspensions. In addition, improvements have been made in the computer control for data storage and for the presentation of data in real-time to the operator.

A thorough review of a variety of the methods mentioned in this chapter was conducted. This review article includes over 300 references dealing with sedimentation, electrical zone sensing methods, optical methods, microscopy, chromatography, and photoncorrelation spectroscopy [19]. A comparison of several different methods (light scattering, electroconductive sensing, and sieving) was conducted on samples in a round-robin test by a task force of the ASTM Committee [20].

It was previously suggested that in dealing with particle size analysis, the laboratory scientist should consider work that is being done in other industries. Ceramics, wastewater, potable water, and catalysts have been mentioned.

In other industries, such as potable water, destabilization of suspensions is desirable. Municipalities want to remove finely suspended matter that does not belong in the final product. In the pharmaceutical industry, one is trying to achieve the opposite effect, namely suspension. The point to be made here is that techniques, such as sedimentation rate and zeta potential, can be applied to many different types of issues. Awareness of techniques that are used to solve problems in other industries can sometimes also be applied to pharmaceuticals.

IV. THE SOLID–LIQUID INTERFACE

A. Wettting

The physical properties of the material being suspended constitute the next area of concern. In light of the general chemistry textbook rule of "like dissolves like," one must consider what factors facilitate the "mixing" of two mutually nonsoluble materials. Similar to principles followed in emulsion science, one tries to promote some degree of interaction by wetting and mechanical agitation.

In preparing a suspension of a powdered substance, the material to be suspended must first be separated into finely divided particles. As part of this process, the particles must be individually wetted.

The wetting process can be subdivided into a series of more discrete steps. The first is wetting of the solid particles by the liquid medium. To do this, the liquid must displace air at the surface of the solid. Any material or substance that facilitates this wetting acts as a surface-active agent. There are many such substances that are commonly used in a variety of pharmaceutical as well as industrial product applications.

The tendency of a solid to be wetted by a liquid is a measure of the interaction of the substances. If the solid surface is hydrophilic, it will be readily wet by water or an aqueous medium. On the other hand, a hydrophobic material will be more easily wetted by an organic or nonpolar liquid. In the pharmaceutical area, one is primarily concerned with aqueous systems or hydroalcoholic mixtures. Since many drug substances are hydrophobic, proper wetting is a necessary first step in the preparation of suspensions of such substances.

To promote the proper wetting of hydrophobic substances, the use of a surface-active agent is recommended. Direct contact between the liquid medium and the solid surface is the first step. Two different degrees of wetting are shown in Fig. 4. At first glance, it is evident that liquid Y has a greater tendency to interact with solid X then liquid Z.

B. Contact Angle

The angle the liquid makes with the solid surface is called the contact angle, θ in Fig. 4. It is defined by the boundaries of the solid surface and the tangent to the curvature of the liquid drop. In part (a) of Fig. 4, it is apparent that the liquid is showing some interaction with the solid surface. The contact angle θ is less than $90°$. In part (b), there is little or no interaction of the liquid with the solid surface, and the contact angle is close to $180°$. As indicated in Fig. 4, these situations are called wetting and nonwetting, respectively.

If the particulate material can be pressed into a wafer, one can measure the angle the liquid phase makes with the "horizontal" tablet surface. The experimental procedure is to place a drop of the liquid on a solid of interest, having first confirmed that the stage on which the solid rests is completely level in all directions. The drop of liquid is generally deposited from a microsyringe. In this way, one can control the volume of the drop. By using an appropriate light source, one shines a beam of light on the drop and examines an inverted image of the drop through a lens with adjustable crosshairs. By

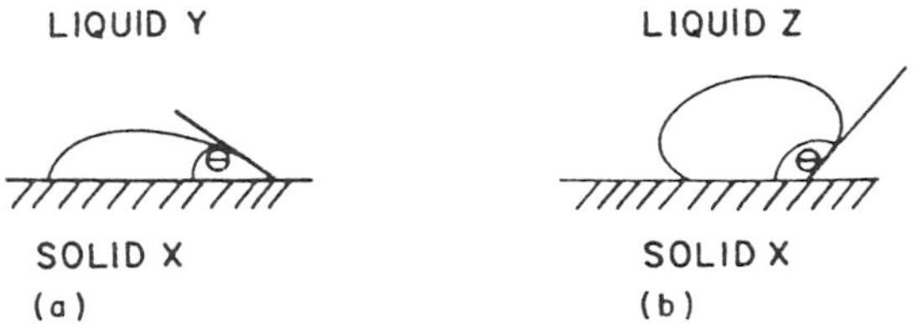

Fig. 4 Wetting of a solid by two liquids with different wetting potential. (a) Wetting, (b) nonwetting.

aligning one crosshair with the horizontal surface and rotating the other until it is tangent to the drop, one can read the contact angle directly off a scale within the lens system. Compressed powder tablets are generally not truly flat, as can be seen through the telescope–lens system. The surface may consist of both crevices and ridges. As a relative tool, however, this technique is applicable if the powder is compressed into a tablet with a high-compression force. This can be accomplished with a Carver press.

Although one could obviously speak of degrees of wetting or partial wetting, as evidenced by contact angles between 0° and 90°, contact angles greater than 90° are classified as nonwetting situations. If, however, the contact angle is 0°, the solid is completely wet by the liquid. If the angle were close to 180°, the solid substance would be described as unwettable by the liquid in question.

Surface tension (γ) is defined as free energy per unit area at an interfacial area. It can also be viewed as a measure of the attractive force between molecules of a liquid. In dealing with liquid, various force methods or shape methods can be used to obtain an estimate of surface tensions. With the duNouy ring method, one measures the force needed to pull a ring of known dimensions from a film or surface of the liquid under study. This is generally accomplished by slowly lifting the ring out of the surface of the liquid under study, while simultaneously recording the torsion required to keep the extended film counterbalanced. Then the investigator measures the force necessary to pull the test ring free from the liquid surface film.

An adaptation of the duNouy technique is the Wilhelmy plate method, in which a plate, rather than an annular ring, is used. A discussion of various methods used for determining surface tension is included in a monograph on emulsions by Becher [21].

Under shape methods, the sessile or pendant drop technique is used. From the dimensions of the drop, one can calculate the surface tension—usually by photographing the drop geometry and then measuring the key distances from the print. This can now be accomplished with more modern techniques such as video cameras. For a solid surface, γ_s is difficult to measure. One can measure the contact angle of liquids of known surface energy on the solid surface in question. By plotting cos θ of the contact angle against γ_{lv}, one can obtain the critical surface tension of the solid by extrapolating to $\theta = 0$ or cos $\theta = 1$. This is shown in Fig. 5, from the work of Fox and Zisman [22].

Since many pharmaceutical substances are hydrophobic, the wetting by aqueous media alone may be insufficient to prepare the preliminary dispersion. One must promote an attraction between the two phases that is greater than the interactions existing within the liquid phase itself. Therefore, the interaction between solid A and liquid B must be greater than both A–A and B–B types of interaction.

In preparing a dispersion or suspension, one is placing an unwetted solid into a liquid phase. Thus, there is an adhesional wetting and an immersional wetting. There also exists a spreading wetting, for a liquid already in contact with a solid. These are described by Shaw, along with free-energy changes associated with immersion of a solid in a liquid [1]. *Adhesive wetting* is defined by the state in which a liquid makes contact with a solid and adheres to it. The degree of wetting is measured by the contact angle. *Immersional wetting* is defined by the state in which a solid, not in contact with the liquid, is completely immersed in it.

For the contact angle, one should keep in mind that the condition of the solid surface is, more often than not, irregular. As such, the use of relative measurements is the rule. Generally, one might use a surfactant to modify the wetting characteristics of the powders. Also, *deflocculation*, defined as the dispersion of primary particles, improves

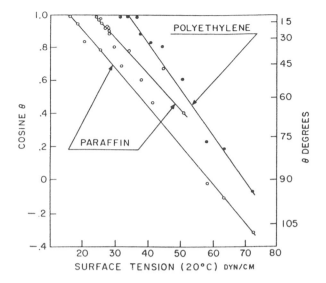

Fig. 5 Cosine of the contact angle versus surface tension for polyethylene and paraffin. (From Ref. 22.)

overall wettability. Surfactants function by lowering the solid–liquid interfacial tension γ_{sl}. For the three types of wetting described by Shaw, a reduction of γ_{sl} always leads to an improvement in wetting. If the contact angle θ is less than 90°, the wetting is spontaneous.

Since a surfactant generally possesses both hydrophilic and hydrophobic character, it is believed that the mechanism of surfactant activity involves the preferential adsorption of the nonpolar hydrocarbon chain by the solid drug surface, which is hydrophobic. Adsorption of the surfactant (onto the solid) can actually promote deflocculation owing to charge repulsion or steric factors. This will be discussed in detail in the next section, dealing with the stabilization of dispersions.

In the measurement of contact angles, one may encounter hysteresis, since the contact angle is larger for an advancing liquid surface than for a retreating (receding) liquid surface. Basically, the advancing angle is that measured when the liquid is advancing over a dry surface; and the receding angle is that measured when the liquid is receding from a wet surface. The process is similar to adsorption and desorption. One measures the angle by either adding or removing a known volume of test liquid with a microsyringe. The needle remains in contact with the drop during the measurement. This is quite observable with impure surfaces or rough surfaces. One needs to be consistent in the measurement technique and look for relative shifts or trends, which then serve as a guide to the selection of appropriate wetting agents. Zografi and Johnson [23] have studied the wetting of pharmaceutical solids and have found that the receding angle is affected by surface roughness more than the advancing angle. For this reason, the advancing contact angle is a more reasonable estimate.

The wet point method, a quick technique for measuring the wettability of a powder, basically consists of measuring the amount of vehicle necessary to just wet all of the powder [24]. In a sense this is quite similar to the process encountered in wet granulation. Generally one measures the amount of a liquid needed to carry a powder through a gauze. The better the wetting agent used, the lower the "wet point" value would be.

For solid–liquid interfaces, the work of adhering a liquid to a dry solid is given by the Dupre equation (see Ref. [23]):

$$W_{sl} = \gamma_{sv} + \gamma_{lv} - \gamma_{sl} \tag{3}$$

where γ_{sv} and γ_{sl} are not directly measurable. When Eq. (3) is combined with the Young equation for a system that is in equilibrium, ($\gamma_{sl} + \gamma_{lv} \cos \theta - \gamma_{sv} = 0$), one arrives at the Young–Dupre equation by substituting for γ_{sl}:

$$W_{sl} = \gamma_{lv} (1 + \cos \theta) \tag{4}$$

Thus, by measuring surface tension and measuring the contact angle between a solid and a wetting liquid, one can obtain the work of adhesion of a liquid to a dry solid.

For spreading of a liquid already in contact with a solid surface, the following relationship exists:

$$S(\text{spreading coefficient}) = W_{sl} - 2 \gamma_{lv} \tag{5}$$

For spreading of a liquid on a solid surface, the work of adhesion between the two substances must be greater than the work of cohesion of the spreading liquid. In Eq. (5), S must be positive for liquid l to spread on solid s.

The S could be considered the free-energy decrease on spreading. Thus, whenever S is positive, there is a decrease in free energy, and spreading will occur.

If one considers Eq. (4) again, W_{sl} equals $2\gamma_{lv}$ when $\cos \theta = 1$ or when $\theta = 0$. If θ were some finite angle, then W_{sl} would be less than $2\gamma_{lv}$, since $\cos \theta$ would be greater than 0 but less than 1.

The spreading coefficient is related to the wetting of solid particles in the initial phase or dispersion or suspension preparation; therefore, it is used as a measure of overall wetting power.

V. PREPARATION

Once the particles have been wetted, they must be separated and distributed uniformly throughout the liquid or suspending medium. The extent to which this is accomplished can be called the degree of dispersion. A solid that is broken down into primary particles without the existence of many twins or aggregates is generally considered to have a good degree of dispersion. This means that, with the use of some mixing device, the particles are in a state dominated by individual particles, wetted and distributed in a uniform way. This does not guarantee that the suspended substance will remain uniformly distributed throughout the liquid medium. The maintenance of this continuous uniform distribution is called the dispersion stability. How the initial suspension or dispersion is maintained over long periods will directly influence the quality of the suspension.

Sufficient agitation of the mixture of solid and liquid must be provided initially to obtain a high degree of dispersion, assuming that wetting is favorable. There are many types of mixing devices available ranging from minimal shear, which can be used to mix two liquids, to high-shear homogenization under moderate pressure. Some of this equipment is also capable of particle size modification. In the laboratory, it is generally sufficient to use moderate shear because of the small quantities of materials used. As the process is developed, in scale-up, higher-shear devices, such as homogenizers, are generally used. However, there are exceptions to this, depending on the suspension in question. Appendix II lists typical mixing devices. To achieve a favorable initial degree of dispersion, it is important to follow several general recommendations. The first is to prepare a vehicle that will eventually support the particles to be suspended. Since all particles that are in suspension will exhibit a tendency to settle or rise in accordance with Stokes' law [Eq. (2)], it is necessary to provide some mechanism to resist this natural tendency. If one examines the general equation for settling velocity, it seems that several options are available to accomplish this. One can reduce particle size, lower the density difference between the suspended particle and the liquid medium ($\rho_s - \rho_l$), or increase the viscosity of the suspending medium. To achieve this, generally some combination of all three approaches can be employed. Although one can use vehicles of many types, the most frequently encountered continuous external phase will certainly be aqueous. In general, a hydrocolloid or some other type of suspending agent is gradually mixed into the liquid medium. This may be preceded by the addition of preservatives, particularly if they are difficult to dissolve. The hydrocolloid may be a water-soluble material, or it could be a finely divided insoluble material, such as a clay or a cellulose derivative. In both examples, the hydrocolloids serve to create a vehicle composed of a suspending agent in the suspending liquid. This is accomplished by the gradual change in the rheological or viscosity characteristics of the liquid phase. These changes, which are discussed later in this chapter, are a result of the hydrocolloid being extended in solution, or of the finely divided material interacting with itself in an aqueous environment to bring about some degree of association that manifests itself as a higher viscosity. This is the base to which the material to be suspended, and any other materials, would eventually be added.

A second general recommendation is to avoid the entrapment of air when adding the various components of a suspension to the liquid medium. Air entrapment may impart increased viscosity to a suspension initially; however, it can be problematic throughout the addition of subsequent components and could result in an ineffective finished suspension. Entrapped air can lead to various potential problems, the most serious being inaccurate drug dosage for medication that is dispensed by volume. In addition, other problems can arise because of entrapped air: namely, those involving rheology, separation, or color inconsistencies. Equipment is available to effectively remove air from such suspensions. Some typical places of deaeration equipment are manufactured by C. Ross and Son and by the Cornell Machine Company.

Third, the use of predispersions of hydrophobic materials in other liquids should be considered, to improve the initial degree of dispersion. Liquids such as glycerin and sorbitol can generally be used in instances where a hydrophobic drug would not be adequately wet. Of course, the use of a surfactant might achieve the same end result. Each case should be considered independently. One can work with small quantities of materials to see which approach, surfactant or predispersion, works best. In this way, one can gain direction toward the best approach for achieving a uniform dispersion.

Finally, the suspension should be examined at various checkpoints in the process. Visual examination should include looking for evidence of foam, undispersed particles, and settling. It is wise to examine samples under a microscope as well, to confirm the general results found during preformulation testing.

Other ingredients that might be included in a typical pharmaceutical suspension could be sucrose or other sweeteners, water-compatible liquids, opacifiers, the material to be suspended, pigments, or flavors, or combinations thereof.

VI. STABILIZATION

Because suspensions are thermodynamically unstable systems, they always tend toward ultimate loss of stability. It is only the apparent stability that one sees at the time of examination of the product. If properly formulated, the suspension should appear uniform.

Suspensions do not form spontaneously, and work has to be expended to achieve the desired degree of dispersion. The suspension may appear to remain stable for a long time; however, thermodynamics dictates a change to a lower energy state. These changes may or may not be reversible. If the system were to find itself in an energy minimum, the change might be irreversible. It would then require too much energy to get out of the energy well or minimum energy state. While the system is thermodynamically unstable, it is the kinetics of change that dictates the usefulness of a suspension. If the change is slow enough relative to the anticipated use or shelf life of a suspension, the thermodynamics may have little practical influence.

If the thermodynamic-driving force is small enough, the rate of change may be so slow that it is indistinguishable over the anticipated shelf life of a particular product. For example, if certain dispersed particles tended to gradually settle and sediment over time, several situations might be anticipated. First, the material might flocculate and settle rapidly. This could be a reversible or an irreversible change, depending on the new energy state of the separated system. Second, the material might settle at an extremely slow rate. This might lead to eventual caking of the suspended material, but the material might appear visually stable over a long period. The third possibility is for an intermediate situation in which the rate of flocculation or coagulation is slower, yet on a time scale that is similar to a reasonable storage time for the product. In a pharmaceutical application, uniformity of product and long-term stability are required to provide accurate dosage rates. Particle size can impinge on the absorption or assimilation of drugs; thus, uniformity is necessary.

In a suspended system, the particles are thermally mobile and may occasionally collide because of their Brownian motion. As the mobile particles approach one another, both attractive and repulsive forces are at work. If the attractive forces prevail, agglomerates can grow in the suspension. This phenomenon is termed *flocculation* or *coagulation* and it represents an unstable system. If repulsive forces dominate, a more stable suspension will result. The balance between these forces determines the overall characteristics of the system. Figure 6 shows photomicrographs of colloidal Avicel* microcrystalline cellulose in various states of dispersion [25]. It is apparent that there are attractive forces operating in the case of the flocculated system.

Hydrophilic agents are often used to impart stability to dispersions and emulsions. A study conducted to examine the stabilization of oil in water emulsions by different hydrocolloids was conducted by Zatz. The breakdown of the emulsions was followed as a function of the hydrocolloid type and concentration [26].

A. Attractive Forces

Among the various types of attractive interaction operating are (a) dipole–dipole forces, (b) dipole-induced dipole forces, (c) London dispersion forces, and (d) electrostatic forces.

---

*Avicel® RC-591 is a registered trademark of FMC Corporation, Philadelphia.

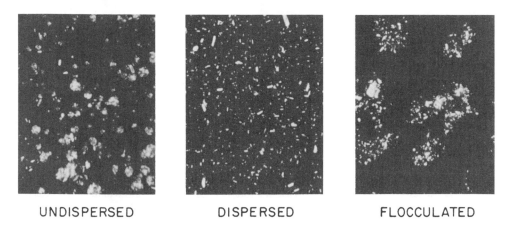

UNDISPERSED   DISPERSED   FLOCCULATED

Fig. 6 Various states of dispersion for the colloidal agent Avicel.

The attractive forces between nonpolar species, commonly called London–van der Waals forces, result from the interaction of electromagnetic dipoles within the particles. This is generally a short-range type of interaction, varying inversely with r^6, where r, in the case of suspensions, is the interparticle distance. The total attractive force between the particles is obtained by summing over all the interactions between all the particle pairs. Obviously this can become a complex mathematical function.

In the simplest case of two spherical particles of radii a_1 and a_2, separated in vacuum by a distance H, the following expression was derived for the interaction energy V_A by Hamaker [27]:

$$V_A = \frac{-A}{12}\left[\frac{y}{x^2 + xy + x} + \frac{y}{x^2 + xy + x + y} + 2\ln\left(\frac{x^2 + xy + x}{x^2 + xy + x + y} \right) \right] \tag{6}$$

where

$$x = \frac{H}{a_1 + a_2}$$

$$y = \frac{a_1}{a_2}$$

A = the Hamaker constant

If a small interparticle separation is assumed so that H is much less than a and x is much less than 1, one arrives at:

$$V_A = \frac{-A}{12}\cdot\frac{1}{2x} = \frac{-Aa}{12H}$$

where a_1 and $a_2 = a$ and $H = 2ax$. Hamaker constants are generally of the order of 10^{-13} to 10^{-12} erg. Some typical values are shown in Table 3.

Table 3   Values of Hamaker Constants

| Material | A_{11} ($\times$ 10^{-13} erg) | |
	Microscopic	Macroscopic
Water	3.3–6.4	3.0–6.1
Silica	50	8.6
Polystyrene	6.2–16.8	5.6–6.4

Source: Ref. 1.

As mentioned previously, this attractive force is additive among particle pairs; therefore, even though the van der Waals attractive force might be small, when the number of particles is high, the sum of the interactions can become quite large. For example, in Fig. 7, one can see one particle interacting with a group of particles separated by some distance *H*. Some of the possible interactions are indicated.

For each particle, one would sum up or integrate over all the interactions experienced. The van der Waals forces, resulting from oscillating dipoles and permanent dipoles, are additive. That is, all the atom pairs on neighboring particles that interact add up to the total attractive force. This can lead to a considerable attractive force. Whereas the potential energy is inversely proportional to the sixth power of the distance of separation, the van der Waals attractive force is inversely proportional to the seventh power of the distance. This is because the product of force and distance is work or energy. For larger particles, the attractive potential energy is inversely proportional to the second power (r^2) of the distance of separation. This attractive potential is more applicable to the pharmaceutical suspensions that are of interest to the formulation scientist. While the formulator may be evaluating the suspension of a macro- or grand scale, the micro- or small-scale interactions, collectively summed up, determine whether aggregation (attraction) or peptization (repulsion) will dominate the system in a kinetic sense. Experimental attempts have been made in recent years to measure the attractive forces between large objects at small distances of separation. Some of these measurements involve the use of mica plates as representative of the surface of large particles [28]. These measurements are generally conducted in electrolyte solutions. The results indicate that the existence of long-range repulsion forces diminishes as the concentration of electrolyte increases, as represented graphically in Fig. 8. A recent effort in the use of this technique was the use of surface force equipment to measure force as a function of surface separation. This is usually conducted with the use of mica surfaces. This technique enables one to study the interactions between adsorbed layers and, thereby, gain some

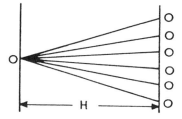

Fig. 7   Interactions among particles separated by distance *H*.

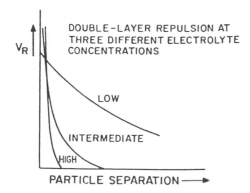

Fig. 8 Repulsive energy as a function of a particle separation at three electrolyte concentrations.

insight into the interactions of different materials. This can be of importance to many suspensions, including biological and medical. A paper on the adsorption of human serum albumin describes the technique [29]. These findings are all improvements to the original DLVO theory [named after its originators, Derjaguin, Landau, Vervey, and Overbeck], which related the balance of attractive and repulsive forces [1,24].

Since suspensions involve a liquid medium, all the foregoing comments and equations must be modified whenever the particles are in the presence of anything other than a vacuum. The interaction energy is then modified by the tendency for the particle to interact with the dispersion medium. Much of this depends on the distance of separation of the particles involved.

Just as there are forces of attraction, as evidenced by agglomerated suspensions, there are repulsive forces, which are also operational in systems that do not show agglomeration, coagulation, or flocculation.

These repulsive forces have a stabilizing influence on suspensions because they work against the aggregation of suspended particles. Repulsive forces can originate from several sources—for example, from electrostatic repulsion or from steric hindrance to the close approach of particles. There are also other sources, such as repulsive hydration forces in the interfacial region. The key requirement for stabilization is that the net repulsive term exceed the net attractive term. The origin of the charge on a suspended particle may be that of the particle itself, or may be due to the interaction of the particle with the liquid medium; or a combination of such. If a polar medium such as water is involved, various electrical interactions can occur.

Functional groups at the surface of a particle can ionize in the presence of a polar liquid. The pH of the aqueous medium typical of suspensions is important in this instance. Low-pH systems will promote a positive charge on the dispersed particle and high-pH systems a negative charge.

B. Adsorption

Other agents, such as protective colloids or polymers, can be adsorbed onto the surface of dispersed particles. This can be accomplished in several ways. The first is by adsorption from solution. In this method, one adds a solution or slurry of the adsorbable species into a slurry of the dispersed particles. Adequate time is provided for the system to equilibrate and to complete the interaction of the adsorbent with the adsorbate. Adsorption of species onto a dispersed particle is responsible for many of the resultant properties of such a system. If the material adsorbed has its own charge, be it positive or negative, the electrostatic repulsion of the like charges contributes to the stability of the dispersion. These additives can also serve as flocculants. Goossens and Luner [30] have studied the effect of agitation on the flocculation of microcrystalline cellulose suspensions with cationic polymers. An increase in suspension stability was found with the extent and degree of agitation.

A second method is by coprocessing a concentrated slurry of colloidal material with a protective colloidal agent and attriting/comminuting the mixture and processing it into a form that will be readily redispersible on contact with an appropriate dispersion medium. Colloidal Avicel microcrystalline cellulose is an example of a coprocessed product [25]. Spray drying and encapsulation represent other coprocessing techniques. As just one example, these techniques are used with flavors and fragrances.

Gums, starches, cellulose derivatives, and polymers can be adsorbed from solution. These materials can be ionized to some extent or nonionized. The degree of protection provided is related to the extent of adsorption and the chain length.

Many polymer molecules have many functional groups and, because of the flexibility of the macromolecule in solution, some of these functional groups could be adsorbed at a solid surface. The possible modes of attachment (polar, hydrogen bonding, etc.) have been described [31]. Depending on the shape of the macromolecule, the thickness of the adsorbed layer can vary. For example, if the chain is coiled into a sphere, the thickness of the adsorbed layer would be approximately the diameter of the coiled macromolecule.

A typical potential energy diagram (Fig. 9) shows the repulsive (V_r) and the attractive (V_a) energy curves for the interaction of two charged particles as a function of interparticle distance. The net or total potential energy curve is also shown. Several key points concerning this graph should be emphasized [32,33].

1. From the curve, it is evident that the attractive potential is predominant at short distances of separation.

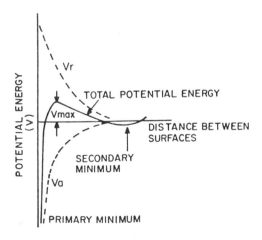

Fig. 9 Potential energy curves for the interaction of two charged surfaces.

2. The potential energy barrier (V_{max}) must be surmounted before contact in the primary energy minimum. This is where one can compare the potential energy with the kinetic energy, kT, where k is the Boltzmann constant (1.38×10^{-16} erg deg^{-1}).

3. At larger distances of separation, there is a secondary minimum. If this is slightly larger than kT, particles might associate to form a loose cluster.

As part of this discussion of potential energy curves, it is appropriate to describe the effect of the charge that is carried by the dispersed particles. As previously mentioned, this can arise from the ionization of surface groups, such as carboxylic acid groups or amine groups. The charge is a function of the pH of the medium. In addition to ionization, adsorption has been mentioned as a route to the introduction of surface charges.

Regardless of origin, charged particles have the potential to move in the presence of an electric field. Their rate of movement, defined as electrophoretic mobility, is generally in the range of 2×10^{-4}–4×10^{-4} cm sec^{-1}, when the potential gradient is 1 V cm^{-1} [34]

The presence of the charge at a solid–liquid interface can be considered to consist of two parts: a region that is held to the surface, so that it moves with the surface; and a more diffuse region or diffuse layer that extends out to the bulk liquid. If the particle is negatively charged, the fixed layer, also known as the Stern layer, will have a positive charge. However, the more diffuse layer, which contains both cations and anions, serves to balance the surface charge.

The primary factor determining the thickness of this "double layer" is the potential energy dropoff. This, in turn, is related to the concentration of electrolyte that may be present. The charge of the ions also plays a role if one considers the equation that describes the thickness of the double layer [35]:

$$\frac{1}{K} = \frac{(DkT)^{1/2}}{2ne^2z^2} \tag{7}$$

where $1/K$ is called the Debye length, D is the dielectric constant of the medium, T is the temperature, k is the Boltzmann constant, n is the concentration of ions in the bulk, e is the electronic charge, and z is the valence.

In water at room temperature, the thickness of the double layer generally ranges from 1.0 to 1000 Å, depending on the concentration of ions in the bulk phase. Figure 10 shows the typical structure of the electric double layer.

The potential is ψ_0 at the surface of the particle and decays to ψ_d, termed the Stern potential, in the fixed or adsorbed layer. It then decays to zero in the diffuse part of the double layer.

If one were to increase the overall electrolyte concentration, the V_{max} barrier would be reduced, promoting flocculation. This is the result of compression of the double layer of charge that surrounds each suspended particle.

If the secondary minimum is small, relative to the kinetic energy, a small amount of energy will be required (e.g., shaking by hand) to reverse the system. Significantly more energy is required to displace the system from the primary energy minimum that is found at small distances of separation.

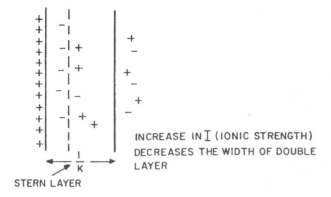

Fig. 10 Diffuse double layer for a positively charged surface.

Again, the double layer of charge consists of a charge localized at the surface of the dispersed particle and a more diffuse layer of opposite sign, which extends away from the particle toward the dispersion medium.

The potential gradient is very dependent on the presence of any electrolytes that may be present in the dispersion medium. The double layer is generally said to have a thickness δ, which takes into account the decay of the potential. Another estimation for the thickness can be calculated from the following equation:

$$\delta \ (\text{in } \text{Å}) = \frac{0.34}{z}\left(\frac{p}{m}\right)^{1/2} \tag{8}$$

where

D = dielectric constant
z = ion valence (same for both anion and cation)
m = concentration of ions (mol L^{-1})

It is apparent from Eq. (8) that the thickness of the double layer will be decreased if the overall ion valence (e.g., $Na^+ \rightarrow Al^{+3}$) and/or ion concentration are increased. This is equivalent to a compression of the double layer of charge.

Since the repulsion between two charged particles depends on the distance between the particles, be they point charges or diffuse double layers, it should be apparent that δ, the double-layer thickness, is a key parameter in the determination of V_R.

Patton [24] has expressed this relationship in the following way:

$$\frac{V_R}{kT} = 0.01Dd \ \zeta^2 \ \ln\left[1 + \exp\left(\frac{-S}{\delta}\right)\right] \tag{9}$$

D = dielectric constant
d = particle diameter (μm)
ζ = zeta potential (mV)
S = separation between surfaces (Å)
δ = double-layer thickness (Å)

Both particle size and zeta potential are directly related to the repulsion potential. Measurements of zeta potential have shown a relationship to dispersion stability such that the higher the magnitude of the zeta potential, the greater stability of the dispersion.

The cell used for the study of colloidal dispersions usually consists of a horizontal tube of circular cross section, with an electrode at each end. It is important that the measurement be taken reasonably quickly, to avoid sedimentation in the cell. More details on the measurement of electrophoretic mobility are found in other sources [36]. Basically, however, electrophoretic mobility is measured by timing individual particles over a certain distance, using a calibrated eyepiece with a scale. Generally, the results of approximately 10–15 timing measurements are averaged. The direct current voltage is adjusted to obtain a velocity that is neither too fast nor too slow, to allow for errors in measurement and Brownian motion, respectively.

From Fig. 8, it can be observed that repulsion potential is generally reduced as the ion concentration increases. This is a result of the compression of the electrical double layer. The charges of added ions or electrolytes serve to diminish the thickness of the double layer. As this occurs, the repulsive forces decrease, and if the particles are able to approach each other closely, the previously mentioned attractive forces will prevail.

The concentration of foreign electrolyte required to cause flocculation decreases as the valence of the coagulating ion increases. For example, less Al^{3+} would be required to flocculate a suspension than Na^+. This has been observed in many instances and is known as the Schulze–Hardy rule. It has been shown that the quantity of electrolyte required to bring about flocculation decreases by a factor of 100 as one goes from a monovalent electrolyte to a divalent one (e.g., Na^+ vs. Mg^{2+}) [37].

Similar to many other chemical occurrences, the repulsive force goes through a maximum before the attractive force takes over. The same situation is found in explanations dealing with reaction mechanisms in chemical kinetics as well as in other physical phenomena, such as fluid flow.

To this point, much of the discussion has centered on the interaction of electrical forces. As previously mentioned, however, adsorbed species may be nonpolar. In such a case, the mechanism of repulsion differs from true elctrostatics. A schematic of several methods of stabilization is shown in Fig. 11 [36]. One can observe that the adsorbed species can extend into the dispersion medium. Part of the protective material is adsorbed at the surface of the suspended particle and another part of the molecule reaches into the bulk liquid.

The adsorbed chains are believed to prevent the close approach of two particles. Interactions between such particles lead to a system with increased order or greater free energy, which is observed as a loss of movement or freedom of movement, respectively, as the polymer chains interact. This implies a more ordered system. In essence, this is energetically unfavorable and, in a sense, constitutes a repulsive force that could stabilize the system. The mechanism centers on the decreased entropy, or increased ordering or alignment, which results from the interaction between two extended adsorbates. The interaction of the dispersion medium with the adsorbates can provide insight into whether flocculation by bridging might occur. If insufficient attraction exists, bridging might occur.

For example, when the chains interact, there is a tendency for a recovery force or a repulsion to manifest itself. This is true as long as there is some affinity or attraction between the adsorbed polymer and the dispersion medium. This type of stabilizing

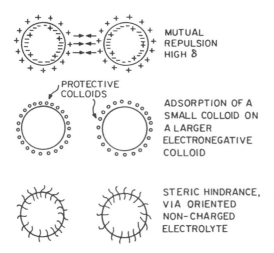

MUTUAL
REPULSION
HIGH δ

PROTECTIVE
COLLOIDS

ADSORPTION OF A
SMALL COLLOID ON
A LARGER
ELECTRONEGATIVE
COLLOID

STERIC HINDRANCE,
VIA ORIENTED
NON-CHARGED
ELECTROLYTE

Fig. 11 Schematic of three methods of stabilization of colloid particles. (From Ref. 36.)

mechanism is more common as the suspension becomes more concentrated. The overlap is too ordered or entropically unfavorable and, therefore, a repulsive force surfaces. Interparticle forces have been discussed in an effort to explain the stability of suspensions of fine particles. The steric repulsion, which arises partly from the repulsion between adsorbed polymer layers, was also examined in an effort to explain the polymer bridging effect [38].

To complete the section on attractive and repulsive forces, it is necessary to include these entropic or steric repulsive forces. The main controlling factor remains the same. The overall repulsion must exceed the attraction so that there exists an energy barrier that is at least several times greater than the thermal energy, designated by the term kT.

Relative to the forces that are involved in dispersions, van Oss maintains that many of the interactions are really consequences of one or several primary forces. These primary forces are van der Waals forces, electrostatic, hydrogen bonding, and Brownian motion-induced interactions. The DLVO theory combines both the van der Waals--London attraction with the electrostatic repulsion between particles. For hydrogen-bonding interactions in water-based dispersions, they can be attractive or repulsive, depending on whether they are viewed as hydrophobic or hydrophilic interactions. Hydrogen-bonding interactions between hydrophobic particles are attractive. Conversely, hydrogen-bonding interactions between similar particles can be repulsive, as a consequence of the interaction of hydration layers. Brownian motion helps keep particles in motion, unless the attraction between two particles can overcome the thermal energy. Particles with a larger surface area have a greater chance of overcoming the repulsive forces of Brownian motions [39].

C. Sedimentation

Some mention has already been made of using sedimentation techniques to measure the particle size distribution of suspended materials. This section describes the effect of sedimentation on both the physical and functional properties of suspensions.

Since adequate and uniform dosage is a prerequisite for any pharmaceutical suspension, the necessity for control of sedimentation is obvious. Because settling velocity is proportional to the second power of the particle radius, it is apparent that agglomerates and flocculates will settle more rapidly than properly dispersed particles. Both gravity and buoyancy are operating on the particle. As a result, one could have either upward or downward movement: "creaming" or "settling," respectively. The determining factor is the difference in density of the suspended particle and the liquid medium. If a flocculate acts as a single particle, the velocity of settling may be greater, since the velocity is proportional to the density difference between the particle and the suspending medium and the size of the particle. Similarly, if there is a particle size distribution of the suspended particles, it is highly likely that the settled material will eventually consist of particles of varying size.

A deflocculated system, that is, one in which the dispersed particles are discrete and in which there is little or no association, might exhibit slow sedimentation of particles over time. The supernatant liquid would be cloudy, and the settled particles might arrange themselves into a hard-packed cake, since the particles have an opportunity to pack. For example, they could settle into a hardened mass, making wetting and subsequent dispersion into primary particles difficult to achieve. Caking requires a high degree of agitation for redispersion. The polydispersity, or range of particle sizes, might have an influence on the tendency toward caking. In some instances, the particles could settle in a manner such that they would not be readily redispersible. This would result in a product lacking in dose consistency because of failure to obtain and maintain a good degree of dispersion, for the reasons mentioned earlier.

When matter is in a dispersed state, the dispersed material will have an equilibrium solubility that varies relative to its particle size. Small particles will have a higher equilibrium solubility than larger particles. As a result, there is a finite tendency for the smaller particles to solubilize. They can subsequently precipitate from solution on the surface of the larger particles. Thus, the larger particles grow at the expense of the smaller particles. This phenomenon is known as Ostwald ripening [43]. Again considering work done in other fields, an adaptation of this phenomenon was observed in paper technology, in which changes in particle size distribution are important in defining the overall qualities and properties of the paper. In a polydisperse system, particles aggregated with larger particles, rather than with identical-sized particles. Thus, the number of smaller particles was reduced. Awareness of this principle leads to a better understanding of the interactions in a suspension [40]. Thus, within certain limitations, it is advisable to keep the differences among the particles to a minimum. If ripening were occurring during sedimentation, a caked deposit might result.

One could prevent this slow settling by building up the viscosity of the suspension medium until the overall settling rate was markedly reduced. This is the area served by thixotropic suspension aids, which provide resistance to flow when the suspension is at rest or at very low rates of shear.

D. Flocculation

An alternative to providing a yield stress that functions against settling is an attempt to achieve some degree of flocculation, which facilitates resuspension.

Particles that associate and settle do not have an opportunity to pack at the bottom of the container or package. As a result, a loose sediment or layer is formed; among colloidal chemists and formulators, this process is called controlled flocculation. It is a method of accepting the reality that settling will occur eventually. From a thermodynamic standpoint, settling is inevitable; the time that it takes is the primary factor in dealing with the stabilization of pharmaceutical products.

If a loose structure or "floc" is formed, it acts as a single particle and commences settling at a faster rate. In some cases, flocs have been known to provide some suspending properties because of their tendency to form networks, which can entrap some suspended particles. The flocs are formed when suspended particles that are allowed to come into contact during motion remain in contact by associating in loose clusters. Generally, these clusters can be ruptured into primary particles by the application of low to moderate shear.

The frequency with which the particles collide is a function of concentration, temperature, the viscosity of the liquid medium, and the physical properties of the particles themselves. With time, as flocculation occurs, the total number of discrete particles is decreased. Thus, the quantity $1/N$, where N is the number of particles, increases with time during flocculation. This quantity is frequently used in equations dealing with the rate of flocculation. Distinctions are made between aggregates and agglomerates.

Flocculates are loosely bound clusters, having an open type of structure. *Aggregates* are more strongly bonded particles and are more difficult to redisperse or resuspend. *Agglomerates* are intermediate between aggregates and flocs.

For flocculation to occur, the repulsive force must be diminished until some attraction prevails. This can be brought about by the introduction of an electrolyte or by bridging between particles.

Electrolytes serve to reduce the effective range of the repulsive forces operating on suspended particles. This is reflected in the overall mobility of the particles. In fact, one can study the acquisition of charge by following the electrophoretic mobility. Formulators of pharmaceutical suspensions attempt to induce flocculation, which can be controlled if it appears likely that a caked sediment would otherwise result. The flocs are soft and easily redispersed with mild agitation, thereby providing a uniform and effective drug dose at the time of administration.

Combining the many separate issues that have been discussed—namely, settling according to Stokes' law, hindered settling, buoyancy forces, rheological yield points, and particle size—it is apparent that many factors contribute to the overall quality of the dispersion. Yet, it is possible that one or several of these parameters could be the decisive one in determining the appearance of the dispersion.

Since many pharmaceutical suspensions are packaged in opaque containers, the separation is not visible to the user. Generally, directions for use indicate that the contents should be shaken before use.

Other methods of bringing about flocculation are coagulation, bridging, and charge neutralization. Bridging generally results from the interaction of an adsorbed species that extends into the bulk medium away from the suspended particle [30]. An example of this is an adsorbed polymer that has groups that could associate with each other through the dispersion medium (e.g., hydroxyl groups). These distances of approach can be influenced by the electrical environment which, in turn, controls the effective repulsion distance. The bridging mechanism generally operates at large distances of separation relative to flocculation by electrolytes. The adsorbed species may be charged or uncharged.

Control measurements made during product development should verify that an adequate and effective dose is available throughout the use of the product. This is an important step in product evaluation while the product is undergoing an accelerated stability test regimen. For example, during the product development program, one should ascertain that pH, viscosity, assay procedure, and appearance, all are satisfactory. These parameters can be evaluated both on in-process samples as well as on the finished dispersion.

However, considering the work that goes into the wetting and subsequent dispersing of the particles that one wishes to suspend, the controlled-flocculation approach seems to be a step in the wrong direction. It might seem preferable to develop a system that, once adequately wetted and dispersed, remains in a deflocculated state with little tendency toward sedimentation. The rate of sedimentation could be extremely slow when compared with the anticipated storage time of the dispersion. Nevertheless, controlled flocculation is used as a method of product stabilization. In contrast, as discussed in the next section, reducing the settling tendency by the addition of rheological agents can obviate the need for flocculation.

VII. RHEOLOGICAL ASPECTS

The rheological behavior of pharmaceutical suspensions is a key factor in assessing the overall performance characteristics of a product. Although the developmental effort to achieve acceptable flow properties can be substantial for a suspension, the consumer is quite aware of product efficacy and elegance. Therefore, the product characteristics should be outlined and achieved early in the product's developmental stage.

This section briefly reviews some fundamental principles of rheology, with emphasis on the principles that influence the functional attributes of pharmaceutical suspensions. In addition, a brief description of some typical suspending agents is provided.

A. Types of Flow

The term *fluidity* describes a material's ability to flow. *Viscosity*, which is defined as the resistance to flow, or the reciprocal of fluidity, is expressed as the ratio between shear stress and shear rate. *Shear stress* (τ) is the ratio of the force used to move one layer of fluid past another compared with the area of material in contact. It is expressed in dynes per square centimeter:

$$\tau = \frac{\text{force (dynes)}}{\text{area (cm}^2)} \tag{10}$$

Shear rate is the ratio of the speed (V) of relative movement of one surface past another to the distance (Y) between the surfaces. Generally, the surfaces are assumed to be flat planes. It is expressed in reciprocal seconds.

$$D = \frac{V(\text{cm sec}^{-1})}{Y(\text{cm})} \tag{11}$$

Viscosity (η) is the ratio of shear stress to shear ratio : $\eta = \tau/D$. Its unit is the poise (P, cP, etc.).

Different pharmaceutical products respond differently to applied shear. Most of the fluids or semisolids encountered are classified as non-newtonian materials. Newtonian fluids will flow under any applied force and exhibit a constant ratio between shear stress and the rate of shear. Plastic, pseudoplastic, dilatant, and thixotropic systems are classified as nonnewtonian.

Briefly, plastic flow requires a minimum shear stress for flow to commence. It is observed in dispersions of finely divided solids in liquids. The minimum stress is designated τ_0 and is often referred to as a yield stress or yield point. The yield stress originates from particle–particle bonds that exist when the suspension is at rest. For the initiation of flow, these bonds must be broken or disrupted. The force necessary to accomplish this is called the yield stress. For a suspension, this characteristic is important in that settling is minimized in systems that possess a yield stress. Once the yield stress has been surpassed, the flow is newtonian and is termed Bingham flow.

Pseudoplastic flow is quite common in pharmaceutical suspensions. In this case, a yield value may not exist, but there is an apparent decrease in viscosity (η) as the rate of shear (D) increases. This is shown by dispersions as well as by some high-molecular-weight polymer solutions. Solutions of hydrocolloids, such as sodium carboxymethylcellulose and other cellulose ethers, show this characteristic.

Dilatant flow is less common and may occasionally be observed in deflocculated dispersions of powders at high volume concentrations. Here, the apparent viscosity increases as the rate of shear increases. This is attributed to the close packing of particles, which during shearing, results in interparticle contact and interaction. This, in turn, manifests itself as an increase in apparent viscosity.

Thixotropic flow is the most unique of all and finds wide application in the pharmaceutical as well as cosmetic, food, and industrial areas. It brings together some of the features previously mentioned. Among the features of thixotropic flow are the following.

1. The material possesses a yield point.
2. A reduction in viscosity occurs on shearing with time.
3. There is a rebuilding of viscosity on standing.
4. The material combines features of both plastic and pseudoplastic flow behavior.
5. There exists a time dependency, which is not common to the other types of flow.

A recent theoretical paper describes the theory of suspensions in terms of the viscoelastic properties of a colloidal dispersion. The theory examines the interactions between dispersed spheres in a newtonian liquid as well as the frictional effects of the liquid medium [41].

In considering the viscosity of pharmaceutical suspensions, the general expectation is for a nonnewtonian system. An approach for the study of concentrated suspensions recently proposed that at some critical concentration of the suspended particle, a cluster or secondary structure is formed throughout the system. The properties of the cluster determine the viscosity of the suspension [42].

B. Important Factors for Suspensions

The flow pattern of a particular suspension can be determined by examining a plot of shear stress versus rate of shear. Figure 12 shows the relationship observed with several types of flow. The slope or $\Delta Y/\Delta X$ of the plot generally determines the type of flow of the system. Here, the change in shear stress divided by the change in shear rate determines the type of flow.

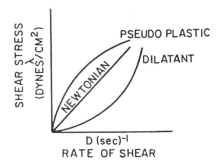

Fig. 12 Flow curves for several types of flow.

Thixotropy is of particular value for pharmaceutical suspensions. During shearing, such as occurs in shaking by hand, the yield stress is exceeded, and the suspension flows. The structure begins to re-form after the cessation of shear. However, it does not re-form immediately. It takes time to rebuild the order or structure that existed when the system was at rest. As long as the system rebuilds itself to a point at which sedimentation is avoided or substantially diminished, one can achieve a pharmaceutical suspension of good quality. The key is the rate at which the structure is rebuilt. This is a function of the nature of the thixotropic agent, its concentration in the vehicle or medium of the suspension, and the amount of agitation before use.

Since it takes time for the structure to rebuild, thixotropic systems are known to show hysteresis, or a difference between upward and downward shear rates during a continuous rheogram (Fig. 13).

Proper formulation design of a suspension requires that one evaluate the characteristics of the product throughout its use cycle. The use of thixotropic agents, such as Veegum, magnesium aluminum silicate, clays, xanthan gum, or colloidal Avicel microcrystalline cellulose, can provide the unique properties needed for an elegant suspension.

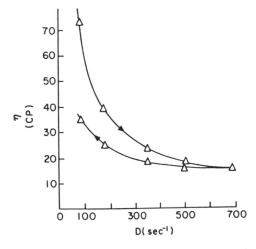

Fig. 13 Typical hysteresis in a rheogram of a thixotrope.

In some cases, combinations of these or other materials provide added benefits, such as resistance to electrolytes. In general, one must also determine the rheological and stability characteristics at temperatures other than normal (ambient), if it is likely that the product will be stored for any length of time at lower or higher temperatures. This should be part of the accelerated-aging protocol for such products. Preferably the rheological characteristics should not be overly sensitive to changes in temperature. Viscosity changes of 10% or more are to be avoided. Some polymeric materials, particularly water-soluble cellulose derivatives, undergo significant viscosity decreases over a 10° (25–35°C) temperature shift. Other materials are less sensitive to such temperature changes. For this, each product must be evaluated separately.

Water-insoluble thixotropic agents generally consist of rod-shaped or irregular particles suspended throughout the medium. When the suspension is at rest, the particles are randomly arranged, providing a three-dimensional network. The yield stress is high enough to overcome any Brownian motion. As the shear rate is increased from the rest position by shaking or pouring, the rod-shaped particles tend to align, with a corresponding reduction in viscosity. On cessation of shear, the particles again rearrange, owing to thermal motion, and structures showing a yield point will be gradually regained.

VIII. EFFECT OF ADDITIVES

A. pH

The correct pH for drug stability is a requirement for all liquid dosage formulations; however, additional considerations need to be addressed for suspensions.

For suspensions that are stabilized primarily by a yield stress mechanism, it is important to consider the optimum pH for the product, since the properties of a suspension, particularly rheology, can be quite dependent on the pH of the system. The viscosity of hydrocolloids is somewhat dependent on pH. At extreme conditions, suspensions of these materials have flocculated. In general, most systems are stable over a pH range of 4–10; however, the viscosity of some materials change as a function of pH. This can be a result of the concept known as the point of zero charge (PZC), that is, the pH at which the net surface charge is zero [35].

For example, some hydrocolloids, such as colloidal Avicel microcrystalline cellulose and some xanthan gums, show a higher viscosity at neutral pH conditions. The difference may not appear to be dramatic, but it can have an effect.

Appendix III lists the characteristics of typical materials used as thickeners or suspending agents. All these materials have some limitations, such as sensitivity to electrolytes. In some instances, one material can serve as a protective colloid for another suspending agent, as with xanthan gum or methylcellulose, which can be used with another agent, such as colloidal Avicel microcrystalline cellulose.

Each particular suspension should be examined for its pH stability with time, because any changes in pH could be indicative of a potential problem.

B. Temperature

The influence of temperature on the preparation and long-term stability of suspensions has already been mentioned. Some suspending agents can tolerate higher temperature during processing. Other materials, such as sodium carboxymethylcellulose, are more sensitive to higher temperatures. Since it is sometimes necessary to heat a suspension preparation to bring about the solubilization of one ingredient (e.g., a preservative), the long-term effect of such a process on the product must be evaluated. The viscosity of suspensions generally decreases with an increase in temperature. How this coefficient of viscosity changes with temperature could be of importance in both the processing and long-term storage of a suspension product. For most liquid materials, viscosity is related to temperature [34] by the following equation:

$$\eta = A \exp \frac{E}{RT} \tag{12}$$

or

$$\ln \eta = \ln A + \frac{E}{RT}$$

where

A is a constant for the liquid
R is the gas constant (1.987 cal deg^{-1} mol^{-1})
E is the activation energy for flow
T is the absolute temperature

For suspensions, one will similarly observe a decrease in viscosity as temperature is increased. However, some materials are much more sensitive than others; therefore, one should understand the changes in rheology as a function of moderate temperature changes ($\pm 20°C$).

C. Additives

Any other materials added to suspensions, such as flavor oils, humectants, or dyes, can impinge on the overall effectiveness and appearance of the product. Ideally, one should strive for a base vehicle that is more tolerant of such additives. Generally, salts provide a destabilizing influence on dispersed particles by bringing about flocculation. Although the details for this type of destabilization are fairly well explained by the previously mentioned DLVO theory [44], the total effect of some types of additives, particularly those that function in a steric role, is more complex.

Additives that adsorb on the surface of a suspended particle can differ quite markedly. Polymeric materials can adsorb at various functional groups. The mode of adsorption depends on the polymer chain and the number of sites available for interaction on the particle itself. Most of the nonelectrolyte polymers promote steric stabilization, which is generally categorized by either entropic stabilization or an osmotic repulsion [31]. The entropic stabilization or change in the ordering of the system has been discussed previously. This stabilization arises from a repulsive force when two adsorbed species try to become associated. The osmotic term represents a driving force to balance any changes that might occur by trying to have two adsorbed species occupy neighboring space. The effect of additives on a suspension can be significant. Not only product appearance, but also product efficacy can be affected. It is necessary to make certain that the additives selected are appropriate and that they do not impair overall product characteristics.

IX. SUMMARY

Some of the factors that are important in preparing a good suspension have been reviewed. Suspensions of various types were classified, and methods of preparation were discussed. The importance of satisfactory wetting and the influence of particle shape and size were also covered by some detail. An extended discussion of the techniques and modifications in particle size analysis has been provided.

The different forces, both attractive and repulsive, that affect suspended particles, were examined. The origin of these forces was also discussed. For a stable dispersion, the repulsive force must exceed the attractive force. Protective colloids or polymers can be adsorbed on the surface of dispersed particles and can play a major role by either charge or steric stabilization mechanisms. The effect of added electrolytes was examined in light of their effect on the repulsive force.

Sedimentation, caking, flocculation, and redispersibility are key performance criteria in suspension preparation.

Finally, the different types of flow that can be encountered in suspension systems were described. The use of rheological additives was emphasized as a means of preventing settling and eventual caking. Yield stress and thixotropy were seen to be two extremely desirable suspension characteristics.

The influence of pH, temperature, and chemical additives on overall suspension quality was considered briefly.

Suspension theory is a field of work in which the experimental techniques are in need of some advancement. New particle-sizing instrumentation and particle analysis techniques have been brought forth in the past few years. Use of these techniques should enable scientists to better understand the mechanisms of flocculation and redispersion.

APPENDIX I

TYPICAL PARTICLE SIZE DEVICES

Sieving Equipment

Tyler Ro-Tap
Alpine Air jet

Sedimentation Equipment

Sartorious sedimentation balance
Cahn sedimentation balance
Micromeritics x-ray sedigraph
Photomicron sizer (Seishen)
Joyce Loebl disk centrifuge

Electrical Sensing Zone Equipment

Coulter Counter
Electrozone Celloscope

Manufacturers of Light-Scattering Equipment

Brookhaven Instruments
Malvern Instruments
Brice-Phoenix
Coulter
Horiba

APPENDIX II

MIXING EQUIPMENT: MANUFACTURERS AND DEVICES

Lightnin' Mixing Equipment Company, Inc. 195 Mount Read Boulevard Rochester, NY 14603	Blender, mixer, aerator, Lightnin' Mixer, portable air mixer, impellers
Charles Ross & Sons Company 710 Old Willets Path Hauppauge, NY 11787	Mixer, emulsifier
Arde Barinco 19 Industrial Avenue Mahwah, NJ 07430	Mixer, blender, emulsifier
Greerco Corporation Executive Drive Hudson, NH 03051	Homogenizer, mixer
Premier Mill Corporation Exeter Industrial Park Birchmont Drive Reading, PA 19606	Dispersator
Caframo Limited P.O. Box 70 Warton, Ontario Appendix III N0H 2T0, Canada	Stirrers

(text continues)

APPENDIX III

PROPERTIES OF TYPICAL HYDROCOLLOIDS

Item[a]	Properties in water	pH stability	Rheology[b]
Methocel	Soluble in cold, insoluble in hot	3–11	Pseudoplastic, η decreases with temperature
Carbopol 934	Wets out	5–11	Plastic flow, significant τ_0
NaCMC Hercules cellulose gum	Soluble hot or cold	4–9	Pseudoplastic, some thixotropy, temperature-dependent
Veegum	Disperses and hydrates	3.5–11	Pseudoplastic, 4% or more for thixotropy, thickens on aging
Xanthan gum (Keltrol)	Dispersible, soluble	3–11	Very pseudoplastic, high η, small τ_0
Sodium alginate	High stirring, dispersible	4–10	Pseudoplastic, η decreases with temperature
Natural gums, guar, tragacanth	Dispersible	4–10	η decreases with aging
Avicel 591	Dispersible	η stable, 4–11	< 1% pseudoplastic, > 1% thixotropic

[a]Methocel, Carbopol, Hercules cellulose gum, and Keltrol are trademarks of Dow Chemical, B.F. Goodrich, Hercules, and Kelco, respectively.
[b]η, viscosity; τ, shear stress (yield).

REFERENCES

1. D. J. Shaw, in *Introduction to Colloid and Surface Chemistry*, 3rd ed., Butterworths, London, 1980.
2. T. Allen, in Powder Technology Series, *Particle Size Measurement*, 2nd ed. (B. Scarlett, ed.), Chapman Hall, London, 1975.
3. H. Heywood, Symposium on particle size analysis, *Inst. Chem. Eng. Supp.*, 25:14, 1947.
4. C. F. Harwood, in *Particle Size Analysis* (J. D. Stockham and E. G. Fochtman, eds.), Ann Arbor Science Publishers, Ann Arbor, MI, 1978, p. 112.
5. W. C. McCrone, L. B. McCrone, and J. Gustav Delly, *Polarized Light Microscopy*, Ann Arbor Science Publishers, Ann Arbor, MI, 1979, p. 100.
6. B. W. Mueller, P. Kleinbudde, T. Oestberg, and T. Waaler, *Pharm. Ind.*, 52, 1967, 1990.

Incompatibility	Advantages	Description	Manufacturer
Electrolytes and surfactants	Good protectors used with other agents, not a primary agent	Methyl ether of cellulose	Dow Chemical Co.
Soluble salts and cationic polyvalent ions	Can suspend up to 10% solids, stable to hydrolysis and high temperature	Carboxyvinyl polymer; high molecular weight	B. F. Goodrich
Di- and trivalent salts	Anionic polyelectrolyte, retards crystal growth, protective colloid	Cellulose ether	Hercules
Flocculation by electrolytes, incompatible with acid drugs	Good suspender, good redispersion	Natural, complex colloidal magnesium aluminum silicate	R. T. Vanderbilt
Cationic and polyvalent ions at high pH	Excellent suspending agent, stable in salts, compatible with nonionics	High molecular weight polysaccharide	Kelco, NJ
Ca precipitate, heavy metal ions, strong acids	Colloidal electrolyte, film-former, newtonian	Polysaccharide from brown seaweed	Kelco, NJ
Rigid specifications		Natural; specifications are important	
Dispersibility affected by electrolytes, sucrose	In dispersion ultimate particle size 0.15 μm, can tolerate glycols and alcohols, compatible with hydrocolloids	Chemically depolymerized wood pulp	FMC Corp.

7. G. Staudinger, M. Hangl, and P. Pechtl, *Particle Charact.*, 3(4), 158, 1986.
8. G. C. Barker and M. J. Grimsom, *Colloids Surf.*, 43, 55, 1990.
9. R. L. Hoffman, *J. Colloid Interface Sci.*, 143, 232, 1991.
10. B. U. Felderhof, *Ber, Bunsen - Ges Phys. Chem.*, 94, 222, 1990.
11. M. J. Groves, *R. Soc. Chem.*, 102 (Part. Size Anal.), 91, 1992.
12. G. Gouesbet, B. Maheu, and G. Grehan, *Pure Appl. Chem.*, 64, 1685, 1992.
13. B. B. Weiner, *R. Soc. Chem.*, 102 (Part. Size Anal.) 173, 1992.
14. T. Stauffer, Horiba. Inst., private communication, 1995
15. J. .J. Cooper, *Ceram. Eng. Sci. Proc.* 12, 133, 1991.
16. A. D. Levine, G. Tchobanoglous, and T. Asano, *Fluid Part. Sep. J.* 4, 89, 1991.
17. A. D. Chin, P. B. Butler, and D. W. Luerkens, *Powder Technol.*, 54, 99, 1988.
18. J. J. Ruan, *ACS Symp. Ser., 492* (Polym. Latexes), 289, 1992.
19. B. V. Miller and R. W. Lines, *Crit. Rev. Anal. Chem.* 20, 75, 1988.
20. W.H. Flank, *Ind. Eng. Chem. Res.*, 26, 1750, 1987.
21. P. Becher, *Emulsions: Theory and Practice,* 2nd ed. Reinhold, New York, 1965, p. 381.
22. H. W. Fox and W. A. Zisman, *J. Colloid Sci.*, 7, 428, 1952.

23.   G. Zografi and B. A. Johnson, *Int. J. Pharm.*, 22, 159, 1984.
24.   T. C. Patton, in *Paint Flow and Pigment Dispersion*, 2nd ed, Wiley, New York, 1979.
25.   Technical Applications Bulletin AVCOL0584P3, FMC Corp., Philadelphia, 1983.
26.   J. L. Zatz and B. K. Ip, *J. Soc. Cosmet. Chem.* 37, 329, 1986.
27.   H. C. Hamaker, *Physica*, 4:1058, 1937.
28.   J. N. Israelachvili and G. E. Adams, *Faraday Trans.* 1, 74:975, 1978.
29.   E. Blomberg, P. M. Claesson, and C. G. Golander, *J. Dispersion Sci. Technol.*, 12, 179, 1991.
30.   J. W. S. Goossens and P. Luner, *Tappi* 59, 89, 1976.
31.   T. Sato and R. Ruch, in Surfactant Science Series, *Stabilization of Colloidal Dispersions by Polymer Adsorption*, Vol. 9 (M. Schick and F. Fowkes, ed.), Dekker, New York, 1980.
32.   K. J. Mysels, *Introduction to Colloid Chemistry*, Wiley-Interscience, New York, 1959.
33.   G. E. VanGils and G. M. Kraay, in *Advances in Colloid Science*, Vol. 1 (E. O. Kraemer, ed.), Wiley-Interscience, New York, 1942.
34.   S. Glasstone and D. Lewis, in *Elements of Physical Chemistry*, 2nd ed., Van Nostrand, Princeton, N.J., 1960.
35.   S. L. Hem, J. R. Feldkamp, and J. L. White, in *The Theory and Practice of Industrial Pharmacy* (L. Lachman, H. A. Lieberman, and J. L. Kanig, eds.), Lea & Febiger, Philadelphia, 1986, p. 110.
36.   T. M. Riddick, in *Control of Colloid Stability Through Zeta Potential*, Vol. 1, Livingston, Wynnewood, PA, 1968.
37.   J. T. G Overbeek, in *Colloid Science*, Vol. 1 (H. Kruyt, ed.), Elsevier, New York, 1952.
38.   K. Furusawa, *Nippon Insatsu Gakkaishi*, 30, 76, 1993.
39.   C. J. van Oss, *J. Dispersion Sci. Technol.*, 12, 201, 1991.
40.   M. Milichovsky, *Sb. Veo. Pr., Vys. Sk. Chem. Technol. Pardubice*, 50B, 467, 1987.
41.   H. Jorquera and J. S. Dahler, *J. Chem. Phys.*, 96, 6917, 1992.
42.   G. A. Campbell and G. Gorgacs, *Phys. Rev. A*, 41, 4570, 1990.
43.   G. A. Hulett, in *Colloid Chemistry*, Vol. 1 (J. Alexander, ed.), Chemical Catalog Co., New York, 1926, p. 637.
44.   P. C. Hiemenz, *Principles of Colloid and Surface Chemistry*, Dekker, New York, 1977.

3

Theory of Emulsions

Stig E. Friberg

Clarkson University, Potsdam, New York

Lisa Goldsmith Quencer

The Dow Chemical Company, Midland, Michigan

Martha L. Hilton

University of Missouri—Rolla, Rolla, Missouri

I. INTRODUCTION

Traditionally, *emulsions* have been defined as dispersions of macroscopic droplets of one liquid in another liquid, with a droplet diameter approximately in the range of 0.5–100 μm [1–3]. A large number of emulsions do, in fact, consist of only two liquids (Fig. 1). The stability of such simple systems is easy to understand from a theoretical point of view; hence, they are chosen for the initial discussion about emulsion stability in this chapter.

However, one must realize that most emulsion formulations used in practice are more complicated [4–6]. This fact made the International Union of Pure and Applied Chemistry (IUPAC) formulate the following definition of an emulsion: "In an emulsion liquid droplets and/or liquid crystals are dispersed in a liquid" [7]. In addition, many "emulsion" formulations also contain solid particles or even three liquids.

With this information in mind, the initial discussion of two-phase systems in this chapter covers only the essentials of the emulsion stability theory. Readers who want a more extensive treatment of two-phase emulsions should read the excellent review by Reiger [8]. In the present chapter, systems with more than two phases will be given more attention because of their special properties. These are determined by the presence and the properties of the "anomalous" phase to a decisive degree. As a matter of fact, emulsions with more than two phases provide useful characteristics that are not found in two-phase emulsions.

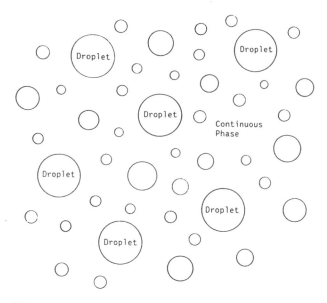

Fig. 1 The majority of emulsions consists of one liquid dispersed in another in the form of macroscopic droplets.

II. GENERAL ASPECTS OF EMULSIONS

An emulsion is formed when two immiscible liquids (usually oil and water) are mechanically agitated [8]. During agitation, both liquids tend to form droplets, but when the agitation ceases, the droplets separate into two phases. If a stabilizing compound, an emulsifier, is added to the two immiscible liquids, one phase usually becomes continuous and the other one remains in droplet form for a prolonged time. Droplets are formed by both phases during agitation and the continuous phase is actually obtained because its droplets are unstable. When water and oil are stirred together, both oil droplets in water and water droplets in oil are formed continuously, and the final result, an oil-in-water (O/W) emulsion, is obtained because the water droplets coalesce with one another much faster than the oil droplets. When a sufficiently large number of water droplets have coalesced, they will form a continuous phase surrounding the oil droplets. This continuous phase is also called the external phase; it surrounds the dispersed (internal) phase (see Fig. 1). This process of forming the continuous phase is rapid, of the order of seconds, and is not relevant to the stability of an emulsion. The stability of an emulsion is a measure of the maintenance of the dispersed droplets. In the long term, these will coalesce with each other and separate as a layer.

The decisive factor in the formation of an emulsion is mechanical agitation [3] and stirrers and extrusion equipment of many different kinds are commercially available. The essential factor in the efficiency of mechanical agitation [9] to produce small droplets is the ratio between the LaPlace pressure and the stress from the shear gradient, the Weber number, We,

$$\text{We} = \frac{\eta Gr}{\gamma} \tag{1}$$

in which η is the viscosity of the continuous phase; G the velocity gradient; r the droplet radius and γ the interfacial tension. The LaPlace pressure is the pressure difference across a curved interface. The general expression is

$$\Delta p = \gamma \left(\frac{1}{r_1} + \frac{1}{r_2} \right)$$

in which Δp is the pressure difference, γ the interfacial tension, and r_1 and r_2 the principal radii. For a sphere $r_1 = r_2$ and

$$\Delta p = \frac{2\gamma}{r}$$

A Weber number in excess of 1 is indicative of the breaking up of droplets. Hence, the velocity gradient (i.e., the intensity of the mechanical agitation) is the essential factor. There is no advantage to stirring for a long time at lower speeds. This factor is even more accentuated when turbulent flow is employed [10]. Now the maximum droplet size is determined by the energy input *per volume and time*. Hence, a short burst of energy is much more efficient than long-time stirring and, what is more important for laboratory practice, emulsification in a fraction of the continuous phase first, followed by dilution, is optimal to form small droplets.

When one of the phases is very viscous, or the material being emulsified is a solid at room temperature, heating is used during agitation to obtain a more efficient dispersion. Margarine production is a typical example of an emulsion preparation in which the emulsification is made at an elevated temperature. The hydrophilic–lipophilic balance (HLB) temperature for emulsification is discussed in another chapter.

The type of emulsion, O/W or W/O, is determined by the phase ratio if these numbers are high. Accordingly, for example, with 5% water and 95% oil, an O/W phase ratio of 19, the emulsion will become W/O, unless extreme measures are taken to ensure the formation of an O/W emulsion. For low-stability emulsions, Smith [11–14] has recently given a complete analysis of rules to select the continuous phase even in complicated systems.

For emulsions with significant stability and with moderate phase ratios (<3), the type of emulsion is decided by several factors [8], such as the order of addition or the type of emulsifier. One phase, when slowly added to the other with agitation, will usually result in the last-mentioned phase being the continuous one. Another factor is preferred solubility of the emulsifier: the phase in which the emulsifier is soluble will most probably be continuous. This phenomenon has nothing to do with the bending energy at the interface; "Bancroft's rule" does not apply to this situation. Bancroft's rule relates the radius of an emulsion droplet to the preferred angle between emulsifier molecules at the oil–water interface; the "wedge effect." However, the average angle between emulsifier molecules in a 1-μm–radius droplet is on the order of 0.01. This value has no influence on the curvature of the droplet. Instead, the importance of the specific solubility of emulsifier for the kind of emulsion formed is that a very soluble emulsifier is a weak protector of a dispersed droplet; it is easily displaced into the droplet at contact with another droplet. This leads to preferential coalescence of the phase in which the emulsifier is soluble. This phase becomes continuous during or immediately after agitation.

This phenomenon is excellently illustrated by the influence of temperature on the relative solubility of a nonionic emulsifier of the structure polyethylene glycol alkyl (aryl) ether in water and hydrocarbon. At low temperatures, the emulsifier is preferentially soluble in water, whereas at high temperatures the solubility is entirely with oil. Hence, low temperatures favor the formation of O/W emulsions and vice versa for high temperatures. The intermediate temperature range is called the HLB temperature by Shinoda [15], who has built a system for emulsifier selection on this phenomenon. The system selects the emulsifier so that the water–oil combination with the emulsifier shows an HLB temperature at approximately 60°C, at which emulsification takes place. Subsequently, immediate and rapid cooling to room temperature results in an emulsion with small droplet size. It should be realized that the extremely low interfacial tension makes the emulsion unstable when retained at the HLB temperature.

The most common types of pharmaceutical or cosmetic emulsions include water as one of the phases and oil or a lipid as the other. An O/W emulsion consists of oil droplets dispersed in a continuous aqueous phase, and a W/O emulsion consists of water droplets dispersed in oil (see Fig. 1). Occasionally, O/W emulsions change into W/O emulsions, and vice versa. This change in emulsion type is called inversion. More complex emulsions are formed when an emulsion is emulsified in the additional liquid that formed the dispersed phase in the original emulsion. A double emulsion is now formed, because the water droplets that are found in the new continuous oil phase themselves contain dispersed oil droplets from the original O/W emulsion (Fig. 2). Such an emulsion is called an oil-in-water-in-oil emulsion, and the notation O/W/O is used. In the same manner, a W/O/W emulsion may be formed. Such double emulsions have found special use as slow-delivery systems and as extraction systems [16,17].

To create the surface between the water and the oil, energy must be added to the system. This added energy is called the *surface free energy,* or the *surface tension,* between the two phases and can easily be measured [18]. This "extra" energy needed to form an emulsion is small compared with the energy required to overcome the viscous forces in the emulsification process [3], but it is important because its variation with added emulsifier is a conveniently measured gauge of the amount of the latter adsorbed to the interface.

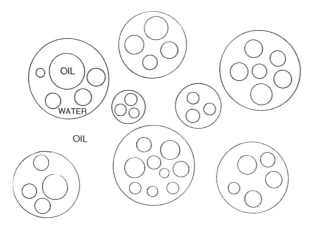

Fig. 2 A double emulsion is formed when the continuous phase (oil) contains droplets (water) which, in turn, contain droplets of the continuous phase (oil).

The surface free energy or the surface tension arises because the attractive forces between similar molecules are greater than between different ones. Hence, as shown in Fig. 3a, the forces on the molecule at the interface are directed toward its own phase. In the interior of the phase, the forces are equal in all directions and cancel each other. This means that energy must be added to bring a molecule from the interior to the surface. If the total surface of the phase is not changed, no energy is spent in bringing one molecule to the surface, since another molecule must leave the surface; consequently, as much energy is gained as lost. An increase in the total surface, on the other hand (e.g., by forming droplets), means that energy must be added because molecules must be brought to the new surface (see Fig. 3b).

Emulsifiers are molecules with one nonpolar hydrocarbon end and one polar end (Fig. 4). As a result of their structure, they are attracted to both the oil phase and the water phase and will preferentially reside at the interface. Their presence causes a reduction of the surface tension and, by measuring it, one can gauge how much emulsifier is present at the interface. This information is all that is obtained from such a measurement; any conclusions that a low interfacial tension per se is an indication of enhanced emulsion stability are not reliable. As a matter of fact, extremely low interfacial tensions lead to instability [19]. The stability of an emulsion is influenced by the charge at the interface and by the packing of the emulsifier molecules, but the interfacial tension at the levels found in the typical emulsion has no influence on it per se.

In a microemulsion, on the other hand, the ultralow interfacial tension is a sine quo non for the stability. The interfacial tension has now reached a level of 10^{-3} mN m^{-1}, and thermodynamic stability is a possibility. The thermodynamic stability of microemulsions is a fascinating subject, but is not a direct route to understanding their preparation.

That subject is better approached from a study of the phenomena of surfactant self-association. An ionic surfactant, such as sodium dodecyl sulfate, is soluble in water, and at low concentration, the surfactant behaves like a salt; the negative dodecyl sulfate ion and the positive sodium ion exist independently of each other. This behavior is changed when the concentration is increased in excess of a certain value, the critical micellization

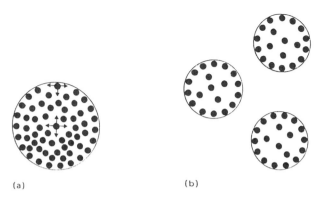

(a)   (b)

Fig. 3 A molecule at the surface is exposed (a) to a resultant force inward while the forces on a molecule interior cancel each other. Bringing more molecules to the surface by forming more droplets (b) means a greater number of molecules at the surface, and energy must be added to bring these molecules there. This is the surface free energy or surface tension.

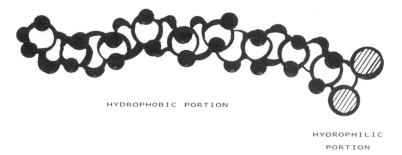

HYDROPHOBIC PORTION

HYDROPHILIC
PORTION

Fig. 4 An emulsifier contains a hydrophobic portion (hydrocarbon and a hydrophilic portion (polar).

concentration (cmc). Approximately all the added surfactant in excess of this concentration forms (frequently spherical) association structures or micelles. In these, the hydrocarbon chains are in the inner part, and the polar groups are positioned at the surface (Fig. 5). The micelle has a diameter of approximately 50 Å. This value is only 1% of the wavelength of visible light, and the micelles cannot be detected visually: the solution is transparent.

Hydrocarbons, long-chain alcohols, esters, carboxylic acids, and other organic compounds, which are poorly soluble in water, may be dissolved in the inner hydrocarbon part of the micelle. This phenomenon is called *solubilization*. In general, micellar solubilization is limited: a maximum solubilization of 10% by weight is a reasonable estimation. Higher solubilization is achieved after changing this micellar solution to a microemulsion, in which the solubilization may reach very high values [20].

The change from micellar solution to microemulsion results from adding a cosurfactant, typically a medium-chain–length alcohol, such as pentanol. The presence of pentanol leads to the formation of microemulsion droplets (Fig. 6), in which the hydrocarbon is located in the center. In the same manner, water or aqueous solutions of water-soluble substances may be dissolved in hydrocarbons to form a water-in-oil (W/O)

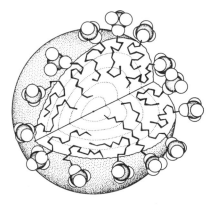

Fig. 5 In a micelle, the hydrocarbon chains form the core of the sphere, whereas the polar groups reside at the surface. (After Gruen, The annual report, Department of Applied Mathematics, Australian National University, 1982).

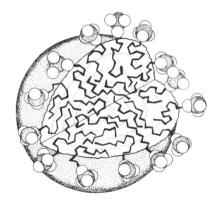

Fig. 6 In a microemulsion droplet, huge amounts of oil may be solubilized. (After Gruen, 1982).

microemulsion, by using a combination of an ionic surfactant and a cosurfactant (Fig. 7).

The important difference between emulsions and microemulsions is the size of the droplets. In a microemulsion, the droplet size is below 0.15 μm, and the entire vehicle appears transparent. The emulsion, with its relatively large droplets, usually several micrometers, is turbid. Thus, it follows that the microemulsion must form spontaneously during preparation; stirring or other mechanical disintegration of a liquid system cannot create such small droplets. This means that both the ratio and the nature of the stabilizers are critical for a microemulsion system. Another important difference between the emulsion and the microemulsion is the longevity of the individual droplets. An emulsion droplet exists as an entity from the time it has been formed until it coalesces with another droplet. A microemulsion droplet, on the other hand, is a dynamic system; it is dissolved after a short time, typically within a fraction of a second, and another droplet is spontaneously formed somewhere else in the system.

Microemulsions require higher amounts of surfactant, in the range of 6–8% by total weight, contrasting with a value of 2–3% for emulsions. This difference means an in-

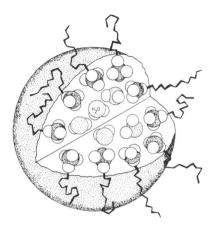

Fig. 7 In a W/O microemulsion the water is solubilized. (After Gruen, 1982).

creased cost for the microemulsion, in the range of 2–3 cents/lb. However, micro-emulsions do replace emulsions in a large number of cases, because of the reduced cost for mixing equipment processing, and even more importantly, because of their stability. An emulsion must be tested for stability, whereas in many situations, a micro-emulsion is thermodynamically stable.

III. STABILITY OF TWO-PHASE EMULSIONS

Two-phase emulsions for pharmaceutical use typically contain an aqueous solution and an oil solution as the two phases. In such a two-phase emulsion, if it is allowed or forced to separate completely, two and only two transparent layers are found. The emulsion always contains more than two components. The aqueous solution may contain water-soluble salts, whereas different organic compounds, including pharmaceutically active ones, may be dissolved into the oil. In addition, emulsifiers, in the form of surfactants or polymers, must be added. However, these compounds are soluble in the water or the oil, or in both, and are found in one or both clear phases when the emulsion is separated. Hence, the two-phase emulsion contains oil droplets dispersed in the water, an O/W emulsion, or vice versa, and the stabilizer is dissolved in one or both of the phases as well as adsorbed to the interface (Fig. 8 and see Fig. 1).

This arrangement means that the stability of the two-phase emulsion is determined by the properties of the interface. The added surfactants or polymers change both the interfacial properties (e.g., interfacial tension) and the properties of the continuous so-

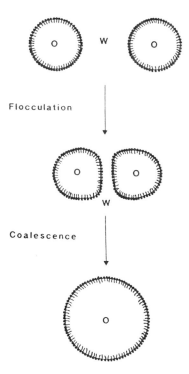

Flocculation

Coalescence

Fig. 8 In flocculation, two droplets become attached to each other, separated by a thin film, whereas in coalescence, the thin film is disrupted and the droplets are united.

lution close to the interface. So, for example, ionic surfactants at the interface give rise to an electric charge that acts at some distance from the interface. In the same manner, loops or tails from adsorbed polymers will occasionally reach out in the solution, giving repulsion forces at a distance from the interface. These two mechanisms of stabilization are the major ones operating in two-phase emulsions and will be discussed in the following sections.

The discussion of the nature of stability of an emulsion must be compared with the question of instability of an emulsion. What happens with an unstable emulsion? The final sign of an unstable emulsion is easy to observe. When an emulsion starts to separate, typically an oil layer appears on top, and an aqueous layer appears on the bottom (Fig. 9). This separation is the final state of an unstable emulsion. It may take months or years to develop, and the detection of earlier phenomena is necessary to remedy the situation in time. This means that attention must be focused on the initial mechanism in the many processes involved in the destabilization of an emulsion.

The first process is flocculation, when two droplets become attached to each other, but are still separated by a thin film of the liquid (Fig. 8). When more droplets are added, an aggregate is formed in which the individual droplets cluster, but retain the thin liquid films between them (Fig. 10a). The emulsifier molecules remain at the surface of the individual droplets during this process, as indicated in Fig. 8. In the final step, coalescence occurs when the thin liquid film between the two droplets is removed, and they form a single large droplet. This process, when continued, leads to larger and larger droplets. The coalescing emulsion is characterized by a wide distribution of droplet sizes, but no clusters are present (see Fig. 10b).

The large droplets cream or sediment much faster than the original small ones; the rate is proportional to the square of the radius

$$v = \frac{2\Delta\rho r^2 g}{9\eta} \qquad (2)$$

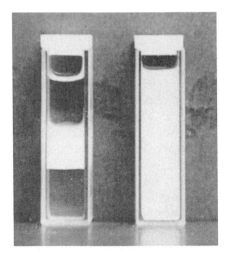

Fig. 9 In destabilization (left), an oil layer or an aqueous layer appear on top and bottom; a stable emulsion (right) shows no layers.

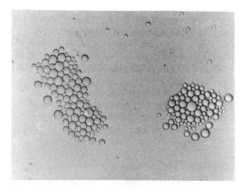

(a)

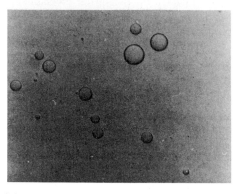

(b)

Fig. 10 In a flocculated system (a), aggregates of droplets are present. In a coalesced system (b), a wide variety of droplet size is found, but no aggregates.

in which v is the sedimentation velocity, Δp the difference in density between the droplet and the continuous phase, g is the gravity acceleration, and η is the viscosity of the continuous phase. Hence, a droplet of 10 times the radius will move 100 times faster and, as a consequence, droplets are collected on top (creaming) or at the bottom (sediment). In fact, these layers are more concentrated emulsions, and the closeness of the droplets result in enhanced flocculation and coalescence. As a consequence, the final state of phase separation, is approached faster owing to the flocculation and coalescence.

Once the sequence of flocculation $\rightarrow$ coalescence $\rightarrow$ sedimentation (creaming) $\rightarrow$ separation, is understood, a fundamental question may be asked: Is a so-called stable emulsion really stable? The answer at first appears simple. Examples of stable emulsions are common phenomena, and emulsions that have been stable for decades are abundant on shelves in formulation laboratories and as commercial products. Countless bottles of milk, cream, skin lotions, turbid shampoos, fruit juices, and soft drinks (colas) serve as an illustration of the ubiquity of stable emulsions. Hence, a *stable* emulsion is more easily described from a practical point of view: it is an emulsion that does not change with time. If a shelf life of 3 years is needed for an emulsion application and the samples preapared last that long without visible changes, the emulsion is considered stable for its intended purpose.

Another question is also important. How does one give a quantitative measure to emulsion stability? The emulsion literature has entertained various arguments for using one of the stages in the chain, discussed in the foregoing as the "true measure of emulsion stability." Such a dispute has very little value. The question about which stage in the destabilization process to use should be entirely decided by the application of the emulsion. Two examples illustrate this fact. For a fluorocarbon emulsion to be used as a blood substitute, the degree of flocculation is the appropriate measure, because aggregates of droplets are not tolerated in the blood vessels, since they may induce clotting. On the other hand, for a beverage emulsion with its natural turbidity, aggregation or coalescence of the oils present, per se, does not influence the consumer's perception of the product. However, phase separation leaving an oily layer around the bottle neck gives a feeling of a greasy bottle and engenders a strong negative reaction from the customer. Here, flocculation is an irrelevant measure of emulsion stability; sedimentation and phase separation are the important criteria.

However, neither type of "stability," as just described, is thermodynamic stability, which is concerned with the free energy of a system. The basic thereom is that a spontaneous change in a system must lead to lower free energy. Hence, if a system is at its lowest free energy, it will not change spontaneously, and if forced to change by an outside influence (stirring, shaking, heating or other), it will return to the level of lowest free energy when left undisturbed. A system at its lowest free energy is thermodynamically stable. Hence, if moved from that state by an external force, it will return to the stable state after the perturbation has ceased. If an emulsion is separated into two phases by centrifugation or other means, it does not reform spontaneously; therefore, emulsions are not thermodynamically stable. An appealing theoretical explanation for the lack of stability is found in the treatment of microemulsions by Ruckenstein [21], who summarized the different terms the sum of which constitutes the free energy of a dispersed system. Table 1 shows this series of terms, which together make up the free energy of the system. The free energy of a system, in whatever form, is equal to the sum of the product of the chemical potential with the molfraction of each compound. For a molecular solution, the chemical potential is influenced by the forces between the molecules (*enthalpic* contributions) and how dispersed the molecules of different kind are (*entropic* contributions). For emulsions or a colloidal solution (see Table 1), the chemical potential is also influenced by the presence of the interface (*surface free energy*), by the forces between droplets (*interdroplet potential*) and by the dispersity of droplets as such (entropic contributions). The important results of this evaluation is that the interfacial free

Table 1   The Free Energy Terms of a
Liquid Dispersed System

Chemical potential of the components
Interdroplet potential
    van der Waals
    Electric double layer
    Adsorbed polymers
Interfacial free energy
    Stretching
    Bending
    Torsion
Entropy from variation in droplet location

Source: Ref. 21.

energy must be extremely small for an emulsion to be thermodynamically stable; values of approximately 10^{-3} mN m^{-1} are needed. This value is found in a microemulsion. Common emulsions, on the other hand, have an interfacial free energy of about 1–10 mN m^{-1}. This value is higher by a factor of 1000 than the maximum value for a thermodynamically stable emulsion, and the emulsions are unstable. Hence, when emulsion stability is estimated, the term is used to describe the retardation of the destabilization process. A stable emulsion separates more slowly than an unstable emulsion. The slowdown may affect the flocculation, the coalescence, or the sedimentation process. This may be due to repulsive forces between the droplets, or it may result from immobilization of droplets owing to increased viscosity, such as gelation of the continuous liquid. These two concepts of emulsion stability are easily understood once the destabilization kinetics of an emulsion have been mastered.

A. Destabilization Kinetics

There is a direct relation between the initial flocculation–coalescence process and the final separation of oil or water from the emulsion. Once coalescence has taken place, the enlarged droplets move faster to the surface (or to the bottom, depending on the relative density of the dispersed and the continuous liquid). Table 2 shows the time it takes for droplets of different radii of a typical oil, with a density of 0.8 g cm^{-3} (800 kg m^{-3}) to move 5 cm in a vertical direction in water, viscosity of 0.01 P. The conclusion is obvious; keeping the droplet size small by preventing flocculation and coalescence is essential to delaying an emulsion's separation. The mathematical treatment of flocculation rates has been gathered in the Appendix to this chapter, and at present, only some useful conclusions will be considered.

An emulsion containing only oil and water, with no added stabilizer, shows extremely fast flocculation and coalescence. As a matter of fact, in an unstabilized emulsion with an oil/water weight ratio of 1 and a droplet radius of 1 μm, the time for half the droplets to flocculate and coalesce, the half-life, is approximately 1 s. Hence, an emulsion that is not protected will be destabilized in a very short time. This is easy to verify by shaking a pure paraffinic oil and water in a test tube. In only seconds oil and water layers will appear. Hence, the emulsion must be made more stable by addition of at least one substance. These added substances, the *stabilizers*, act to slow the flocculation and coalescence of the droplets by preventing their movement through the in-

Table 2 Time for a Droplet to Move 5 cm in Vertical Direction[a]

$r(\mu m)$	t
100	11.5 s
10	10 min
1	32 h
0.1	133 d
0.01	36 yr

[a]Density difference = 200 kg m^{-3}; viscosity = 0.01 P.

creased viscosity of the continuous phase, or by protection of the droplets through the establishment of some form of energy barrier between them.

B. Increase of Viscosity

The flocculation rate of an emulsion is inversely proportional to the viscosity of the continuous phase [see Eq. (2)]. An increase of the viscosity from 0.01 P (water at room temperature) to a value of 100 P (very thick syrup) reduces the flocculation rate by factor of 10,000. This appears impressive, but in reality, is not of much importance. Such a change would increase the half-life of the previously mentioned emulsion to approximately 3 h, a less than useful value.

Hence, if there is no stabilization from forces between the droplets, stable emulsions require gelation of the continuous medium. Such action changes the character of the emulsion, in principle, from a liquid to a more pastelike consistency. However, a polymeric thickener for the continuous phase may give such small rigidity that it is not observed when handling the emulsion, but it may be sufficient to prevent the droplets from moving. A polymer giving a highly thixotropic solution, with short breakdown and buildup times, is useful for such applications. Addition of this type of polymer is the optimal way of retaining the appearance of a liquid emulsion. The polymers used for this purpose are natural gums or synthetic polymers. Some of these are listed in Table 3, which shows that the natural gums are mainly polysaccharides for which the thickening power critically depends on several factors, such as pH, electrolyte content, and the presence of specific cations. Among the synthetic polymers the example of two cross-linked carboxyvinyl polymers should be noticed, because they give a yield value (cause rigidity) at low concentrations.

Both the natural gums and the synthetic polymers in Table 3 are water-soluble, and they stabilize only O/W emulsions. The water droplets dispersed in an oil phase are unstable and coalesce immediately, because the polymer is restricted to the aqueous phase and does not form a protective barrier in the oil phase. On the other hand, the oil droplets dispersed in the aqueous phase are prevented from flocculation and subsequent coalescence by the rigidity imparted to the aqueous phase by the polymer. Clay particles also act as viscosity enhancers. The members of the bentonite family, derived from montmorilonites, swell in water and strongly enhance the viscosity at pH values in excess of 6. One should realize that the gelation of the continuous phase does not necessarily mean that the emulsion is perceived as a gel. The yield value may be so low that the gravity forces, when tilting the container or pouring the emulsion, easily overcome the yield value and the emulsion behaves similar to a liquid. However, gravity forces on the individual droplets is so vanishingly small, approximately 10^{-3}–10^{-16} N, that the droplets are immobilized. However, for applications in which the emulsion must retain a very low viscosity, the stability must be enhanced by an energy barrier between the droplets.

C. Energy Barrier

An energy barrier between emulsion droplets means that they experience repulsion when they approach each other. The formula for the influence of this barrier on the flocculation rate and the half-life time is given in the Appendix at the end of this chapter. The formula is not easy to interpret directly, but a few examples help illustrate how the

Table 3 Natural Gums and Synthetic Polymers

Source	Name	Comment
Tree exudate	Gum arabic (acacia)	Essentially neutral polysaccharide
	Gum ghatti	Essentially neutral polysaccharide
	Karaya	Essentially neutral polysaccharide
	Tragacanth	Essentially neutral polysaccharide
Seaweed	Agar, carrageenan	Sulfated polysaccharide
	Alginates	Acidic polysaccharide
Seed extracts	Locust bean	Essentially neutral polysaccharide
	Guar	Essentially neutral polysaccharide
	Quince seed	Essentially neutral polysaccharide
Synthetic (fermentation)	Xanthan gum	Essentially neutral polysaccharide
Cellulose	Methyl-; hydroxyethyl-; hydroxypropyl ether	Neutral polysaccharide
	Carboxymethyl ether	Anionic polysaccharide
Collagen	Gelatin	Amphoteric protein
Synthetic	Polyoxyethylene polymer	Neutral
	Carboxyvinyl polymer (cross-linked)	Anionic

Source: Ref. 8

barrier functions. Table 4 shows the change of half-life of an emulsion when energy barriers of different heights are introduced in the system. The half-life of an emulsion is the time it takes for one-half of the original droplets to disappear through flocculation. [The method of calculation is given in the Appendix; see Eqs. (7)–(10)]. An unprotected emulsion has a half-life of about 1 s, and adding a barrier of a few kiloteslas (kT; 4.1×10^{-14} erg $= 4.1 \times 10^{-21}$ J) is not of much use, since it increases the half-life to only a few hours, which is not sufficient for most applications. However, increasing the barrier to 20 kT results in a half-life of 4 years, which is sufficient for a great number of applications. A barrier of 50 kT gives a half-life of more than 10,000 times the age of the universe, obviously stable enough for any purpose. The last example is an impressive show of stability of an emulsion, but it must be emphasized that even such an emulsion is not thermodynamically stable. It will over trillions of years move slowly,

Table 4 Influence of Barrier Height on Half-Life

$W(kT)$	$t_{1/2}$
0	0.8 s
5	38.2 s
10	1.55 h
20	3.91 yr
50	4.17×10^{13} yr

but steadfastly, to its destabilization and separation. In 1 cm³ of such an emulsion, it takes, on the average, 2 days for the first pair of droplets out of the total number of 100 billion to coalesce.

In contrast, a thermodynamically stable emulsion would not change with time and would, if separated by centrifugation, form again spontaneously. Thermodynamic stability means reversibility; but, since separated emulsions never reform spontaneously, they are not thermodynamically stable. With this important distinction clarified, the different kinds of barriers available in emulsion technology can be described.

1. *Examples of Energy Barriers*

There are several methods for creating an energy barrier between two droplets. For the simple emulsion now being treated, two kinds of barriers are essential; namely, the electric double layer and stearic repulsion from adsorbed polymers. An ionic surfactant adsorbed at the interface of an oil droplet in water orients the polar group toward the water. Some counterions of the surfactant (e.g., the sodium ion in sodium dodecyl sulfate) will separate from the surface and form a diffuse cloud reaching out into the continuous phase (Fig. 11). Hence, a charged droplet surface shows a diffuse layer of counterions extending from it. The surface charge plus the counterions are called the *electric double layer*. When the counterions start overlapping at the approach of two droplets, a repulsive force results (see Fig. 11). The repulsion from the electric double layer is well known because it plays a decisive role in the theory of colloidal stability that is called DLVO, after its originators Derjaguin, Landau, Vervey, and Overbeek [22,23]. The theory provided a quantum leap forward in the understanding of colloidal stability, and its treatment dominated the colloid science literature for several decades.

A second type of barrier arises from the action of a polymer adsorbed at the oil–water interface. If its polar–nonpolar constituents are balanced, it will reach into the continuous phase with tails and loops. These parts in the continuous phase require space to attain all possible conformations and, within this space, will not tolerate the presence of or parts of another polymer molecule adsorbed to another droplet. Hence, if a second drop should approach within a short distance, the polymer restricts its conformation, causing a strong repulsion force.

2. *DLVO Theory*

Before discussing some details of DLVO theory, it is necessary to point out the practical limitations to its application. The DLVO theory was originally introduced for suspensions of solid particles, which differ from droplets in being rigid. However, emulsion droplets retain their shape during the initial part of the flocculation and, for this process, the theory developed for spherical particles is applicable. During the coalescence process, the interactions between two flat plates are suitable for the calculations. For both of these cases, it is absolutely essential to realize that the theory is useful for O/W (oil-in-water) emulsions, but for W/O (water-in-oil) systems its applicability is highly doubtful [24]. The essential value of the DLVO theory for emulsion technology lies in its ability to relate the stability of an O/W emulsion to the electrolyte content of the continuous phase. In summary, the theory says that the electric double-layer repulsion will stabilize an emulsion where the electrolyte concentration in the continuous phase is less than a certain value. It is essential to realize that, if an emulsion is stable at salt concentrations in excess of this value, the stabilization is due to phenomena other than the electric double-layer repulsion. The fact that the electric double-layer repulsion is

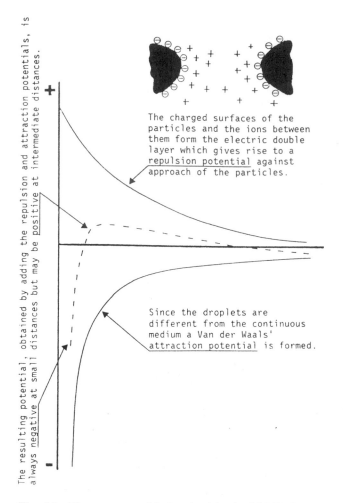

The charged surfaces of the
particles and the ions between
them form the electric double
layer which gives rise to a
<u>repulsion potential</u> against
approach of the particles.

Since the droplets are
different from the continuous
medium a Van der Waals'
<u>attraction potential</u> is formed.

Fig. 11   The two potentials involved in the DLVO theory are from an overlap of the electric double layer (top line) and from the van der Waals interaction (lower line). A sufficient positive value of the total potential (dashed line) gives colloidal stability (top part). Addition of salt (bottom part) reduces the electric repulsion potential, the total potential is negative, and no stabilization takes place.

of no importance when the concentration of counterions in an added salt exceeds a certain value, is understood if the total interaction between two emulsion droplets is taken into consideration (see Fig. 11).

When two droplets approach each other (see Fig. 11 top to bottom), the counterions forming the diffuse part of the electric double layer (see Fig. 11 bottom) begin to overlap. This overlap means that the electric potential (the work done to bring one electric charge from a long distance to the point observed) between the droplets is increased which, in turn, means that more energy must be added with reduced distance between the droplets. An increase in energy with reduced distance means a repulsive force between the droplets. (The force is equal to the negative value of the slope of the curve.)

At the same time, there is always an attractive force between emulsion droplets, and this force becomes stronger with reduced distance between them. A negative force means a negative potential between the droplets (see Fig. 11).

The interaction between droplets is decided by the total potential (e.g., the sum; with signs of the two potentials in Fig. 11 top). In this example, the energy from the electric double-layer is numerically greater than the van der Waals potential for a certain distance range, and the sum of the two energies becomes positive. This means that the resulting force is repulsive. On the other hand, for small distances, the resulting energy is always negative, and the particles will spontaneously move toward each other, if they, for one reason or another, come that close. These interactions may be easily understood if one consideres one droplet as a stationary ball at distance zero, whereas the other is rolling along the total energy curve with gravity acting on it. The ball must be pushed up the hump (energy must be added); but, once it is over the top, it will roll by itself.

A positive range of the "hump" in Fig. 11 top, is insufficient to ensure stability of an emulsion. The droplets are in constant movement, and the maximum value of the positive energy in Fig. 11 top, must have a minimum value to prevent a sufficient number of them from exceeding the maximum value. One or two droplets will always happen to move fast enough to exceed the maximum and, hence, stability is best described as the half-life of the emulsion, for example, the time when half the droplets have coalesced [see Appendix, Eq. (10)]. Table 4 shows that a barrier height of 20 kT is sufficient for most particle emulsion systems. This energy maximum cannot be measured directly. It must be estimated from the electric surface potential, which can be estimated from the so called zeta or ζ-potential which, in turn, can be determined experimentally with commercial instruments. For O/W emulsions with low electrolyte content in the aqueous phase, a ζ-potential of ± 30 mV (the sign is not relevant as a negative potential will stabilize as well as a positive one) is sufficient to bring the energy maximum to this level.

The relative value of the two potentials also explains why the electric stabilization disappears entirely for an added electrolyte for which the concentration of the electric double-layer counterions exceeds a certain value. Addition of an electrolyte to the continuous phase causes a reduction of the electric double-layer repulsion potential (see Fig. 11 bottom), whereas the van der Waals potential remains essentially unchanged. Hence, a maximum in the total potential is reduced more with increased electrolyte concentration and, at a certain value, the maximum barrier height is reduced to a level at which the stability is lost, according to Table 4. This change of the total potential for emulsion droplets with salt concentration is pronounced. For example, a change of NaCl concentration from 0.1 to 0.101 M typically causes a reduction of the total potential by more than 100 kT. In light of the drastic change of stability that occurs in moving below a potential barrier of 20 kT (see Table 4), one may easily accept that the change from a stable to an unstable emulsion takes place at a well-defined electrolyte concentration.

Calculations of the relative height of the barrier with electrolyte content are scientifically interesting, but of limited value in daily formulation efforts. The essential information for daily practice may be formulated very simply. An O/W emulsion can be stabilized by the repulsion from the electric double-layer only if the aqueous phase contains monovalent counterions at a concentration less than 0.1 M, divalent ones at less than 0.01 M, or trivalent ones at less than 0.001 M (the Schultz–Hardy rule). For these cases, a ζ-potential of 30 mV or greater will provide the stability that the electric double-layer can offer. For electrolyte content higher than these values, or in an O/W emulsion or for W/O emulsion in general, the ζ-potential has no importance for stability, and other stabilizing mechanisms must be found.

In the same manner, if an emulsion is to be destabilized, the addition of salts is useful to remove the stabilizing influence of the electric double-layer. However, if the emulsion remains stable at electrolyte contents higher than those cited in the preceding paragraphs, the stability is not due to electric double-layer repulsion. Hence, it may be economically advantageous to find the real reason for the stability to be able to take optimal counteraction instead of swamping the emulsions with electrolyte.

3. *Adsorption of Hydroxy Complex Ions*

Aluminum ions are trivalent and should be powerful destabilizing agents. A concentration of only 10^{-3} M reduces the electric double-layer repulsion potential (see Fig. 11) to an extent that it is equal to or less than the van der Waals attraction potential. Hence, there is no stabilization by the electric double layer. Investigations on the stability of latices [25] have confirmed the prediction, but only for pH values below 3.5. At pH values above this limit, the latex actually showed improved stability at an aluminum ion concentration of 10^{-3} M; as a matter of fact, the latices remained stable at aluminum salt additions higher than that. A diagram (Fig. 12) of the stability limits versus aluminum ion concentration and pH value explains that result [25]. With increased pH values, destabilization requires lower concentrations of aluminum ions, but such destabilization takes place only over a limited concentration range. Concentrations higher than this range now lead to restabilization. The charge of the latex particles is positive in this high concentration stability range, whereas the original latex was covered by a negative charge. The explanation to this obvious deviation from the Schulze–Hardy rule for alumninum as well as some other multivalent metal ions is because the hydroxy complexes formed by these ions in a certain pH range are adsorbed extremely strong to the latex surface. The amount adsorbed is not only sufficient to enhance the reduction of

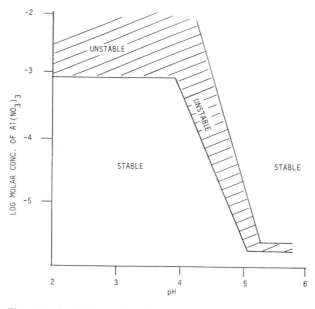

Fig. 12 Stability regions for a polystyrene latex in the presence of an aluminum salt.

the electric double-layer repulsion potential (see Fig. 11), but actually recharges the surface to the opposite sign.

4. *Polymer Stabilization*

Thus far, polymers have been used comparatively less than the common surfactants to stabilize emulsions. The limited use is not due to lack of performance; publications in the area point to excellent stabilization of emulsions by polymers [26–28]. Application probability is limited because the adsorption of polymers to emulsion droplets has not been well understood, especially since small changes in polymer structure or in solvent properties may lead to drastic changes in adsorption. A polymer may be adsorbed in the form of loops, tails, and trains (Fig. 13). The stabilizing action depends on the presence of sufficiently long tails or loops, as explained in Fig. 14. The stabilizing action of the protruding part of the polymer is extremely efficient [28]; a single loop or tail gives a barrier of approximately 20 kT. With literally thousands of such chains adsorbed to one emulsion droplet, the stabilization should be excellent. The limited application of polymers as emulsion stabilizers, despite such excellent stabilization, calls for an explanation. In short, what is the problem?

One problem is the sensitivity of the adsorption to the properties of the polymer versus the environment. This has been described in an excellent manner by Clayfield and Lumb in early calculations of polymer conformation at an interface [29]. They compared the fraction of adsorbed polymer as a function of its total adsorption energy (which equals the number of adsorbing groups times their individual adsorption energy), at constant molecular weight. Their results (Fig. 15) showed that the range of adsorption energy for useful polymer stabilization was extremely narrow. For adsorption energies lower than the optimal range (see Fig. 15), the polymer does not adsorb at all, and there is no stabilization from adsorbed polymer. With adsorption energies in excess of the optimal range (see Fig. 15), all groups of the polymer are adsorbed; it now lies flat at the interface. Such adsorption is without stabilization effect, because the protective action reaches only a short distance into the continuous medium. Figure 14 explains why such a state offers no stabilization. At short distances, the van der Waals potential has already reached such large negative values that the flocculated state is permanent. The potential well is so deep that the droplets remain attached to each other. For the same reason, a minimum molecular weight is necessary to obtain stability, because the protective action of the polymer must reach far out to prevent the van der Waals potential from becoming dominant.

The problems encountered with copolymers possessing statistically distributed surface-binding groups are severe, and it appears difficult to synthesize such a polymer that would have general application. The solution to the problem lies with a different kind

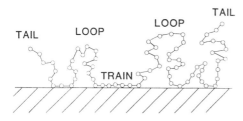

Fig. 13 A polymer can be adsorbed in the form of trains, loops, and tails.

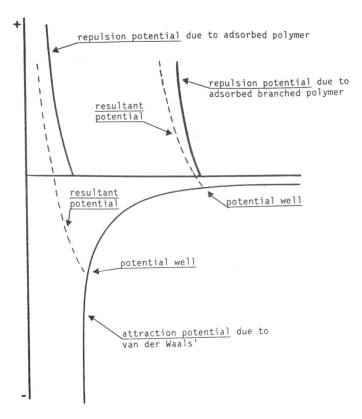

repulsion potential due to adsorbed polymer

repulsion potential due to
adsorbed branched polymer

resultant
potential

resultant
potential

potential well

potential well

attraction potential due to
van der Waals'

Fig. 14 The chain length of an adsorbed polymer must be sufficient to prevent the van der Waals potential from creating too deep a minimum.

of polymer, the so-called block copolymers, consisting of one block of one polymer to which two or more blocks of a different polymer are attached. These two polymers are chosen to be selectively soluble in the aqueous and oil phase, respectively. With sufficient molecular weight in the polymer part that is soluble in the continuous phase, excellent stability is achieved. Table 5 provides examples of commercially available copolymers that have found use as emulsion stabilizers.

D.   Stability Testing

The dilemma for the formulator of an emulsion is that the success of a formulation effort or approach can be judged only after a long time. If a shelf life of 1 year is needed, in principle, it is necessary to wait 1 year to find out whether a number of samples prepared by a variety of formulations or formulation approaches are still intact. Such a long waiting period is not practical, and there is a great need for methods to estimate the stability shortly after preparation.

The room temperature instability of an emulsion under unperturbed conditions emanates from two phenomena. The droplets bounce against each other owing to their constant movement. During the course of this diffusion, they sediment toward the bottom of the vessel if they are heavier than the continuous phase, or cream toward the

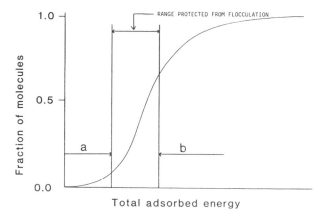

Fig. 15 With too small an adsorption energy, the polymer will not adsorb at the interface (a). Too high an adsorption (b) leads to a train type of adsorption alone. Stabilization is achieved only in the limited range between the two.

top if lighter. The sedimentation or creaming brings the droplets closer together, enhancing the number of collisions (proportional to the square of the number of droplets per unit volume). In addition, the sedimentation (creaming) per se increases the number of collisions, because huge droplets move faster than small ones. The driving force for sedimentation or creaming is proportional to the droplet volume (the radius cubed), whereas the resistance to the droplet movement is proportional to the radius, and the stationary speed is proportional to the radius squared. With these facts in mind it is obvious that any method that enhances one or both of these factors will effect faster destabilization.

Table 5 Some Commercially Available Polymers

Compound	Source	Stabilizer for emulsion type	
		O/W	W/O
Carboxymethylcellulose	Courtaulds		X
Methylhydroxyethylcellulose	Hoechst	X	
Hydroxypropylmethyl cellulose ether	Courtaulds	X	
Polyethylene oxide	Union Carbide	X	
Polyvinyl alcohol	Revertex	X	
Copolymer of 12-hydroxystearic acids with polyalkylene (usually ethylene) glycol	ICI Paints	X	X
Fatty acid-modified polyethylene glycol esters	ICI Paints	X	
Polyolefin-modified polyester	ICI Paints	X	
Alk(en)yl-substituted mono- and dicarboxyl acids and anhydrides	ICI Paints	X	
Acrylic polyethylene glycol graft polymer	ICI Paints	X	
Polymethylvinyl ether/maleic anhydride	G.A.F.	X	
Polyacrylic acid (high molecular weight)	B. F. Goodrich	X	

The easiest way to accelerate the number of collisions is to heat the sample. The enhanced thermal motion of the droplets will increase the collision rate and speed up the destabilization rate. This effect may be quantified. The diffusion coefficient is proportional to the absolute temperature and, in principle, it should be possible to calculate the shelf life at room temperature from determinations at higher temperatures. Unfortunately, the changed number of collisions is not the only effect of increased temperature. In addition, heat reduces the protective action of adsorbed surfactants, enhances the mutual solubility of the components, changes the electric double layer, lowers the adsorption of stabilizers, and causes other effects. With all these factors being influenced, a general rule for the influence of increased temperature cannot be expected to be valid for all kinds of stabilizers. Instead, an empirical evaluation of the shelf life to be expected from such tests must be made for each category of emulsions. In industrial practice, it is considered reasonable to use the time for destabilization at 45°C multiplied by 4 to give an estimate of the shelf life at room temperature. In pharmaceutics a factor of 2 is used in the same manner for solid preparations at 37°C.

However, accelerated testing is not always reliable, and the formulator better utilizes earlier experience with the same kind of emulsions before a suitable temperature level for accelerated testing for a new system can be established. Some emulsions in which the emulsifier displays temperature-dependent transitions must be treated differently. Anyone will realize that trying to relate the shelf life at room temperature with the emulsion's behavior at the HLB temperature for a preparation stabilized by a nonionic emulsifier of the polyethylene glycol type is a completely fruitless endeavor. All such emulsions are extremely unstable at the HLB temperature.

The second factor, sedimentation, may be accelerated by centrifugation, but attempts to relate the rate of phase separation during centrifugation to shelf stability have not justified expectations. The phase separation seen during such forced sedimentation does not subject the product to gravitational stresses it will never encounter in practice and may give completely erroneous results.

The best evaluation of an emulsion's stability is probably to determine its particle size distribution frequently during the first few weeks of storage. If there is no change in the size distribution, the formulator may be at least hopeful for the stability of the product. An increasing number of huge droplets, giving the long "tail" of the distribution toward large sizes, is a bad sign indeed. Such an emulsion invariably becomes unstable with time. An even and narrow size distribution is not a guarantee for stability, but such an emulsion may be stable.

One aspect of stability that is frequently neglected, but may be of pronounced importance, is the ability of the emulsion to remain stable during transport and handling. This property is called the *shake stability* and is tested by shaking the emulsion in the final package. The shaking process involves two mechanisms for destabilization. At first, the movement of the emulsion in the package causes a shearing action; that is, droplets are moved with different speeds and, hence, collide more often. Second, the shaking process spreads the emulsion along the walls of the container at regular intervals. This latter phenomenon causes no instability if the continuous phase of the emulsion will be destabilized because a thin film of dispersed phase forms along the container surface and slowly moves to the bottom or top of the container, depending on its relative density compared with the continuous phase. New film is continuously formed and the dispersed phase separates into a bottom or top layer. The emulsion has separated. Instability of the type just described depends on the surface properties of the container, including the inside of the cap or cover, and it is not only wise, but necessary, to check this find of stability when selecting the final package.

The only stability that can be determined with advantage in an accelerated manner is the freeze–thaw stability. When an emulsion is stored under freezing and thawing conditions, the destabilizing action is concentrated in the freezing and thawing periods. Long storage under frozen conditions per se does not cause structural changes (as a matter of fact, some systems that are difficult to stabilize are stored frozen to avoid destabilization). A good opinion about the stability under varying temperature at such low levels that freezing may occur is obtained by studying the emulsion tolerance against repeated freeze–thaw cycles at short intervals. Special equipment that automatically varies the temperature between set limits is commercially available. The temperature variation is usually between $-20°C$ ($-4°F$) and $25°C$ ($77°F$), and the time at each temperature is 1 h.

Recently, Karbstein and Schubert [30] have calculated the middle-term stability—a few weeks—from the influence of double-layer repulsion on coalescence kinetics. The calculations integrated the nonlinear, coupled differential equations for coalescence and sedimentation at a set number of layers and obtained surprising agreement with experimental results for emulsion with 10% oil.

E. Summary of the Stability of Two-Phase Emulsions

Stability of two-phase emulsions may be obtained in several ways. For O/W systems, the electric surface potential formed by an adsorbed ionic surfactant is useful if it is sufficiently high and if the electrolyte content does not exceed 0.1 M (monovalent counterions), 0.01 M (divalent counterions), and 0.001 M (trivalent counterions). Caution is necessary in the presence of metal salts, which form hydroxy complexes. These complexes may adsorb extremely strongly to an interface and may recharge a negative surface to become positive, restabilizing it against other positive counterions. Polymers are excellent stabilizers for emulsions, especially block copolymers for which the adsorption sensitivity to the condition of the environment is removed.

IV. STABILITY OF THREE-PHASE EMULSIONS

Three-phase emulsions are more common than is generally believed. Many pharmaceutical and cosmetic lotions and creams consist not only of the water and the oil phase, as described in the earlier sections, but may contain other additional phases. The difference between a two-phase emulsion and systems with more than two phases is easy to understand. A two-phase emulsion will separate into two clear layers, with one interface between them. The emulsions discussed in this section separate into three phases (three layers), which means that two interfaces are found at separation. Such three-phase emulsions exist *nolens volens* in formulations, and knowledge about their properties is necessary to understand the sometimes puzzling behavior of these emulsions. In addition, a discussion of their properties is justified, because they provide opportunities to formulate emulsions with properties outside the scope of normal two-phase emulsions.

Several examples of three-phase emulsions are provided in the following treatment, but three main categories have been chosen in which the third phase is, respectively, a solid, a liquid, or a liquid crystal. These three cases impart different properties to the emulsion and, together, provide a chart of the manner in which the three-phase emulsions both enlarge our knowledge of emulsions as such and exemplify the specific properties to be found in emulsions.

A. Third Phase a Solid

Solid particles are often part of an emulsion formulation, and the simultaneous stabilization of both an emulsion and a suspension often causes problems. In fact, the solid particles may be used to stabilize an emulsion and can serve as an aid, rather than an encumbrance, in the formulation efforts. The key factor for the use of particles as a stabilizing agent is their ability to be wetted by the two phases. They will stabilize the emulsion if they are located at the interface between the two liquids (Fig. 16). At the interface they serve as a mechical barrier to prevent the coalescence of the droplets. If they are electrically charged against a continuous aqueous phase, the electric double layer will further assist in the stabilization against flocculation. This latter kind of stabilization has been treated in the section on two-phase emulsions. In this section the mechanical action against coalescence will be the focus of attention.

The protection against coalescence (see Fig. 16) is based on the energy to expel the particles from the interface into the dispersed droplets [31]. This energy depends on the contact angle and is easily calculated for spherical particles located at the oil–water interface. The expression is [4].

$$\Delta E = \pi r_p^2 \gamma_{o/w} (1 - \cos \theta)^2 \tag{3}$$

in which ΔE is the energy to expel a spherical particle with radius r from the interface into the phase by which it is predominantly wet and toward which its contact angle is θ (Fig. 17); $\gamma_{o/w}$ is the interfacial tension between the oil and water phases. The value for ΔE should grow continuously as θ increases to a value of 180°C. This is theoretically correct, but experimental investigations [15] have shown 90° to be a practical maximum. Higher values probably lead to the expulsion of the particle into the continuous phase.

These energies are of a magnitude to make solid paritcles efficient stabilizers; their repulsive force significantly exceeds that of the van der Waals force. Assuming the contact angle to be constant during expulsion from the interface, the combined van der Waals and wetting force becomes

$$\frac{dE}{dh} = 2\pi\gamma_{o/w}(h - r\cos\theta) \tag{4}$$

in which h is the distance perpendicular to the interface that the particle has moved from its equilibrium position.

Figure 18 is drawn for paritcles of 50 Å radius action on a flat interface of size 10^4 Å^2. The total force is repulsive even for contact angles of 60°, and for 90° angles

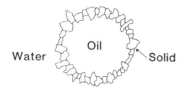

Fig. 16 Solid particles stabilize an emulsion when they are adsorbed at the interface.

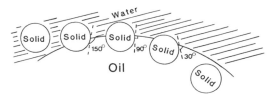

Fig. 17 The contact angle at the oil–water–solid line determines the stabilizing action.

the repulsion force is extremely strong. Hence, the stabilization is excellent, bearing in mind that thousands of such particles are adsorbed on one emulsion droplet.

The essential information from Eq. (3) and from Fig. 18 is that the protection energy from adsorbed solid particles is rapidly lost with reduced contact angle. When this happens, the particle is spontaneously moved toward the interior of the droplet (see Fig. 16), and its complete expulsion into the droplet requires less energy. Figure 19 shows that the energy to displace one particle into the dispersed droplets from its location at the interface, is reduced to half its value with a contact angle change from 90° to 75°. An angle decrease to 60° leads to an energy value only one-fourth of that of 90°. These values make it evident that the contact angles must be observed rather carefully to obtain a value close to 90°. Equipment is available to measure the contact angle, but di-

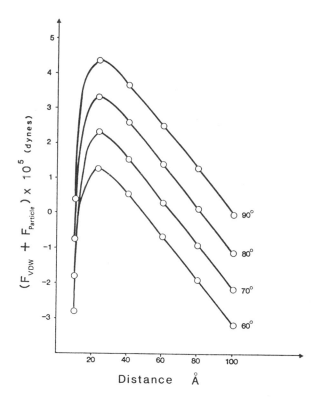

Fig. 18 The combination of wetting forces, $F_{particle}$, and van der Waals, F_{VDW}, becomes strongly repulsive for high-contact angles.

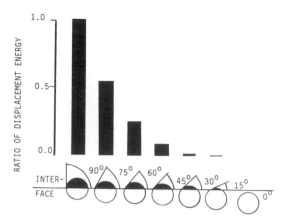

Fig. 19 The protective action of a spherical solid particle is rapidly lost with reduced contact angle.

rect visual observation is sufficient to obtain good results. The following experimental procedure is practical to obtain good stability.

The solid particles are assumed to be heavier than the aqueous phase which, in turn, is assumed to be heavier than the oil. The particles, which must be small ($\ll 0.1\ \mu$m), are put into a small container and evened out to give a surface that is even with the top of the walls of the container. No attempt should be made to pack or press the particles to obtain a more even surface. If the particles are soft, such treatment will change the surface properties of the particles. If that happens, the results will be erroneous because the contact angle depends on the surface properties. Hence, a change of the surface properties means a change of contact angle, and a small change of contact angle means a marked reduction of the stabilization energy (see Fig. 19). The container with the particles is placed on the bottom of a vessel with parallel walls (a container with powder may have to be rocked gently to remove the air from between the particles), and oil is poured in the vessel. This oil must have exactly the same composition as that in the emulsion formulation. Optimal results are obtained by bringing the oil with *all* added components into contact with the aqueous phase, also with all its components, to obtain equilibrium before the experiment. The separated oil phase is used in the vessel, and a drop of the aqueous phase is placed on the powder with a syringe or pipette. The contact angle between the droplet and the solid (Fig. 20) determines which correction should be made to obtain optimum stabilizing by the solid particles.

The first case, a contact angle of 90° between the water and the solid material (see a, Fig. 20) is trivial. It means that the solid particles are optimally useful to stabilize the emulsion with no further treatment. This does not happen often, but is gratefully received when it does. A contact angle smaller than 90° between the water and the solid particles (see b, Fig. 20) means that the interfacial free energy is too great between the solid material and the oil. To increase the contact angle between the aqueous phase and the powder, an oil-soluble surface-active agent must be added. This surfactant should not be water-soluble at all, and it should bind *strongly* to the solid surface. Such a surfactant will bind strongly to the solid–liquid interface, and a low concentration in the oil phase will be sufficient to reduce the interfacial free energy at the oil–solid inter-

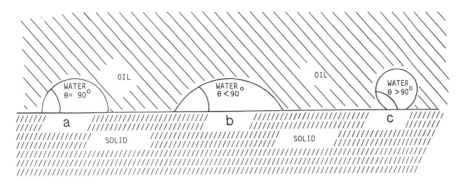

Fig. 20 An oil–water–solid contact angle of $\theta = 90°$ means that the particles as such are optimal stabilizers (a). If the contact angle toward water is less than 90° (b), an oil-soluble surfactant is added. If θ exceeds (c), a water-soluble surfactant is added to reduce the interfacial free energy between water and the solid, reducing θ.

face. Use of as low a concentration as possible is essential, because higher concentrations also lower the interfacial tension at the water–oil interface. A reduction of the O/W interfacial tension has a disadvantage: it makes the contact angle θ more sensitive to small differences between $\gamma_{w/s}$ and $\gamma_{o/s}$ (Fig. 21). After a certain concentration of surfactant in the oil phase has brought the contact angle to 90°, the process is repeated, but now with the amount of surfactant added to the oil before the phases are brought into contact. The contact angle is usually not 90° because of hysteresis, and the amount needed for the unrestricted reading of surfactant is adjusted further in the correct direction [4]. If the water droplet does not spread and its contact angle is in excess of 90° (see c, Fig. 20) the surfactant is added to the aqueous phase. The adjustments are identical with the ones described for the oil phase.

However, an added surfactant will also adsorb at the oil–water interface and reduce the value of $\gamma_{o/w}$. Such a reduction results in a reduced stabilization energy [see Eq. (3)], and it would be an advantage to avoid additional surfactant. Hence, for emulsions produced in huge quantities or repeated batches, a change of the surface of the solid particles through a chemical reaction is worthwhile. A small contact angle in the aqueous phase means too great an interfacial energy between the oil phase and the solid particles.

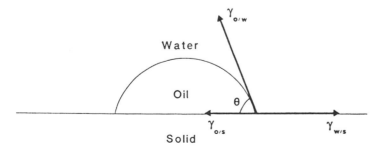

Fig. 21 A reduction of $\gamma_{o/w}$ makes, the θ very sensitive to small differences between $\gamma_{o/s}$ and $\gamma_{w/s}$.

The surface of the solid particle must be made more hydrophobic, which may be achieved by esterification of polar groups on the particle surface, by silanization, or by similar processes. In the opposite case, a large contact angle toward the aqueous phase is corrected by making the particle surface more polar through oxidation, hydrolysis, or other reactions.

Research in the area of particle-stabilized emulsions has been scant. This condition will most certainly change in the future. There are a great number of problems to be investigated, and diverse phenomena will have to be clairifed. A common problem in formulation is the dispersion of a solid drug in a liquid, and great pains are often taken to prevent sedimentation of the particles. A combination of an emulsion with solid particles, the latter adsorbed to an emulsified droplet, adds two stabilizing factors. First, the emulsion droplets will keep the particles dispersed; second, with the dispersed liquid droplets lighter than the continuous liquid–droplet–particle combination, the droplets may approach a density similar to that of the liquid and reduce sedimentation. Another common problem is the combination of proteins and oils in an emulsion. Solid protein particles are excellent stabilizers. Not to be forgotten, for example, is in fact, known since ancient times, that mustard powder is a good stabilizer for mayonnaise and similar products.

B.   Third Phase a Liquid

The third-phase case has been well known for 30 years [15] for nonionic surfactants of the polyethylene glycol alkylaryl ether type. It is a very useful case because it allows low-energy emulsification [32] by using the strong temperature dependence of the colloidal association structures in water–surfactant–hydrocarbon systems. The basic background follows: At low temperatures, below the cloud point (the temperature above which a nonionic surfactant of this kind ceases to be water-soluble at low concentrations), these surfactants are preferentially water-soluble; hence, they are heavily partitioned toward the aqueous phase in an emulsion. At high temperatures, well above the cloud point, the surfactant's solubility in water is extremely small, and it is then partitioned almost entirely into the oil. At some intermediate temperature, the HLB temperature [33] or the phase inversion temperature (PIT) [15], a third phase, the surfactant phase, [34] appears between the oil and the water (Fig. 22). This phase is an isotropic liquid phase, slightly grayish in appearance.

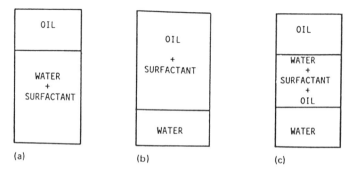

Fig. 22   Water, hydrocarbon, and a nonionic surfactant form two phases at (a) low and (b) high temperature. In a small temperature range between (a) and (b), three liquid phases are found (c) in the HLB temperature range.

The key to low-energy emulsification is to emulsify at this HLB temperature and to follow this by *rapid* cooling to about 25°–30°C, if an O/W emulsion is desired. For an O/W emulsion to be used at room temperature, the HLB temperature should be approximately 55°C. A W/O emulsion requires the opposite condition: the HLB temperature should be lower than the room temperature by the same amount (e.g., an HLB temperature close to 0°C) [15].

With this background information, the following process is used for the selection of the emulsifier. Equal amounts of the oil and the aqueous phases with all the components of the formulation preadded are mixed with 4% of the emulsifiers to be tested in a series of samples. The samples are left thermostated at 55°C to separate, for an O/W emulsion (at +5°C for an W/O emulsion). After complete separation, the emulsifiers that give systems separating into three transparent layers are selected for emulsification and determination of emulsion stability; the rest, giving two phases, are discarded. At this stage one fact cannot be overemphasized. An emulsion separation into one oil phase on top and one aqueous phase on the bottom part *separated by an emulsion layer is not a three-phase system*. To find whether there are two layers or three, the central emulsion layer must be separated. The top transparent layer is first removed to a separate test tube with a tight screw cap. The emulsion layer is removed, heated to 95°C (screw cap), then frozen to –20°C and returned to 55°C to separate. The oil layer that is separated is added to the original one, any aqueous layer separated is added to the original test tube and any remaining emulsion heated and frozen again until it is completely separated when stored at 55°C.

The emulsifiers giving separation into three layers are used for emulsification to find which ones give the most stable emulsion. The emulsions are extremely unstable at the HLB temperature [15], and cooling to room temperature must be rapid. This can be achieved by spreading the emulsion in a thin layer on a cold plate or by letting it pass through cold rollers. For an O/W emulsion with a sufficiently low O/W volume ratio, the following method may be useful. Before emulsification, an amount corresponding to half the total emulsion is removed from the aqueous phase and cooled close to 0°C. The remaining part of the emulsion is emulsified at 55°C and stirred directly into the cooled aqueous part. The average droplet size of these emulsions is less than 1 μm with very little stirring. With these small droplets the stability is good and can be improved further by addition of small amounts of an ionic surfactant ($\cong$0.05–0.1%).

The water-in-oil emulsions are prepared by emulsification at a temperature close to 0°C, followed by immediate and rapid heating to room temperature. For these emulsions the O/W ratio is usually greater than 1. Rapid heating is obtained by removing part of the oil phase and heating to 55°C or higher. Here the entire phases are mixed rapidly to avoid partial formation of an O/W emulsion, which happens when the emulsion formed at low temperatures is gradually added to the hot oil.

These emulsions have long been known [15], and low-energy emulsification has been promoted by Lin and others in a series of papers [32–34]. One of the more interesting future developments is in the area of separation using microemulsions. By using a temperature change of only 25°C, instead of the normal solvent extraction—with its expensive distillation processes to remove solvent—obviously has economic advantages [35]. The extraction process of hydrocarbons contains several specific features [36], which have been treated theoretically [37]. The latest development is to apply these procedures in the separation of products from biotechnological processes.

C. Third Phase a Liquid Crystal

In addition to micelles and microemulsion droplets (see Figs. 5–7), surfactants may form liquid crystals, of which the one with a layered structure (Fig. 23) is the most important for emulsion science. Micelles and microemulsion droplets are microscopic entities within a solution; a liquid crystal is a separate phase, which comes out of solution. A liquid crystal is not a true crystal. In a lamellar crystal, the hydrocarbon chains are packed with crystalline order and the diffusion is limited as in a solid. In a liquid crystal, the chains are in a liquid state (but with preferred orientation), and the diffusion *along the layers* is of the same magnitude as in a liquid.

The introduction of liquid crystals as a stabilizing element for emulsions occurred in 1969, when it was found that the sudden stabilization at emulsifer concentration in excess 2.5% of a water–*p*-xylene emulsion, by a commercial octaethylene glycol nonylphenyl ether, was due to the formation of a liquid crystalline phase in the emulsion [38]. Later investigations confirmed the strong-stabilizing action of these structures [39].

The essential features of such emulsions are:

1. The structure of the liquid crystal
2. Its stabilizing action
3. The specific applications of such emulsions
4. Useful surfactants

The identification of the liquid crystal is primarily based on its anisotropic optical properties. This means that a sample of this phase will look radiant when viewed against a light source placed between crossed polarizers. An isotropic solution is black under such conditions (Fig. 24, left), whereas the liquid crystal system is radiant (see Fig. 24, right). The structure of the phase may be identified by optical microscopy in which the lamellar liquid crystal has a pattern of oil streaks and Maltese crosses (Fig. 25a), whereas the hexagonal array of cylinders give a different optical pattern (see Fig. 25b). Small-angle x-ray diffraction patterns also distinguish between these two varieties. The lamellar phase has a ratio of 1, 2, 3, 4 . . . between the interlayer spacings, whereas the hexagonal

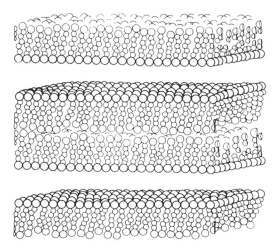

Fig. 23 In a lamellar liquid crystal the surfactants form double layers separated by their water layers.

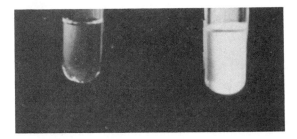

Fig. 24 The liquid crystal is radiant between crossed polarizers (right), whereas an isotropic solution (left) appears black.

array of cylinders has ratios 1, 3, 4. . . . The presence of the liquid crystals may also be detected directly in the emulsion by using optical microscopy. An emulsion without a liquid crystal shows only the two phases (Fig. 26a), whereas the liquid crystal is conspicuous from its radiance in polarized light (see Fig. 26b).

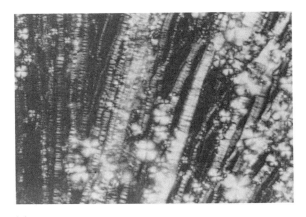

(a)

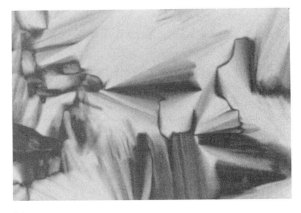

(b)

Fig. 25 Optical patterns of (a) a lamellar and (b) hexagonal liquid crystal.

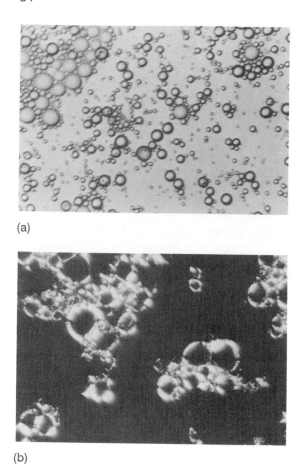

(a)

(b)

Fig. 26 An emulsion with only two liquids (a) shows only the droplets. (b) An emulsion containing a liquid crystalline layer also shows the characteristic optical patterns in polarized light.

The stabilizing action of liquid crystals is limited to protection against coalescence (e.g., short distance action). It serves in four manners.

1. The lamellar structure leads to a strong reduction of the van der Waals forces during the coalescence step. The mathematical treatment of this problem is fairly complex [40] and will not be treated in this chapter, but the diagram of the van der Waals potential (Fig. 27) illustrates the phenomenon [41].

    Without the liquid crystalline phase, coalescence takes place over a thin liquid film in a distance range at which the slope of the van der Waals potential is steep (huge van der Waals force). With the liquid crystal present, coalescence takes place over a thick film, and the slope of the van der Waals potential is small (small force). One should also realize that the liquid crystal is highly viscous, and it is no surprise that an emulsion with a viscous film of liquid crystal combined with a small compressive force exhibits enhanced stability against coalescence in comparison with a two-phase system.

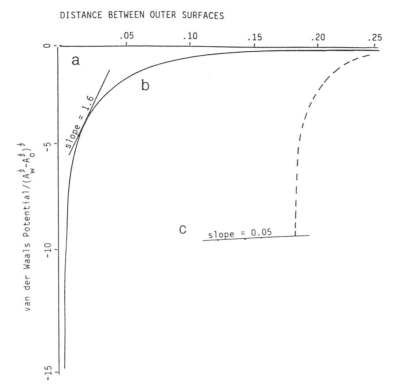

DISTANCE BETWEEN OUTER SURFACES

Fig. 27 During coalescence, the van der Waals force in a system with liquid crystals (slope of dashed line) is much smaller than in the system with monomolecular layers of surfactant.

2. The network of liquid crystalline leaflets [42] hinders the free mobility of the emulsion droplets and makes a stabilization contribution similar to that of increasing the viscosity of the continuous phase (two-phase emulsions).

3. The high-energy dissipation during emulsification gives rise to the formation of vesicles. They most certainly serve as stabilizers, but no systematic investigatoins of this effect have yet been reported.

4. The final consideration of the stability of these three-phase emulsions is probably the most important one. Small changes in emulsifier concentration lead to drastic changes in the amounts of the three phases. As an example, consider the points 1–3 in Fig. 28. At point 1, with 2% emulsifier, 49% water, and 49% oil, 50% oil phase and 50% aqueous phase are the only phases present. At point 2 the emulsifier concentration has been increased to 4%. Now the oil phase constitutes 47% of the total, and the aqueous phase is reduced to 29%. The remaining 24% is the liquid crystalline phase. The importance of these numbers is best perceived by a calculation of thickness of the protective layer of the emulsifier (point 1) and of the liquid crystal (point 2). The 2.0% added surfactant, which would add a protective film of only 0.07 μm to emulsion droplets of 5 μm if all of it were adsorbed, has now been transformed to 24% of a viscous phase. This phase would form a very viscous film

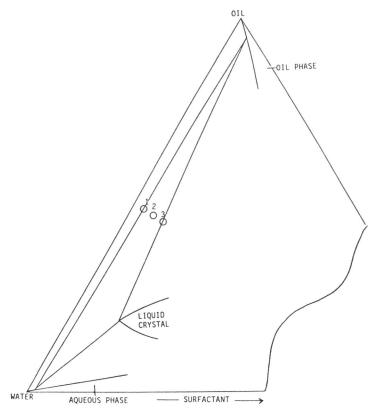

Fig. 28 The nature of the emulsion is completely changed from an oil and water system at 2% emulsifier to an oil and liquid crystal system at 7% emulsifier.

0.85 μm thick. The protective coating is more than ten times thicker than one from the surfactant alone. The reason for this unusual phenomenon is that the thick viscous film contains only 7% emulsifier; whereas the rest is 75% water and 18% oil. At point 3, the aqueous phase has now disappeared, and the entire emulsion consists of 42.3% oil and 57.5% liquid crystalline phase. The stabilizing phase is now the major part of the emulsion.

The first application of these systems is high-internal-ratio emulsions (O/W emulsions with high content of oil) is apparent in light of the fact that the liquid crystals stabilize against coalescence, but offer no protection against flocculation. In a high-internal-ratio emulsion, the dispersed phase occupies a large share of the total volume. An emulsion of this kind consists of very close-packed droplets, and flocculation is unavoidable. The structure often consists of a single aggregate of flocculated droplets that slide against one another to achieve mobility. Protection against coalescence now becomes the essential characteristic of the emulsion, and the structures involving liquid crystals are useful.

The second application involves dissolution of substances that are only sparingly soluble in any solvent. It takes advantage of the fact that the lamellar liquid crystal is the only possible association structure for a wide range of the packing ratios, R [43,44] whree

$$R = \frac{v}{a_0 l} \tag{5}$$

v = volume of the hydrocarbon
a_0 = cross-sectional area occupied by the head group
l = length of the surfactant

A perfect lamellar liquid crystal should have a packing ratio of 1, but geometric considerations show the lamellar structure to be the only one for R values in the range from 1 to 0.5. Lamellar liquid crystals with $R = 0.5$ are far from their lowest free energy, providing a potential for dissolution of substances that otherwise are very difficult to dissolve. In a first example, published in 1984, the solubility of hydrocortisone was increased by more than 200% [45]. This characteristic will probably find several interesting applications in the future.

A third application is concerned with spontaneous emulsification, a phenomenon treated by Groves in a series of articles [46]. A fourth application, which has been investigated by Frank [47], is in systems for delayed drug delivery. The relevance of using a lamellar liquid crystal to delay drug delivery should be seen against the diffusion rates in a lamellar liquid crystal [48]. The diffusion rate parallel to the layers is of the same magnitude as in a liquid, but perpendicular to the layers a value three orders of magnitude smaller is found. Hence, a lamellar liquid crystal covering an emulsion droplet could be expected to have a decisive influence on the mass transfer across the interface.

The conditions for surfactants to be useful to form liquid crystals exist when the R value is in the range 0.5–1. This means that double-chain surfactants are eminently suited, and lecithin is a natural choice [42]. Combinations of a monochain ionic surfactant with a long-chain carboxylic acid or alcohol yield lamellar liquid crystals at low concentrations, but suffer the disadvantage of the hydrophobic part being too soluble in the oil phase. A combination of long-chain carboxylic acid plus an amine of equal chain length suffers less from this problem because of extensive ionization of both amphiphiles.

In summary, three-phase emulsions have as yet been investigated in only a preliminary manner. There is no doubt that, in the future, when their properties are better known, they will be used extensively for drug delivery systems. Not only may a liquid crystal dissolve more of some substances that are only poorly soluble in liquid solvents, but the delivery rate of drugs from them may be varied and controlled. The first developments to use liquid crystals as a matrix for solvents to enhance transdermal transport have now been initiated. It appears highly probable that new and interesting applications will be found in the future.

APPENDIX: FLOCCULATION KINETICS OF SPHERICAL PARTICLES OR DROPLETS

The flocculation kinetics of particles or droplets is well illustrated by a system with the simplest possible form of dispersed particles (spherical), the simplest interparticle interaction (particles stick when they touch, but there are no other distance-dependent forces between them), and the simplest size distribution (all particles of equal size).

The flocculation range now depends only on the diffusion of particles

$$dn/dt = (-16\pi Da)n^2 = \left(-\frac{8kT}{3\eta}\right)n^2 \tag{6}$$

where

dn/dt = flocculation rate (particles per second and volume unit)
a = radius of droplet
D = diffusion coefficient for one droplet
n = number of particles per volume unit
k = Boltzmann constant
T = absolute temperature
η = viscosity of continuous medium

The flocculation rate is proportional to the square of the number of droplets per unit volume, to the radius of the droplets, and to their diffusion coefficient. The second version of the equation is obtained from the first by the use of Einstein's relation $Df = kT$ (f = friction coefficient for a droplet) and Stokes' law $f = 6\pi\eta a$.

Equation (4) shows extremely fast flocculation rates for an emulsion. In 1 cm^3 of an emulsion with equal amounts of water and oil and a droplet radius of 1 µm, the flocculation would be of the magnitude of 10^{11} particles per second; that is, a great majority of the droplets would flocculate within the first second.

The half-life ($t_{1/2}$; the time needed for half of the original number of particles to flocculate) is obtained as follows:

$$t_{1/2} = \frac{3\eta}{8kTn} = 9.0 \times 10^{10}\,\eta \tag{7}$$

If an energy barrier of height W (expressed in kT units) is introduced between the particles, the flocculation rate is reduced by a factor and now becomes

$$\frac{dn}{dt} = -\frac{8kT}{3\eta}\,n^2/2a\int_{2a}^{\infty}\frac{e^w}{l^2}\,dl \tag{8}$$

where l is the distance between centers of droplets.

If the influence of the barrier is restricted to within a distance of one radius from the surface of the droplet, then

$$2a\int_{2a}^{\infty}\frac{e^w}{l^2}\,dl = \frac{1}{3}(e^2 + 2) \tag{9}$$

This is the factor by which the flocculation rate is reduced. A barrier of 20 kT reduces the flocculation rate from approximately 100 billion droplets per second per cubic centimeter in an emulsion without a barrier to approximately 1,000 droplets per second per cubic centimeter for a barrier of 20 kT.

The half-life gives a better illustration of the barrier. It now becomes:

$$t_{1/2} = \frac{\eta(e^w + 2)}{8ktn} \tag{10}$$

One milliliter of an emulsion with the oil/water ratio of 1 and a droplet radius of 1 μm contains approximately 10^{11} droplets, and without an energy barrier, $t_{1/2}$ equals 0.08 s. With no energy barrier, the collision rate is entirely determined by the diffusion rate of the droplets. There is no interaction between them when they approach one another, and each collision leads to immediate coalescence because no repulsive forces are involved. The presence of a barrier has a drastic influence on the coalescence rate and, hence, on $t_{1/2}$. Table 4 is a good illustration of this influence.

REFERENCES

1. J. T. Davies, in *Recent Progress in Surface Science*, Vol. 2 (J. F. Daniells, K. G. A. Pankhurst, and A. C. Riddiford, eds.), Academic Press, New York, 1964, p. 129.
2. P. Becher, *Emulsions: Theory and Practice*. Reinhold, New York, 1965, p. 1.
3. P. Sherman, ed., *Emulsion Science*. Academic Press, New York, 1968.
4. S. E. Friberg, ed., *Food Emulsion*. Marcel Dekker, New York, 1976.
5. P. Becher, ed., *Encyclopedia of Emulsion Technology*, Vol. 2. Marcel Dekker, New York, 1985.
6. K. Shinoda, and S. E. Friberg, *Adv. Colloid Interface Sci.*, 4:281 (1975).
7. International Union of Pure and Applied Chemistry, *IUPAC Manual of Colloid and Surface Chemistry*. Butterworths, London, 1971.
8. M. M. Rieger, Emulsions, in *Theory and Practice of Industrial Pharmacy*, 3rd ed. (L. Lachman, H. A. Lieberman, J. L. Kanig, eds.) Lea & Febiger, Philadelphia, 1986, p. 502.
9. E. S. R. Gopal, in *Emulsion Science* (P. Sherman, ed.), Academic Press, New York, 1968, p. 1.
10. P. Walstra, in *Encyclopedia of Emulsion Technology*, Vol. 1 (P. Becher, ed.) Marcel Dekker, New York, 1983, p. 57.
11. D. H. Smith and K.-H. Lim, *J. Phys. Chem.*, 94:3746 (1990).
12. D. H. Smith, G. L. Covatch, and K.-H. Lim, *Langmuir* 7:1585 (1991).
13. K. H. Lim and D. H. Smith, *J. Dispersion Sci. Technol.*, 11:529 (1990).
14. D. H. Smith, J. S. Reckley, and G. K. Johnson, *J. Colloid Interface Sci.*, 151:3831 (1992).
15. K. Shinoda and H. Arai, *J. Phys. Chem.*, 68:3485 (1964).
16. A. F. Brodin, D. R. Kavaliunas, and S. G. Frank, *Acta Pharm. Suec.*, 15:1 (1978).
17. J. W. Frankenfield, W. J. Asher, and N. N. Li, *Recent Developments in Separation Science*, Vol. 4. CRC Press, Boca Raton, FL 1978.
18. R. Defrey and G. Petré, in *Surface and Colloid Science*, Vol. 3 (E. Matijević, ed.) Wiley-Interscience, New York, 1971, p. 27.
19. K. Madani and S. E. Friberg, *Prog. Colloid Polym. Sci.*, 65:164 (1978).
20. M. Podzimek and S. E. Friberg, *J. Dispersal Sci. Technol.*, 1:341 (1980).
21. E. Ruckenstein, *J. Dispersal Sci. Technol.*, 2:1 (1981).
22. B. Derjaguin and L. D. Landau, *Acta Physicochim. USSR*, 14:633 (1941).
23. E. J. W. Vervey and J. T. G. Overbeek, *Theory of the Stability of Lyophobic Colloids*. Elsevier, Amsterdam, 1948.
24. W. Albers and J. T. G. Overbeek, *J. Colloid Sci.*, 15:489 (1960).
25. E. Matijević, *Pure Appl. Chem.*, 53:2167 (1981).
26. J. T. C. Boehm and J. Lyklema, in *Theory and Practice of Emulsions Technology* (A. L. Smith, ed.) Academic Press, New York, 1976, p. 23.
27. D. E. Graham and M. C. Phillips, in *Theory and Practice of Emulsion Technology* (A. L. Smith, ed.) Academic Press, New York, 1976, p. 75.
28. D. H. Napper, *Polymeric Stabilization of Colloidal Dispersion*. Academic Press, New York, 1983.
29. E. J. Clayfield and E. C. Lumb, *Macromolecules*, 1:133 (1968).

30. H. Karbstein and H. Schubert, *Chem. Eng. Technol.*, 66:99 (1994).
31. J. H. Schulman and I. Leja, *Trans. Faraday Soc.*, 50:598 (1954).
32. T. J. Lin, *J. Soc. Cosmet. Chem.*, 29:117 (1978).
33. H. Saito and K. Shinoda, *J. Colloid Interface Sci.*, 35:359 (1971).
34. S. E. Friberg and I. Lapczvnska, *Prog. Colloid Polym. Sci.*, 56:16 (1975).
35. T. D. Flaim and S. E. Friberg, *Separation Sci. Technol.*, 16:1467 (1981).
36. S. E. Friberg, M. Mortensen, and P. Neogi, *Separation Sci. Technol.*, 20:285 (1985).
37. P. Neogi, M. Kim, and S. E. Friberg, *Separation Sci. Technol.*, 20:613 (1985).
38. S. E. Friberg, L. Mandell, and M. Larsson, *J. Colloid Interface Sci.*, 29:155 (1969).
39. S. E. Friberg, and K. Larsson, in *Advances in Liquid Crystals*, Vol. 2. Academic Press, New York, 1976, p. 173.
40. P.-O. Jansson and S. E. Friberg, *Mol. Cryst. Liquid Cyst.*, 34:75 (1976).
41. S. E. Friberg, P.-O. Jansson, and E. Cederberg, *J. Colloid Interface Sci.*, 55:614 (1976).
42. B. W. Barry, *Adv. Colloid Interface Sci.*, 5:37 (1975).
43. J. N. Israelachvili, D. J. Mitchell, and B. W. Ninham, *J. Chem. Soc. Faraday Trans, 2*, 76:1525 (1976).
44. D. J. Mitchell and B. W. Ninham, *J. Chem. Soc. Faraday Trans. 2*, 77:601 (1981).
45. S. Wahlgren, A. L. Lindstrom, and S. E. Friberg, *J. Pharm. Sci.*, 73:1484 (1984).
46. M. J. Groves and H. S. Yalabik, *Pharm. Technol.*, 2:21 (1977).
47. S. G. Frank, *Acta Pharm. Suec.*, 15:1 (1978).
48. G. Lindblom and H .Wennerström, *Biophys. Chem.* 6:167 (1977).

4

Theory of Colloids

John W. Vanderhoff

Lehigh University, Bethlehem, Pennsylvania

I. INTRODUCTION

The use of colloids in the pharmaceutical sciences has grown rapidly over the last several decades and is expected to accelerate in the future. One area of importance is the newly developed polypeptide chemotherapeutic agents and their delivery in the form of colloidal dispersions by convenient methods of administration.

A second area is the use of colloidal dispersions for drug delivery, which was reviewed recently [1]. Most studies have used irreversible colloidal systems, such as emulsions, suspensions, and liposomes, but others have used micellar systems [2]. These four colloidal systems, as well as polymer microspheres, are important ways of delivering drugs, both orally and parenterally. Several investigators have noted that the administration of drugs in oils or emulsions increased their biological availability [3]. Various mechanisms may contribute to such enhanced absorption, including prolonged gastric residence of the drug and reduced intestinal motility, stimulation of bile salts leading to favorable drug–bile salt interactions, and enhanced lymphatic transport. Interfacial adsorption of drugs and emulsion systems may also play a role in the enhanced oral absorption of insulin and heparin after intraduodenal administration of such dispersions [4,5]. More recently, the preferential absorption of lipsome-containing drugs by the reticuloendothelial system, notably the liver and spleen, has stimulated interest in examining other colloids for the targeting of drugs to specific body organs. Both simple and multiple emulsion systems have already found considerable use in cancer chemotherapy [1].

A third area of importance is the use of colloidal systems as pharmaceutical excipients, product components, vehicles, and carriers. Water-based polymer latexes have found application in a wide range of pharmaceutical-coating applications. The latexes used are primarily copolymers of methacrylic acid or 2-trimethylammoniummethyl methacrylate with acrylate or methacrylate esters. These latexes provide a series of synthetic polymers, with water solubilities ranging from insoluble, to slowly soluble, to pH-dependent (enteric) soluble, to completely soluble, all from concentrated aqueous dispersions without organic solvents.

These latexes have been accepted more rapidly abroad than in the United States because they are prepared from liquid monomers and, hence, contain residual monomer, as well as the residues of emulsifiers, initiators, and buffers. A newer class of colloidal dispersions, known as pseudolatexes (false latexes), has been developed even more recently. These dispersions have all of the characteristics of a true latex in terms of colloidal stability, particle size, high solids concentration, and film-forming ability, but they are not made by emulsion polymerization; rather, they are made by direct emulsification of preexisting polymers by mechanical means, as will be described later in this chapter. Thus, these pseudolatexes are totally free from monomer; they are generally regarded-as-safe (GRAS) status polymers and emulsifiers, and they are even acceptable in food applications. A commercial ethylcellulose pseudolatex has found a range of applications in pharmaceutical development, from taste-masking to controlled-release coatings [6,7]. Latex and pseudolatex dispersions have also been used as unique vehicles for drug and chemical entrapment [8–14].

In addition, the principles of colloidal science govern many practices in industrial pharmacy.

1. The milling of pharmaceuticals to (a) decrease their particle size and increase their surface area; (b) increase their rate of dissolution; (c) increase their rate of absorption; (d) increase the rate of drying of their powders; (e) improve the texture, taste, and rheology of their suspensions [15].
2. The preparation of emulsions and suspensions of pharmaceuticals, in particular, the use of emulsifiers (a) in the preparation and stabilization of these emulsions and suspensions; (b) the importance of the surface or interfacial tension and its experimental measurement; (c) the origins and effects of the surface charge on stabilization; (d) the forces between the particles and the state of their aggregation; (e) the mechanisms of crystal growth by Ostwald ripening, polymorphic transformation, and temperature cycling; (f) the wetting of powders by emulsifier solutions; (g) the absorption of emulsifiers at the solid–liquid interface [16].
3. The coating of pharmaceutical tablets to (a) mask the taste, odor, and color of the drug; (b) provide physical and chemical protection of the drug; (c) control the release of the drug; (d) protect the drug from the gastric environment of the stomach (enteric coatings); (e) incorporate another drug in the coating to produce sequential drug release and avoid chemical incompatibilities [17].
4. The microencapsulation of drugs to (a) convert liquid drugs to a solid; (b) alter their colloidal and surface properties; (c) protect drugs from the environment; (d) control their release rate (18). The preparation of microcapsules by (a) air suspension; (b) coacervation-phase separation; (c) multiorifice centrifugation; (d) pan coating; (e) spray drying and spray congealing; (f) solvent evaporation; (g) polymerization [18].
5. The solubilization, complexation, and hydrotropy of drugs in emulsifier solutions [19].
6. The preparation and stabilization of pharmaceutical suspensions, in particular, (a) the wetting of the solid particles by emulsifier solutions; (b) the repulsive and attractive forces between the particles and their combination to give sta-

bility or flocculation; (c) the clustering of the particles in open or closed network aggregates; (d) the sedimentation rate of the dispersed particles; (e) the crystal habit and structure factors; (f) the preparation of suspensions by precipitation or dispersion; (g) the rheology of the suspensions; (h) the evaluation of suspension stability and sedimentation volume; (i) the evaluation of the electrokinetic properties [20].

7. The preparation and stabilization of pharmaceutical emulsions, in particular, (a) the relation between droplet stabilization, interfacial tension, interfacial film properties, and the repulsion and attraction between droplets; (b) the classification of emulsions as oil-in-water or water-in-oil types; (c) the classification according to microemulsions, macroemulsions, and miniemulsions; (d) the factors involved in emulsion stability, such as heat, phase inversion, and time; (e) the use of auxiliary emulsifiers, such as finely divided solids and hydrophilic colloids; (f) the evaluation of emulsion instability, creaming, flocculation, and coalescence; (g) the evaluation of emulsion shelf life as a function of aging, temperature increase or decrease, centrifugation, and agitation [21].

8. The preparation of pharmaceutical aerosols, in particular, (a) the aerosol components such as product concentrate, propellant, container, valve, and actuator; (b) the choice of propellant according to its vapor pressure, environmental acceptability, and the possibility of interaction with the product; (c) the different types of product formulations, such as solutions, water-based systems, suspensions, dispersions and foams, including aqueous stable, nonaqueous stable, quick breaking, and thermal foams; (d) stability testing of the aerosol components [22].

All of these operations and forms of matter are governed by the same underlying principles of colloidal science. The purpose of this chapter is to review these principles, in particular, (a) the adsorption of ionic surfactants and the electrostatic stabilization of colloidal sols and dispersions; (b) the adsorption of nonionic surfactants and the steric stabilization of colloidal sols and dispersions; (c) the preparation of pseudolatexes by emulsification. The emphasis of this chapter will be on polymer latexes, but the principles described are equally applicable to all colloidal dispersions, emulsions, suspensions, foams, and aerosols prepared by dispersion, emulsification, coating, and encapsulation.

II. ELECTROSTATIC STABILIZATION OF LATEXES

A. General Introduction

1. *Colloidal Nature of Latexes*

A *colloidal dispersion*, by definition, is a two-phase system that comprises a dispersed phase and a dispersion medium. The overall physicochemical properties of the colloidal dispersion are determined by (a) the chemical and physical nature of the dispersed phase; (b) the chemical and physical properties of the dispersion medium; (c) the nature of the interaction at the interfaces between air and the dispersion medium, and the dispersed phase and the dispersion medium.

The dispersed phase in a latex comprises spherical polymer particles, usually with average diameters of 200–300 nm. The dispersion medium is water that contains various water-soluble compounds (nonaqueous latexes will not be considered here). The properties of the aqueous phase are determined by the type and concentration of dissolved compounds (simple electrolytes, surfactants, polyelectrolytes) and the pH.

In a latex, the interfacial area between the aqueous phase and air is small; however, it controls such important practical properties as wetting and foaming during formulation and application, as well as the stability of latex foams. The interfacial area between the polymer particles and the aqueous phase is large because of the small size of the particles and the inverse proportionality of the specific surface area to the particle diameter. Thus, the smaller the particle size, the greater the contribution of its surface properties and the less the contribution of its bulk properties to the overall colloidal behavior of the latex. A knowledge of the chemical composition of the dispersed phase allows speculation on the mode of stabilization of the particles. The nature of the interface between the polymer particles and aqueous phase determines many important properties of the latex system, such as stabilization–destabilization, rheology, and particle movement in an electrical field.

2. *Stabilization–Destabilization of Latexes*

Colloidal dispersions have a true interface, with a defined interfacial tension γ between the dispersed particles and the dispersion medium. The state of the colloidal dispersions is characterized by the excess free energy G of the system:

$$dG = \gamma dS \tag{1}$$

where S is the specific surface area. In the thermodynamic sense, all colloidal dispersions of small-particle size are unstable because the system tends to minimize its excess free energy (and, hence, its large specific surface area) by aggregation of the small particles. This aggregation may comprise flocculation (clustering together) or coalescence (fusion). Hence, the particle size increases with decreasing excess free energy unless there is an energy barrier between the particles to prevent them from aggregating. With this energy barrier, flocculation-stable and coalescence-stable colloidal dispersions may be distinguished. Figure 1 shows schematically the processes occurring during the formation and destruction of these colloidal dispersions [23].

The colloidal stability of a latex that comprises colloidal particles undergoing Brownian motion is defined by its resistance to a change in the state of the system. Precautions are taken in the preparation of latexes to ensure good colloidal stability during polymerization, storage, and application. The term *good colloidal stability* means that little or no particle aggregation has occurred in the latex between preparation and use. The aggregation is a kinetic phenomenon; in practice, the colloidal stability is assessed by measuring the rate of aggregation of the latex particles. Thus, the stability of a latex is a relative parameter that depends on the application for which the latex is intended and the method by which colloidal stability is determined. Many latexes have excellent colloidal stability; their particles show no tendency to aggregate, even after years of aging.

In a colloidal dispersion, the Brownian motion results in frequent collisions between particles. The stability of these dispersions is determined by the interaction between the particles during collision. There are two types of interactions: attraction and repulsion. When attraction predominates, the particles adhere after collision and aggregate. When repulsion predominates, the particles rebound after collision and remain individually dispersed.

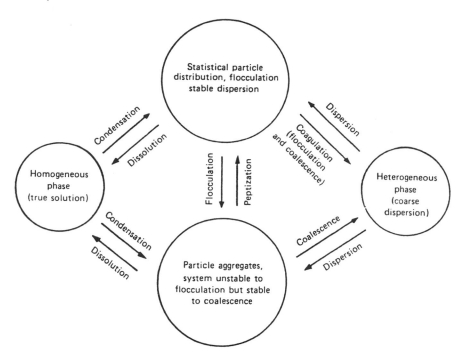

Fig. 1 Schematic diagram of the processes involved in the production or destruction of dispersed systems. (From Ref. 23.)

In a latex, the attractive forces of interaction are mainly the van der Waals forces that arise when particles are dispersed in a medium with a different dielectric constant. Therefore, a latex can be stable only when the repulsive forces are sufficiently strong to outweigh the van der Waals attraction. These repulsive forces operate by one or both of the following mechanisms: (a) electrostatic repulsion, which arises from the presence of an ionic charge on the surface of the particles; (b) steric repulsion, which arises from the presence of uncharged molecules on the surface of the particles, and which, by enthalpic or entropic changes, prevents aggregation of the particles. The latter case is unusual in that the latexes that are thermodynamically unstable are stabilized by thermodynamic means.

The objective of this section is to discuss the principles determining the electrostatic stabilization of latexes that derive their electrostatic charge from the adsorption of surfactants.

B. Adsorption of Surfactants

Surfactants play a key role in the preparation, formulation, and application of latexes. In emulsion polymerization, the type and concentration of surfactant determines the mechanism of particle nucleation and the number of particles nucleated and, thereby, the rate of polymerization. Surfactants are also essential for the stabilization of the latex system during preparation, stripping to remove monomer, formulation, storage, shipping, and finally, application. In these functions, the underlying fundamental property of the surfactant is its adsorption at the various interfaces of the latex.

Most of the surfactant in a latex is adsorbed at the particle–water interface; only small fractions are adsorbed at the water–air interface or remain in the bulk aqueous phase as solute surfactant. The surfactant adsorbed at the particle–water interface plays an important role in determining the overall latex properties. Thus, a knowledge of the adsorption of surfactants in a latex is necessary to understand its colloidal properties.

1. *Classification of Surfactants*

Surfactant molecules comprise a hydrophobic "tail" and a hydrophilic "head." These surfactants can be classified into four categories according to the charge of the head: (a) anionic surfactants (e.g., alkyl carboxylates, sulfates, and sulfonates; alkylaryl sulfonates, alkyl phosphates); (b) cationic surfactants (e.g., alkyl quaternary nitrogen bases, amines, and nitriles; and nonquaternary nitrogen bases); (c) nonionic surfactants, including alkylaryl-polyoxyethylene adducts; (d) ampholytic surfactants, such as those containing both amino and carboxylic acid groups.

An annual listing of commercial surfactants [24] includes several thousand different products. The selection of a surfactant for a given application has often been a trial-and-error process, involving the screening of hundreds of surfactants. A more systematic approach is the hydrophile–lipophile balance (HLB) system [25–27]. Most anionic and nonionic surfactants have HLB values in the range of 1–20. An HLB value of 1 indicates that the surfactant is soluble in oil; an HLB value of 20, that it is soluble in water. Surfactants with low HLB values are good stabilizers for water-in-oil emulsions; surfactants with high HLB values are good stabilizers for oil-in-water emulsions. Aqueous latexes are in the latter category. Ross et al.[28] demonstrated that the HBL value of a surfactant can be correlated with a fundamental physical property: the spreading coefficient of the dispersed phase on the surface of the surfactant solution in the dispersion medium.

The HLB system has been used to select surfactants for the emulsion polymerization of vinyl monomers [29,30]. Polystyrene and poly(vinyl acetate) latexes of optimum stability were prepared using surfactants of HLB 14–15 and 16–17.5 in their respective emulsion polymerization processes [29]. The particle size and viscosity of the latexes varied strongly with the surfactant HLB and the composition of the surfactant mixture used to reach a given HLB [29]. In poly(styene-*co*-butyl acrylate) emulsion copolymerization, the surfactant HLB values were correlated with the percentage conversion, latex particle size, and copolymer molecular weight [30].

Some practical surfactant systems are mixtures of two or more surfactants of the same or different types. These surfactant mixtures often have surface properties different from the single parent surfactants. These differences are due to specific interactions (e.g., the complexation or phase transitions that occur when the two surfactants are mixed) [31].

2. General Features of Surfactant Adsorption

Above a certain critical concentration, surfactant molecules form aggregates of 50–100 molecules in water. These aggregates are called *micelles*, and the concentration at which they first appear is called the *critical micelle concentration* (*CMC*). A dynamic equilibrium exists between the surfactant molecules in the micelles and in the bulk aqueous phase. In a latex, the surfactant molecules also adsorb at the particle–water and water–air interfaces; consequently, another dynamic equilibrium exists between the surfactant molecules adsorbed at the interfaces and those in the bulk aqueous phase. The overall equilibrium condition of the surfactant concentration in any latex can be represented by Eq. (2):

$$\text{Micellar surfactant} \xleftrightarrow{\quad k_1 \quad} \text{solute surfactant} \xleftrightarrow{\quad k_2 \quad} \text{absorbed surfactant} \quad (2)$$

where k_1 and k_2 are constants that depend on the surface composition and structure of the particles, as well as the activity of the surfactant molecules.

The adsorption of surfactant molecules on the latex particles is a thermodynamic process driven by the decrease in the overall free energy of the system. The interaction forces involved in surfactant adsorption are van der Waals forces. These interaction forces are weak; therefore, the surfactant molecules can desorb easily from the particle surface. This ease of adsorption and desorption of physically adsorbed surfactant is important in latex-coating compositions in which the latexes are blended with colloidal dispersions of pigments or fillers, which also have large specific surface areas; the desorption of surfactant molecules from the latex particles and the readsorption on the pigment or filler particles often causes significant flocculation of the latex particles.

The amount of surfactant adsorbed per unit area of the latex particle surface, as well as the extent of surface coverage, are important fundamental properties of the latex system. The variation of the amount of surfactant adsorbed per unit surface area over a range of bulk surfactant concentrations constitutes the adsorption isotherm. The Gibbs adsorption equation is a thermodynamic expression that relates the surface concentration of the surfactant to the surface tension and the bulk activity of the adsorbate (32). Thus, it can be used to determine the surface concentration and, consequently, the adsorption isotherm, of the surfactant. In the absence of electrolytes in the latex (e.g., as in cleaned latexes), the adsorption isotherm is given by:

$$\Gamma = -(1/2\,RT)\left(\frac{\partial \gamma}{\partial \ln C} \right) \quad (3)$$

where Γ is the concentration of surfactant molecules adsorbed at the surface, γ the surface tension of the latex, C the bulk concentration of surfactant (assuming that the activity of the ions is equivalent to their bulk concentration, which is valid for dilute solutions), R the gas constant, and T the temperature. In the presence of excess electrolyte, the adsorption isotherm is given by:

$$\Gamma = -\left(\frac{1}{RT} \right)\left(\frac{\partial \gamma}{\partial \ln C} \right) \quad (4)$$

A comparison of the two equations shows that small concentrations of electrolyte given an increase in the amount of surfactant adsorbed per unit area of the latex particle surface at a given surfactant concentration. This increase was verified experimentally for the adsorption of several surfactants on polystyrene and poly(methyl methacrylate) latex particles as a function of electrolyte concentration [33,34].

3. *Determination of Adsorption Isotherms of Surfactants*

Adsorption isotherms of a surfactant on a latex particle surface are usually defined indirectly (e.g., by determination of the change in bulk surfactant concentration in the aqueous phase after the added surfactant has been allowed to equilibrate with the latex particles. The concentration of surfactant adsorbed on the latex particle surface is determined from the difference between the bulk surfactant and the total surfactant concentrations. In practice, the conductivity or surface tension of the dilute latex–surfactant system is determined as a function of added surfactant concentration [33–42]; the attainment of the critical micelle concentration in the aqueous phase is taken as the point at which the latex particle surface is saturated with surfactant molecules. This method, known as the soap titration method of Maron et al. [37–40], is used to determine (a) the cross-sectional area of the adsorbed surfactant molecule on the surface of the latex particles, provided that the particle size is known; (b) the average (volume–surface area) particle size, provided that the cross-sectional area of the surfactant molecule is known; (c) the percentage surface coverage of the latex particles with the surfactant.

The serum replacement method developed to clean latexes for characterization has been used to determine adsorption isotherms of surfactants [43–46]. The latex is confined in a filtration cell with a semipermeable Nuclepore membrane, and double-distilled, deionized water is pumped through the latex to replace the serum. This method allows complete recovery of the serum, as well as the determination of the concentration profile of the desorbing surfactant in the effluent stream by conductance, spectrophotometric absorption, or refractive index measurements. To determine the adsorption isotherm, a known amount of surfactant is added to a cleaned latex, and the concentration profile of the surfactant in the effluent stream is determined. A material balance between added and desorbed surfactant gives the adsorption isotherm. This method has been applied to measure the adsorption isotherms of ionic and nonionic surfactants on the particle surfaces of different latexes. In a recent modification [47], a surfactant solution of known concentration is pumped through the latex confined in a filtration cell and the surfactant concentration in the effluent stream is measured.

Most adsorption isotherms of conventional surfactants on latex particle surfaces are of the Langmuir type. The number of surfactant molecules n adsorbed per unit surface area at a given bulk concentration C is given by:

$$\frac{1}{n} = \left(\frac{1}{N}\right) + \left(\frac{1}{CNb}\right) \tag{5}$$

where N is the number of surfactant molecules adsorbed per unit surface area at the saturation point (i.e., the plateau of the adsorption isotherm) and b is the Langmuir constant, which is related to the free energy of adsorption ΔG^0 of a surfactant molecule by the equation:

$$b = k \exp\left(\frac{\Delta G^0}{RT}\right) \tag{6}$$

where k is a constant. A plot of $1/n$ versus $1/C$ allows the determination of the cross-sectional area of the surfactant molecule on a given substrate $(1/N)$ at the saturation point, which is a fundamental property of the surfactant–substrate system

4. *Factors Affecting Adsorption of Surfactant on Latex Particles*

The adsorption isotherm of surfactant molecules on latex particles is influenced by the following factors:

a. The Interaction Between the Particle Surface and the Surfactant Molecules

The physical and chemical nature of the polymer particles plays an important role in determining the adsorption isotherms of surfactants. The cross-sectional area of the adsorbed surfactant molecules on the latex particle surface increases with increasing hydrophilicity of the surface [33,34,46]. A correlation was found between the saturation adsorption of a surfactant molecule and the polymer–water interfacial tension and the polarity of the polymer surface [48,49]. The saturation cross-sectional area of sodium lauryl sulfate on the latex particle surface decreased with increasing polymer–water interfacial tension and increasing polarity of the particle surface. In the adsorption of anionic and nonionic surfactants on polystyrene latex particles, the adsorption decreased with decreasing hydrophobicity of the surfactant (i.e., with increasing HLB value) [47,50]. The optimum HLB ranges for maximum adsorption of nonionic surfactants on polystyrene and poly(vinyl acetate) latex particle surfaces were 13–14 and 16–17, respectively [50], consistent with the optimum HLB values of surfactants found to give stability during emulsion polymerization [29].

This interaction between the particle surface and the surfactant is important in emulsion polymerization, in particular, the particle nucleation step. In semicontinuous poly(vinyl acetate-*co*-*n*-butyl acrylate) emulsion copolymerization, the average particle size increased, and the polydispersity decreased, with decreasing *n*-butyl acrylate content in the polymer [51,52]. An explanation was given in terms of the mechanism of particle nucleation and the effect of copolymer composition at the particle surface on the surfactant adsorption and the stability of the particles formed initially. It was proposed that particle formation was predominantly due to initiation in the aqueous phase, followed by coalescence of the smaller-sized particles. With comonomer mixtures rich in the more hydrophobic *n*-butyl acrylate, the closer packing of the surfactant molecules on the *n*-butyl acrylate-rich surface would give small particles with a high concentration of adsorbed surfactant and, therefore, better stability against coalescence; thus, the average particle size would be smaller and the particle size distribution would be broader. With conomer mixtures rich in the more hydrophilic vinyl acetate, the looser packing of the surfactant molecules on the vinyl acetate-rich surface would give small particles, with a low concentration of adsorbed surfactant and a relatively hydrophilic surface and, therefore, poorer stability against coalescence; thus, the average particle size would be larger and the particle size distribution would be narrower.

Swelling of the latex particles with monomer or other organic solvents also affects the cross-sectional area of the adsorbed surfactant molecules. The magnitude of this effect depends on the hydrophilicity of the solvent–polymer mixture at the particle–water interface which, in turn, depends on the nature of the polymer, the solvent, and the polymer/solvent swelling ratio. The cross-sectional area of potassium oleate at saturation was 40% larger for polystyrene latex particles swollen with benzene (solvent/polymer ratio 0.33) than for the unswollen particles [34]; the cross-sectional area was only 15% larger for particles swollen with styrene in the same ratio. The cross-sectional area of sodium lauryl sulfate adsorbed on polystyrene particles swollen with benzene (ratio 0.35) was 37% larger than for the unswollen particles; in contrast, that of the same surfactant on poly(methyl methacrylate) particles swollen with benzene (ratio 0.46) was 37% smaller than for the unswollen particles. The poly(methyl methacrylate)–benzene-swollen surface was more hydrophobic (less polar) than the poly(methyl methacrylate) surface alone.

This effect has important implications in emulsion polymerization in which there is a continuous desorption of surfactant molecules from the particle surface, as the monomer/polymer ratio decreases continuously during the polymerization, particularly during the latter stages. Similar effects were found for latexes formulated with plasticizers.

Specific interactions between the surfactant molecules and the surface of the latex particles (e.g., charge neutralization, complexation, and solubilization) cause major changes in the adsorption isotherm. The anionic particle surface groups provide specific sites for the head-to-head adsorption of cationic surfactants by charge neutralization; after complete neutralization of the anionic groups, the adsorption reverts to the tail-to-tail type, and the charge on the particles is reversed [35]. Both complexation and solubilization affected the adsorption isotherms of sodium lauryl sulfate on poly(vinyl acetate) latex particles [50,53]; apparently, strong interactions between the absorbed sodium lauryl sulfate and the poly(vinyl acetate) gave a solubilized polymer–surfactant complex [50,53,54]. The particle size affected the cross-sectional area at saturation for some surfactant–latex systems [34,55]; the cross-sectional area of potassium oleate on polystyrene latex particles decreased from 0.452 nm^2 on 178-nm–diameter particles to 0.360 nm^2 on 43-nm–diameter particles. Urban [55] found similar results for the adsorption of potassium oleate on polystyrene latex particles and for the recalculated data of Willson et al. [56] for potassium oleate on poly(butadiene-*co*-styrene) particles.

b. The Mutual Interaction Between Surfactant Molecules in the Adsorbed Layer

The charged heads of the ionic surfactant in the adsorbed layer repel one another because of electrostatic repulsion, with the result that the packing is less dense (i.e., the cross-sectional area is increased). The addition of anionic surfactant in mixture with nonionic surfactant gave a smaller cross-sectional area of the anionic surfactant [36]; the nonionic surfactant molecules apparently acted as a shield to reduce the electrostatic repulsion between the adsorbed anionic surfactant molecules and, thereby, enhance their adsorption. Similar effects were found in the behavior of surfactant mixtures in solution and adsorbed at interfaces [57]; mixed micelles and mixed monolayers of anionic and nonionic surfactants showed a strong deviation from ideal behavior.

The chain length of the surfactant molecule plays an important role in determining its adsorption isotherm on a given substrate. In a homologous series of surfactants, the longer the chain length, the lower is the equilibrium concentration at which the saturation adsorption is attained. Also, the number of surfactant molecules adsorbed per unit area at saturation is expected to be independent of surfactant chain length; however, the chain length was found [35,37] to affect the packing density of surfactants on the particle surface, presumably because of the lateral interaction among adsorbed surfactant molecules and the physical orientation of the surfactant molecules on the surface.

c. The Interaction Between the Ions in the Bulk Solution with the Adsorbed Layer

An increase in the ionic strength of the bulk solution usually gives an increase in the number of surfactant molecules adsorbed per unit area and, thus, a decrease in the cross-sectional area of the surfactant molecule at saturation [33–35]. The addition of electrolytes reduces the electrostatic repulsion between the ionic heads of the surfactant molecules in the adsorbed layer and, thus, results in closer packing.

A practical problem associated with this type of interaction is the possible under-estimation of the concentration of adsorbed surfactant. As the concentration of adsorbed surfactant approaches saturation, the charged surface may expel ionic surfactant molecules. Thus, the bulk solution concentration may be an erroneous measure of the adsorption isotherm. Studies of the temperature effect on the adsorption of surfactants showed that there is a small, but significant, increase in the cross-sectional area of the adsorbed ionic surfactant (0.05 nm^2) with an increase in temperature from $25°$ to $70°$C [34,55].

C. Electrostatic Stabilization

The electrostatic stabilization of colloidal systems was described quantitatively and independently by Deryaguin and Landau [58], and Verwey and Overbeek [59]. The resultant theory is known as the Deryaguin–Landau–Verwey–Overbeek (DLVO) theory. A colloidal dispersion is stable when the potential energy of repulsion arising from the approach of charged particles exceeds the inherent attractive energy between the particles over a given distance of separation. According to the DLVO theory, the interaction between colloidal particles is given by the superposition of the electrostatic repulsion and the van der Waals attraction. The details are described by Verwey and Overbeek [59] and others [23,60–64].

1. *Electrostatic Repulsion*

a. Origin of the Charge on the Colloidal Particle Surface

The basic principles behind the electrostatic stabilization of a colloidal dispersion is the accumulation of charges at the surface of the particles. There are several mechanisms for this accumulation of charge:

1. Preferential adsorption of potential-determining ions [60]; for example, silver iodide particles adsorb an excess of Ag$^+$ or I$^-$ ions, depending on their relative concentration in the equilibrium solution. The Ag$^+$ or I$^-$ ions are called potential-determining ions, and the surface potential of the particles is constant and independent of the presence of an indifferent electrolyte.
2. Ion deficiencies in the crystal lattice or interior of the particles [65]; for example, the charge on mineral clay particles arises from the isomorphic replacement of a Si^{4+} ion inside the solid lattice by an Al^{3+} ion, resulting in a deficit of charge. This charge is constant and dependent on the presence of an indifferent electrolyte.
3. Adsorption of ionized surfactants; for example, carbon black particles or latex particles acquire a negative charge by adsorption of anionic surfactant.
4. Adsorption of ions from the medium [66,67]; for example, OH$^-$ ions from the aqueous phase are preferentially adsorbed on nonionogenic colloidal particles owing to the ion-induced dipole interaction.
5. Dissociation of ionogenic surface groups is the charge-determining mechanism for various oxides and latex particles; for example, silica particles acquire a negative charge by dissociation of surface silanol groups [68], and latex particles by dissociation of surface sulfate groups introduced by the persulfate-ion initiator [69] or carboxyl groups introduced by copolymerization of carboxyl-containing monomers.

6. Contact electrification or electron injection [67,70,71]. In a dispersed system comprising two nonconducting phases, the phase of lower dielectric constant acquires a negative charge owing to electron injection from the phase of higher dielectric constant; for example, nonionogenic cleaned polystyrene latex particles may acquire a negative charge from the injection of electrons from the aqueous phase into the polymer phase. This contact charge exchange is attributed to the overlap between the distribution of acceptor states of the polystyrene particles with the distribution of the donor states of the water.

A colloidal dispersion becomes unstable if the particles lose their charge. The *zero point of charge* is defined as the pH at which the surface charge is zero; the *isoelectric point*, as the pH at which the electrophoretic mobility is zero. A zero point of charge is expected for origins of charge *1, 2, 4,* and *5*. The zero point of charge of silver iodide is 5.5 (the value of pAg). Alkaline alumina has a zero charge at a high pH; acidic silica, at a low pH. The isoelectric point is similar to the zero point of charge; however, these two parameters may be different when nonpotential-determining ions are adsorbed on the particle surface, as in origin of charge *3*.

b. Diffuse Electric Double Layer

The surface charge of a colloidal particle is compensated by an equivalent number of ions of opposite charge that accumulate in the medium near the particle surface. The surface and counterion charges together constitute the electric double layer. The counterions are attracted to the particle surface electrostatically; they also tend to diffuse away from the surface because their concentration in the bulk solution is lower than that near the surface. This combination of electrostatic attraction and diffusion results in the formation of a counterion cloud around the particle, with a defined distribution of counterions as a function of distance from the surface, which is known as the *diffuse electric double layer*.

The thickness of the double layer is given by the Debye length l/κ, where κ for symmetric electrolytes is

$$\kappa = \left(\frac{8\pi n z^2 e^2}{\varepsilon kT} \right)^{1/2} \tag{7}$$

where n is the number of ionized groups, z their valency, e the elementary charge, ε the dielectric constant, k the Boltzmann constant, and T the absolute temperature. Thus, the Debye length is an inverse function of both the square root of the electrolyte concentration and the valence of the electrolyte.

The charge at the particle surface gives rise to two electrostatic potentials relative to a point in the bulk solution: the surface potential (ψ_0), which exists at the surface, and the Stern potential (ψ_δ), in the diffuse double layer at a distance δ from the surface. Neither of these two potentials has been measured experimentally. A third potential is the zeta potential which exists in the diffuse double layer at a distance from the surface outside the Stern layer; this potential can be measured experimentally by electrophoresis as the potential at the shear plane where the double layer parts when the particle moves in an electric field. The relation between the theoretical surface and Stern potentials, and the experimental zeta potential, is unknown; however, the zeta potential is usually taken as a good approximation of the potential across the diffuse part of the electric double layer.

When two particles approach one another, their electric double layers interact so that work must be performed to bring the particles closer together. The repulsive energy V_R at a given interparticle distance is the work that must be performed to bring the particles to that point. It is difficult to develop an exact expression for the variation of V_R with interparticle distance; however, many approximate expressions have been developed [72]. For small potentials ($\psi_0 < 50$ mV):

$$V_R = \left(\frac{\varepsilon a \psi_0}{\kappa^2} \right) \ln[1 + \exp(-\kappa H_0)] \tag{8}$$

where a is the particle radius and H_0 the distance of separation between the two particles.

For higher surface potentials:

$$V_R = \left(\frac{64 \pi \eta kTa}{2} \right) \gamma^2 \exp(-\kappa H_0) \tag{9}$$

where:

$$\gamma = \frac{\{\exp[(ze\psi\gamma/2kT) - 1]\}}{\{\exp[(ze\psi\delta/2kT) + 1]\}} \tag{10}$$

All approximations show that the repulsive energy V_R is a function of the quantity κH_0 and that it decays exponentially with increasing distance of separation between the particle surfaces.

2. van der Waals Attraction

To explain the phenomenon of coagulation requires that there be an attractive force between the particles. Moreover, the magnitude and range of action of this attractive force must be comparable with those of the electrostatic repulsion force. These requirements are met by the total attractive van der Waals forces between the particles, which are obtained by summation of the London dispersion forces between all atom pairs in the particles. These dispersion forces arise from the charge fluctuations in an atom associated with the motion of electrons, which produces a time-dependent dipole moment. A phase difference in the fluctuating dipoles leads to mutual attraction. Neglecting retardation effects, the expression for the attractive energy V_A between two particles of radius a at a distance of separation H_0 for $a \gg H_0$ is

$$V_A = \frac{A * a}{12 H_0} \tag{11}$$

where $A*$ is the effective Hamaker constant describing the attraction between the particles and the dispersion medium. This simple equation for V_A is not valid at separation distances greater than 10 nm; beyond this range, allowance must be made for the retardation effects that are caused by the finite time required for the electromagnetic wave to travel from one atom to the other atom in which it is inducing a dipole. Schenkel and Kitchener [73] have developed empirical equations for the calculation of attractive energies with corrections for the retardation effect. Hamaker constants have been determined experimentally for several types of particles; the data from different sources show considerable disagreement [74]. Fowkes developed a simple method to calculate the Hamaker constant from surface tension data (75): the surface tension γ is divided into a dispersion contribution γ_d and a contribution from other forces, such as dipole–dipole attractions; the Hamaker constant is then calculated from γ_d.

3. Total Energy of Interaction

The DLVO theory states that the total energy of interaction between colloidal particles is given by the sum of the attraction and repulsion energies:

$$V_T = V_A + V_R \tag{12}$$

Figure 2 shows the total interaction energy curve for a stable colloidal system. At very small distances, the Born repulsion between adjoining electron clouds predominates, and the net interaction is repulsion. At small distances, the van der Waals attraction predominates over the electrostatic repulsion (the Born repulsion being negligible), and the net interaction is attraction in the deep potential energy minimum V_p. At greater distances, the electrostatic repulsion energy falls off more rapidly (exponential decay), with increasing separation distance, than the van der Waals attraction energy (power law), and the net interaction is attraction in the shallow secondary minimum V_S. At intermediate distances, the electrostatic repulsion predominates, and the net interaction is repulsion with the maximum potential V_m.

The stability of a colloidal system is defined by the height of the maximum in the potential energy curve. This potential energy barrier must be surmounted if the colloidal particles are to approach each other sufficiently closely to fall into the deep primary minimum of irreversible coagulation. The value of V_m necessary to prevent this irreversible coagulation is considered to be about 10–20 kT, which corresponds to a zeta potential of about 50 mV; such a system is considered kinetically stable. If the secondary minimum is deep enough (about 5 kT or greater), the particles coagulate, but the coagulation is weak and reversible. Aggregation in the secondary minimum usually does

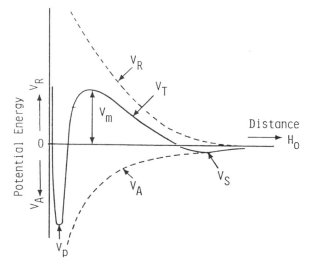

Fig. 2 Variation of the attraction and repulsion energies and the total energy of interaction between two colloidal particles with interparticle distance.

not occur with small colloidal particles because the energy minimum is of the same order as the mean thermal energy of the particles, and the aggregation is easily reversed by Brownian motion. Polystyrene latex particles of 10-μm diameter aggregate in the secondary minimum [73], and the reversibility of aggregation of other polystyrene latex particles has been shown by optical microscopy combined with high-speed cinematography [76].

The attraction energy arises from long-range van der Waals forces; hence, it does not vary significantly with changes in the parameters of the colloidal dispersion. In contrast, the repulsion energy varies significantly with changes in the surface potential of the particles and the valence of the electrolyte in the bulk solution. Consequently, in many practical applications, the stability of the colloidal dispersion is determined by the magnitude of the repulsion energy.

The DLVO theory describes the basic phenomena related to colloidal stability. Over the past 40 years, much theoretical and experimental research on colloidal stability has been carried out to confirm and extend the basic concepts of the DLVO theory. The theoretical work comprises the development of more detailed models to evaluate both V_A and V_R. The experimental work includes measurement of the van der Waals attraction forces and the electrostatic repulsion forces, the rate of coagulation and the critical coagulation concentration, and the electrophoretic mobility and zeta potential, to gain information on the electrical properties of the particle surface.

D. Coagulation and Flocculation of Latexes

According to the DLVO theory, colloidal particles coagulate whenever their kinetic energy is sufficient to surmount the potential energy barrier V_m. Thus, the coagulation of colloidal particles may be accelerated in two ways: (a) by reducing the height of the potential energy barrier; (b) by increasing the kinetic energy of the particles.

1. *Coagulation by Simple Electrolytes*

The reduction of the height of the potential energy barrier is usually accomplished by addition of substances that (a) neutralize the particle charge or cause the loss of the hydration layer; (b) compress the double layer; (c) cause the surfactant to desorb from the particle surface. The substances used to coagulate latexes include electrolytes, which reduce the thickness of the double layer, such that attraction predominates over repulsion. The efficiency of coagulation is sensitive to the valence of the counterion; the concentration of counterions required for coagulation decreases drastically with increasing valence. In carboxyl-containing latexes, the addition of divalent metal ions causes the formation of insoluble nonionized metallic salts, with resultant collapse of the double layer and coagulation of the latex; the addition of strong acids gives similar results owing to the formation of the nonionized carboxyl groups. The addition of trivalent metal ions results in the precipitation of fine metal hydroxide particles that compete with the latex particles for their surfactant. Other substances that can cause coagulation are water-miscible organic solvents (e.g., alcohols or acetone), which reduce the dielectric constant of the medium and dehydrate the stabilizing layer; and polymer-miscible organic solvents (e.g., benzene or carbon tetrachloride), which swell the latex particles, increase the volume fraction of the dispersed phase, and soften the particles, so that collisions may no longer be elastic. The addition of surfactants of opposite charge causes coagulation by charge neutralization.

a. Kinetics of Coagulation

The coagulation of colloidal particles proceeds by three different mechanisms: (a) Brownian or diffusion-controlled coagulation; (b) agitation-induced or mechanical coagulation; (c) surface coagulation. von Smoluchowski [77] derived the following expression for diffusion-controlled coagulation:

$$\frac{-dN}{dt} = \left(\frac{k_o}{W}\right)N_0^2 \qquad k_0 = 8\pi DR \qquad \qquad [13]$$

where $-dN/dt$ is the rate of disappearance of N primary particles, N_0 the initial number of particles per unit volume, k_0 the rate constant for diffusion-controlled rapid coagulation (i.e., where every particle–particle collision leads to coagulation), D the diffusion coefficient of a single particle, R the collision radius (often taken as $2a$), and W the stability ratio.

The stability ratio W represents the retardation factor of the slow coagulation (i.e., when only a fraction of the particle–particle collisions leads to coagulation) compared with rapid coagulation. The stability ratio is related to the height of the maximum of the total potential energy curve of Fig. 2 by [78]

$$W = 2a\int_0^\infty \exp\left(\frac{V_T}{kT}\right)\left\{\frac{dH_0}{(H_0 + 2a)}\right\}^2 \qquad \qquad (14)$$

For $V_T = 0$, $W = 1$, which is the condition for rapid coagulation. The rate constant k for slow coagulation is thus given by

$$k = \frac{k_0}{W} \qquad \qquad (15)$$

Thus, the value of W can be determined experimentally from the rate constants for rapid and slow coagulation.

The rate of coagulation (i.e, the rate of particle disappearance) is measured at different electrolyte concentrations by turbidimetry or light-scattering measurements. The data are usually given as the variation of log W with log electrolyte concentration C_e as shown in Fig. 3. The following information can be obtained from the log W–log C_e plots:

1. The slope of the descending leg is proportional to $(a\gamma^2/z^2)$, which shows the dependence of the stability on particle radius, surface potential, and electrolyte valence. In contrast with the dependence on the square of the particle radius expected from theory, the experimental stability of latexes was either independent of particle radius [79] or decreased with increasing particle radius [80].

2. The intersection of the two lines representing slow and rapid coagulation is taken as the critical coagulation concentration (CCC). By using an approximation of the DLVO theory, the critical coagulation concentration was found to be proportional to (γ^4/A^2z^6), which relates it to the surface potential, Hamaker constant, and electrolyte valence. Thus, the Hamaker constant can be obtained from the experimental determination of the critical coagulation concentration. Also, the dependence of the critical coagulation concentration on counterion valence can be determined experimentally and compared with the theoretical prediction of the inverse sixth-power dependence; according to the

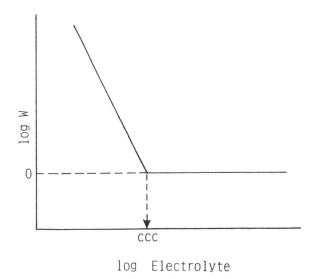

log Electrolyte

Fig. 3 Variation of log stability factor with log electrolyte concentration.

Schultze–Hardy rule, the ratio of critical coagulation concentrations for monovalent, divalent, and trivalent counterions should be in the ratio of 1:0.016:0.0014.

Experimental determinations show that the critical coagulation concentration did indeed follow the sixth-power dependence of the Schultze–Hardy rule for latex particles of high-surface-charge density. For latex particles of low-surface-charge density (e.g., cleaned latex particles), however, the dependence was on the second power of the counterion valence, rather than the sixth-power [80]. This lower-power dependence has a theoretical basis in the DLVO theory [66].

b. Coagulation by Hydrolyzable Cations

Multivalent cations often undergo hydrolysis and oligomerization in aqueous solution to give species of different net charge and adsorptive properties. The extent and nature of the hydrolysis of the cation is strongly pH-dependent. If the hydrolysis increases the charge of an ion, the coagulating power is increased; if the hydrolysis decreases the charge, the coagulating power is decreased. Hydrolyzed species often exhibit strong specific adsorption on latex particles; these species, in sufficient concentration, can even reverse the sign of the charge on the latex particles and redisperse the flocculated particles. Matijevic et al. [81–83] studied this coagulation phenomenon extensively using tri- and tetravalent polynuclear cations (e.g., Al^{3+}, La^{3+}, Sc^{3+}, Th^{4+}, or Hf^{4+}).

c. Mechanical and Surface Coagulation

Some colloidal dispersions (e.g., latexes and iron oxide sols) that are stable indefinitely when left undisturbed coagulate rapidly when subjected to mechanical agitation or sparging with gas bubbles. Heller et al. [84–88] postulated that this coagulation occurred at the water–vapor interface, and they developed a quantitative theory of surface coagulation, assuming that the adsorption of primary particles at the water–vapor interface follows a Langmuir adsorption isotherm and that the coagulation follows second-order kinetics. The latex stability must be below a critical level for surface coagulation to occur. Substances that adsorb preferentially at the water–vapor interface and, thus, reduce the number of particles adsorbed there also render the latex immune to this type of coagulation. Heller et al. proposed several reasons why colloidal particles that were stable in bulk became unstable at the water–vapor interface: (a) the dielectric constant of the liquid at or near the surface is lower than that in the bulk solution; (b) the electric double layer of a particle adsorbed at the surface is asymmetric; (c) the electrolyte is redistributed between the surface and the bulk solution.

2. *Flocculation by Polymers*

Both synthetic and natural water-soluble polymers are used as flocculants for electrostatically stabilized colloidal dispersions. These polymers flocculate stable colloidal dispersions in concentrations as low as 0.1–1.0 lb polymer per ton suspended solids; the large flocs settle rapidly and are easily filtered and washed; moreover, the supernatant phase is clear. Examples of natural polymer flocculants include unmodified and modified gelatin, starches, proteins, and gums. Examples of synthetic polymer flocculants include (a) anionic polymers, such as partially hydrolyzed polyacrylamide and poly(styrene sulfonate); (b) cationic polymers, such as polyamines, poly(dimethylaminoethyl methacrylate), and polyethyleneimine; (c) nonionic polymers, such as polyacrylamide, methylcellulose, poly(vinyl alcohol), and poly(ethylene oxide); (d) amphoteric polymers, such as partially hydrolyzed poly(acrylamide-*co*-dimethylaminoethyl methacrylate) [89].

a. Flocculation with Anchored Polymer Molecules

Several mechanisms have been proposed that require the adsorption of the polymer flocculant on the surface of the colloid particles.

Charge neutralization [91,95]. Polymers of charge opposite in sign to the colloidal particles adsorb on their surface by electrostatic attraction and neutralize their charge. The result is both compression of the electrical double layer by the added polyelectrolyte (ionic strength effect) and the loss of part of the electrical double layer by specific interaction (surface charge density effect). Both effects decrease the electrostatic repulsion and flocculate the colloidal dispersion. Thus, this mechanism of flocculation is relatively insensitive to the molecular weight of the polymer.

Polymer bridging. The polymer bridging mechanism [90,92–94,96,97,102–105], involves the adsorption of a single polymer molecule on more than one colloidal particle to form polymer bridges and destabilize the dispersion (Fig. 4). One argument that supports this mechanism is that negatively charged colloidal particles can be flocculated with anionic polyeletrolytes. The efficiency of flocculation by bridging is enhanced when (a) each polymer molecule has more than two adsorbable segments; (b) the polymer

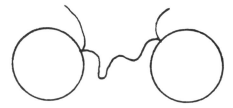

Fig. 4 Flocculation of two colloidal particles by bridging with a single polymer molecule.

molecules are rigid, extended, and long enough to adsorb on more than two particles; (c) the amount of polymer added is considerably less than the maximum amount that can be adsorbed on the colloidal particles, so that there is a greater chance that a single adsorbed polymer molecule extends from one particle to another. Thus, flocculation by bridging occurs most efficiently over a narrow range of low polymer concentrations in which the surface coverage of the particles is less than one-half the saturation value. As a result, this type of flocculation is critically sensitive to the molecular weight of the polymer.

Another mechanism of flocculation by bridging [106] involves the interaction of polymer molecules adsorbed on different particles to cause flocculation (Fig. 5). The efficiency of flocculation by this mechanism is enhanced when (a) the polymer molecules are very long: (b) the affinity of the interacting polymer molecules is great; (c) the surface coverage of the colloidal particles is so high that few adsorption sites are unoccupied.

Interaction between polymer and adsorbed surfactant.   Schlueter [100] studied the agglomeration of potassium oleate-stabilized poly(styrene-*co*-butadiene) rubber latex by poly(ethylene oxide) and postulated that the poly(ethylene oxide) formed a complex with the anionic surfactant that increased the sensitivity of the particles to electrolyte. Saito and Fujiwara [101] postulated that poly(acrylic acid) formed in insoluble complex with nonionic surfactant, which in the presence of electrolyte caused the flocculation of an acrylic copolymer latex.

b.   Flocculation with Free Polymer Molecules

Several mechanisms have been proposed that do not require the adsorption of polymer flocculant on the surface of the colloidal particles.

Polymer network.   The polymer network theory [98,99] comprises the formation of a network of polymer flocculant molecules in solution that entraps the colloidal particles and, thus weighted, subsides, leaving a clear supernatant layer. The polymer molecules, whether randomly coiled or extended and rigid, are bound together by associative bonds at various points along the polymer chains to form a network that extends throughout the solution. These associative bonds may be hydrogen bonds, interchain cross-links by di- and trivalent metal ions, van der Waals bonds, or other types. This network must form quickly after the polymer flocculant solution is mixed with the colloidal dispersion. The colloidal particles, moving about with their characteristic Brownian motion, become enmeshed or entrapped in this newly formed network. The attachment of a colloidal particle to the polymer network increases its aggregate mass considerably;

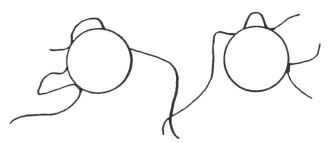

Fig. 5   Flocculation of two colloidal particles by bridging with two or more polymer molecules.

as more and more particles become attached, the mass increases to the point where the network begins to subside, entrapping more particles and sweeping the aqueous phase clear of unattached particles.

   Depletion flocculation.   The addition of a given concentration of polymer to a stable colloidal dispersion often results in the flocculation of the dispersion [85,86]. This type of flocculation does not require the adsorption of the polymer molecules on the surface of the colloidal particles. Instead, the flocculation is the result of the expulsion or depletion of the free polymer molecules from the interparticle region, which leads to an effective attraction between the colloidal particles, causing their flocculation. Feigin and Napper [108] coined the term *depletion flocculation* to describe this phenomenon and developed a theoretical treatment of it [107] based on earlier work by Asakura and Oosawa [109], who demonstrated that the average segment density of polymer molecules near a particle surface is less than in the bulk solution. Others [110,111] showed that sterically stabilized polystyrene latex particles were flocculated by the addition of poly(ethylene oxide) and also developed a theoretical treatment [112] that comprised the construction of a three-component latex particle–solvent–polymer phase diagram and analyzed the stability or instability behavior of the dispersions in terms of the free energy of flocculation, which is equal to zero at the instability boundary line.

   Vrij [113] predicted, on theoretical grounds, that a system comprising a mixture of sterically stabilized particles and polymer molecules would show phase separation. DeHek and Vrij [114] also showed that lyophilic silica particles dispersed in cyclohexane were flocculated by addition of polystyrene; the system separated into a lower silica-rich layer and an upper layer of polystyrene solution in cyclohexane. More recently, Sperry et al. [115] confirmed the depletion flocculation of acrylic copolymer and polystyrene latexes stabilized by hydroxyethyl cellulose.

   Walz and Sharma [116] used a force balance approach to calculate the depletion force between two changed spheres in a solution of charged spherical macromolecules and found that the depletion effect can either enhance the stability of the colloidal dispersion or induce flocculation.

   These principles are applicable to the flocculation of latexes by water-soluble polymers, not only in the treatment of wastewater-containing latex particles, but also in the use of polymers in the preparation, poststabilization, and formulation of latexes. Generally, latexes are flocculated by low concentrations of water-soluble polymers and stabilized by higher concentrations; an example of the classic sensitization–stabilization effects of protective colloids on colloidal sols. In latex preparation, the concentration of water-soluble polymer is relatively high at low conversions, but decreases with increasing conversion, so that flocculation is unlikely. In latex poststabilization, the first increments of added water-soluble polymer are in low concentration relative to the latex polymers; hence, flocculation is possible, even though the intended outcome is stabilization. In latex formulation, the water-soluble polymer may be added as one of the components of the system (e.g., a pigment dispersion prepared using a water-soluble polymer dispersant or a water-soluble polymer added to the coating composition to adjust its viscosity) so that flocculation is possible.

3.   *Diffusion-Controlled Versus Agitation-Induced Cogulation*

Theories have been developed for diffusion-controlled and agitation-induced coagulation. The von Smoluchowski theory of diffusion-controlled coagulation [77] assumed that, in a stable colloidal sol comprising uniform-sized primary particles, each primary particle acts as a center to which other particles diffuse and flocculate, and that all particle–particle collisions result in flocculation and coagulation; however, only a certain proportion of the particle–particle collisions result in flocculation and coagulation because of the potential energy barrier between the particles. The theory for agitation-induced coagulation [117,118] shows that the probability of collision J of a central particle i of N particles per cubic centimeter with another particle j is

$$J = (4/3)N(R_{ij})^3 \left(\frac{du}{dz} \right) \tag{16}$$

where R_{ij} is the collision radius and (du/dz) is the velocity gradient. This equation is difficult to test experimentally because the velocity gradient varies from one part of the sample to another; however, the probability of agitation-induced coagulation can be related to that of diffusion-controlled coagulation [118], which is

$$I = 4\pi D_{ij} R_{ij} N \tag{17}$$

where I is the probability of diffusion-controlled (Brownian) collisions. The ratio of these probabilities is given by

$$\frac{J}{I} = \frac{\eta(R_{ij})^3 (du/dz)}{2kT} \tag{18}$$

where η is the viscosity of the medium and k the Boltzmann constant.

For a colloidal sol of 0.1-μm–particle size and a velocity gradient of 1 s^{-1}, the ratio J/I is about 10^{-3}; that is, initially, the agitation-induced coagulation is negligible compared with the diffusion-controlled coagulation; however, as the coagulation proceeds and the particle aggregates grow in size, J/I increases; for example, at an average diameter of about 1 μm, the contributions of diffusion-controlled and agitation-induced coagulation are about the same, and J/I is about 1; at an average diameter of about 10 μm, the contribution of agitation-induced coagulation is much greater than that of diffusion-controlled coagulation and J/I is much greater than unity.

The foregoing estimated J/I ratios show that, for an agitated industrial coagulation that proceeds from a small primary particle size to large aggregates, the predominant mechanism shifts from diffusion-controlled coagulation to agitation-induced coagulation, and the growth of aggregates by agitation-induced coagulation is autoaccelerating.

The literature contains many examples of attempts to reconcile agitation-induced coagulation with diffusion-controlled coagulation, (e.g., Van de Ven and Mason [119] Zeichner and Showalter [120,121] developed trajectory analyses for two-sphere models in a shear field).

E. Summary

The stability of colloidal sols against flocculation or coagulation usually results from electrostatic or steric stabilization. The electrostatic stabilization is based on the presence of charges on the surface of the colloidal particles. When two particles approach one another, the interaction of their electric double layers results in a positive change in the free energy of interaction which, in turn, results in repulsion between the two particles.

The electrostatic stabilization has been described quantitatively by the DLVO theory. The coagulation of electrostatically stabilized latexes results from the addition of substances that destroy their stabilizing mechanism or increase their kinetic energy by temperature or agitation, which increases the probability of particle–particle interaction at small separation distances.

III. STERIC STABILIZATION OF LATEXES

A. Introduction

Steric stabilization refers to the prevention of flocculation of colloidal particles by the adsorption of nonionic polymer molecules [122]. The term *protection* was used earlier to denote the stabilization by naturally derived molecules [123]. Steric stabilization may be distinguished from protection by the absence of any electrostatic component in steric stabilization. Napper [124] pointed out that the term *steric* as used in this context has a broad thermodynamic connotation, rather than the usual organic chemical meaning.

Steric stabilization may be combined with electrostatic stabilization (e.g., in the case of stabilization by polyelectrolytes and ionogenic comonomeric surfactants). Sterically stabilized colloidal dispersions are more stable to added electrolytes, mechanical shear, and freezing-and-thawing than comparable electrostatically stabilized dispersions. Another advantage of steric stabilization is that it functions well in both aqueous and nonaqueous systems.

Even though steric stabilization has been traced back to the oldest technology known to mankind, that of ancient Egypt [125], only recently has an understanding of the mechanism by which adsorbed polymers stabilize colloidal particles been developed. Steric stabilization is the subject of several excellent review articles [126–132] and a comprehensive monograph [133], with a special section on the preparation of sterically stabilized latexes.

B. Adsorption of Polymers on Latex Particles

The adsorption of polymers on colloidal particles is important in flocculation and stabilization. Naturally occurring polymers have long been used as surfactants. Synthetic polymers have also been used as surfactants; these can be tailor-made for a specific function (e.g., homopolymers or random copolymers for flocculating agents and block or graft copolymers for stabilizers). These tailor-made polymer surfactants include anionic, cationic, nonionic, and amphoteric types, according to the functionality of the stabilizing polymer molecule.

1. *General Features of Polymer Adsorption*

The general features of the solution properties of polymer surfactants and their adsorption on colloidal particles are as follows:

1. The molar critical micelle concentrations of polymer surfactants are much lower than those of conventional low molecular weight surfactants because of the high molecular weight of the polymer molecules.
2. The adsorption of polymer surfactants occurs only if the adsorption energy at the interface is sufficient to compensate for the loss of entropy of the poly-

mer molecules on leaving the bulk solution and adsorbing on the particle surface. Here, the adsorption of polymers is similar to that of conventional low molecular weight surfactants. For the polymer molecules, however, the loss of entropy (increase in free energy) is due to the restriction of the three-dimensional random coil on the two-dimensional particle surface.

3. The extent of adsorption of polymer molecules on any substrate is determined by the polymer–solvent and solvent–surface interactions. A complicating factor is the conformation of the adsorbed polymer molecule on the surface. The number of conformations that a polymer molecule can adopt at an interface increases rapidly with increasing molecular weight and is a strong function of the flexibility of the polymer molecule. These conformations largely determine the configurational entropy and enthalpy of adsorbed polymer molecules, and these, in turn, are needed to calculate the extent of adsorption.

4. The larger the polymer molecule, the greater is the number of possible adsorption contacts per molecule. This results in a large net adsorption energy for polymer molecules, even if the energy of individual contacts is low.

5. The amount of the polymer adsorbed per unit area is far greater than that required for the monolayer adsorption of monomer molecules. Jenckel and Runbach [134] proposed a model to explain this phenomenon, in which each polymer molecule is attached to the surface by a sequence of adsorbed segments (trains), separated by sequences that extend into the solution (loops).

6. Because of their large size, the polymer molecules in solution diffuse to the surface slowly, which accentuates the importance of the porosity of the adsorbent.

7. There is a high probability that, owing to their topological nature, the adsorbed polymer molecules remain in a metastable entangled conformation at the surface, rather than adopting the conformation of lowest energy.

2. *Theoretical Considerations of Polymer Adsorption*

Several theories have been developed to describe the adsorption and conformation of polymer molecules on the colloidal particle surface [135–140]. Most of these theories are based on the following assumptions: (a) the structure of a polymer molecule can be represented by a flexible chain of segments; (b) all or some of these segments can absorb on the particle surface; (c) the particle surface is plain and structureless; (d) an adsorbed polymer molecule consists of alternating trains of segments in contact with the surface and loops of segments extending away from the surface. Some theories treated the adsorption of isolated polymer molecules without consideration of interactions with other adsorbed polymer molecules. Other theories made assumptions about excluded volume effects [141], polymer–solvent interactions [142], and the distribution of surface adsorption sites.

The main objectives of these theories was to predict the dependence of the concentration of polymer adsorbed per unit area, the fraction of polymer segments in trains, and the thickness of the adsorbed layer on polymer concentration, molecular weight, structure, polymer–solvent interaction, temperature, and energy of adsorption. Thus, the problem was to calculate the most probable configuration of the adsorbed polymer molecule and, hence, its chemical potential. Equating this potential to the chemical potential of the polymer molecules in the bulk solution gives the adsorption isotherm.

For an isolated adsorbed polymer molecule, theory predicts that (a) the distributions of train and loop sizes are broad; (b) low adsorption energies favor longer loops and shorter trains; high energies, shorter loops and longer trains; (c) the number of segments in contact with the surface increases with an increase in energy, sharply when the adsorption energy is low and much less rapidly when it is high; (d) the lengths of the loops and trains are independent of the molecular weight; (e) greater flexibility of the polymer molecules favors shorter loops and trains.

For polymer adsorption at low surface coverage (neglecting adsorbed polymer–polymer interactions) (a) the adsorption is proportional to the solution concentration, and the logarithm of the initial gradient of the adsorption isotherm is proportional to the polymer molecular weight; (b) for a given differential free energy of adsorption between the solvent molecules and the polymer segments, there is a critical flexibility for the polymer molecule below which no adsorption occurs; similarly, for a given degree of flexibility, there is a critical differential free energy of adsorption (which is lower with increasing flexibility); (c) just above the critical value of the free energy of adsorption, the fraction of segments adsorbed in trains increases rapidly before leveling off at higher values of the free energy of adsorption; at these higher values of differential free energy, the average loop size is small and the average train length is large; (d) the number of segments adsorbed in trains is proportional to the molecular weight at constant flexibility and differential energy of adsorption.

For polymer adsorption at higher surface coverage (at which adsorbed polymer–polymer interactions are important): (a) the adsorption of polymer rises steeply at low solution concentrations and then levels off, although no horizontal plateau is reached and the gradient remains positive; (b) the adsorption of segments in trains reaches a limiting value and then slowly increases with increasing solution concentration because of the increasing number of segments in loops; (c) the higher the polymer molecular weight, the greater is the concentration of polymer adsorbed in the near-plateau region, owing to the increased volume of the polymer in the loops; (d) at the θ point (the point at which the second virial coefficient of the polymer molecule in the solvent is zero), the size of the loops increases with increasing polymer molecular weight. The mean square distance of the segments from the surface $<z^2>$ is approximately proportional to the polymer molecular weight. The better the solvent relative to a θ solvent, or the more flexible the polymer molecule, the smaller is the limiting value of $<z^2>$ and the concentration of polymer adsorbed. For high molecular weight polymers adsorbed from better than θ solvents, the isotherms resemble Langmuir isotherms. The limiting adsorption arises from the mutual repulsion of polymer loops, giving rise to an osmotic effect.

The segment density distribution of the adsorbed polymer molecules normal to the interface is of special importance in the theory of steric stabilization. Hoeve [140] calculated this distribution for an adsorbed homopolymer of loops and trains, using random-flight statistics, and showed that there was a discontinuity in the distribution at a distance from the interface corresponding to the thickness of the trains, beyond which the segment density fell exponentially with distance. Meier [143] developed an equation for the segment density distribution of a polymer molecule with a single terminally adsorbed tail. Hesselink [144,145] corrected Meier's theory and developed a theory for the segment density distribution of homopolymers and random copolymers adsorbed with single tails and loops.

3. *Experimental Techniques of Polymer Adsorption*

The most important characteristic of polymer adsorption relative to stabilization and flocculation of latexes is the structure of the adsorbed layer. The properties of this layer are defined by (a) the adsorption density; (b) the fraction of segments in trains; (c) the segment density distribution normal to the interface; (d) the thickness of the adsorbed layer; (e) the net interaction energy between the surface and the polymer molecules. The experimental techniques used in the determination of these parameters are described in detail in two books [146,147] and outlined in a review article [132].

The adsorption density is usually determined from the concentrations in bulk solution before and after adsorption. The fraction of segments in trains is determined by shifts in the infrared adsorption spectra of adsorbed polymer molecules in bulk solution, by laser Raman spectroscopy, or by ^1H or ^{13}C nuclear magnetic resonance spectroscopy. The segment density distribution normal to the interface is determined by direct measurement of the interaction force between particles with adsorbed layer as a function of distance of separation. The thickness of the adsorbed polymer layer is usually measured by hydrodynamic techniques (e.g., viscosity, photon correlation spectroscopy, ultracentrifugation, electrophoresis, and ellipsometry) that give the distance of the plane of shear from the interface. The net interaction energy between the surface and the adsorbed polymer molecules is measured by microcalorimetry.

The effects of experimental parameters such as the polymer concentration, molecular weight, solvency, and temperature, on the adsorption isotherms of polymers on latex particles have been described (see Refs. 148–157].

C. Preparation of Sterically Stabilized Latexes

The most effective steric stabilizers comprise two parts: (a) one that is insoluble in the dispersion medium and anchors the stabilizer to the particle surface; (b) another that is soluble in the dispersion medium and imparts stability. The stabilizers that provide the best stability are graft copolymers with insoluble backbones and soluble sidechains, or block copolymers with soluble and insoluble blocks. These polymer molecules can be anchored to the particle surface, either physically or chemically. The physically anchored stabilizer can be displaced from the particle surface by the approach of another particle, which may lead to flocculation. Unlike the physically anchored stabilizer, the chemically anchored stabilizer cannot desorb from the particle surface at the approach of another particle; thus, it can impart better stability to the colloidal dispersion. The physically anchored stabilizer can impart good stability, however, if the particle surface is completely covered to prevent lateral movement of the stabilizer with the approach of another particle.

The monograph by Barrett [133] describes the two general methods of preparation of sterically stabilized latexes: (a) the generation of latex paraticles in the presence of the steric stabilizer, which may be prepared beforehand or in situ; (b) the addition of steric stabilizer to an already prepared latex as a poststabilizer.

D. Types and Origins of Steric Stabilization

Our knowledge of the forces that can lead to short-range repulsion in sterically stabilized dispersions is still uncertain; however, Napper [124,125,158] used the second law of thermodynamics to identify these basic mechanisms of steric stabilization: (a) entropic stabilization; (b) enthalpic stabilization; (c) combined enthalpic–entropic stabilization. According to the second law of thermodynamics, the change in the Gibbs free energy of close approach ΔG_R for two sterically stabilized particles is

$$\Delta G_R = \Delta H_R - T\Delta S_R \tag{19}$$

where ΔH_R is the change in enthalpy, ΔS_R the change in entropy, and T is the temperature. At constant temperature and pressure, the change in the Gibbs free energy must be negative for the close approach of the particles (i.e., flocculation) to be thermodynamically feasible; conversely, it must be positive for the particles to be stable. Table 1 gives the three different mechanisms of steric stabilization and the ways of obtaining a positive ΔG_R for each of them [124].

1. Entropic Stabilization

Entropic stabilization arises when the change in entropy opposes flocculation and the product of the temperature and the entropy change outweighs the change in enthalpy. Since $T\Delta S_R$ usually decreases with decreasing temperature, the enthalpy and entropy terms become equal and flocculation occurs. Thus, entropically stabilized dispersions are characterized by their tendency to flocculate after cooling.

A typical entropically stabilized latex comprises poly(methyl methacrylate) particles dispersed in *n*-heptane and stabilized with a chemically bound poly(methyl methacrylate)–poly(12-hydroxystearic acid) graft copolymer [159]. To prepare the graft copolymer stabilizer, glycidyl methacrylate was condensed with poly(12-hydroxystearic acid) to form a macromonomer, which was then copolymerized with methyl methacrylate to form a "comb" or feather-like polymer comprising a linear poly(methyl methacrylate) with poly(12-hydroxystearic acid) side chains. This graft copolymer readily adsorbs on the poly(methyl methacrylate) latex particles nucleated in its presence. Moreover, heating the system in the presence of a base catalyst covalently bound the comb polymer to the particle surface. Table 2 gives other examples of entropic (and enthalpic) stabilizers [159].

Napper [124] attributed the repulsion between entropically stabilized latex particles on close approach to a decrease in the configurational entropy of the chain on interpenetration or compression coupled with a corresponding decrease in entropy of mixing of the polymer segments with solvent. The solvency of the dispersion medium for the stabilizing chains is an important parameter in sterically stabilized latexes. According to Fischer [161], then later, Ottewill [127,162], the solvent must be a better than θ solvent for the stabilizing chains for the dispersion to be stable. In θ solvents, the polymer molecules behave as if they are noninteracting point molecules; consequently, ΔG_R is zero and the dispersion is unstable.

Table 1 Three Types of Steric Stabilization

ΔH_R	ΔS_R	$(\Delta H_R)/T(\Delta S_R)$	Stability type
Negative	Negative	< 1	Entropic
Negative	Positive	< 1	Enthalpic
Positive	Negative	$\lesssim 1$	Combined enthalpic–entropic

Source: Ref. 124.

Table 2 Classification of Steric Stabilizers

| Stabilizer | Dispersion medium | | Dispersion type | Ref. |
	Type	Example		
Poly(lauryl methacrylate)	Nonaqueous	*n*-Heptane	Entropic	163
Poly(12-hyroxy stearic acid)	Nonaqueous	*n*-Heptane	Entropic	163
Polystyrene	Nonaqueous	Toluene	Entropic	170
Polyisobutylene	Nonaqueous	*n*-Heptane	Entropic	171
Poly(ethylene oxide)	Nonaqueous	Methanol	Entropic	166
Polyisobutylene	Nonaqueous	2-Methylbutene	Enthalpic	169
Poly(ethylene oxide)	Aqueous	0.48 *M* $MgSO_4$	Enthalpic	164,167
Poly(vinyl alcohol)	Aqueous	2 *M* NaCl	Enthalpic	158
Poly(methacrylic acid)	Aqueous	0.02 *M* HCl	Enthalpic	168
Poly(acrylic acid)	Aqueous	0.2 *M* HCl	Entropic	168
Polyacrylamide	Aqueous	2.1 *M* $(NH_4)_2SO_4$	Entropic	168
Poly(vinyl alcohol)	Mixed	Dioxane/water	Combined	158
Poly(ethylene oxide)	Mixed	Methanol/water	Combined	166

Source: Ref. 151.

As stated earlier, entropically stabilized latexes can be flocculated by reducing the $T\Delta S_R$ term (i.e., by cooling the latex). Another method is to increase the ΔH_R term at constant temperature, which can be achieved by adding a nonsolvent to the dispersion medium. The poly(methyl methacrylate) latex particles stabilized with the poly(methyl methacrylate)–poly(12-hydroxystearic acid) graft copolymer stabilizer can be flocculated by addition of nonsolvent ethanol to the *n*-heptane medium.

2. *Enthalpic Stabilization*

Enthalpic stabilization arises when the change in enthalpy opposes flocculation and outweighs the product of the temperature and the change in entropy. When an enthalpically stabilized dispersion is heated, $T\Delta S_R$ usually increases more than ΔH_R, and at the θ temperature, the two terms become equal. Thus, in contrast with entropically stabilized dispersions, enthalpically stabilized dispersions are characterized by their tendency to flocculate on heating.

A typical enthalpically stabilized latex comprises poly(vinyl acetate) particles dispersed in water and stabilized with a physically adsorbed poly(ethylene oxide)–poly(vinyl acetate) or –poly(methyl methacrylate) block copolymer [164]. These block copolymers readily adsorb on the poly(vinyl acetate) latex particles nucleated in their presence, with the poly(vinyl acetate) or poly(methyl methacrylate) blocks serving as anchors and the poly(ethylene oxide) blocks servicing as stabilizing chains. Table 2 gives other examples of enthalpically stabilized latexes.

Napper [124] attributed the repulsion between enthalpically stabilized particles on close approach to the release of hydrogen-bonded water molecules (water of hydration) from the poly(ethylene oxide)-stabilizing chains, with the energy (about 0.5 kT/mol) required to break the hydrogen bonds corresponding to the repulsive energy barrier for stabilization. Thus, the more highly hydrated ions, such as Li^{+1}, Mg^{+2}, and Ca^{+2}, should be more effective flocculants, and the more poorly hydrated ions, such as Rb^{+1} and

Cs^{+1}, poorer flocculants. Experimentally, the reverse was found [143], which suggests that flocculation is not merely the result of dehydration of the poly(ethylene oxide) chains, but more likely, the effect of the electrolyte on the association properties of water and the change in solvency with its addition, to make the dispersion medium a solvent for the stabilizing chains.

3. *Combined Enthalpic-Entropic Stabilization*

Both the change of enthalpy and the change of entropy oppose flocculation if ΔH_R is positive and ΔS_R is negative. In this case, flocculation would not occur, at least at practical temperatures, because the θ temperature would be negative. Examples of latexes stabilized by combined enthalpic–entropic stabilization are rare. Napper and Netschey [158,166] described a few poly(vinyl acetate) latexes stabilized by this mechanism (see Table 2).

E. General Considerations of Steric Stabilization

1. The general term *steric stabilization* encompasses enthalpic, entropic, and combined enthalpic–entropic stabilization.

2. Enthalpic stabilization is more common for aqueous latexes, and entropic stabilization is more common for nonaqueous latexes [172]; however, the preparation of aqueuos entropically stabilized latexes [168] and nonaqueous enthalpically stabilized latexes [169] has been reported [150].

3. A given polymer may stabilize latex particles by different mechanisms in different media (e.g., poly(ethylene oxide) is an enthalpic stabilizer in water and an entropic stabilizer in methanol; see Table 2.

4. Napper, along with Evans and Davison [158,164,167–169], found a strong correlation between the critical flocculation point of sterically stabilized latexes with the θ point of the stabilizer in the dispersion medium. In contrast, Osmond et al. [173] argued that this correlation was fortuitous and an artifact of the method of determining the θ point. In return, Napper [160] argued that the correlation was observed independently of the method used to determine the θ point.

5. This correlation between the critical flocculation point and the θ point is observed only if the surface of the latex particle is fully covered by stabilizer; in dispersion media that are better than θ solvents, flocculation occurs at less than full surface coverage, perhaps because of lateral movement of the stabilizer, desorption of poorly anchored stabilizer, or bridging of the particles by the stabilizer chains.

6. If the stabilizer chain is anchored to the latex particle surface at too many points (multipoint anchoring), the best stability is observed in media that are poorer than θ solvents (rather than θ solvents) for the stabilizing chains; this behavior was observed [174] at low pH for aqueous latex particles with carboxylic acid surface groups stabilized by poly(ethylene oxide); this phenomenon, which is called "enhanced" steric stabilization [78], was explained by Smitham and Napper (175) in terms of two different effects that contribute to the stability in poorer than θ solvents: (a) the "loopy" conformation of the polymer that results in small segment densities in the outer regions of the stabilizing layer and, hence, a decrease in the total steric attraction of the par-

ticles; (b) the changes in the thermodynamic parameters governing the segment–solvent interactions.

7. Sterically stabilized latexes can be flocculated by a change in temperature or pressure, or by the addition of a nonsolvent for the stabilizer molecules.

8. The θ point should be independent of the molecular weight of the stabilizer, because it is a measure of the magnitude of the segment–solvent interaction; Evans and Napper [176] showed that a 1000-fold change in the molecular weight of poly(ethylene oxide) scarcely altered the θ temperature or the critical flocculation temperature of poly(ethylene oxide)-stabilized latexes.

9. Napper [163,167] also showed that the critical flocculation point is essentially independent of the latex particle size, the polymer composition, and the composition of the anchor polymer, which is insoluble in the dispersion medium.

F. Quantitative Theories of Steric Stabilization

The determination of the steric repulsion force as a function of the particle separation distance is not as quantitative as that of the electrostatic repulsion and van der Waals attraction forces. Certainly, the steric repulsion force is of shorter range than the electrostatic and van der Waals forces; moreover, it increases rapidly with decreasing distance of separation [177].

The total energy of interaction V_T between two colloidal particles stabilized by both electrostatic and steric repulsion is

$$V_T = V_R + V_A + V_S \tag{20}$$

where V_R is the electrostatic repulsion energy, V_A the van der Waals attraction energy, and V_S the steric repulsion energy. Both V_R and V_A can be calculated according to the DLVO theory after modification to take into account the presence of the adsorbed polymer layer on the surface of the particles. The main effect of this adsorption was a decrease in the Stern potential and, hence, the electrostatic repulsion [128,179]; its effect on the energy of attraction between colloidal particles has been treated by Vold [180] and Ottewill [128]; the increase in the thickness of the adsorbed layer results in a drastic decrease in the attraction between the particles, and, hence, a considerable increase in stability.

Napper [160] noted that the magnitude of the van der Waals attraction forces between the latex particles stabilized by polymer molecules of molecular weight greater than 10^4 are negligibly small. Consequently, he concluded that the mechanism of flocculation of sterically stabilized latexes can be explained by the attraction between polymer molecules in slightly poorer than θ solvents, rather than the van der Waals attraction forces between the particles, in the mechanism for electrostatically stabilized latexes.

Several theories have been proposed over the past 30 years to account quantitatively for the steric stabilization term V_S in Eq. (20), but no clear picture of the underlying physical principles has yet emerged. A review of the state of the art can be found in several publications [126–132,180]. All attempts to calculate the magnitude of V_S were based on model-dependent statistical thermodynamic theories. Most models involve polymer molecules anchored (irreversibly attached) to the particles and projecting into, and being dissolved by, the dispersion medium. Three different approaches were used to calculate V_S.

1. *The Entropy Theory Approach*

The collision of two particles with adsorbed polymer layers is elastic in the same sense that rubber is elastic. These elastic collisions result in the loss of configurational entropy of the adsorbed polymer molecules, which is used to calculate the free-energy change, assuming that the enthalpy effects are negligible. Mackor [181] and Mackor and van der Waals [182] considered the simplest case of a rigid rod attached to a flat plate and capable of free rotation about the point of attachment. Clayfield and Lumb [183–187] allowed for the flexibility of this attached rod by computer simulation. Osmond et al. [173] asserted that this was the best approach developed thus far, but Napper [160] disagreed on the grounds that the Clayfield and Lumb approach lacked the physical meaning of the loss of entropy and failed to predict the incipient flocculation near the θ point, which was observed experimentally.

2. *The Fischer Solvency Approach*

The solvency approach was first described by Fischer [161] and later applied to steric stabilization calculations by Ottewill [127]. When two particles with adsorbed polymer layers undergo Brownian collision, the chemical potential of the solvent in the interaction zone decreases, thereby establishing a gradient between the solvent in this zone and that in the external dispersion medium. The net result is that solvent in the external dispersion medium diffuses into the interaction zone, thus forcing apart the polymer chains and the particles on which they are adsorbed.

3. *The Combined Entropy–Solvency Approach*

All recent theories agreed that both the entropy and the solvency approaches should be combined to account for the steric stabilization forces. Meier [188] combined the Mackor and Clayfield-Lumb entropy approaches with the Fischer solvency approach; he assumed that repulsion is due to two phenomena: (a) the loss in configurational entropy (the elastic term which Hesselink et al. [189] referred to as the volume restriction effect); (b) the possible change in the free energy of mixing of polymer segments and solvent as the segment density increases in the interaction zone (the mixing term, which Hesselink et al. [189] referred to as the osmotic pressure effect). The elastic term was estimated from the diffusion equation; the mixing term using the Flory-Krigbaum theory (190) for the mixing with solvent molecules of the randomly oriented polymer molecules, for which the centers of gravity are fixed in space. Meier used an incorrect derivation of the segment density distribution function and, thus, underestimated the mixing contribution.

Hesselink et al. [189,191] corrected Meier's error and extended the calculation for both tails and loops of the adsorbed polymer molecules to give the repulsive potential energy ΔG_R:

$$\Delta G_R = \Delta G_{VR} + \Delta G_M \tag{21}$$

where ΔG_{VR} is the free energy change due to volume restriction, and ΔG_M the free energy change due to mixing. The final equation is:

$$\Delta G_R = \underbrace{2\nu k T V_{(i,d)}}_{\Delta G_{VR}} + \underbrace{2(2\pi/9)^{3/2}\nu^2 kT(\alpha - 1) <r^2>^{1/2} M_{(i,d)}}_{\Delta G_M} \tag{22}$$

where α is the intramolecular expansion parameter for the polymer in free solution (equal to the ratio of perturbed to unperturbed end-to-end distances of the free polymer molecule ($\alpha = 1$ for a good solvent and $\alpha < 1$ for a poor solvent); $<r^2>^{1/2}$ is the root-mean-square end-to-end length of the polymer molecule; v the number of molecules per unit surface area; d the distance between two plates; i the number of segments per tail; X the average number of segments per loop; $V_{(i,d)}$ the volume restriction function; $M_{(i,d)}$ the mixing function.

Hesselink et al. [189] tabulated numerical functions of $V_{(i,d)}$ and $M_{(i,d)}$. Their calculations predicted that (a) the stability–instability boundary of sterically stabilized latexes depends on the molecular weight of the stabilizer molecules; (b) stability should be observed in poorer than θ solvents; (c) there should be no correlation between the critical flocculation point and the θ point. These conclusions were challenged by Evans and Napper [176] on the grounds that the theoretical predictions were in disagreement with their experimental results. Napper [165] and Evans and Napper [192] attributed this discrepancy to "an insidious difficulty that intrudes when the entropy and solvency theories are combined" (i.e., the osmotic term calculated by Hesselink et al. incorporated the effect of the volume restriction term).

Osmond et al. [173] argued against this explanation of the discrepancy and asserted that Hesselink et al. and Evans and Napper, actually compared different modes of flocculation behavior: Evans and Napper were concerned with incipient phase separation-type flocculation; Hesselink et al. were concerned with predicting the conditions for weak pseudosecondary minimum flocculation in which the long-range van der Waals forces are still strong enough to cause coagulation. Later, Napper [160] agreed that his previous explanation of the discrepancy between his experimental results and the predictions of Hesselink et al. was incorrect, but not for the reasons presented by Osmond et al. [173]; instead, he attributed the discrepancy to the use of the segment density distribution function that extended to infinity, which in the theory of Hesselink et al. gave a significant elastic contribution at separation distances that, in Napper's opinion, obviated any correlation between the θ point and the critical flocculation point, and would be strongly dependent on molecular weight, as predicted by the calculations of Hesselink et al.

Both Napper [160] and Osmond et al. [173] agreed that the main problem in the calculation of the steric stabilization forces lies in the development of the model and the method of computation of both the mixing and the elastic terms within the interaction zone between the two particles without artificial separation. Both had high hopes that the newly developed theoretical calculations by Dolan and Edwards [193,194] offered significant potential in the calculation of the steric stabilization forces.

Figure 6 shows the potential energy–distance curve for sterically stabilized particles, assuming the potential energy curves are additive [195]. The net interaction at small distances is repulsion, in contrast with the attraction observed for the combination of electrostatic repulsion with London–van der Waals attraction; with increasing distance, this repulsion decreases, sharply at first, and then more slowly, to zero. The electrostatic repulsion barrier can be reduced by addition of electrolyte and, at high electrolyte concentrations, the double layer is compressed to a minimum. If the addition of electrolyte has no effect on the steric stabilization layer, the potential energy–distance curve would be the same as for sterically stabilized neutral particles, as shown in Fig. 7 [195]. The net interaction at small distances is repulsion, which decreases sharply to a shallow minimum of attraction.

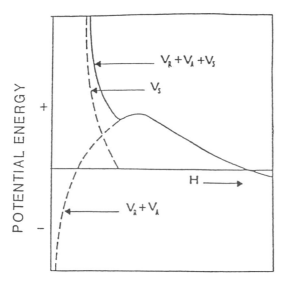

Fig. 6 Potential energy–distance of separation curve for combined steric and electrostatic stabilization. (From Ref. 195.)

G. Flocculation of Sterically Stabilized Latexes

The flocculation of sterically stabilized latexes differs from that of electrostatically stabilized latexes in many respects: (a) Electrostatically stabilized latexes are sensitive to electrolytes; sterically stabilized latexes are not. (b) For electrostatically stabilized latexes, the effectiveness of the counterions in flocculation increases with increasing valence, according to the Schulze–Hardy rule; for sterically stabilized latexes, counterions

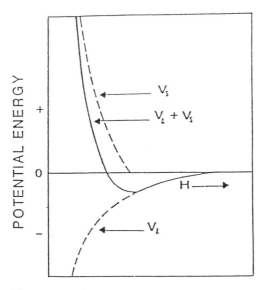

Fig. 7 Potential energy–distance of separation curve for steric stabilization of neutral particles. (From Ref. 195.)

of higher valence are usually less effective in flocculation. (c) Sterically stabilized latexes often flocculate on cooling or heating; electrostatically stabilized latexes are generally much less sensitive to temperature, although they may coagulate on heating.

According to Napper's classification of sterically stabilized latexes, flocculation may be induced by (a) changing the temperature at constant pressure; (b) changing the pressure at constant temperature; (c) changing both the temperature and pressure; (d) adding nonsolvent (including salt) at constant temperature and pressure.

For well-anchored stabilizers that fully cover the particle and do not exhibit multipoint anchoring, Napper found a strong correlation between the critical flocculation point and the θ point for the stabilizing chains in free solution.

Latex particles stabilized with high molecular weight polymers cannot approach each other closely enough for the van der Waals dispersion attraction to be significantly greater than the thermal energy; therefore, these dispersion forces have a negligible effect in inducing flocculation; instead, the flocculation is due to the attraction between the polymer molecules in the poorer than θ-solvent.

Sterically stabilized latexes may be flocculated by addition of a low concentration (10–20 ppm) of a second polymer; homopolymers or simple random copolymers are best suited as flocculants; water-soluble polymers used as flocculants include natural polymers, such as starch and gums, and synthetic polymers, such as polyacrylamide.

There are two main mechanisms for the flocculation of colloidal sols by polymers: (a) charge neutralization; that is, the loss of all or part of the electrical double layer by specific interaction of the surface charge with a polyelectrolyte or other ions (surface charge density effect) and the compression of the double layer by added electrolyte (ionic strength effect); (b) polymer bridging; that is, the adsorption of one or more segments of a polymer molecule on two or more particles, which is favored by linear high molecular weight polymers; bridging occurs at low surface coverages because there is free surface available for the adsorption of loops of polymer molecules adsorbed on other particles.

Feigin and Napper [196] found experimentally that mixing sterically stabilized latexes resulted either in heterosteric stabilization or heteroflocculation. Heterosteric stabilization was observed on mixing latexes stabilized by incompatible polymers; heteroflocculation, on mixing latexes stabilized by compatible polymers, especially those that coprecipitate or coacervate. The importance of this finding lies in the possibility of selective flocculation of mixed latexes.

Croucher and Hair [197] found that polyacrylonitrile latex particles stabilized by poly(α-methyl styrene) in *n*-butyl chloride flocculated on both heating and cooling; the upper and lower critical flocculation temperatures correlated with the θ temperatures associated with the lower and upper critical solution temperatures (LCST and UCST) of poly(α-methyl styrene) in *n*-butyl chloride, respectively. They also suggested [198] that this correlation indicated that the phenomenon that causes phase separation in polymer solutions also causes flocculation in nonaqueous sterically stabilized dispersions. Croucher and Hair [198] analyzed the incipient flocculation behavior of sterically stabilized latexes in terms of the free volume theories of polymer solutions and were able to predict both the temperature and pressure dependence of the incipient flocculation.

Chen [199] prepared cross-linked polystyrene miniemulsion latexes using azobis-(2-methylbutyronitrile) initiator to avoid the surface sulfate end-groups resulting from the use of persulfate-ion initiator; these latexes were used as seed latexes for the incorporation of polyether structures by covalent bonding. The best stability to added electrolyte was obtained with a tail-structured latex (critical flocculation concentration 80 mM NaCl at room temperature; ca. 2000 mM at 60°C); a train-loop-train, structured latex with 22 ethylene oxide units in the loop was slightly less stable (critical flocculation concentration 60 mM at room temperature; 3 mM at 60°C).

Sung and Piirma [200] used sulfate-capped alkyl polyoxyethylene emulsifiers with an alkyl chain length of 12 or 15 and a polyoxyethylene chain length of 3, 7, 9, or 15 to prepare polystyrene latexes and found that the stabilization mechanism switched from primarily electrostatic to steric between 9 and 15 ethylene oxide units.

Einarson and Berg [201,202] found that the stability of polystyrene latexes stabilized by low molecular weight ethylene oxide–propylene oxide block copolymers was both electrostatic and steric. Ethylene oxide–propylene oxide triblock copolymers of the shortest chain length gave only marginal stability, requiring only sufficient electrolyte to collapse the electric double layer; long chain lengths gave robustly stable latexes, requiring the reduction in polymer solvency that occurs at high electrolyte concentrations.

Li and Caldwell [203] determined the surface density and layer thickness of poly(ethylene oxide) and ethylene oxide–propylene oxide triblock copolymers on different-sized polystyrene particles by sedimentation field-flow fractionation, field-flow fractionation, and photon correlation spectroscopy.

Adachi et al. [204] studied the flocculation of polystyrene latex with poly(ethylene oxide) and developed a reproducible method of mixing by end-over-end rotation. The initial flocculation was several times faster than the rapid coagulation because of the electrolyte; this enhancement, which was dependent on the time of incubation, was ascribed to an increase in the collision radius of the particles. The estimated thickness of adsorbed polymer at the initial stage correlated with the size of the free polymer coil in bulk solution, rather than the equilibrium thickness of the adsorbed layer. The formation of poly(ethylene oxide) clusters influenced the rate of flocculation. The abrupt cessation of flocculation was ascribed to steric stabilization, which was limited by transport of polymer toward the particle surface.

Tamai et al. [205] studied the flocculation of polystyrene and poly(styrene-*co*-acrylamide) latexes stabilized with adsorbed human serum albumin as a function of electrolyte concentration and pH. No flocculation of the human serum albumin-coated latexes was observed with NaCl; with $MgCl_2$ and $CaCl_2$, the latexes flocculated at concentrations greater than 3 mM; bridging by divalent cations was suggested as the mechanism. The better stability of the human serum albumin-coated poly(styrene-*co*-acrylamide) latexes to the three cations was ascribed to steric stabilization; these latexes flocculated at pHs below the isoelectric point.

Nonaqueous systems were also studied. Dawkins and Shakir [206] studied nonaqueous dispersions of poly(vinyl acetate) in *n*-alkanes stabilized with diblock poly(styrene-*b*-ethylene oxide–propylene oxide); the stability in a *n*-heptane–propanol mixture was determined as a function of temperature by viscosity measurements; the thickness of the adsorbed layer at 25, 35, and 45°C was greater than the dimensions of the free copolymer chains in solution. Shin et al. [207] studied the stability of magnetite dispersions in kerosene containing Tween and Span emulsifiers; the Tween acted as a primary stabilizer to provide the anchor group and the Span, as a secondary stabilizer that adsorbed on the surface of the magnetite particles.

Systems other than latexes were also studied. Rogan et al. [208,209] studied the stability of calcite dispersions, with 0–28 mg poly(acrylic acid) per gram of calcite, by viscosity, electrophoretic mobility, and ionic concentration. The stability at low levels (< 2 mg/g) was explained by the DLVO theory and ascribed to electric double-layer repulsion; at higher levels (2–6 mg/g), the stability was ascribed to electrosteric repulsion and, at still higher levels (> 6 mg/g), to steric stabilization. Biggs and Healy [210] studied the adsorption of poly(acrylic acid) on zirconia particles, by atomic force microscopy, as a function of pH; the size of the adsorbed polyelectrolyte increased with increasing pH; the segment–surface affinity decreased and segment–segment repulsion increased; the data at low pH was used to estimate the size of the uncharged collapsed polymer coil at the interface. Giersig and Mulvaney [211] found that the equilibrium distance between gold particles in a two-dimensional lattice was the same as the dimensions of adsorbed steric stabilizers, which suggested steric, rather than electrostatic repulsion.

Gallego et al. [212] studied, theoretically, a one-component sterically stabilized colloidal dispersion using the Scheutjen-Fleer lattice model for interaction of two surfaces with grafted polymer chains; the results supported the temperature dependence of the short-range steric repulsion and, thereby, the polymer layer thickness. Zhulina and Borisov [213] studied, theoretically, the steric stabilization of dispersions by uncharged polymer chains grafted to the colloidal particles with neighboring coils overlapped, to form a single stabilizing layer. Rodrigues and Mattice [214] used a cubic lattice to study the steric stabilization by diblock polymers and found that the steric stabilization was enhanced by an increase in molecular weight of the soluble block and an increase in the quality of the solvent for the soluble block.

H. Summary

Latexes are stabilized against coagulation or flocculation by electrostatic or steric stabilization. Electrostatic stabilization arises from the presence of charges on the latex particle surface; steric stabilization, from the presence of physically adsorbed or chemically bound nonionic polymer molecules.

The basic mechanism of steric stabilization is not well understood, and a complete quantitative theory has not yet been developed; however, when two particles approach each other, the interaction of the adsorbed polymer layers leads to a positive change in the free energy of the two interacting particles and, thus, the repulsion between them. Sterically stabilized latexes may be flocculated by changing the temperature or pressure, adding nonsolvent, or adding a low concentration of a second polymer.

IV. PREPARATION OF LATEXES BY DIRECT EMULSIFICATION

A. Introduction

To comply with governmental restrictions on the emission of solvents to the atmosphere, the coatings industry has developed replacements for organic solvent-based coatings to decrease or eliminate solvent emissions, including water-based coatings, high-solids coatings, powder coatings, electrodeposition coatings, and radiation-cured coatings. Presently, water-based coatings are among the most promising candidate systems for functionality, effectiveness, convenience, and economics.

Water-based polymers used in the formulation of coatings can be divided into three categories, according to the state of subdivision of the polymer: (a) latexes (i.e., colloidal dispersions of polymer particles characterized by low viscosities, which are independent of the molecular weight of the polymer); (b) polymer solutions (i.e., molecular dispersions of polymer molecules characterized by high viscosities, which increase strongly with increasing polymer molecular weight and concentration; (c) water-solubilized polymers (i.e., dispersions intermediate in size between the colloidal particles of the latexes and the polymer molecules of the solutions, and characterized by intermediate properties).

Latexes that are used in water-based coatings can be divided into three categories [215], according to their origin and method of preparation: (a) natural latexes, which are the metabolic products of various plants and trees; (b) synthetic latexes, which are prepared by emulsion polymerization of their corresponding monomers; (c) artificial latexes, which are prepared by dispersion of the bulk polymer in an aqueous medium.

Until recently, the artificial latexes were the least important of the three categories and were typified by aqueous dispersions of reclaimed rubber, butyl rubber, and stereoregular rubbers, such as *cis*-1,4-polyisoprene. Since emulsion polymerization is limited to water-immiscible monomers that can be polymerized by free-radical, vinyl-addition polymerization, latexes of polymers that cannot be prepared by this method can be prepared only by dispersion of bulk polymer in an aqueous medium (e.g., by emulsification of the fluid polymer in water). This section describes the preparation of artificial latexes (or pseudolatexes) of interest to the pharmaceutical industry by direct emulsification in water.

B. Preparation of Oil-in-Water Emulsions

1. *Principles of Emulsification*

The emulsification of an oil in water is the result of two competing processes: the dispersion of the bulk oil phase into droplets and the coalescence of the droplets to form the bulk phase. Coalescence is favored over dispersion from the point of view of the free energy. Thus, the coalescence of droplets must be prevented or delayed if the dispersion of droplets is to be stable. The efficiency of this complex dynamic emulsification is determined by the relative efficiencies of formation and stabilization of droplets, which are determined by (a) the intensity and duration of agitation; (b) the type and concentration of surfactants; (c) the mode of addition of the surfactant, and the oil and water phases; (d) the density ratio of the two phases; (e) the temperature. Much work has been done to correlate these parameters with the stability and droplet size of the emulsions [216–221].

The droplet size decreases with increasing intensity of agitation. Many different types of emulsification equipment are available [e.g., mixers, colloid mills, or homogenizers]. Also used are ultrasonifiers, which convert electrical energy to high-frequency mechanical energy, and electric dispersers, in which the oil streaming through a capillary is subjected to a high positive potential, breaking the stream into droplets that are collected in an immiscible medium [204]. One interesting feature of electric dispersion is the uniformity of the emulsion droplet size [222,223].

With increasing surfactant concentration, the emulsion droplet size decreases owing to the decrease in the oil–water interfacial tension, to a low plateau value. There are several guidelines to the choice of the surfactant [215]: (a) It must have a specific molecular structure, with polar and nonpolar ends; (b) it must be more soluble in the water phase so that it is readily available for adsorption on the oil droplet surface; (c) it must adsorb quickly on the droplet surface with the polar end of the molecule oriented toward the water phase and the nonpolar end toward the oil phase; (d) it must adsorb strongly and not be easily displaced when two droplets collide; (e) it must reduce the interfacial tension to 5 dynes/cm or less; (f) it must impart a sufficient electrokinetic potential to the emulsion droplets; (g) it must work in small concentrations; (h) it should be relatively inexpensive, nontoxic, and safe to handle. A wide variety of commercial surfactants fulfill these requirements.

Selection of a surfactant from the many available is not an easy task, however. Selection by trial and error is costly and impractical. One empirical selection system proposed by Griffin [25–27,224] (and mentioned earlier) is the HLB system. The HLB is the hydrophile–lipophile balance of the surfactant. Most of the common anionic and nonionic surfactants have HLB values in the range of 1–20; an HLB value of 1 indicates oil solubility; an HLB value of 20, indicates water solubility. Thus, the HLB system is essentially a means of selecting surfactants with the proper solubility.

The temperature has only an indirect effect on emulsification that is attributed to its effect on viscosity, surfactant absorption, and interfacial tension. An increase in the density difference between the oil and water phases results in a decrease in droplet size owing to the different velocities imparted to the two phases during emulsification.

2. *Emulsion Droplet Size*

The emulsification of an oil in water by mechanical shear usually gives average droplet sizes in the range of 2–5 μm, and, at best, as small as 1 μm. The emulsions have broad distributions of droplet sizes, so that an emulsion with an average droplet size of 1 μm contains some droplets as small as 0.5 μm and some as large as 5 μm. In contrast, most coatings latexes have average particle sizes in the range 100–300 nm, about five- to tenfold smaller than droplets prepared by emulsification.

This five- to tenfold difference in particle size between latexes prepared by emulsion polymerization (100–300 nm) and the smallest droplet sizes that can be prepared by emulsification (1000 nm) is critical because it encompasses the critical particle size for settling or creaming of most polymer latexes; for example, a monodisperse polystyrene (density 1.050 g/ml) latex of 800-nm diameter sedimented after standing within 1–3 months, whereas similar latexes of 200- to 500-nm diameter never settled [225]. Thus, the first requirement for an artificial or pseudolatex to be used for coatings is that it must be shelf-stable (i.e., the particles must not sediment or cream within a given time).

The critical size for settling may be calculated from the criterion of Overbeek [226], which states that colloidal particles that settle at a rate of only 1 mm in 24 h, according to Stokes' law, will never settle in practice, because the Brownian motion of the particles and the chance thermal convection currents arising from small temperature gradients in the sample offset the settling. The Brownian motion, which results from the unbalanced collisions of solvent molecules with the colloidal particles, increases in intensity with decreasing particle size. The convection currents depend on the sample size and the storage conditions.

The rate of settling or creaming of spherical particles according to Stokes' law is

$$\text{Rate of settling or creaming} = \left(\frac{D^2}{18\eta}\right)(d_p - d_m)g \tag{23}$$

where D is the particle diameter, η the viscosity of the medium, d_p and d_m the densities of the particles and the medium, respectively, and g the gravitational constant.

Substituting the foregoing sedimentation rate of 1 mm in 24 h [226] into Eq. (23) gives values of the critical particle size for settling. Figure 8 shows the variation of log-critical particle size with log-density difference between the particles and the medium as a function of viscosity of the medium calculated from this equation.

For polystyrene latex particles in water, the density difference is 0.05 g/ml, and the viscosity of the medium is about 1 cps; therefore, from Fig. 8, the critical particle diameter for settling is 650 nm. This calculated size is in good agreement with the foregoing experimental observations [225] that monodisperse polystyrene latex particles of 800 nm diameter settled within 1–3 months and that particles of 500 nm diameter or smaller never settled.

Since most of the polymers to be emulsified to form artificial or pseudolatexes have densities in the range 1.10–1.15 g/ml, their critical particle diameters for settling would be 300 nm or smaller. Therefore, it is critical whether the emulsification process produces droplets of 1000 nm or 200 nm diameter.

The artificial or pseudolatexes used for coatings must form continuous films after drying under given conditions. The forces exerted on the latex particles during drying are those arising from the water–air and polymer–water interfacial tensions [227,228]. The maximum shear modulus of a polymer particle that can coalesce with drying from an aqueous latex is calculated to be about 1600 psi for a particle diameter of 100 nm

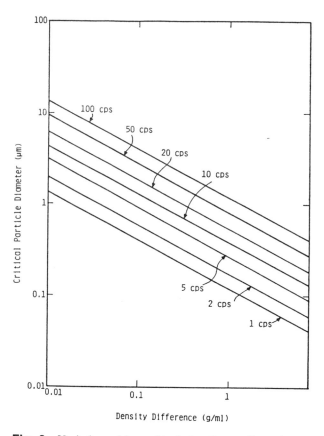

Fig. 8 Variation of log critical size for settling with log density difference as a function of medium viscosity.

at 30-dynes/cm surface tension [229]. This maximum shear modulus decreases inversely with increasing particle size (i.e., the maximum shear moduli for coalescence for particle diameters of 1,000 nm and 10,000 nm are 160 and 16 psi, respectively). Thus, the larger the latex particle size, the softer must be the polymer for the particles to coalesce after drying. If the shear modulus of the polymer is too high for the latex particle size, the coalescence will be incomplete, and the film properties will be poor.

C. Latexes Prepared by Conventional Emulsification

1. *Conventional Methods of Preparing Artificial Latexes*

Polymers, such as polyurethanes, epoxy resins, polyesters, polypropylene, ethylcellulose, and stereoregular rubbers, cannot be prepared by free radical-initiated, vinyl-addition emulsion polymerization. An alternative method for the preparation of latexes of these polymers is the emulsification of polymer (or a solution of the polymer) in water by using conventional surfactants and emulsification methods. The emulsification methods for the preparation of latexes from polymer solutions have been reviewed by Warson [230] and Blackley [215], who described three different methods for the preparation of artificial latexes by emulsification.

1. *Direct emulsification* [231–234]. The liquid polymer or polymer solution in a volatile water-immiscible organic solvent (or mixture of solvents) is emulsified in water that contains surfactant by using conventional emulsification methods, and the emulsion is steam-distilled to remove the solvent (if used).
2. *Inverse emulsification* [235–238]. The liquid polymer or polymer solution in a volatile water-immiscible organic solvent (or mixture of solvents) is compounded with a long-chain fatty acid (e.g., oleic acid) using conventional rubber-mixing equipment and mixed slowly with a dilute aqueous base, to give a water-in-polymer emulsion, which then inverts to a polymer-in-water emulsion as more aqueous base is added; the emulsion is then steam-distilled to remove the solvent (if used).
3. *Self-emulsification* [239–241]. The polymer molecules are modified chemically by the introduction of basic (e.g., amino) or acidic (e.g., carboxyl) groups in such concentration and location that the polymer undergoes self-emulsification without surfactant after dispersion in acidic or basic solution.

With all three methods, the emulsification may be carried out at elevated temperatures to lower the viscosity of the polymer or polymer solution.

The latexes prepared by direct or inverse emulsification have average particle sizes in the range 1–10 µm, with a small-particle–sized tail extending to about 0.5 µm. These sizes are about five- to tenfold larger than the 100- to 300-nm–average particle size of commercial coating latexes prepared by emulsion polymerization. This five- to tenfold difference in particle size is responsible for the inferior film properties and poor shelf stability of these latexes made by direct or inverse emulsification, when compared with those prepared by emulsion polymerization. Consequently, a substantial decrease in the average particle size of latexes prepared by direct or inverse emulsification would be an important contribution to the development of water-based coatings.

The average particle size of polymer emulsions prepared by direct or inverse emulsification of polymer solutions would be reduced by removal of the solvent. However, this solvent removal is usually insufficient to make the average particle size smaller than the critical size for settling; for example, a polymer emulsion of 10:90 polymer/solvent ratio and average particle size 1 μm would have an average diameter of 460 nm after removal of the solvent (provided no agglomeration of the particles occurred). Further dilution of the polymer solution would be impractical; even the 10:90 polymer/solvent ratio places a heavy burden on the economics of the process.

Self-emulsification gives average particle sizes as small as 100 nm, much smaller than the other two methods and fully competitive with those produced by emulsion polymerization; however, the hydrophilic functional groups of the polymer make the coating films water-sensitive. Moreover, the concentration and location of the functional groups is critical: with too low a concentration or improper location of the functional groups, the polymer is not self-emulsifiable; with too high a concentration, the polymer forms a polymer solution on emulsification–neutralization. Thus, although self-emulsification gives average particle sizes that are competitive with those produced by emulsion polymerization, its applications are limited by the water sensitivity of the films.

B. Emulsification Using Mixed Emulsifer Systems

1. *Emulsion of Monomers Using Mixed Emulsifier Systems*

Generally, it is not possible to prepare oil-in-water emulsions with average droplet sizes smaller than about 1 μm using practical concentrations of anionic surfactants, such as sodium lauryl sulfate. However, it was recently shown [242–248] that fluid, opaque, thermodynamically unstable styrene-in-water emulsions of 100- to 200-nm–average droplet size were prepared by simple stirring, by using 0.5–2% of the sodium lauryl sulfate–cetyl alcohol mixed emulsifier system. Similar cationic styrene emulsions were prepared with the hexadecyltrimethylammonium bromide–cetyl alcohol mixed emulsifier system, and similar anionic and cationic styrene emulsions were prepared using sodium lauryl sulfate- or hexadecyltrimethylammonium bromide–*n*-decane mixed emulsifier systems [248]. These emulsions were called *miniemulsions* to distinguish them from *microemulsions*, which are viscous, translucent, thermodynamically stable emulsions of 8- to 80-nm–average droplet size prepared using 15–25% anionic emulsifier–alcohol mixtures [249–251], and the conventional emulsions or *macroemulsions*, which are fluid, opaque thermodynamically unstable emulsions of 1- to 10-μm–average droplet size, prepared with 0.5–2% of surfactants such as sodium lauryl sulfate.

Thus, miniemulsions differ from both microemulsions and macroemulsions. Outwardly, the miniemulsions resemble macroemulsions; they are fluid and opaque, and are prepared by using low concentrations of emulsifier; however, their average droplet sizes are only slightly larger than those of microemulsions (and are well below the critical size for settling or creaming) and their shelf-lives are correspondingly longer. Microemulsions, which consist of oil solubilized in micellar emulsifier solutions, are stable in the thermodynamic sense; miniemulsions and macroemulsions are not. The mixed emulsifier systems are also different: those of the microemulsions use anionic or cationic emulsifiers in mixture with alcohols, such as pentanol, hexanol, or heptanol; those of the miniemulsions use anionic or cationic emulsifiers in mixture with higher alcohols, such as lauryl alcohol or cetyl alcohol. Moreover, the order of addition of the ingredients is different: the preparation of miniemulsions requires a specific order of addition of the ingredients; the order of addition is immaterial in the preparation of microemulsions. Thus, these miniemulsions represent a new and important technology that can be used in the preparation of pharmaceutical emulsions.

Several mechanisms have been proposed for the emulsification and stabilization of oil-in-water microemulsions with mixed emulsifier systems [249–255]. For the microemulsions, the most common method of preparation is to dissolve the alcohol in the oil phase and then emulsify this solution in the aqueous emulsifier solution. For the miniemulsion, however, the required method of preparation is to disperse the cetyl alcohol in the aqueous sodium lauryl sulfate solution and stir for 30–90 min at 60°C to form the emulsifier–fatty alcohol complex, then emulsify the styrene in this solution by stirring for 30 min, to give a stable emulsion of 100- to 200-nm–average droplet size [242]. Addition of the cetyl alcohol as a solution in styrene gives the same 1-μm or greater average droplet size obtained with sodium lauryl sulfate alone.

2. *Preparation of Latexes by Miniemulsification*

Mixed emulsifier systems, comprising a conventional surfactant and a cosurfactant, were used in the preparation of a wide variety of polymer latexes [256–260]. The polymer was dissolved in a solvent (or mixture of solvents) to lower its viscosity to a level suitable for emulsification. Two general emulsification procedures were used, according to whether the cosurfactant was added to the aqueous phase or to the oil phase.

1. *Addition of cosurfactant to the aqueous phase*: Table 3 gives a typical recipe used in this process. The emulsifier solution was prepared by stirring the hexadecyltrimethylammonium bromide–cetyl alcohol mixture in the water for 30–90 min at 60°C; the Epon 1001 solution in toluene and methyl isobutyl ketone mixture was then added, and the mixture was stirred for another 30 min, to give a crude emulsion of 1- to 50-μm–droplet size; this crude emulsion was then homogenized in the Manton–Gaulin Submicron Dipserser or ultrasonified to an average droplet size of 100–200 nm; the solvent was then removed by vacuum steam distillation.
2. *Addition of cosurfactant to the oil phase*: Table 4 gives a typical recipe used in this process. The *n*-decane was dissolved in the poly(vinyl butyral) solution in a toluene/*n*-butanol/ethanol mixture at room temperature, and the sodium lauryl sulfate was dissolved in the water at 60°C. The crude emulsion was then prepared by stirring the poly(vinyl butyral) solution containing the *n*-decane into the water phase containing the sodium lauryl sulfate for 30 min, to give a crude emulsion, which was then homogenized and distilled under vacuum to remove the solvent.

The particle size distributions of the latexes prepared according to the recipes of Tables 3 and 4 are shown in Figs. 9 and 10, respectively. Table 5 gives the particle

Table 3 Recipe for Emulsification of Epon 1001

Ingredient	Parts
Epon Resin 1001[a]	31.25
50:50 toluene/methyl isobutyl ketone mixture	93.75
Hexadecyltrimethylammonium bromide	0.78
Cetyl alcohol	1.73
Water	300.0

[a]Epichlorhydrin/bisphenol A epoxy prepolymer; MW 900; Shell Chemical Co.
Source: Ref. 256.

Table 4 Recipe for Emulsification of Poly(vinyl butyral)

Ingredient	Parts
Butvar B-79[a]	10.0
75:20:5 toluene/*n*-butanol/ethanol mixture	90.0
Sodium lauryl sulfate	0.60
n-Decane	1.00
Water	300.0

[a]Poly(vinyl butryal); MW $3.8–4.5 \times 10^4$; Monsanto Co.
Source: Ref. 256.

sizes of other latexes prepared by direct emulsification by the mixed emulsifier systems. It is clear that these mixed emulsifier systems gave average particle sizes of 100–200 nm, similar to those of latexes prepared by emulsion polymerization. This mini-emulsification procedure can be applied to any fluid polymer or polymer solution in a water-immiscible solvent of viscosity 10^4 cps or less and free from gels [256]. Examples of such polymers include polystyrene, poly(vinyl acetate), epoxy resins, epoxy resin-curing agents, ethylcellulose, cellulose acetate phthalate, polyesters, alkyd resins, rosin derivatives, synthetic natural rubbers, poly(vinyl butyral), and silicones. Fully cured and air-drying polyurethane latexes can also be prepared by miniemulsification [257,258, 260,261].

The factors that determine the particle size of latexes produced by miniemulsification are (a) the ratio of fatty alcohol to surfactant in the mixed emulsifier; (b) the total concentration of mixed emulsifier; (c) the chain length of the fatty alcohol; (d) the viscosity of the polymer solution; (e) the type of solvent or mixture of solvents.

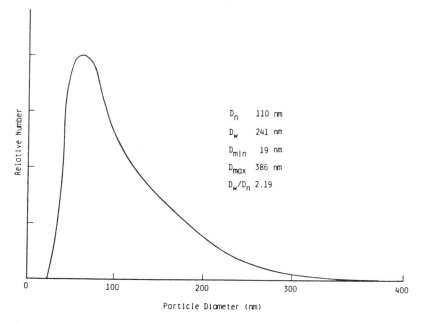

Fig. 9 Particle size distribution of Epon 1001 pseudolatex prepared according to Table 3. (From Ref. 256.)

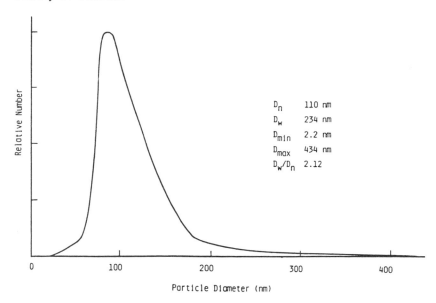

Fig. 10 Particle size distribution of poly(vinyl butyral) pseudolatex prepared according to Table 4. (From Ref. 256.)

The same polymer can be used to produce both anionic and cationic latexes, provided that the polymer molecules do not contain charged groups. For polymer molecules containing charged cationic or anionic groups, only one type of latex with the same net charge can be prepared by emulsification.

The variation of pseudolatex particle size with emulsification method has been determined [262]. Table 6 gives the composition of an Ebecryl 810 miniemulsion, and Table 7 gives the particle size as a function of ultrasonification time (Bronson Sonic Power Co. Model W-350; power level 7; 50% duty cycle; assisted by magnetic stirring bar). The particle sizes were measured by photon correlation spectroscopy (Nicomp Particle Size Analyzer).

Table 5 Latexes Prepared by Direct Emulsification (Sodium Lauryl Sulfate Emulsifier)

Polymer	Cosurfactant	D_n	D_w	D_w/D_n	D_{min}	D_{max}
Epon 1001	n-Decane	122	273	2.24	46	487
Ethylcellulose	Cetyl alcohol	180	696	3.88	6	912
Ethylcellulose	n-Decane	135	445	3.29	5	709
Polystyrene (MW 3.5×10^4)	Cetyl alcohol	115	223	1.94	5	326
Polystyrene (MW 3.5×10^4)	n-Decane	83	421	5.09	3	653
Polystyrene (MW 2.0×10^4)	Cetyl alcohol	165	460	2.78	31	718
Poly(vinyl butyral)	n-Decane	110	241	2.19	19	386

Source: Ref. 256.

Table 6 Recipe for Emulsification of
Ebecryl 810

Ingredient	Parts
Ebecryl 810[a]	24.0
Water	36.0
Sodium lauryl sulfate	20 mmol[b]
Hexadecane	60 mmol[b]
Water	75.0

[a]Ebercryl 810 polyester prepolymer with acrylate functionality plus monomer; visc. 550 cps 25°C; Radcure.
[b]Based on water.

This sample was also emulsified using the Sorvall Omni-Mixer, which operates at speeds up to 16,000 rpm. Table 8 shows that the particle size decreased to a minimum with shearing time at 16,000 rpm and then increased. The emulsion sample was immersed in an ice-water bath to control the temperature increase, which tended to destabilize the emulsion.

This sample was also emulsified using the Microfluidics Model MP 110-A (Microfluidics Corp.). The 425-ml samples were ultrasonified for 2 min, then charged to the inlet valve at 80 psi and pumped to the high-pressure interaction chamber at 6000–8000 psi; here, the emulsion was split into two streams, which impinged on the orifice "plate" to break up the dispersed phase by shear and collision forces; the two streams were then brought together and forced through a small orifice at high velocity (30,000 cm/s). This produced a combination of shear, cavitation, and collision forces, resulting in the breakup of the droplets to a submicroscopic size. The reaction chamber was wrapped in an ice bag to remove the heat generated by the shearing and high-speed fluid movement. The viscosity of the sample increased with each pass, indicating that the particle size had decreased; the final particle size was about 60 nm.

For larger samples, the Manton–Gaulin Submicron Disperser (Model 15M; Gaulin Corp.), which uses a mechanism similar to the Microfluidics instrument, can be run continuously at a rate of about 1 L/min. Table 9 gives the recipe for the emulsification of a polyketone resin, and Table 10 gives the particle sizes attained using the Manton–Gaulin Submicron Disperser. The heat generated by this homogenization made chilling with ice water necessary. Each batch of emulsion was ultrasonified in 600-ml aliquots for 2 min and then passed through the Manton–Gaulin Submicron Disperser at 1800 psi for the first pass and 7500 psi for the second pass.

Table 7 Pseudolatex Particle Size and Ultrasonification Time

Ultrasonification time (min)	Particle size (nm)
1	260
2	241
3	241
4	214

Table 8 Particle Size and Shearing Time in the Omni-Mixer

Shearing time (min)	Particle Size (nm)
5.0	420
10.0	390
20.0	325
30.0	290
40.0	370
50.0	352
60.0	395

Table 11 summarizes the particle sizes of the polyketone resins prepared by emulsifications in different mixers (exception: the Omni-Mixer used Ebecryl 3700-25R, a low molecular weight epoxide prepolymer with vinyl functionality; Radcure). The Manton–Gaulin Submicron Disperser and the Micrfluidizer gave the smallest particle sizes, which were both well below the critical size for settling.

E. Formation and Stabilization of Miniemulsions

Shinoda and Friberg [251] summarized two different points of view on the formation and stabilization of emulsions using mixed emulsifier systems. The first point of view was based on the interfacial aspects, according to which the role of the long-chain alcohol was to lower the interfacial tension between the oil and water phases. This lowering of the interfacial tension was attributed to the formation of a fluid bimolecular interfacial film of the emuslifier and long-chain alcohol between the oil and the water phases; this film ensured the efficient use of the energy applied to disperse the oil phase to fine droplets [263–265]. The stability of the emulsion was attributed to the formation at the oil–water interface of a complex, that prevented the oil droplets from coalescing [266,267]. According to this view, the complex formation at the oil–water interface resulted in either an increase in the strength of the interfacial film against rupture during collisions of the droplet, or a decrease in the movement of the surfactant away from the points of contact between the colliding oil droplets, both of which should enhance the stability [268,269].

Table 9 Recipe for Miniemulsification of Polyketone Resin

Ingredient	Parts
Polyketone resin[a]	40.0
1:1 Toluene-methyl isobutyl ketone mixture	60.0
Water	60.0
Sodium lauryl sulfate	20 mmol[b]
Cetyl alcohol	80 mmol[b]

[a]Polyketone resin (Lawter International)
[b]Based on water

Table 10 Particle Size of Polyketone Resin
Pseudolatexes (Manton-Gaulin)

Number of passes	Particle size (nm)
2	206
4	170
6	139

These views on the role of the complex formation in the stabilization of micro-emulsions were criticized [270], and it was declared that the complex formation has "no influence whatsoever on the emulsion stability" [271]. This conclusion was based on a nuclear magnetic resonance spectroscopic investigation [271], which showed that the specific interaction between the surfactant and fatty alcohol molecules was weak at a low water content and vanished at the higher water content used in the emulsification. This weak interaction between the surfactant and the fatty alcohol molecules was used as an argument against the strength of the interfacial layer and its role in the stabilization of the emulsion.

Nevertheless, hexadecyltrimethylammonium bromide has been shown, by electron microscopy and electron diffraction, to form a crystalline complex with cetyl alcohol that was not formed by either component alone [272,273]. The formation of this complex was time-dependent, and the degree of crystallinity was greatest for the 1:3 hexadecyl-trimethylammonium bromide/cetyl alcohol molar ratio. The stability of the emulsions was also highest for the same molar ratio of the two components. These results suggest that the emulsion droplets were stabilized by an adsorbed hexadecyltrimethylammonium bromide–cetyl alcohol complex; however, more work is required to confirm this mechanism.

The second point of view was based on the solubilization aspects, according to which the association of surfactant, cosurfactant, and water caused the solubilization of relatively large volumes of the oil phase, which could be predicted from phase diagrams [274–277]. The stability of the emulsion was attributed to the presence at the oil–water interface of liquid crystals, with ordered arrays of ionic surfactant, fatty alcohol, and water molecules [255,278,279]. The presence of these liquid crystals at the oil–water interface reduced the van der Waals energy available for coalescence of the oil droplets, thereby enhancing the stability of the emulsion [280].

The use of the mixed emulsifier system reduced the oil–water interfacial tension to a very low value, which gave emulsions of fine droplet size after mechanical shear.

Table 11 Particle Size of Polyketone Resin Pseudolatexes
(Different Mixers)

Mixer	Particle size (nm)
Ultrasonification (2 min)	506
Omni-Mixer (10 min)	393
Manton–Gaulin (6 passes)	139
Micro-Fluidizer (5 passes)	60

However, these emulsions are unstable in the thermodynamic sense, and the fine droplets can recombine into the bulk oil phase by either collision of the droplets and rupture of the oil–water interface, followed by coalescence, or degradation by diffusion of the oil through the aqueous phase from the smaller droplets to the larger droplets [281]. Obviously, in the present miniemulsification system, which gave stable emulsions of 100- to 200-nm–average diameter, the mixed emulsifier system enhanced the stability of the emulsion droplets against degradation by collision or diffusion or both.

This excellent stability was attributed [282] to the elimination of emulsion coalescence by diffusion; the incorporation in the oil phase of a cosurfactant (e.g., cetyl alcohol or *n*-decane) of such low water solubility that it could not diffuse from the smaller droplets through the water phase to the larger droplets. This concept was based on earlier work [281] on the degradation by diffusion of fine oil–water emulsion droplets; the solubility of the oil droplets in water increased with decreasing droplet size; however, the addition of low concentrations (< 1%) of a noninteracting low molecular weight compound, with much lower solubility in water than the oil phase, enhanced the stability of the system undergoing molecular diffusion. In this case, the rate of degradation of the emulsion was governed by the diffusion rate of the less-soluble compound. The changes in the emulsion system occurred only as fast as the changes in distribution of the slowest diffusing component. The degradation rate of an oil–water emulsion was retarded by a factor given by the ratio of the partition coefficient of the less water-soluble component to the partition coefficient of the more water-soluble component [283]. The higher the ratio of the partition coefficients, the more efficient was the less-soluble component in stabilizing the oil–water emulsion.

F. Preparation of Latexes by Emulsion Polymerization

The annual production of artificial or pseudolatexes is small compared with that of latexes produced by emulsion polymerization. The purpose of this chapter is not to describe emulsion polymerization in detail, but to give a brief description of it for reference [see Ref. 284 for a more complete description].

There are many families of latexes made by emulsion polymerization, each of which is a major industry: polybutadiene, poly(butadiene-*co*-styrene), poly(butadiene-*co*-acrylonitrile), and polychloroprene for synthetic rubber; poly(styrene-*co*-butadiene) for paints, paper coatings, carpet backing, and nonwoven fabrics; poly(vinyl acetate) and vinyl acetate copolymers for adhesives and paints; acrylate and methacrylate ester copolymers for paints and nonwoven fabrics; poly(vinyl chloride) and vinyl chloride copolymers for plastisols and coatings; vinylidene chloride copolymers for barrier coatings; polyethylene and ethylene copolymers for adhesives and paints; polytetrafluoroethylene and related fluorinated polymers for low-friction coatings; polyacrylamide, acrylamide copolymers, and derivatives for flocculation, sludge treatment, and enhanced oil recovery.

The preparation of latexes by emulsion polymerization is both a science and an art. It is a science in the sense that the kinetics of free–radical-initiated vinyl-addition polymerizations are superimposed on the heterogeneous latex system. It is an art in the sense that it uses a recipe that comprises water, monomer, emulsifier, initiator, and other ingredients, and the quality of the latex produced depends on small variations in the polymerization parameters as well as the skill of the operator.

Emulsion polymerization constitutes emulsfication of a water-immiscible monomer in a continuous water medium, using an oil–water emulsifier, and polymerization, using a water-soluble or oil-soluble initiator to give a colloidal dispersion of polymer particles in water. The average size of these particles is usually 100–300 nm, in contrast with the original droplet size of 1–10 μm. Thus, the mechanism of polymerization is not simply one of polymerization of the monomer droplets, but involves some mechanism of particle nucleation.

Therefore, the emulsion polymerization can be divided into particle nucleation and particle growth stages. The particles are nucleated by some appropriate mechanism and grow until the supply of monomer or free radicals is exhausted. The particle nucleation and particle growth stages occur concurrently or at least overlap (i.e., the particle growth stage begins with the nucleation of the first particle). In the particle nucleation stage, the number of particles N formed depends on (a) the type and concentration of emulsifier, (b) the rate of radical generation, (c) the type and concentration of electrolyte, (d) the temperature, (e) the type and intensity of agitation, (f) other parameters that are not well understood. Thus, the particle nucleation stage is sometimes difficult to reproduce in consecutive experiments.

In contrast, the particle growth stage is tractable and reproducible. As a first approximation, the rate of polymerization R_p is proportional to the number of particles N and the number–average degree of polymerization, to N divided by the rate of radical generation R_i. This unusual dependence of R_p and X_n on N (which is in contrast with the inverse variation of R_p and X_n with R_i in mass, solution, and suspension polymerization) is known as *emulsion polymerization kinetics* and requires two criteria: the free radicals must be segregated, and the number of *loci* available for segregation must be within a few orders of magnitude of the number of free radicals existent in the system. In emulsion polymerization, growing polymer radicals in adjacent particles are unable to terminate with one another because of the intervening aqueous phase, and the values of N may easily reach 10^{14}/ml of water, within a few orders of magnitude of the number of existent free radicals.

The many mechanisms proposed for the nucleation of polymer particles can be divided into four main categories, according to the *locus* of particle nucleation: (a) monomer-swollen emulsifier micelles [285–287]; (b) adsorbed emulsifier layer [288]; (c) aqueous phase [289–293]; (d) monomer droplets [242,243,294].

The particle nucleation stage can be avoided by *seeding*; that is, by polymerizing monomer with controlled amounts of emulsifier and initiator in a previously prepared latex, so that the seed particles grow in size, without the nucleation of a new crop of particles. Thus, the difficult-to-reproduce particle nucleation stage is obviated, and the polymerization begins at the tractable growth stage.

There are three types of emulsion polymerization processes: (a) *batch*, in which all ingredients are added to the polymerization reactor, and the mixture is heated with stirring to the polymerization temperature; (b) *semicontinuous* or *semibatch*, in which neat or preemulsified monomer (and sometimes initiator and emulsifier) are added continuously or incrementally to the reaction mixture at the polymerization temperature; (c) *continuous*, in which all ingredients are added continuously to one part of the polymerization system, and partially or completely converted latex is removed continuously from another part; the polymerization system may constitute a single continuous stirred-tank reactor, a series or cascade of continuous stirred-tank reactors, a loop or tube reactor, or a combination of any of the foregoing systems.

Seeded emulsion polymerization can be used with batch, semicontinuous, or continuous polymerization to give the desired value of N. In batch or semicontinuous polymerization, seeding ensures batch-to-batch reproducibility of the final particle size; in the continuous emulsion polymerization, it ensures the reproducibility, not only of the final particle size, but also of the conversion of the exit stream. Seeded emulsion polymerization is equally adaptable to emulsion homopolymerization or copolymerization. Moreover, two-stage or multi-stage polymerization can be used to produce core-shell or structured latex particles; the variation of the batch, semicontinuous, or continuous process types, as well as the parameters of the polymerization, can be used to control the extent of grafting between the different stages of the polymerization. The versatility of this seeding process has resulted in its wide use in industry to give excellent batch-to-batch reproducibility and to tailor the latex to the specific application.

G. Latexes for Pharmaceutical Coatings

Several types of latexes have been developed for use in coating pharmaceutical pills and tablets to protect them and to control the breakdown of the pills and tablets in the stomach or intestine.

Roehm Tech Inc. (formerly Roehm Pharma) offers 30% aqueous dispersions of: (a) Eudragit E30D, a 67:33 poly(ethyl acrylate-*co*-methyl methacrylate) latex, prepared by emulsion polymerization [295]; (b) Eudragit NE30D, a neutral poly(ethyl acrylate-*co*-methyl methacrylate) latex, prepared by emulsion polymerization; (c) Eudragit L30D-55, a 50:50 poly(ethyl acrylate-*co*-methacrylic acid) latex, prepared by emulsion polymerization [296]; (d) Eudragit RL30D, a pseudolatex, prepared by self-emulsification of a 31:63:6 poly(ethyl acrylate-*co*-methyl methacrylate-*co*-2-trimethylammoniumethyl methacrylate) in water [296]; (e) Eudragit RS30D, a pseudolatex, prepared by self-emulsification of a 32:65:3 poly(ethyl acrylate-*co*-methyl methacrylate-*co*-2-trimethyl-ammoniumethyl methacrylate) in water [297]. The Eudragit E30D and RL30D pseudo-latexes were recommended for rapid-disintegrating coatings, and Eudragit L30D and RL30D, for sustained-release coatings.

Colorcon Inc. offers (a) Surelease, a 25%-solids dibutyl sebacate-plasticized ethyl-cellulose pseudolatex, prepared by inverse emulsification using oleic acid in the polymer phase and ammonia in the water phase to form ammonium oleate emulsifier in situ [298,299]; (b) Coateric, a dry concentrate, containing poly(vinyl acetate phthalate), plasticizer, and pigment, which is dispersed in water to form a pseudolatex [300]; (c) Opadry, a dry concentrate containing ethylcellulose, plasticizer, and pigment developed for both aqueous and organic solvent systems [301]; (d) Opadry II, a further development of Opadry that gives higher-coatings solids and shorter-coating times [302]; (e) Opaspray, a dry concentrate for spraying from aqueous or organic systems [303]. Surelease pseudolatex was recommended for sustained-release coatings; Coateric pseudo-latex, for enteric coatings [304].

FMC Corporation offers (a) Aquacoat, a 30%-solids ethylcellulose pseudolatex, prepared by miniemulsification using the sodium lauryl sulfate–cetyl alcohol mixed emulsifier system; this pseudolatex is entirely made up of materials on the FDA list of safe materials for use in pharmaceutical film coatings and foods [305]; (b) Aquateric aqueous enteric coating, a redispersible cellulose acetate phthalate pseudolatex, prepared by miniemulsification using the poly(propylene oxide-*b*-ethylene oxide)–acetylated mono-glyceride mixed emulsifier system [306]; Aquateric powder, formed by spray-drying Aquateric pseudolatex, can be redispersed in water to reconstitute the pseudolatex. Both Aquacoat and Aquateric pseudolatexes have average particle sizes of about 200 nm and a broad distribution of particle sizes (range 50–3000 nm). Aquacoat pseudolatex is recommended for controlled-release coatings when plasticized (e.g., with dibutyl sebacate or triethyl citrate), and for water-soluble films when formulated with an equal amount of hydroxypropylmethylcellulose. Aquateric pseudolatex also requires plasticization (e.g., with diethyl phthalate or triethyl citrate) and is recommended exclusively for enteric coatings.

Other pseudolatexes of pharmaceutically acceptable water-insoluble polymers can also be made using the same process employed by FMC Corporation. These include pseudolatexes of cellulose acetate and hydroxypropylmethylcellulose phthalate. A non-spray-dried, liquid Aquateric pseudolatex (30% solids) could be used as an alternative to the spray-dried Aquateric powder, but storage of this latex at 5°C would be required to prolong its shelf life.

Many studies on the use of latex and pseudolatex coatings have been published. Banker and Peck [6] were the first to describe pseudolatexes as a new class of coatings for pharmaceutical products; they noted that these pseudolatexes gave the first water-based solvent-free controlled-release and enteric coatings comprising material on the FDA list of safe materials for use in pharmaceutical film coatings and foods. Onions [307] and Porter and Hogan [308] reviewed the use of pseudolatexes as tablet coatings. Chang et al. [309] reviewed the preparation of latexes and their use as coatings to provide sustained-release theophylline pellets. Also, Lehmann [310] described the preparation of methacrylic acid copolymer latexes and their use as controlled-release coatings.

Several investigators have studied the physical properties of latexes and pseudo-latexes. Zhang and Zhang [311] studied the particle size distribution, viscosity, and pH of acrylic latexes used for this purpose. De-Smidt and Crommelin [312] studied the diffusional transport of latex particles, using dynamic light scattering and microviscosity, and related these properties to latex stability. Bodmeier and Chen [313,314] studied the chemical stability of pseudolatexes containing polymers that are prone to hydrolysis.

Other investigators studied the factors influencing film performance. Guo et al. [315] investigated the mechanical and transport properties of pseudolatex films and offered a new hypothesis for the mechanism of film formation (the coalescence was known to be time- and temperature-dependent). Bodmeier and Paeretakul [316] studied the effect of curing temperature on the drug release and the morphological properties of ethylcellulose pseudolatex-coated beads; both retardation and enhancement of the rate of release were observed, according to the curing conditions used.

Numerous reports have described the formulation and processing parameters that influence the performance of the latex- and pseudolatex-coated pharmaceutical products. Bodmeier and Paeratakul [317] described the leaching of water-soluble plasticizers from latex and pseudolatex films and their influence on drug release rates; the leaching rates varied considerably, according to the latexes and pseudolatexes studied, as well as with plasticizer concentration, the nature of the drug that was coated, and whether or not there were other soluble components in the film. Hutchings et al. [318] also studied the influence of plasticizers and media pH on drug release from ethylcellulose pseudolatex-coated pellets; the effect of plasticizer solubility and concentration was determined in a model that used six plasticizers at three concentration levels; the mechanical strength of the latex and pseudolatex films was influenced by plasticization. Bodmeier and Paeratakul [319] described these effects for both wet and dry films; the effects of curing were also described, as were the relations between the mechanical film properties and the rate of release by dissolution.

Coated beads are commonly used in oral controlled-release. Bodmeier and Paeratakul studied the process and formulation variables that affect drug release from beads coated with several pseudolatex systems; they attributed the pH-dependent drug release that was observed in one coating composition to the presence of sodium lauryl sulfate. Bianchini and Veechio [320,321] studied the effect of drug loading and particle size on drug release from pseudolatex-coated beads; the smallest particle size and the higher drug concentrations gave the fastest release rates; the effect of adding more soluble plasticizers, or a small amount of soluble polymer or surfactant, were also evaluated as a means of further controlling dissolution release.

The compression of pseudolatex-coated pelletized materials into tablet compacts was also investigated [322]; the ethylcellulose pseudolatex coating contained additives to give a highly plasticized, elastic film; compression resulted in a substantial loss of the controlled-release properties.

Water-based *enteric*-coating systems have also been reported. Plaizer-Vercammen and Suenens [323] reviewed the use of a cellulose acetate phthalate pseudolatex as an enteric coating; they described the thickness of the plasticized coating required to give 3-h resistance in gastric fluid. Chang [324] compared the rheological and enteric properties of organic solvent solutions of polymer, aqueous ammonium salt solutions, and a pseudolatex system. Chang et al. [325] described the preparation and evaluation of a shellac pseudolatex as an aqueous enteric coating; a range of products was produced, and both the controlled-release and enteric performance of the products were reported.

The use of latex and pseudolatex dispersions to produce controlled-release coatings is rapidly growing. Much of this work by pharmaceutical companies is proprietary or is covered by patents. Chang et al. [326,327] described the formulation and processing variables and effects of acrylic copolymer pseudolatexes. Harris et al. [328] described the use of a pseudolatex coating applied in a rotor-granulator, overcoated with a water-soluble film, and cured in the same apparatus; this process resulted in a stable film coating, with reproducible drug-release profiles. Kelbert and Bechard [329] described a cellulose acetate pseudolatex, modified with flux enhancers, to produce controlled-release products. These reports describe the wide range of polymers used as colloidal dispersions and the wide variety of coating methods used to achieve controlled- and sustained-release. Pseudolatexes and latexes are also being used as granulating agents and binders, as an alternative to polymer solvent solutions, or as an alternative to conventional aqueous hydrophilic polymer solutions. Adikwu and Ossai [330] described a pseudolatex-granulating system that provided rapid drug release, and Patel et al. [331] described an ethylcellulose latex used as a binder for granulation that produced a controlled-release product.

Since latexes and pseudolatexes combine high concentrations with low viscosities, and their particle sizes are in the colloidal range and thus their surface areas are enormous, they can be used to entrap, incorporate, or serve as a solvent phase for drugs. Such systems can be used as drug delivery systems, either by themselves or fabricated into films or other structures. Therefore, it is not surprising that these latexes and pseudolatexes are finding application in ophthalmic and transdermal drug delivery. Gurny et al. [332,333] described the use of pseudolatexes for opthalmic drug delivery, as well as the concept and development of ophthalmic pseudolatex systems using the pH of the eye to trigger release; they also developed a pseudolatex prolonged drug delivery system for the treatment of glaucoma. Vyas et al. also described a pseudolatex system for controlled release of isosorbide dinitrate [334], albutenol (salbutamol) [335], and pilocarpine [336].

The use of latexes and pseudolatexes in transdermal applications has also grown. The 3M nitroglycerin patch used a dispersion containing nitroglycerin, which also served as the adhesive for the patch. Vyas et al. [337] described the development and characterization of a pseudolatex-based transdermal drug delivery system for diclofenac; this system reportedly maintained a constant and effective plasma level for 24 h. Thassu and Vyas [338] also described a pseudolatex-based transdermal mucolytic delivery system. Jain et al. [339] described an effective controlled transdermal delivery system for ephedrine, based on an acrylic copolymer latex; plasma–time profiles were reported for both an oral control form and a transdermal patch. Finally, the application of latexes and pseudolatexes in new biodegradable systems is growing in importance. Banker and Peck [6] were the first to describe biodegradable, injectable latexes for controlled release of potent drugs; they described controlled-release biodegradable systems for direct installation in the brain. Coffin and McGinity [340] described the effects of surfactant system, temperature, pH, and particle size on the chemical stability of biodegradable poly(D,L-lactide) and other polymers in aqueous dispersion form; pseudolatexes prepared with nonionic surfactants were the most stable, and some of these systems showed only small changes in weight-average molecular weight after 350 days of storage. Jalil [341] reviewed various biodegradable polymers and their different physical forms, including pseudolatexes, and assessed the long-term parenteral drug delivery of various classes of drugs.

The foregoing review of the ongoing work in the use of latexes and pseudolatexes as coatings in controlled-release and targeted-drug delivery applications is not intended to be all-inclusive, but is offered to provide an appreciation for the ongoing research in the field, and for the expanding drug delivery approaches that these unique systems offer.

H. Summary

Water-based latex coatings are suitable replacements for solvent-based pharmaceutical coatings because of their economic and environmental advantages. Latexes of polymers that cannot be prepared by emulsion polymerization can be prepared by direct emulsification of their polymer solutions; however, the average particle sizes of the latexes prepared by conventional emulsification are about five to ten times greater than the 100- to 300-nm–average particle size of latexes prepared by emulsion polymerization; the larger particle size allows settling of the latex particles and gives poorer film properties.

Recently, a new emulsification process has been developed, which is based on the use of mixed emulsifier systems that comprise a conventional surfactant and a cosurfactant with a very low water solubility. Practical concentrations of the mixed emulsifiers were used to prepare a wide variety of polymer latexes by direct emulsification, which were stable and had average particle sizes of 100–200 nm, the same size range as the latexes prepared by emulsion polymerization.

REFERENCES

1. S. S. Davis, *Pharm. Technol.*, 11:110 (1987).
2. A. T. Florence and M. N. Gillam, *J. Pesticide Sci.*, 6:429, 1975.

3. E. S. Gerard, D. G. Kaiser, and J. G. Wagner, *Clin. Pharmacol. Ther.*, 7:610 (1966).
4. R. H. Engel and S. J. Riggi, *J. Pharm. Sci.*, 58:1372 (1969).
5. R. H. Engel and M. J. Fahrenbach, *Proc. Soc. Exp. Biol. Med.*, 129:772 (1968).
6. G. S. Banker and G. E. Peck, *Pharm. Technol.*, 5(4):55 (1981).
7. G. S. Banker (to Purdue Research Foundation), *U.S. Patent 4,330,338* (1982).
8. G. S. Banker, in *Polymeric Delivery Systems* (R. J. Kostelnik, ed.). Gordon and Breach, New York, 1978, p. 25.
9. R. Gurny, S. P. Simmons, G. S. Banker, R. Meeker, and R. D. Myers, *Pharm. Acta Helv.*, 54:349 (1979).
10. R. Gurny, N. A. Peppas, D. D. Harrington, and G. S. Banker, *Drug Dev. Ind. Pharm.*, 7:1 (1981).
11. W. Yang and G. S. Banker, *Drug Dev. Ind. Pharm.*, 8:27 (1982).
12. A. B. Larson and G. S. Banker, *J. Pharm. Sci.*, 65:838 (1976).
13. G. S. Banker (to Purdue Research Foundation), *U.S. Patent 3,608,063* (1971).
14. G. S. Banker and H. Goodman (to Purdue Research Foundation), *U.S. Patent 3,629,392* (1971).
15. E. L. Parrott, in *The Theory and Practice of Industrial Pharmacy* (L. Lachman, H. A. Lieberman, and J. L. Kanig, eds.). Lea & Febiger, Philadelphia, 1986, p. 21.
16. S. L. Hem, J. R. Feldkamp, and J. L. White, in *The Theory and Practice of Industrial Pharmacy* (L. Lachman, H. A. Lieberman, and J. L. Kanig, eds.). Lea & Febiger, Philadelphia, 1986, p. 100.
17. J. A. Seitz, S. P. Mahta, and J. L. Yeager, in *The Theory and Practice of Industry Pharmacy* (L. Lachman, H. A. Lieberman, and J. L. Kanig, eds.). Lea & Febiger, Philadelphia, 1986, p. 346.
18. J. A. Bakan, in *The Theory and Practice of Industrial Pharmacy,* (L. Lachman, H. A. Lieberman, and J. L. Kanig, eds.). Lea & Febiger, Philadelphia, 1986, p.412.
19. J. C. Boylan, in *The Theory and Practice of Industrial Pharmacy* (L. Lachman, H. A. Lieberman, and J. L. Kanig, eds.). Lea & Febiger, Philadelphia, 1986, p. 462.
20. N. K. Patel, L. Kennon, and R. S. Levinson, in *The Theory and Practice of Industrial Pharmacy* (L. Lachman, H. A. Lieberman, and J. L. Kanig, eds.). Lea & Febiger, Philadelphia, 1986, p. 479.
21. M. M. Reiger, in *The Theory and Practice of Industrial Pharmacy* (L. Lachman, H. A. Lieberman, and J. L. Kanig, eds.). Lea & Febiger, Philadelphia, 1986, p. 502.
22. J. J. Sciarra and A. J. Cutie, in *The Theory and Practice of Industrial Pharmacy* (L. Lachman, H. A. Lieberman, and J. L. Kanig, eds.). Lea & Febiger, Philadelphia, 1986, p. 589.
23. H. Sonntag and K. Strenge, *Coagulation and Stability of Disperse Systems* (Trans. by R. Kondor) Halsted Press, New York, 1972.
24. *McCutcheon's Detergents and Emulsifiers, North American Edition,* MC Publishing, Glen Rock NJ, 1987.
25. W. C. Griffin, *J. Soc. Cosmet. Chem.*, 1:311 (1949).
26. W. C. Griffin, *Am. Perfum. Essent. Oil. Rev.*, 65(6):26 (1955).
27. W. C. Griffin, *Off. Dig. Fed. Paint Varnish Prod. Clubs*, 28, June (1956).
28. S. Ross, E. S. Chen, P. Becher, and H. J. Ranauto, *J. Phys. Chem.* 63:1681 (1959).
29. G. G. Greth and J. E. Wilson, *J. Appl. Polym Sci.*, 5:135 (1961).
30. M. P. Merkel, M. S. Thesis, Lehigh University, 1982.
31. E. H. Lucassen-Reynders, in *Anionic Surfactants* (E. H. Lucassen-Reynders, ed.) Marcel Dekker, New York, 1981, p. 1.
32. J. W. Gibbs, *Collected Works*, Vol. 1, 2nd ed. Longmans, New York, 1928, p. 219.
33. T. R. Paxton, *J. Coll. Interface Sci.*, 31:19 (1969).
34. I. Piirma and S. R. Chen, *J. Coll. Interface Sci.*, 74:90 (1980).
35. P. Connor and R. H. Ottewill, *J. Coll. Interface Sci.*, 37:642 (1971).

36. R. J. Orr and L. Breitman, *Can. J. Chem.*, 38:668 (1960).
37. S. H. Maron, M. E. Elder, and I. N. Ulevitch, *J. Coll. Sci.*, 9:89 (1954).
38. S. H. Maron, M. E. Elder, and C. Moore, *J. Coll. Sci.*, 9:104 (1954).
39. S. H. Maron and M. E. Elder, *J. Coll. Sci.*, 9:263 (1954).
40. S. H. Maron, M. E. Elder, and I. N. Ulevitch, *J. Coll. Sci.*, 9:382 (1954).
41. Z. Pelzbauer, V. Hynkova, M. Bezdek, and F. Krabak, *J. Polym. Sci.*, C16:503 (1967).
42. H. J. van den Hul and J. W. Vanderhoff, in *Polymer Colloids* (R. M. Fitch, ed.). Plenum, New York, 1971, p. 1.
43. S. M. Ahmed, *Ph.D. dissertation*, Lehigh University, 1978.
44. S. M. Ahmed, M. S. El-Aasser, F. J. Micale, G. W. Poehlein, and J. W. Vanderhoff, in *Solution Chemistry of Surfactants* (K. L. Mittal, ed.). Plenum, New York, 1979, p. 853.
45. S. M. Ahmed, M. S. El-Aasser, G. H. Pauli, G. W. Poehlein, and J. W. Vanderhoff, in *Journal of Colloid. and Interfac. Science, 73*:388, 1980.
46. S. M. Ahmed, M. S. El-Aasser, F. J. Micale, G. W. Poehlein, and J. W. Vanderhoff, in *Polymer Colloids II* (R. M. Fitch, ed.). Plenum, New York, 1980, p. 265.
47. B. Kronberg, L. Kall, and P. Stenius, *J. Dispersion Sci. Technol.*, 2:215 (1981).
48. B. R. Vijayendran, *J. Appl. Polym. Sci.*, 23:733 (1979).
49. V. I. Yeliseyeva and A. V. Zuikov, in *Emulsion Polymerization* (I. Piirma and J. L. Gardon, eds.). *ACS Symp. Ser.*, 24:62 (1976).
50. B. R. Vijayendran, T. Bone, and C. Garjria, in *Emulsion Polymerization of Vinyl Acetate* (M. S. El-Aasser and J. W. Vanderhoff, eds.). Applied Science, London, 1981, p. 253.
51. M. S. El-Aasser, T. Makgawinata, S. Misra, J. W. Vanderhoff, C. Pichot, and M. F. Llauro, in *Emulsion Polymerization of Vinyl Acetate* (M. S. El-Aasser and J. W. Vanderhoff, eds.). Applied Science, London, 1981, p. 215.
52. T. Makgawinata, M. S. El-Aasser, J. W. Vanderhoff, and C. Pichot, *Acta Polym.*, 32:583 (1981).
53. S. M. Ahmed, *M. S. thesis*, Lehigh University, 1981.
54. H. Arai and S. Harin, *J. Coll. Interface Sci.*, 30:312 (1969).
55. P. C. Urban, *J. Dispersion Sci. Technol.*, 2:233 (1981).
56. E. A. Willson, J. R. Miller, and E. H. Rowe, *J. Phys. Coll. Chem.*, 53:357 (1949).
57. C. P. Kurzendorfer, J. J. Schwunger, and H. Lange, *Ber. Bunsenges. Phys. Chem.*, 82:962 (1978).
58. B. V. Deryaguin and L. D. Landau, *Acta Physicochim. USSR*, 14:633 (1941).
59. E. J. W. Verwey and J. T. G. Overbeek, *Theory of the Stability of Lyphobic Colloids*. Elsevier, New York, 1948.
60. H. W. Kruyt, *Colloid Science*, Vol. I. Elsevier, New York, 1952.
61. D. H. Napper and R. J. Hunger, in *Hydrosols*, MTP Int. Rev. Sci., Phys. Chem., Surface Chem. Colloids (M. Kerker, ed.). Ser 1, Vol. 7, Butterworths, London, 1972, p. 225.
62. J. Lyklema, in *Molecular Forces and Colloidal Stability*, Proc. Intermolecular Forces, Vatican City, 1966, Contr. 7; ibid., *Pontif. Acad. Sci. Scripta Varia*, 31:181 (1967).
63. J. T. G. Overbeek and A. van Silfhout, in *Van der Waals Forces Between Macroscopic Objects*, Proc. Intermolecular Forces, Vatican City, 1966, Contr. 6; ibid., *Pontif. Acad. Sci. Scripta Varia*, 31:143 (1967).
64. R. H. Ottewill, in *Emulsion Polymers and Emulsion Polymerization* (D. R. Bassett and A. E. Hamielec, eds.). *ACS Symp. Ser.*, 165:31 (1981).
65. H. van Olphen, *An Introduction to Clay Colloid Chemistry*. Interscience, New York, 1963.
66. H. A. Abramson, *Electrokinetic Phenomena*, Chemical Catalog, New York, 1934.
67. A. A. Kamel, C. M. Ma, M. S. El-Aasser, F. J. Micale, and J. W. Vanderhoff, *J. Dispersion Sci. Technol.*, 2:215 (1981).
68. R. K Iler, *The Colloid Chemistry of Silica and Silicates*. Cornell University Press, Ithaca, 1955.
69. J. W.Vanderhoff and H. J. van den Hul, *J. Macromol. Sci. Chem.*, A7:677 (1973).

70. A. Cohen, *Ann. Physik,* 66:217 (1898).

71. F. M. Fowkes and F. W. Hielscher, *Preprints ACS Org. Coat. Plast. Chem. Div.,* 42:169 (1980).

72. R.H. Ottewill, in *Polymer Colloids,* NATO Advanced Study Institute, University of Trondheim, 1975.

73. J. H. Schenkel and J. A. Kitchener, *Trans. Faraday Soc.,* 56:161 (1960).

74. J. Lyklema, *Adv. Coll. Interface Sci.,* 2:65 (1968).

75. F. M. Fowkes, *Ind. Eng. Chem.,* 56:40 (1964).

76. R. M. Cornell, J. W. Goodwin, and R. H. Ottewill, *J. Coll. Interface Sci.,* 71:254 (1979).

77. M. von Smoluchowski, *Physik. Ann.,* 17:557, 585 (1916); ibid. *Z. Physik. Chem.,* 92:129 (1917).

78. H. Reerink and J. T. G. Overbeek, *Disc. Faraday Soc.,* 18:74 (1954).

79. R. H. Ottewill and J. N. Shaw, *Disc. Faraday Soc.,* 42:154 (1966).

80. W. C. Wu, *Ph.D. dissertation,* Lehigh University, 1977.

81. L. J. Stryker and E. Matijevic, *Adv. Chem.,* 79:44 (1968).

82. E. Matijevic, A. B. Levit, and G. E. Janauer, *J. Coll. Interface Sci.,* 28:10 (1968).

83. E. Matijevic and C. G. Force, *Kolloid Z. Z. Polym.,* 255:33 (1968).

84. W. Heller and J. Peters, *J. Coll. Interface Sci.,* 32:592 (1970).

85. J. Peters and W. Heller, *J. Coll. Interface Sci.,* 33:578 (1970).

86. W. Heller and W. B. de Lauder, *J. Coll. Interface Sci.,* 35:60 (1971).

87. W. Heller and J. Peters, *J. Coll. Interface Sci.,* 35:300 (1971).

88. W. B. de Lauder and W. Heller, *J. Coll. Interface Sci.,* 35:308 (1971).

89. B. Vincent, *Adv. Coll. Interface Sci.,* 4:193 (1974).

90. T. W. Healy and V. K. LaMer, *J. Phys. Chem.,* 66:1835 (1962).

91. J. Gregory, *Trans. Faraday Soc.,* 65:2260 (1969).

92. H. E. Ries and B. C. Meyers, *Science,* 160:1449 (1968).

93. H. E. Ries and B. C. Meyers, *J. Appl. Polym. Sci.,* 15:2023 (1971).

94. A. P. Black and M. C. Vilaret, *J. Am. Water Works Assoc.,* 61:209 (1969).

95. J. Gregory, *J. Coll. Interface Sci.,* 42:448 (1973).

96. A. S. Teot, *Ann. N. Y. Acad. Sci.,* 155:593 (1969).

97. A. S. Teot and S. L. Daniels, *Environ. Sci. Technol.,* 3:825 (1969).

98. J. W. Vanderhoff, in *Proc. Chem. Inst. Canada 'Flocculation and Dispersion Symposium,"* Toronto, 1974, p. 173.

99. J. W. Vanderhoff, paper presented at 51st Colloid and Surface Science Symp., Grand Island, New York, 1977.

100. H. Schlueter, in *Copolymers, Polyblends and Composites* (N. A. J. Platzer, ed.). *ACS Adv. Chem. Ser.* 142:99 (1975).

101. S. Saito and M. Fujiwara, *Colloid Polym. Sci.,* 255:1122 (1977).

102. R. A. Ruehrwein and D. W. Ward, *Soil Sci.,* 73:485 (1952).

103. A. S. Michaels, *Ind. Eng. Chem.,* 46:1485 (1954).

104. A. S. Michaels and O. Morelos, *Ind. Eng. Chem.,* 47:1801 (1955).

105. W. F. Linke and R. B. Booth, *Trans. Am. Inst. (Metall.) Eng.,* 217:364 (1959).

106. P. Somasundaran, T. W. Healy, and D. W. Fuerstenau, *J. Coll. Interface Sci.,* 22:599 (1966).

107. R. I. Feigin and D. H. Napper, *J. Coll. Interface Sci.,* 75:525 (1980).

108. R. I. Feigin and D. H. Napper, *J. Coll. Interface Sci.,* 74:567 (1980).

109. S. Asakura and F. Oosawa, *J. Polym. Sci.,* 33:183 (1958).

110. F. K. R. Lin-In-On, B. Vincent, and F. A. Waite, *ACS Symp. Ser.* 9:165 (1975).

111. C. Cowell, F. K. R. Li-In-On, and B. Vincent, *J. Chem. Soc., Faraday Trans.,* 174:337 (1978).

112. B. Vincent, P. F. Luckham, and F. A. Waite, *J. Coll. Interface Sci.,* 73:508 (1980).

113. A. Vrij, *Pure Appl. Chem.,* 48:471 (1976).

114.   H. DeHek and A. Vrij, *J. Coll. Interface Sci.,* 70:592 (1979).

115.   P. R. Sperry, H. B. Hopfenberg, and N. L. Thomas, *J. Coll. Interface Sci.,* 82:62 (1981).

116.   J. Y. Walz and A. Sharma, *J. Coll. Interface Sci.,* 168:485 (1994).

117.   M. von Smoluchowski, *Z. Physik. Chem.* 92:155 (1917); Tuorila, *Kolloidchem. Beihefte,* 24:1 (1927), H. Mueller, *Kolloidchem Beihefte,* 27:223 (1928).

118.   J. T. G. Overbeek, in *Colloid Science,* Vol. 2 (H. R. Kruyt ed.). Elsevier, New York, 1952, p. 290.

119.   T. G. M. Van de Ven and S. G. Mason, *J. Coll. Interface Sci.,* 57:505, 517 (1976).

120.   G. R. Zeichner and W. R. Showalter, *AIChE J.,* 23:243 (1977).

121.   G. R. Zeichner and W. R. Showalter, *J. Coll. Interface Sci.,* 71:237 (1979).

122.   W. Heller and T. L. Pugh, *J. Chem. Phys.,* 22:1778 (1954).

123.   H. Freundlich, *Colloid and Capillary Chemistry,* Methuen, London, 1926, p. 589.

124.   D. H. Napper, *I&EC Prod. Res. Dev.,* 9:467 (1970).

125.   D. H. Napper, *Proc. R. Aust. Chem. Inst.,* 327, Nov (1971).

126.   B. Vincent, *Adv. Coll. Interface Sci.,* 4:193 (1974).

127.   R. H. Ottewill, in *Nonionic Surfactants* (M. J. Schick, ed.). Marcel Dekker, New York, 1967, p. 627.

128.   R. H. Ottewill, in Specialist Periodical Report, *Chem. Soc. Coll. Sci.,* Vol. 1, 1973, p. 173.

129.   D. H. Napper and R. J. Hunter, in *MTI Int. Rev. Sci.* Ser. I, Vol. 7. (M. Kerker, ed.). Butterworths, London, 1972, p. 225.

130.   D. H. Napper and R. J. Hunter, in *MTI Int. Rev. Sci.* Ser. II, Vol. 7. (M. Kerker, ed.). 1973. Butterworths, London, p. 161.

131.   J. Lyklema, *Adv. Coll. Interface Sci.,* 2:65 (1968).

132.   B. Vincent, *Adv. Coll. Interface Sci.,* 4:193 (1974).

133.   K. Barrett, *Dispersion Polymerization in Organic Media,* John Wiley, New York, 1975.

134.   E. Jenkel and B. Runbach, *Z. Elektrochem.* 55:612 (1951).

135.   H. L. Frisch, R. Simha, and E. R. Eirich, *J. Chem. Phys.,* 21:365 (1953).

136.   E. R. Gilliland and E. B. Gutoff, *J. Phys. Chem.,* 64:407 (1960).

137.   W. I. Higuchi, *J. Phys. Chem.,* 65:487 (1961).

138.   W. C. Forsman and R. Hughes, *J. Chem. Phys.,* 38:2130 (1963).

139.   A. Silverberg, *J. Phys. Chem.,* 66:1872 (1962).

140.   C. A. J. Hoeve, *J. Chem. Phys.,* 43:3007 (1965).

141.   C. A. J. Hoeve, *J. Polym. Sci.,* C30:361 (1970).

142.   C. A. J. Hoeve, *J. Polym. Sci.,* C34:1 (1971).

143.   D. J. Meier, *J. Phys. Chem.,* 71:1861 (1967).

144.   F. T. Hesselink, *J. Phys. Chem.,* 73:3488 (1969).

145.   F. T. Hesselink, *J. Phys. Chem.,* 75:65 (1971).

146.   M. Rosoff, in *Physical Methods in Macromolecular Chemistry,* Vol. 1 (B. Carroll, ed.). Marcel Dekker, New York, 1969, p. 1.

147.   R. R. Stromberg, in *Treatise on Adhesion and Adhesives,* Vol. 1 (R. L. Patrick, ed.). Marcel Dekker, New York, 1967, p. 69.

148.   A. Silberberg, *J. Polym. Sci.,* C30:393 (1970).

149.   S. G. Ash, *Colloid Science,* Vol. 1, Chap. 3, Chem. Soc., London, 1973.

150.   J. G. Brodnyan and E. L. Kelley, *J. Polym. Sci.,* C27:263 (1969).

151.   F. L. Saunders, *J. Coll. Interface Sci.,* 28:475 (1968).

152.   M. J. Garvey, T. F. Tadros, and B. Vincent, *J. Coll. Interface Sci.,* 49:57 (1974).

153.   W. Norde and J. Lyklema, *J. Coll. Interface Sci.,* 66:266 (275), 277, 285, 295 (1978).

154.   T. V. den Boomgaard, T. A. King, T. F. Tadros, H. Tang, and B. Vincent, *J. Coll. Interface Sci.,* 66:68 (1978).

155.   J. M. G. Lankveld and J. Lyklema, *J. Coll. Interface Sci.,* 41:454, 466, 475 (1972).

156. T. F. Tadros, in *Theory and Practice of Emulsion Technology* (A. L. Smith, ed.), Academic Press, New York, 1976, p. 281.
157. D. Eagland and G. C. Wardlaw, *Coll. Polym. Sci.*, 256:1079 (1978).
158. D. H. Napper, *Kolloid Z.Z. Polym.*, 234:1149 (1969).
159. D. W. J. Osmond and D. J. Walbridge, *J. Polym. Sci.*, C30:381 (1970).
160. D. H. Napper, *J. Coll. Interface Sci.*, 58:390 (1977).
161. E. W. Fischer, *Kolloid Z.*, 160:120 (1958).
162. R. H. Ottewill and T. Walker, *Kolloid Z. Z. Polym.*, 227:108 (1968).
163. D. H. Napper, *J. Trans. Faraday Soc.*, 64:1701 (1968).
164. D. H. Napper, *J. Coll. Interface Sci.*, 29:168 (1969).
165. D. H. Napper, *J. Coll. Interface Sci.*, 33:384 (1970).
166. D. H. Napper and A. Netschey, *J. Coll. Interface Sci.*, 37:528 (1971).
167. D. H. Napper, *J. Coll. Interface Sci.*, 32:106 (1970).
168. R. Evans, J. B. Davison, and D. H. Napper, *J. Polym. Sci.*, B10:449 (1972).
169. R. Evans and D. H. Napper, *J. Coll. Interface Sci.*, 52:260 (1975).
170. A. Doroszkowski and R. Lambourne, *J. Coll. Interface Sci.*, 43:97 (1973).
171. F. Bueche, *J. Coll. Interface Sci.*, 41:374 (1972).
172. R. H. Ottewill, *Annu. Rep. Progr. Chem.* (Chem. Soc., London) A66:212 (1969).
173. D. W. J. Osmond, B. Vincent, and F. A. Waite, *Coll. Polym. Sci.*, 253:676 (1975).
174. J. W. Dobbie, R. Evans, D. V. Gibson, J. B. Smitham, and D. H. Napper, *J. Coll. Interface Sci.*, 45:557 (1973).
175. J. B. Smitham and D. H. Napper, *Coll. Polym. Sci.*, 257:748 (1979).
176. R. Evans and D. H. Napper, *Kolloid Z.Z. Polym.*, 251:409 (1973).
177. L. M. Barclay and R. H. Ottewill, in *Faraday Soc. Special Disc. Symp. Thin Liquid Films and Boundary Layers*, No. 1, Univ. of Cambridge, 1970, p. 169.
178. A. Watanabe, F. Tsuji, and S. Ueda, *Kolloid Z.*, 39:193 (1963).
179. M. J. Vold, *J. Coll. Interface Sci.*, 16:1 (1961).
180. P. Bagchi, *J. Coll. Interface Sci.*, 47:86 (1974).
181. E. J. Mackor, *J. Coll. Interface Sci.*, 6:492 (1951).
182. E. J. Mackor and J. H. van der Waals, *J. Coll. Interface Sci.*, 7:535 (1952).
183. E. J. Clayfield and E. C. Lumb, *J. Coll. Interface Sci.*, 22:269 (1966).
184. E. J. Clayfield and E. C. Lumb, *J. Coll. Interface Sci.*, 22:28 (1966).
185. E. J. Clayfield and E. C. Lumb, *J. Coll. Interface Sci.*, 47:6 (1974).
186. E. J. Clayfield and E. C. Lumb, *J. Coll. Interface Sci.*, 47:16 (1974).
187. E. J. Clayfield and E. C. Lumb, *J. Coll. Interface Sci.*, 49:489 (1974).
188. D. J. Meier, *J. Phys. Chem.*, 71:1861 (1967).
189. F. T. Hesselink, A. Vrij, and J. T. G. Overbeek, *J. Phys. Chem.*, 75:2094 (1971).
190. P. J. Flory, *Principles of Polymer Chemistry*, Cornell University Press, Ithaca, NY, 1953.
191. F. T. Hesselink, *J. Phys. Chem.*, 75:65 (1971).
192. R. Evans and D. H. Napper, *Kolloid Z.Z. Polym.*, 251:329 (1973).
193. A. K. Dolan and S. F. Edwards, *Proc. R. Soc. Lond. Ser.*, A337:509 (1974).
194. A. K. Dolan and S. F. Edwards, *Proc. R. Soc. Lond. Ser.*, A343:427 (1975).
195. H. M. H. M. Scheutjens and G. J. Fleer, *J. Phys. Chem.*, 84:178 (1980).
196. R. I. Feigin and D. H. Napper, *J. Coll. Interface Sci.*, 67:127 (1978).
197. M. D. Croucher and M. L. Hair, *Macromolecules* 11:874 (1978).
198. M. D. Croucher and M. L. Hair, *J. Phys. Chem.*, 83:1712 (1979).
199. W.-C. Chen, *Ph.D. dissertation*, Lehigh Univ., 1992.
200. A.-M. Sung and I. Piirma, *Langmuir*, 10:1393 (1994).
201. M. B. Einarson and J. C. Berg, *J. Coll. Interface Sci.*, 155:165 (1993).
202. M. B. Einarson and J. C. Berg, *Langmuir*, 8:2611 (1992).
203. J. T. Li and K. D. Caldwell, *Polym. Mater. Sci. Eng.*, 65:27 (1991).
204. Y. Adachi, H. A. Cohen-Stuart, and R. Fokkink, *J. Coll. Interface Sci.*, 167:346 (1994).

205. H. Tamai, T. Oyanagi, and T. Suzawa, *Colloid Surf.*, 57:115 (1991).
206. J. V. Dawkins and S. A. Shakir, *ACS Symp. Ser.* 492 432 (1992).
207. H. G. Shin, H. M. Jang, and T. O. Kim, *Yoop Hakhoechi*, 27:684 (1990).
208. K. R. Rogan, A. C. Bentham, G. W. A. Beard, I. A. George, and D. R. Skuse, *Prog. Colloid Polym. Sci. (Trends in Colloid and Interface Science VIII)*, 97:97 (1994).
209. K. R. Rogan, A. C. Bentham, I. A. George, and D. R. Skuse, *Colloid Polym. Sci.*, 272:1175 (1994).
210. S. Biggs and T. W. Healy, *J. Chem. Soc. Faraday Trans.*, 90:3415 (1994).
211. M. Giersig and P. Mulvaney, *J. Phys. Chem.*, 97:6334 (1993).
212. L. J. Gallego, M. J. Grimson, C. Rey, and M. Silbert, *Colloid Polym. Sci.*, 270:1091 (1992).
213. E. B. Zhulina and O. V. Borisov, *Makromol. Chem. Makromol. Symp. (German-USSR Symp. Polym. Sci. 4th)* 44:274 (1990).
214. K. Rodrigues and W. L. Mattice, *Polym. Prepr. (Am. Chem. Soc.), Div. Polym. Chem.*, 32:269 (1991).
215. D. C. Blackley, *High Polymer Latices*, Vol. 1, Maclaren, London, 1966.
216. S. Berkman and G. Egloff, *Emulsion and Foams*, Reinhold, New York, 1941.
217. R. M. K. Cobb, *Emulsion Technology* (H. Bennett, ed.), Chemical Publishing, New York, 1946.
218. P. Becher, *Emulsions, Theory and Practice*, 2nd ed., Reinhold, New York, 1965.
219. L. H. Princen, in *Treatise on Coatings* Vol. I, Part III (R. R. Myers and J. S. Long, eds.). Marcel Dekker, New York, 1972, p. 77.
220. S. Friberg and G. La Force-Gillberg, in *Recent Advances in Emulsion Technology, Repr. Progr. Appl. Chem.*, 58:715 (1973; publ. 1975).
221. F. Harusawa and T. Mitsui, *Prog. Org. Coatings* 3(2):177 (1975).
222. M. A. Nawab and S. G. Mason, *J. Coll. Sci.*, 13:179 (1958).
223. A. Watanabe, K. Higashitsuji, and K. Nishizawa, *J. Coll. Interface Sci.*, 64:278 (1978).
224. W. C. Griffin, in *Encyclopedia of Chemical Technology*, 2nd ed., Vol. 8, John Wiley, New York, 1965, p. 117.
225. J. W. Vanderhoff, H. J. van den Hul, R. J. M. Tausk, and J. T. G. Overbeek, in *Clean Surfaces: Their Preparation and Characterization for Interfacial Studies* (G. Goldfinger ed.). Marcel Dekker, New York, 1970, p. 15.
226. J. T.G. Overbeek, in *Colloid Science*, Vol. I (H. R. Kruyt, ed.). Elsevier, New York, 1952, p. 80.
227. J. W. Vanderhoff, H. L. Tarkowski, M. C. Jenkins, and E. B. Bradford, *J. Macromol. Chem.*, 1:361 (1966).
228. J. W. Vanderhoff, *Br. Polym. J.*, 2:161 (1970).
229. G. L. Brown, *J. Polym. Sci.*, 22:423 (1956).
230. H. Warson, *The Applications of Synthetic Resin Emulsions*, Benn, London, 1972.
231. D. Aelony and H. Wittcoff (to General Mills, Inc.), *U.S. Patent 2,899,397* (1959).
232. A. L. Miller, S. B. Robison, and A. J. Petro (to Esso Res. Eng. Co.), *U.S. Patent 3,022,260* (1962).
233. H. Schnoering, J. Witte, and G. Pampus (to Farbenfabriken Bayer AG), *Ger. Offen. 2,013,359*, 1971; *Chem. Abstr.*, 76:26187k (1972).
234. O. W. Burke, Jr., *U.S. Patent 3,652,482* (1972).
235. W. Cooper (to Dunlop Rubber Co.,. Ltd.), *U.S. Patent 3,009,891* (1961).
236. F. L. Saunders and R. R. Pelletier (to Dow Chemical Co.), *U.S. Patent 3,642,676* (1972).
237. M. Date and M. Wada (to Toyobo Co. Ltd.), Japan 73 06,619 (1973); *Chem. Abstr.*, 80:38097b (1974).
238. S. P. Suskind, *J. Appl. Polym. Sci.*, 9:2451, 1965.
239. W. J. Fuller, *Paint Varnish Prod.*, 58(7):23 (1968).
240. P. Judd (to W. R. Grace & Co.), *British Patent 1,142,375* (1969); *Chem. Abstr.*, 70:69355g (1969).

241. D. Dieterich, W. Keberle, and R. Wuest, *J. Oil Col. Chem. Assoc.* 53:363 (1970).
242. J. Ugelstad, M. S. El-Aasser, and J. W. Vanderhoff, *J. Polym. Sci.*, B11:503 (1973).
243. J. Ugelstad, F. K. Hansen, and S. Lange, *Makromol. Chem.*, 175:507 (1974).
244. A. R. M. Azad, J. Ugelstad, R.M. Fitch, and F. K. Hansen, *ACS Symp. Ser.*, 24:1 (1976).
245. J. Ugelstad, K. Herder-Kaggerud, F. K. Hansen, and A. Berge, *Makromol. Chem.*, 180:737 (1979).
246. J. Ugelstad, F. K. Hansen, and K. Herder-Kaggerud, *Faserforsch. Textiltechn. E. Polym. Forsch.*, 28:309 (1977).
247. F. K. Hansen, E. Baumann-Ofstad, and J. Ugelstad, in *Theory and Practice of Emulsion Technology* (A. L. Smith, ed.). Academic Press, London, 1976, p. 13.
248. M. S. El-Aasser and J. W. Vanderhoff, *unpublished research*, Lehigh University, 1972.
249. J. H. Schulman and E. G. Cockbain, *Trans. Faraday Soc.*, 36:651 (1940).
250. J. H. Schulman and D. P. Riley, *J. Coll. Sci.*, 3:383 (1948).
251. K. Shinoda and S. Friberg, *Adv. Coll. Interface Sci.*, 4:281 (1975).
252. J. T. Davies and D. A. Haydon, *Proc. 2nd Int. Conf. Surface Activity*, London, 1:417 (1957).
253. B. W. Barry, *J. Colloid Interface Sci.*, 28:82 (1968).
254. L. M. Prince, *J. Soc. Cosmet. Chem.*, 21:193 (1970).
255. S. Friberg and L. Rydhaug, *Kolloid Z. Z. Polym.* 244:235 (1971).
256. J. W. Vanderhoff, M. S. El-Aasser, and J. Ugelstad (to Lehigh University), *U.S. Patent 4,177,177* (1979).
257. M. S. El-Aasser, J. D. Hoffman, C. Kiefer, H. Leidheiser, Jr., J. A. Manson, G. W. Poehlein, R. Stoisits, and J. W. Vanderhoff, *Final Report AFML-TR-74-208, Water-Base Coatings, Part I*, July 1973–August 1974 (dated November 1974).
258. Y. N. Chou, L. M. Confer, K. A. Earhart, M. S. El-Aasser, J. D. Hoffman, J. A. Manson, S. C. Misra, G. W. Poehlein, J. P. Scolare, and J. W. Vanderhoff, *Final Report AFML-TR-74-208 Water-Base Coatings, Part II*, February 1975–November 1975 (dated 1976).
259. M. S. El-Aasser, G. W. Poehlein, and J. W. Vanderhoff, *Preprints, ACS Org. Coat. Plast. Chem. Div.*, 37(2):92 (1977).
260. M. S. El-Aasser, S. C. Misra, J. W. Vanderhoff, and J. A. Manson, *J. Coatings Technol.*, 49 (635):71 (1977).
261. J. W. Vanderhoff, M. S. El-Aasser, and J. D. Hoffman (to Lehigh University), *U.S. Patent 4,070,323* (1978).
262. K. Gan, *Ph.D. dissertation*, Lehigh University, 1995.
263. J. H. Schulman, W. Stockenius, and L. M. Prince, *J. Phys. Chem.*, 63:1677 (1959).
264. W. Gerbacia and H. L. Rosano, *J. Colloid Interface Sci.*, 44:242 (1973).
265. L. M. Prince, *J. Colloid Interface Sci.*, 23:165 (1967).
266. J. H. Schulman and E. G. Cockbain, *Trans. Faraday Soc.*, 36:651 (1940).
267. E. G. Cockbain and T. S. McRoberts, *J. Colloid Sci.*, 8:440 (1958).
268. P. H. Elworthy, A. T. Florence, and J. A. Rogers, *J. Colloid Interface Sci.*, 35:43 (1971).
269. G. W. Hallworth and J. E. Carless, *J. Pharm. Pharmacol.*, 25(Suppl.):78 (1971).
270. S. Friberg, *Kolloid Z. Z. Polym.*, 244:333 (1971).
271. S. Friberg, L.Mandell, and P. Ekwall, *Kolloid Z.Z. Polym.*, 233:955 (1969).
272. Y. J. Chou, *Ph.D. dissertation*, Lehigh University, 1978.
273. Y. J. Chou, M. S. El-Aasser, and J. W. Vanderhoff in *Polymer Colloids II* (R. M. Fitch, ed.). Plenum, New York, 1980, p. 599.
274. P. A. Winsor, *Trans. Faraday Soc.*, 44:376 (1948).
275. G. Gillberg, H. Lehtinen, and S. Friberg, *J. Colloid Interface Sci.*, 33:40 (1970).
276. P. Ekwall, L. Mandell, and K. Fontell, *J. Colloid Interface Sci.*, 33:40 (1970).
277. K. Shinoda and H. Kunieda, *J. Colloid Interface Sci.*, 42:381 (1973).
278. S. Friberg, L. Mandell, and M. Larsson, *J. Colloid Interface Sci.*, 29:155 (1969).
279. S. Fukushima, M. Yamaguchi, and F. Harusawa, *J. Colloid Interface Sci.*, 51:548 (1975).
280. S. Friberg and P. O. Jansson, *J. Colloid Interface Sci.*, 55:614 (1976).

281. W. I. Higuchi and J. Misra, *J. Pharm. Sci.*, 51:459 (1962).
282. J. Ugelstad, *Makromol. Chem.*, 179:815 (1978).
283. S. S. Davis and A. Smith, in *Theory and Practice of Emulsion Technology* (A. L. Smith, ed.). Academic Press, New York, 1976.
284. J. W. Vanderhoff, *J. Polym. Sci., Polym. Symp.*, 72:161 (1985).
285. W. D. Harkins, *J. Am. Chem. Soc.*, 69:1428 (1947).
286. W. V. Smith and R. H. Ewart, *J. Chem. Phys.*, 16:592 (1948).
287. W. V. Smith, *J. Am. Chem. Soc.*, 70:3695 (1948); 71:4077 (1949).
288. S. S. Medvedev. *Ric. Sci. Supl.* 25:897 (1955); in *International Symposium on Macromolecular Chemistry*, Prague, Pergamon, New York 1957, p. 174.
289. W. J. Priest, *J. Phys. Chem.*, 56:1077 (1952).
290. B. Jacobi, *Angew. Chem.*, 64:539 (1952).
291. R. Patsiga, M. Litt, and V. Stannett, *J. Phys. Chem.*, 64:801 (1960).
292. C. P. Roe, *Ind. Eng. Chem.*, 60:20 (1968).
293. R. M. Fitch, in *Polymer Colloids* (R. M. Fitch, ed.). Plenum, New York, 1971, p. 73.
294. D. P. Durbin, M. S. El-Aasser. G. W. Poehlein, and J. W. Vanderhoff, *J. Appl. Polym. Sci.*, 24:703 (1979).
295. *Eudragit E30D Prospectus (Info ED-1/e); Eudragit E, Technical Application Pamphlet (Info ED-12/e,* Roehm Tech, Malden, MA.
296. *Eudragit L30D, Prospectus (Info LD-1/e); Eudragit L, Technical Application Pamphlet (Info LD-12/e),* Roehm Pharma, Malden, MA.
297. *Eudragit RL/RS Dispersions, Provisional Leaflet,* Roehm Pharma, Malden, MA.
298. D. E. Leng, W. L. Sigelko, and F. L. Saunders (to Dow Chemical Co.), *U.S. Patent 4,502,888,* 1985.
299. *Surelease PTB 9-90,* Colorcon, Inc., West Point, PA.
300. *Coateric P-T-23 (3/87),* Colorcon Inc., West Point, PA.
301. *Opadry PB-7-87,* Colorcon Inc., West Point, PA.
302. *Opadry II PTB-806-01 (9-89),* Colorcon Inc., West Point, PA.
303. *Opaspray Concentrate,* Colorcon Inc., West Point, PA.
304. *Surelease 0601 Aqueous Controlled Release Coating System,* Colorcon Inc., West Point, PA.
305. *Aquacoat Aqueous Polymeric Dispersion,* FMC Corporation, Philadelphia, PA.
306. *Aquateric Aqueous Enteric Coating,* FMC Corporation, Philadelphia, PA.
307. A. Onions, *Manuf. Chemist,* 57(Mar):55, 57, 59 (1986).
308. S. C. Porter and J. E. Hogan, *Pharm. Int.,* 5(May):122 (1984).
309. R. K.Chang, C. H. Hsiao, and J. R. Robinson, *Pharm. Technol.,* 11(Mar):56 (1987).
310. K. Lehmann, *Acta Pharm. Technol.,* 31(2):96 (1985).
311. J. S. Zhang and X. Zhang, *J. China Pharm. Univ.,* 23:272 (1992).
312. J. H. De-Smidt and D. J. Crommelin, *Int. J. Pharm.,* 77:261 (1991).
313. R. Bodmeier and H. Chen, *Drug Dev. Ind. Pharm.,* 17(13):1811 (1991).
314. R. Bodmeier and H. Chen, *Drug Dev. Ind. Pharm.,* 19:521 (1993).
315. J. H. Guo, R. E. Robertson, and G. L. Amidon, *Pharm. Res.,* 10:405 (1993).
316. R. Bodmeier and O. Paeratakul, *Drug Dev. Ind. Pharm.,* 20:1517 (1994).
317. R. Bodmeier and O. Paeratakul, *Drug Dev. Ind. Pharm.,* 18:1865 (1992).
318. D. Hutchings, S. Clarson, and A. Sakr, *Int. J. Pharm.,* 104:203 (1994).
319. R. Bodmeier and O. Paeratakul, *Pharm. Res.,* 11:882 (1994).
320. R. Bianchini and C. Veechio, *Bol. Chim. Farmac.,* 128:373 (1989).
321. R. Bianchini and C. Veechio, *Farmaco,* 44:645 (1989).
322. S. R. Bechard and J. C. Lerouox, *Drug Dev. Ind. Pharm.,* 18:1927 (1992).
323. J. Plaizer-Vercammen and G. Seunens, *STP Pharm. Sci.,* 1:307 (1991).
324. R. K. Chang, *Pharm. Technol.,* 14(Oct):62 (1990).
325. R. K. Chang, G. Iturrioz, and G. W. Luo, *Int. J. Pharm.,* 60(Apr 30):171 (1990).

326. R. K. Chang and C. Hsiao, *Drug Dev. Ind. Pharm.*, 15:187 (1989).
327. R. K. Chang, J. C. Price, and C. Hsiao, *Drug Dev. Ind. Pharm.*, 15:161 (1989).
328. M. R. Harris, I. Ghebre-Sellassie, and R. U. Nesbitt, *Pharm. Technol.*, 10(Sept.):102 (1986).
329. M. Kelbert and S. R. Bechard, *Drug Dev. Ind. Pharm.*, 18:519 (1992).
330. M. U. Adikwu and A. O. Ossai, *STP Pharma Sci.*, 4:190 (1994).
331. M. R. Patel, M. C. Gohel, and J. S. Desai, *Drug Dev. Ind. Pharm.*, 19:439 (1992).
332. R. Gurny, *Pharm. Acta Helv.*, 56(4–5):130 (1981).
333. H. Ibrahim, C. Bindschaedler, E. Doelker, F. Buri, and R. Gurny, *Int. J. Pharm.*, 77(Nov 15):211 (1991).
334. S. P. Vyas, S. Ramchandraiah, C. P. Jain, and S. K. Jain, *J. Microencapsulation*, 9:347 (1992).
335. S. P. Vyas, C. P. Jain, S. Gupta, and A. Uppadhayay, *Drug. Dev. Ind. Pharm.*, 20:101 (1994).
336. S. K. Jain, S .P. Vyas, and V. K. Dixit, *Drug Dev. Ind. Pharm.*, 20:1991 (1994).
337. S. P. Vyas and P. J. Gogoi, *Drug Dev. Ind. Pharm.*, 17:1041 (1991).
338. D. Thassu and S. P. Vyas, *Drug Dev. Ind. Pharm.*, 17:561 (1991).
339. S. K. Jain, S. P. Vyas, and V. K. Dixit, *J. Controlled Release* 12(May): 257 (1990).
340. M. D. Coffin and J. W. McGinity, *Pharm. Res.*, 9:200 (1992).
341. R. U. Jalil, *Drug Dev. Ind. Pharm.*, 16:2353 (1990).

BIBLIOGRAPHY

Adamson, A. W., *Physical Chemistry of Surfaces,* 5th ed., Wiley-Interscience, New York, 1990.

Aveyard, R. and D. A. Haydon, *An Introduction to the Principles of Surface Chemistry*, Cambridge, London, 1973.

Bikerman, J. J., *Surface Chemistry*, 2nd ed., Academic Press, New York, 1958.

Davies, J. T. and E. K. Rideal, *Interfacial Phenomena*, 2nd ed., Academic Press, New York, 1963.

Defay, R., I. Prigogine, A. Bellemans, and D. H. Everett, *Surface Tension and Adsorption*, John Wiley, New York, 1966.

El-Aasser, M. S., Electrostatic stabilization and aggregation of electrostatically stabilized latexes, in *Advances in Emulsion Polymerization and Latex Technology*, Vol. 1, 26th Annual Short Course, Lehigh University, June 1995.

Goddard, E. D. and K. P. Ananthapadmanabhan (eds.), *Interactions of Surfactants with Polymers and Proteins*, CRC Press, Boca Raton, FL, 1993.

Harkins, W. D., *The Physical Chemistry of Surface Films*. Reinhold, New York, 1952.

Jungermann, E. (ed.), *Cationic Surfactants*, Surfactant Science Series, Vol. 4., Marcel Dekker, New York, 1970.

Kruyt, H. R., *Colloid Science,* Vol. 1, Elsevier, New York, 1952.

Lyklema, J., in *Molecular Forces and Colloidal Stability, Proc. Intermolecular Forces, Vatican City,* 1966, Contr. 7; *ibid., Pontif. Acad. Sci. Scripta Varia*, 31:181 (1967).

McBain, J. W., *Colloid Science,* Reinhold, New York, 1950.

Mirnik, M., Ion exchange theory of coagulation and its experimental verification, Croat. Chem. Acta., 42:161 (1970).

Moilliet, J. L., B. Collie, and W. Black, *Surface Activity*, 2nd ed., van Nostrand, Princeton, 1961.

Mukerjee, P. and A. Anavil, in *Adsorption at Interfaces*, ACS Symp. Ser. 8: 107 (1975).

Mysels, K. J., *Introduction to Colloid Chemistry*, Interscience, New York, 1959.

Napper, D. H., and R. J. Hunger, Hydrosols, in *MTP. Int. Rev. Sci., Phys. Chem., Surface Chem. Colloids* (M. Kerker, ed.). Ser. 1, Vol. 6, Butterworths, London, 1972, p. 225.

Ottewill, R. H., *Prog. Colloid Polym. Sci.*, 59:14 (1976).

Ottewill, R. H., *J. Colloid Interface Sci.*, 58:357 (1977).

Overbeek, J. T. G., *J. Colloid Interface Sci.*, 58:408 (1977).

Overbeek, J. T. G. and A. Van Silfhout, *Van der Waals forces between macroscopic objects*, in *Proc. Intermolecular Forces, Vatican City*, 1966, Contr. 6; *ibid.*, *Pontif. Acad. Sci. Scripta Viaria*, 31:143 (1967).

Rosen, M. J., *Surfactants and Interfacial Phenomena*, John Wiley, New York, 1978.

Santore, M. M., Adsorption of polymeric molecules and steric stabilization of latexes, in *Advances in Emulsion Polymerization and Latex Technology*, Vol. 1, 26th Annual Short Course, Lehigh University, June 1995.

Schwartz, A. M., J. W., Perry, and J. Berch, *Surface Active Agents and Detergents*, Vol. 2, Interscience, New York, 1958.

Shaw, D. J., *Introduction to Colloid and Surface Chemistry*, Butterworths, London, 1966.

Shinoda, K., T. Nakagawa, B. Tamamushi, and T. Isemura, *Colloidal Surfactants*, Academic Press, New York, 1963.

Sonntag, H. and K. Strenge, *Coagulation and Stability of Disperrse Systems* (Trans by R. Kondor). Halsted Press, New York, 1972.

Van de Ven, T. G. M., *Colloidal Hydrodynamics*, Academic Press, San Diego CA, 1989.

van Dolsen, K. M. and M. J. Vold, in *Adsorption from Aqueous Solution, ACS Adv. Chem. Ser.* 79:145 (1968).

Voyutskii, S. S., The causes of the stability of emulsions, Russ Chem. Rev. (Engl. transl.), 30:556 (1961).

5

Rheological and Mechanical Properties of Dispersed Systems

Galen W. Radebaugh

Parke-Davis Pharmaceutical Research, Warner-Lambert Company, Morris Plains, New Jersey

I. INTRODUCTION

The response of pharmaceutical materials to an externally applied stress or strain is reflected in their rheological and mechanical properties. The study of the response is referred to as rheology and the application of measurement techniques and instrumentation is referred to as rheometry or viscometry. *Rheology*, by definition, is the study of the flow and deformation of matter. All pharmaceutical materials undergo flow or deformation when subjected to externally applied stress or strain. This includes pharmaceutical systems such as free-flowing elixirs, ointments and creams, foams, and compacted powders.

Pharmaceutical systems undergo flow and deformation in all phases of production and use. Misjudgment or miscalculation of flow and deformation in product formulation or stability testing may lead to not only an inelegant, unstable, or therapeutically deficient product, but may also cause extensive damage to manufacturing and packaging equipment [1]. Of the many pharmaceutical systems, none is subjected to more consumer scrutiny and evaluation than the group consisting of oral suspensions, ointments, creams, pastes, gels, and foams. This is also the group of pharmaceutical systems that has undergone the greatest amount of research and testing. In generations past, a formulator would describe the properties of these systems in terms such as slip, body, or rubout. Today the formulator has more exacting terms to use, such as compliance or modulus. Quantitative parameters can now be measured that relate the structural properties of the pharmaceutical system to end-use performance.

Of particular importance are the parameters that describe the viscoelastic properties of a system. The deformation of any pharmaceutical system can be arbitrarily divided into two types: spontaneously reversible deformation, called *elasticity*; and irreversible deformation, called *flow*. Many classic testing procedures failed to address viscoelastic phenomena and applied idealized newtonian behavior to all systems. Since newtonian describes only idealized behavior, it becomes important to measure those parameters most relevant to the system. The most relevant rheological measurements are those that can be most closely related to end-use performance. For example, viscosity is the most commonly measured parameter, even though the measured amount of viscosity is a function of the test procedure. Soci and Parrott [2] demonstrated that the clinical effectiveness of nitrofurantoin suspension could be extended by increasing the viscosity of the suspension. Ludwig et al. [3] showed that viscosity strongly affects the retention time of polymeric suspensions in the precorneal area of human eyes. Likewise, Pennington et al. [4] found that the clearance rate of colloidal solutions from the nasal cavity could be decreased by increasing their viscosity. A similar result was observed by DiColo and others [5] for the percutaneous absorption of benzocaine. Radebaugh et al. [6] developed new properties of deformation that were capable of differentiating the properties of puncture and shear in polymeric coatings used to taste-mask granules used in pediatric chewable tablets.

This chapter not only explains viscosity, but also describes parameters that define viscoelasticity and other mechanical properties. In addition, it provides references to rheological test techniques that the scientist can use to characterize pharmaceutical systems. There are many techniques and a greater number of types of equipment to measure rheological properties. The burden is on the pharmaceutical scientist to select those techniques that provide the most relevant information that will allow him to predict the effect of rheological changes on end-use performance.

II. FUNDAMENTALS

The elementary rheological properties of most materials can be described in terms of at least three parameters: stress, strain in solids or its liquid equivalent (shear rate), and time. A basic understanding of these parameters and their interaction is essential to the measurement and interpretation of all rheological data. To illustrate the following definitions, some simple problems are included to demonstrate the principles of rheological practices.

A. Stress

There are two types of stress: normal stress and shear stress. Without invoking advanced mathematics, the two can be explained in the following way. If a unit cube (Fig. 1) is

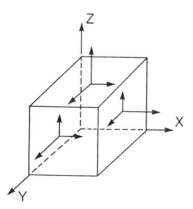

Fig. 1 Force components acting on a cubic volume element.

acted on by a force F tangential to a surface, all the faces of the cube (except the base) will be slightly displaced. The *stress* is defined as the internal force acting on the area A of the cube (i.e., F/A). The force is internal, since it acts to balance out the applied force and keeps the cube in equilibrium. Without the balancing of forces the cube would disintegrate. There are 18 components of stress, one perpendicular to each of the 6 faces of the cube and 12 shear components, 2 perpendicular to each other in each of the 6 faces. Since the forces on the opposite sides of the cube are equal, there are only 9 independent stress components. The component perpendicular to a plane on which the force acts is a *normal stress* (tension out of and compression into the plane). A stress component tangential to a plane is a *shear stress*. The unit of stress in units of the Système International d'Unités (SI units) is the pascal, Pa (1 pascal = newton (N) m^{-2} = 10 dyne cm^{-2}). In the centimeter-grams-second (CGS) system, the unit is the dyne per square centimeter (dyn/cm^2). The symbols for stress adopted by the Society of Rheology [7] are σ for shear stress and σ_E for elongational stress. However, much of the scientific literature uses F, (p) [8], or σ for shear stress.

B. Strain

Strain is the relative deformation of a solid body in response to a stress. There are two major types of strain, elongational or compression strain and shear strain. For small elongation strains, the strain ε is

$$\varepsilon = \frac{\Delta l}{l} \tag{1}$$

where Δl is the change in length of the material and l is the original length before the stress was applied; Δl will be negative if the sample is being compressed. Note that there are no units associated with strain.

Shear strain is deformation produced when successive layers are forced to slide over one another without changing thickness h of the sample. An illustration of this parameter is the displacement of a deck of cards (Fig. 2). The shear strain is $\delta l/h$ and is sometimes denoted as $\tan \gamma$, since $\delta l/h$ equals the tangent of γ. For small angles $\tan \gamma = \gamma$, in radians. Shear strain is unitless.

Problem 1: The upper surface of a gelatin film 1 cm thick is displaced by 0.05 cm. Determine the shear strain (γ) for the film.

Solution: $\tan \gamma = \dfrac{0.05}{1} = 0.05$

To show that $\tan \gamma$ for this small angle is indeed equal to γ, calculate $\tan^{-1}\gamma = 0.05$ in radians. The answer is 0.049996, which varies from 0.05 by 0.08%.

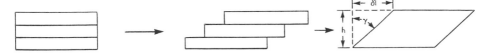

Fig. 2 Illustration of shear strain.

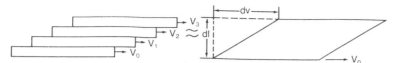

Fig. 3 Illustration of shear rate.

Liquids cannot be strained per se; that is, one cannot elongate or shear strain a liquid for any finite time before the liquid relieves the strain by flowing away. However, if parallel layers or a liquid are moving in the same direction at different velocities (Fig. 3), a velocity gradient dV/dl can be maintained indefinitely. This gradient is called the shear rate. The symbol for shear rate is γ, D, or S. The unit for shear rate is reciprocal seconds (s^{-1}).

Problem 2: Kostenbauder and Martin [9] calculated the approximate shear rate for spreading a layer of ointment 0.2 cm thick on the surface of the skin by using a 6-cm stroke at four strokes per second. What was the calculated shear rate?

$$\text{Solution: } \dot{\gamma} = \frac{V}{l} = \frac{6\text{-cm stroke}^{-1} \times 4 \text{ strokes}^{-1}}{0.2 \text{ cm}}$$

$$= \frac{24 \text{ cm}^{-1}}{0.2 \text{ cm}} = 120^{-1}$$

C. Time

Time is the third important parameter that affects the rheological properties of material. Shear rate itself has units of reciprocal time. Many so-called viscoelastic materials are affected by both stress and time; that is, the response to stress depends on both the magnitude of the stress and the length of time the material is subjected to the stress. Many liquids are affected by shear rate and time. These effects will be covered later in this chapter (see Sec. III.C).

D. Poisson's Ratio

Poisson's ratio μ is an elastic constant obtained from a tensile stress–strain test in which a deformation force is applied two-dimensionally. It is defined for small elongations as the decrease in width of the specimen per unit width, divided by the increase in length per unit length on the application of a tensile force. When Poisson's ratio is equal to 0.5, the volume of the specimen remains constant while being deformed. This condition of constant volume holds for typical pharmaceutical systems, such as liquids and semisolids.

III. ELASTICITY AND VISCOSITY

A. Hookeian and Newtonian Systems

Two very important relationships are derived from the interactions between stress and either strain or shear rate. The first is Hooke's law, which states that within elastic limits, the ratio of stress to stain in an elastic material is constant. No real material is elastic at all stresses. At some point the material will yield or fail. The proportionality constant between stress and tensile strain is known as Young's modulus E, or the elastic modulus. The corresponding constant for shear stress and strain is the shear modulus G.

$$E = \frac{\text{tensile stress}}{\text{tensile strain}} = \frac{\sigma_E}{\varepsilon} \tag{2}$$

$$G = \frac{\text{shear stress}}{\text{shear strain}} = \frac{\sigma}{\gamma} \tag{2a}$$

The units of measure for the moduli are the same as those for stress, that is, pascals or dynes per square centimeter, since strain is unitless. Engineers use kilogram force per square meter or pounds per square inch (psi). The reciprocals of E and G are sometimes used. The reciprocal of the elastic modulus E is known as the tensile compliance D. The reciprocal of the shear modulus G is known as the shear compliance J.

A similar relationship for liquids was discovered by Newton, who related shear stress to shear rate with the proportionality constant, η, which is defined as viscosity. The relationship is described mathematically in Eqs. (3) and (3a).

$$\frac{F}{A} = \sigma = \eta \frac{V}{l} = \eta \dot{\gamma} \tag{3}$$

or

$$\eta = \frac{\sigma}{\dot{\gamma}} = \frac{\text{shear stress}}{\text{shear rate}} \tag{3a}$$

Viscosity is a measure of a liquid's resistance to flow. As the value of η decreases; less and less stress is required to maintain $\dot{\gamma}$ at a constant value. The converse also is true: as η increases, σ must increase to maintain a constant shear rate.

The SI unit for viscosity is the pascal-second (Pa-s). In the CGS system, it is poise (P). One pascal-second = 10 poise = 10 dyn-s cm^{-2}.

Problem 3: A shear stress of 1×10^3 dyn cm^{-2} is required to maintain a shear rate of 100 s^{-1}; that is, 100/s. What is the viscosity of the fluid being sheared?

Solution: $\eta = \dfrac{\sigma}{\dot{\gamma}} = \dfrac{\text{shear stress}}{\text{shear rate}} = \dfrac{1 \times 10^3 \text{ dyn cm}^{-2}}{100^{-1}} = \dfrac{10 \text{ dyn-sec}}{\text{cm}^3}$

$= 10 \text{ P} = 1 \text{ Pa-s}$

Note: A shear rate of 100 s^{-1} is a little more than the shear rate of pouring water from a bottle.

Graphically, the properites of a newtonian liquid are portrayed by a straight line that passes through the origin and has a slope equal to the viscosity (Fig. 4). An elastic solid is described in an analogous way, the slope being the elastic (tensile or shear) modulus or Young's modulus (Fig. 5).

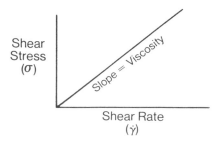

Fig. 4 Rheological behavior of a newtonian liquid.

B. Nonnewtonian or Generalized Newtonian Liquids

Very few, if any, liquids are truly newtonian; very few, that is, exhibit a direct proportionality between shear stress and shear rate at all shear rates, or a constant viscosity at all shear rates. However, a number of low molecular weight liquids can be considered newtonian for all practical purposes. Typical newtonian liquids include water,
alcohols, glycerin, and true solutions. Emulsions suspensions, dispersions, and polymer
solutions or melts are generally nonnewtonian, as though this is dependent on concentration; that is, the higher the concentration the more likely the material is nonnewtonian.

Nonnewtonian liquids can display a wide range of behaviors. The essential characteristics of a nonnewtonian liquid is that the viscosity is not directly proportional to
the shear rate. In other words, the viscosity changes with shear rate. Some nonnewtonian
liquids also show time dependencies. It is often difficult to differentiate a nonlinear
behavior from a time dependency with a single experiment. Time dependency will be
covered in Section III.C.

1. Bingham or Plastic Flow

There are several types of nonnewtonian rheological behavior that can be described by
relatively simple mathematical equations. A pure Bingham liquid is probably the simplest of these (Fig. 6a). An ideal Bingham flow requires an initial stress, the yield stress
σ_y, before it starts to flow. Once it has started to flow, its behavior corresponds to that
of a newtonian liquid. This type of behavior is known as *plastic flow* and may be expressed mathematically by Eq. (4):

$$\sigma - \sigma_y = U\dot{\gamma} \quad \text{or} \quad U = \frac{\sigma - \sigma_y}{\dot{\gamma}} \tag{4}$$

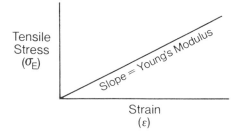

Fig. 5 Rheological behavior of an ideal elastic solid.

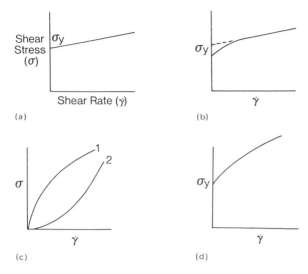

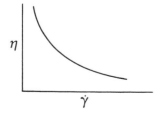

Fig. 6 Typical nonnewtonian responses: (a) ideal Bingham flow, (b) real Bingham flow, (c) pseudoplastic flow, and (d) pseudoplastic flow imposed on Bingham flow.

where σ_y is the yield point, $\dot{\gamma}$ is the shear rate, σ is the shear stress, and U is the plastic viscosity, which is equal to the slope of the flow curve. At stress less than the yield stress the material behaves as an elastic solid.

Problem 4: Show that the viscosity (η) of a Bingham material actually decreases as the shear rate increases. Graph η as a function of shear rate.

Solution: Remember that the viscosity η always equals shear stress over shear rate. Until the shear stress becomes greater than the yield stress (σ_y), the viscosity (η) is undefined, since $\dot{\gamma}$ equals zero. At very low shear rates ($\dot{\gamma} \to 0$), η is relatively large; for example, if $\sigma = 1000$ dyn cm^{-2} and $\dot{\gamma} = 1$ s^{-1} , then the viscosity is 1000 dyn-s cm^{-2} = 1000 P = 100 Pa-s. At high shear rates the viscosity becomes relatively small; for example, if $\sigma = 2000$ dyn cm^{-2} and $\dot{\gamma}$ is 100 s^{-1}, the viscosity is 20 dyn-s cm^{-1} = 20 P = 2 Pa-s. The plastic viscosity approaches U as $\dot{\gamma} \to \infty$. Graphically this behavior is illustrated in Fig. 7. The value of U, the plastic viscosity, is constant over this range.

Fig. 7 The viscosity (η) of a Bingham liquid.

In real Bingham liquids, the transition from a stationary liquid to a flowing liquid is not nearly as abrupt as that illustrated in Fig. 6a. Figure 6b illustrates the behavior of a real Bingham liquid. The yield point for this type of liquid is extrapolated from the linear portion of the curve to the shear stress axis. The yield point is often used to characterize the rheology of creams and suspensions. Plastic flow (i.e., Bingham flow), is normally associated with flocculated or coagulated particles in concentrated solutions. The flocculated particles add an increased degree of structure to the system. The yield point is a measure of the degree of flocculation, since an increase in structure requires a greater stress to initiate motion in the system.

2. *Pseudoplastic Flow*

Many emulsions, dispersions, and polymeric solutions have rheological properties that can be represented by the two curves of Fig. 6c. For these two curves, the slope at any given point is the apparent viscosity of the liquid; that is, the viscosity is changing continuously. the viscosity is shear stress over shear rate and is constant only for varying shear rates in newtonian liquids.

Curve 1 in Fig. 6c illustrates the rheological behavior known as *shear thinning*. The slope of the curve and, therefore, the viscosity is high initially and decreases with increasing shear rate, thus the name shear thinning. Curve 2 illustrates the opposite behavior, which is appropriately known as *shear thickening*. In shear thickening, the viscosity is low for low shear rate and increases with increasing shear rate.

Shear thinning, a result of a varying shear rate, should not be confused with thixotropy. *Thixotropy* is the reversible loss of viscosity, as a function of time, at a constant shear rate. *Reversible* means that the viscosity will return to its original value with time in the absence of agitation. In a similar way, negative thixotropy is a reversible increase in viscosity, as a function of time, at a constant shear rate. More will be said about these phenomena in connection with time-dependent phenomena (see Sec. III.C).

The reader should also be familiar with rheomalaxis or rheodestruction. *Rheomalaxis* is the permanent loss of viscosity owing to shearing. There is no rebuilding of the structure responsible for viscosity in the material. An example of rheomalaxis is the permanent loss of viscosity of a high molecular weight polymer solution subjected to high shear rates. High shear rates are capable of breaking covalent bonds in polymers. The resulting lower molecular weight polymer will show a decreased solution viscosity.

Many shear-thinning and shear-thickening liquids behave according to the "power law." One of the several representations of the power law to given in Eq. (5):

$$\dot{\gamma} = \psi\sigma^N \tag{5}$$

where ψ and N are constants characteristic of the material and $\dot{\gamma}$ and σ are shear rate and shear stress, respectively.

If the two curves in Fig. 6c are plotted on a logarithmic scale on both axes, the curves become straight lines (see Problem 6 for a single curve). Power law liquids with N greater than 1 are shear thinning, whereas those with N less than 1 are shear thickening. When $N = 1$ and $\psi = 1/\eta$, η is the newtonian viscosity. Not all shear thinning and shear thickening materials obey the power law equation.

Problem 5: Another common form of the power law is $\sigma = k\dot{\gamma}^\eta$, where $\eta = 1/N$ and $k = \psi^{-1/N}$. Show that this equation is equivalent to Eq. (5).

Solution: Make the substitutions in the second equation; that is, $\eta = \psi^{-1/N}\dot{\gamma}^{1/N}$. Put this equation in a logarithmic form, that is, $\log \sigma = (-1/N)\log \psi + (1/N)\log \dot{\gamma}$, and

Solve for $\log \dot{\gamma}$: $\log \dot{\gamma} = N \log \sigma + \log \psi$
Solve for $\log \dot{\gamma}$ in Eq. (5): $\log \dot{\gamma} = N \log \sigma + \log \psi$

The two equations are identical. Q.E.D.

The logarithmic equation is of the form $y = mx + b$, the equation of a line; in this case, $y = \log \dot{\gamma}$, N equals the slope (m), $x = \log \sigma$, and b equals the intercept (i.e., $\log \psi$). Therefore, the values for N and ψ in Eq. (5) can be easily determined from a plot of data of $\log \sigma$ versus $\log \psi$. Alternatively, a pocket calculator capable of performing linear regressions can quickly determine N and ψ for a set of measured values of shear stresses at given shear rates. The two parameters, N and ψ, can be used to characterize a given material, just as a yield point and slope can be used for a Bingham material.

Problem 6: Shear stresses were measured at six different shear rates for a lotion. The values were as follows:

$\dot{\gamma}$ (s^{-1}):	1	10	30	50	80	100
σ(dyn/cm^2):	9.78	43.0	87.1	121.0	163.7	188.9

(a) Plot $\dot{\gamma}$ versus σ; (b) calculate the viscosity at each shear rate; (c) plot the appropriate logarithmic curve and determine the values for ψ and N; (d) state whether the lotion is shear thickening or shear thinning and tell why.

Solution: a. See Fig. 8.
b. $\eta = \sigma/\dot{\gamma}$; therefore:

$\dot{\gamma}$ (s^{-1}):	1	10	30	50	80	100
σ (dyn cm^2):	9.78	43.0	87.1	121.0	163.7	189
η (dyn-s cm^{-2}):	9.78	4.3	2.90	2.42	2.05	1.89

c. See Fig. 9. The linear regression of $\log \dot{\gamma}$ versus $\log \sigma$ gives a slope of 1.555 and an intercept of -1.540; therefore, $N = 1.56$, and $\psi = 10^{-1.540} = 0.0288$.
d. Since the value of N is 1.56, which exceeds 1, the material is shear thinning. This can also be determined from answer b, which indicates that the viscosity of the lotion is becoming lower with an increasing shear rate.

Dilatancy is a phenomena best defined and illustrated by an example. Anyone who has walked along a beach knows that if the feet are placed gently on wet sand they will sink. However, if one steps on the same sand very rapidly, the sand will become rigid. Materials that behave in this way are called dilatant. The mechanism is as follows. The grains of sand in the undisturbed state are close-packed. When the sand is vigorously agitated, the water no longer fills all the interstices. The sand appears to become dry because its volume has increased. It is the *increase in volume* that makes dilatancy dif-

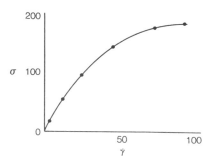

Fig. 8 Shear rate versus shear stress.

ferent from shear thickening. Dilatancy is not a synonym for shear thickening, since normal shear thickening is not accompanied by a volume change.

Dilatancy can take place when the ratio of solid phase to the liquid phase is large. This may occur in paints, inks, mineral slurries, or concentrated starch pastes. One must be very careful when milling dilatant materials, since they tend to solidify suddenly. Motors can become overheated rapidly because of the great, and often sudden, increase in viscosity of the material being stirrred. The flow curve for a dilatant material resembles curve 2 in Fig. 6c, but exhibits a much more rapid increase in slope with increasing shear rate.

3. *Non-Bingham Flow*

Figure 6d illustrates a material that initially behaves like a Bingham material; that is, it possesses a yield point, but after yielding, it behaves like a power law material. The simplest mathematical model for this type of material is known as the Herschel–Bulkley model and is given in Eq. (6):

$$\sigma = \sigma_y + k\dot{\gamma}^n \tag{6}$$

where $k\dot{\gamma}^n$ is defined as in Problem 5. Again the parameters in the equation (i.e., σ_y, + k, and n) characterize the rheological properties of the material.

C. Time-Dependent Phenomena

The term *thixotropy* was mentioned briefly in the preceding section. Thixotropy is a phenomena that occurs very frequently in dispersed systems. It is defined as a revers-

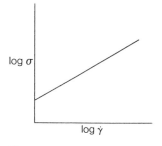

Fig. 9 Log shear rate versus log shear stress.

ible, time-dependent decrease in viscosity at a constant shear rate. As a rule, a thixo-tropic material is a dispersion that shows an isothermal gel–sol–gel transformation. A gel is a colloidal system that possesses a yield point, whereas a sol is a colloidal sys-tem that does not possesses a yield point. The mechanism of thixotropy is the break-down and re-forming of the gel–sol–gel structure.

Figure 10a shows the shear stress in a thixotropic material as a function of time at several shear rates. If shearing is continued long enough, the shear stress becomes con-stant. The significance of thixotropy as a time effect as well as a shear rate effect is frequently not made clear. Thus, thixotropy is often confused with shear thinning.

Figure 10b shows the results of a typical experiment conducted on a thixotropic material. An initial shear rate of $\dot{\gamma}$ produces a shear stress of A. After a period at a shear rate of $\dot{\gamma}_1$, the shear stress will decrease to B. An increase in shear rate to $\dot{\gamma}_2$, will raise the shear stress to point C, where a loss of shear stress will again occur. This process may be repeated many times until a complete up-curve has been generated. The process is then reversed by decreasing the shear rate in steps and maintaining shearing times equal to those used in the up-curve. Figure 10b shows a rise in the shear stress as the shear rate is decreased (H to I in the down-curve). This effect is not always seen, since some materials will not regain their structure while under shear. Figure 11 shows thixotropic loops for materials sheared for two different time intervals. Curve A results from short shear times, whereas curve B is observed during long-time shearing. The formation of a thixotropic loop is the accepted criterion of thixotropy. A pure shear-thinning fluid will not show a loop. These curves were constructed from data generated by the type of experiment shown in Fig. 10b. Instruments that generate a continuously changing shear rate are available. The area enclosed within the up-curve and the down-curve is known as a thixotropic hysteresis loop.

Care must be taken to avoid long shearing times, which produces irreversible changes, and to maintain constant temperatures during the experiment. Temperature changes can produce spurious results, since shear stress at a constant shear rate, is also a function of temperature. Whorlow [8] presents a detailed explanation of the measure-ment and precautions for examining thixotropic materials.

Thixotropy is quite common, but pure thixotropic materials are unusual. Usually the thixotropic nature of a material is superimposed on another rheological behavior. Idson [10] shows curves similar to those in Fig. 12 for the thixotropic effect superimposed on a Bingham material, a pseudoplastic material, and a dilatant paste. Examples of com-mon thixotropic materials are gelatin, mayonnaise, latex paint, and many emulsion sys-tems.

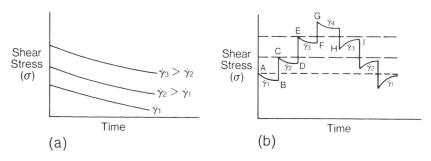

Fig. 10 Thixotropy: (a) individual shear rates as a function of time and (b) composite curve with varying shear rates.

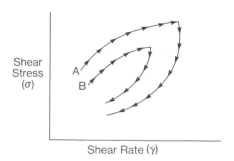

Fig. 11 Thixotropic loops at short (A) and long (B) times of shear.

1. *Quantitation of Thixotropy*

Several methods have been proposed for the quantitation of thixotropy. The area of the hysteresis loop has been mentioned as one way of measuring thixotropy. However, as shown in the preceding section, the area of hysteresis loop is very much dependent on the time taken to make the measurement as well as the maximum shear rate. As Whorlow [8] states, "There is no reason to suppose that two materials which give identical loops in a 15 second sequence of speed changes would necessarily give identical loops in a 5 second sequence."

Sherman [11] indicates that it is "possible for the hysteresis loop to be an artifact." He cites the effects of viscous heating and inertial forces as a source of the artifact. Viscous heating is the heat produced by the physical interaction of the liquid and the measuring device. Changing the inertia of a liquid can also convert mechanical energy to heat energy. When energy is added to a liqiud that is not adequately cooled, the temperature of the liquid increases. Herein, the hysteresis is due to the change in temperature of the liquid and is not a true hysteresis, which requires a constant temperature.

There is one condition in which a thixotropic material will yield a consistent curve. When the up-curve loss in shear stress with time (A–B in Fig. 13a) and the down-curve recovery of shear stress (E–F) both approach the same respective limiting value for a number of shear rates and shear stresses, then a plot of these equilibrium shear stresses versus their respective shear rates will yield an equilibrium hysteresis curve (see Fig. 13b). Such a curve obviously has no hysteresis loop and is also rarely found in nature.

Despite all the possible pitfalls in making hysteresis loop measurements, the method is commonly used to characterize materials of many different types. One method for

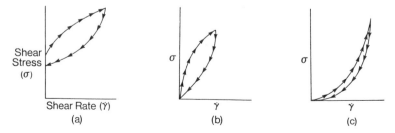

Fig. 12 Thixotropic behavior superimposed on nonnewtonain responses. (a) on a Bingham material, (b) on a pseudoplastic material, and (c) on a dilatant paste.

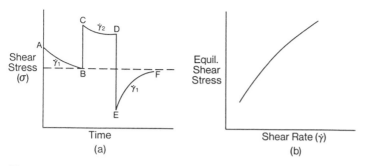

Fig. 13 Equilibrium hysteresis curves.

quantitating thixotropic behavior in Bingham (plastic) materials is to measure the plastic viscosity U of the down-curves for two values of shearing times (t_1 and t_2). Figure 14 shows the shearing sequence for this determination. The uppermost down-curve (A) occurs when the shear rate is immediately reversed after it reaches its maximum value. Down-curve B occurs when the maximum shear rate is applied for time t_1 before reversing, and down-curve C occurs when the maximum shear rate is applied for time t_2. Note that in a Bingham material, the down-curve as well as the up-curve are linear (after the extrapolated yield point). The slope of each down-curve is the plastic viscosity U for each condition of shearing time. From this type of experiment, a thixotropic coefficient B is calculated: this is the rate of breakdown of structure with time at constant shear rate and is calculated as follows:

$$B = \frac{U_B - U_C}{\ln(t_2/t_1)} \tag{7}$$

where U_B and U_C are the plastic viscosities of the down-curves after t_1 and t_2 shearing times, respectively. Since the choice of the maximum shear rate is arbitrary, the same objections raised for hysteresis loops can be raised here.

A second measure of thixotropy in Bingham materials is the so-called coefficient of thixotropic breakdown M, shown in Eq. (8).

$$M = \frac{2(U_1 - U_2)}{\ln(\dot{\gamma}_2/\dot{\gamma}_1)^2} \tag{8}$$

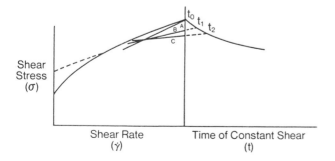

Fig. 14 Graphic method for determining the thixotropic coefficient B.

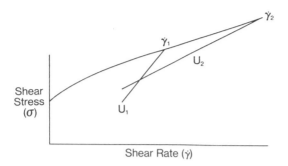

Fig. 15 Experimental curve for determining the "coefficient of thixotropic breakdown."

where U_1 and U_2 are the plastic viscosities for two separate down-curves having maximum shear rates of $\dot{\gamma}_1$ and $\dot{\gamma}_2$, respectively (Fig. 15). The original relationship, derived by Green and Weltmann [12] was based on an empirical finding that the area of the thixotropic hysteresis curve was proportional to the revolutions per minute (rpm) of their viscometer. In Eq. (8), $\dot{\gamma}_1$ and $\dot{\gamma}_2$ were originally angular velocities ω_1 and ω_2, not shear rates. This equatoin has been stated incorrectly in several references. The method is again faulted because the values of $\dot{\gamma}_1$ and $\dot{\gamma}_2$ are arbitrary.

2. *Complex Thixotropic Curves*

In a previous section, the superimposed effect of thixotropy on classic rheological curves was described (see Fig. 12). Not all thixotropic materials are so well behaved. Boylan [13] demonstrated some of the abnormalities of thixotropy in his study of white petrolatum USP, as shown in Fig. 16a, which is typical of a "bulge"-type hysteresis curve.

Boylan explained the shape of the curve in terms of the breakdown in structure of the three components of white petrolatum: normal paraffins, isoparaffins, and cyclic paraffins. Normal paraffins can align themselves in the direction of the shear. Isoparaffins and cyclic paraffins do so less readily. The unaligned iso- and cyclic paraffins provide the initial "body" to the up-cruve until, at high shear rates, all the paraffins align and disentangle. The disentangled chains remain that way during the down-curve and, therefore, yield a much flatter curve.

Ober et al. [14] demonstrated the classic "spur"-type thixotropic curve (see Fig. 16b) in a study of a procaine penicillin gel. The spur value Y is the point at which rapid breakdown or consolidation of structure is taking place. The authors showed that peni-

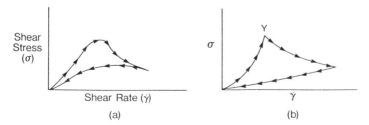

(a)   (b)

Fig. 16 (a) Bulge-type curve and (b) spur-type curve. (Adapted from a, Ref. 13 and b, Ref. 14.)

cillin gels that behave in this manner formed intramuscular deposits after injection. These deposits intended to prolong blood levels of the drug.

Carboxymethylcellulose solutions also tend to give rheograms that contain spur points. The mechanisms by which bulges and spurs occur are usually not obvious and continue to be controversial.

3. *Negative Thixotropy and Rheopexy*

Negative thixotropy or antithixotropy is a time-dependent increase in viscosity at constant shear. Dispersions that show negative thixotropy typically contain between 1 and 10% solids (in contrast with dilatant systems, which contain more than 50 vol% solids). Negative thixotropy is *not* the same as dilatancy, which is shear rate-dependent.

There is some disagreement about the equivalence of negative thixotropy and rheopexy. *Rheopexy* has been defined as negative thixotropy, on one hand, and, on the other hand, as "a phenomenon in which a sol forms a gel more readily when gently shaken or otherwise sheared than when allowed to form the gel while the material is kept at rest" [15]. In the latter definition of a rheopectic system, the gel is the equilibrium form, whereas in antithixotropy, the equilibrium state is the sol [16].

The first definition uses a phenomenological approach; that is, during the rheological measurement, the material under study shows an increase in viscosity as a function of time. The second mechanistic definition requires specific information on the (generally unknown) mechanism of the phenomenon. Therefore, for practical purposes, the first definition is more direct, and rheopexy and negative thixotropy may be used interchangeably. Magnesia magma and clay suspensions may show negative thixotropy, but very few other materials are known to show this phenomenon.

D. Viscoelasticity

1. *Modeling of Rheological Behavior and Simple Viscoelasticity*

a. Modeling Elements

To understand complex rheological behavior more clearly, the use of mechanical models is sometimes useful. The simplest model for elasticity is the ideal spring (Fig. 17a), since, by definition, it obeys Hooke's law. This model is known as a Hooke body or a hookeian element. The corresponding newtonian body or element is called a dashpot (see Fig. 17b). A dashpot comprises a piston inside a cylinder filled with a fluid of viscosity, η. As the piston is moved through the fluid, the fluid between the piston and cyl-

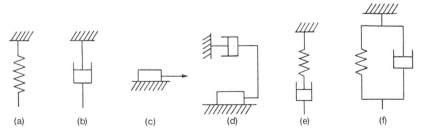

(a) (b) (c) (d) (e) (f)

Fig. 17 Various elements used in modeling rheological behavior: (a) hookeian, (b) newtonian, (c) Saint-Venant body, (d) model for Bingham plastic, (e) Maxwell element, and (f) Voigt or Kelvin element.

inder walls is sheared, thereby producing a stress proportional to the viscosity of the fluid. When the force applied to the piston becomes zero, the piston stops and does not return to its starting point. A hookeian element does return to its starting point as the force becomes zero.

By using one additional element, known as the Saint-Venant body or element most elementary rheological systems can be modeled. The Saint-Venant body (see Fig. 17c) is a weight lying on a flat surface. The weight will not move until a force large enough to overcome the static friction of the weight–surface interface is applied. Once the static friction has been overcome, the weight will move at a constant velocity under the influence of a constant force.

The parallel combination of the Saint-Venant body and the newtonian body (see Fig. 17d) models the behavior of a Bingham plastic. The dashpot cannot move and, therefore, cannot add to the stress until the Saint-Venant body moves. Once the Saint-Venant body has started to move, the dashpot moves. The total force observed for the system is the force to overcome the Saint-Venant body plus the force to shear the fluid in the newtonian element. This behavior is exactly the same as that of a Bingham plastic. The yield point of the Bingham plastic is modeled by the Saint-Venant body. The linear plastic viscosity U is modeled by the newtonian element. (See Fig. 6a for the flow characteristics of a Bingham plastic.) If power law fluids are used in the dashpot instead of newtonian fluids, behavior such as that shown in Fig. 6d is modeled.

Two other models, the Maxwell model and the Voigt or Kelvin model, are useful for modeling the rheological behavior known as viscoelasticity. Viscoelasticity may be viewed as a combination of viscous and elastic properties. A good example for illustrating viscoelastic properties is polymethylsiloxane, an organic silicone polymer used in making "silly putty." When rolled into a sphere and dropped, this material will bounce like a rubber ball. When left undisturbed, this material will deform to a puddle under the influence of gravity. Other examples of viscoelastic materials are molten polymers, chewing gum, and most gels.

b. Stress Relaxation and the Maxwell Model

The Maxwell body or element consists of a newtonian element in series with a hookeian element (see Fig. 17e). The Maxwell element is used to model a property of viscoelasticity known as stress relaxation. *Stress relaxation* is the change in stress under a constant strain as a function of time.

Example: A strip of viscoelastic plastic 10 cm long is instantaneously strained to 10.05 cm. The stress to maintain the strain is recorded after 1, 5, 10, 20, 60, and 600 s. The stress is plotted versus time to give a stress relaxation curve (Fig. 18).

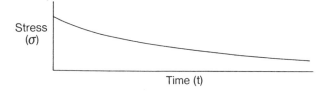

Fig. 18 Stress relaxation curve.

The Maxwell model behaves exactly as the example. At zero time the total stress is supported by the spring. As the dashpot slowly extends, less and less stress is supported by the spring, which contracts. After a long enough period, all the stress is relieved by the flow of the dashpot, at which time the stress becomes zero.

The mathematical expression for the stress as a function of time is

$$\sigma = \gamma_0 G^{(-Gt/\eta)} \tag{9a}$$

for shear stress relaxation and for tensile stress relaxation is

$$\sigma_E = \varepsilon_0 E^{(-Et/\eta)} \tag{9b}$$

where σ or σ_E is the stress, γ_0 or ε_0 is the initial shear or tensile strain. G or E is the shear or elastic modulus, and η is the viscosity of the fluid in the dashpot.

The ratios η/G and η/E are known as the relaxation time, that is, the time for the stress to fall to $1/e$ of its initial value, where e is the base of the natural logarithm.

Mathematically, the strain as a function of time is given in Eq. (10) for shear strain and tensile strain respectively:

$$\gamma = \frac{\sigma}{G} + \frac{\sigma t}{\eta} \quad \text{or} \quad \varepsilon = \frac{\sigma_E}{E} + \frac{\sigma_E t}{\eta} \tag{10}$$

c. Creep and the Voigt Model

The second model is known as the Voigt or Kelvin model, which models fairly solid materials. The Voigt element consists of a newtonian element in parallel with a hookeian element (see Fig. 17f). The Voigt model is useful in modeling the viscoelastic property known as creep. *Creep* is the change in strain under a constant stress as a function of time.

Example: A viscoelastic plastic 10 cm long is subjected to a stress of 1 kPa. The strain is measured at 1, 5, 10, 30, 60, and 600 s. The strain is plotted versus time to give a creep curve (Fig. 19).

Again the Voight model follows the behavior of the example. The applied stress is shared between the elements, since each experiences the same strain; that is, both elements are extended the same distance that is controlled by the spring. The final strain

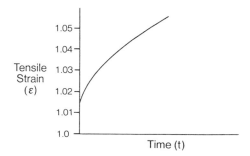

Fig. 19 Creep curve.

is limited by the elongation limit of the spring. The shear strain as a function of time is given by Eq. (11).

$$\dot{\gamma} = \frac{\sigma_0}{G}[1 - \exp(-Gt/\eta)] \qquad (11)$$

For creep the ratios η/E and η/G are known as the *retardation time* τ, the time required for strain to relax to $1/e$ of its initial value when the stress is removed. Tensile strain as a function of time is determined by inserting the corresponding tensile parameters into Eq. (11). The stress at a constant strain, for a Voight model, is totally due to the hookeian element and is defined in Eq. (12).

$$\sigma = \gamma_0 E = \text{constant} \qquad (12)$$

Real viscoelastic materials are not accurately modeled by any of these models, but the models facilitate analysis of the processes of creep and stress relaxation. Combinations of Maxwell and Voigt elements are capable of closely modeling real viscoelastic materials.

2. *Complex Viscosity*

A brief phenomenological description of viscoelastic behavior was given in the preceding section. It is apparent that stress, strain, and shear rate (time) are involved in the rheological behavior of viscoelastic materials. In practice, stress is not always directly proportional to strain, but may be related to it in a more complicated way. Abnormalities in time occur whenever stress is a function of both stress and strain rate. When only time abnormalities exist, the behavior is known as *linear viscoelastic*: that is, stress is proportional to strain but varies with time. The theories and mathematics of nonlinear viscoelastic material are beyond the scope of this text. All viscoelastic behavior in this text is assumed to be of the linear type.

a. **Dynamic Measurements**

The effect of transient loading of viscoelastic materials (i.e., creep and stress relaxation) was also desribed in the preceding section. Transient loading measures relatively long relaxation and retardation times; that is, minutes to hours. For a number of pharmaceutically important materials, the rheological effects of interest happen in fractional seconds to a few minutes. For phenomena of such short duration, dynamic or periodic motions of the material are used. Such as sinusodial motions. A dynamic experiment at a frequency ω (rad s^{-1}) is quantitatively equivalent to a transient experiment at $1/\omega$ (s rad^{-1}). If an elastic element is loaded in a periodic way, or any other way, for that matter, the stress will always be in phase with the strain. That is, the stress will be zero when the strain is zero and the stress will be at a maximum when the strain is at a maximum. At any time the ratio of stress to strain will be constant (Fig. 20a).

The newtonian element responds in an entirely different way to a periodic shear. It is fundamental that a liquid responds to a strain rate not a strain. A newtonian liquid exhibits the highest stress when subjected to the highest shear rate. In Fig. 20b, the ordinate of the graph is strain (not strain rate), whereas the slope of the sine curve at any point is the shear rate. The shear rate is at a maximum when the shear strain crosses the time axis. As would be expected, the shear stress also reaches a maximum when the shear rate is maximum (see lower curve in Fig. 20b). The fact that the shear stress,

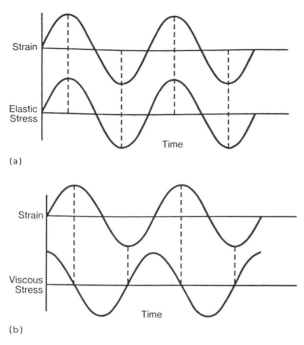

(a)

(b)

Fig. 20 (a) Tensile stress in phase with strain (elastic response) and (b) shear stress 90° out of phase with strain (viscous response).

which is a cosine curve, appears to become negative at regular intervals should not confuse the argument. The apparent negative values are actually positive stresses in the opposite direction; for example, either a push or a pull requires the absolute value of a force, a positive number. For a newtonian element, the stress is said to be 90° out of phase with the strain. That is, if the time axis were marked off in degrees, the maximum stress would occur 90° before and 90° after the maximum strain.

b. Complex Numbers

Electronic engineers use a mathematical tool, known as an imaginary or complex number, to analyze the phase relationships between voltage, current, resistance, and impedance. The rheologist uses the same technique to analyze the relationship between the *elastic modulus* and the *viscous modulus* in a viscoelastic material.

Complex numbers are the sum of a real part and a so-called imaginary part. The imaginary part is composed of a real number multiplied by i, $i = \sqrt{-1}$. A typical complex number could be $73.5 \pm 14.3i$. The presence of i prevents one from combining the 14.3 with the 73.5. This property is just what is needed to separate the elastic modulus from the viscous modulus in the mathematics of viscoelastic material. The so-called complex modulus G^* is expressed as a complex number in Eq. (13).

$$G^* = G' + iG'' \tag{13}$$

where G' is the elastic shear modulus and G'' is the viscous modulus.

There is nothing imaginary, in the usual sense of the word, about these systems. The use of i is merely a tool to keep the in-phase and out-of-phase components separated. The easiest way to demonstrate this is to use a graphic method. One normally labels a graph with the coordinates X and Y. When graphing imaginary numbers, Y became the i axis (Fig. 21). The in-phase component is plotted on the X axis and the out-of-phase component is plotted on the i axis. The complex modulus G is the vector sum of G' and G'' [see Eq. (14)]

$$|G*| = \sqrt{(G')^2 + (G'')^2} \tag{14}$$

The phase angle δ is given by $\tan \delta = G''/G'$:

$$\tan \delta = \frac{G''}{G'} \quad \text{or} \quad \delta = \tan^{-1} \frac{G''}{G'} \tag{15}$$

Experimentally, $G*$ is measured as a torque (or compression–tension), and δ is measured as the phase angle between the elastic and viscous components. The individual components are then calculated by the following equation:

$$G' = |G*| \cos \delta \tag{16a}$$

$$G'' = |G*| \sin \delta \tag{16b}$$

Problem 8: An instrument capable of making dynamic measurements (sinusoidally) determines that $G* = 5.0 \times 10^2$ dyn cm^{-2}, and the phase angle (δ) as 45°. What are the values of G' and G''?

Solution: Both the cosine and the sine of 45° are $1/\sqrt{2} = 0.707$.

Therefore: $G' = G'' = G* \sin \delta = G* \cos \delta = 5.0 \times 10^2$ dyn cm$^{-2} \times 0.707 = 3.535 \times 10^2$ dyn cm^{-2}.

To check this value Eq. (14) can be used:

$$|G*| = [(G')^2 + (G')^2]^{1/2} = [(3.235 \times 10^2 \text{ dyn cm}^{-2})^2$$

$$+ 3.535 \times 10^2 \text{ dyn cm}^{-2})^2]^{1/2}$$

$$= 5 \times 10^2 \text{ dyn cm}^{-2}$$

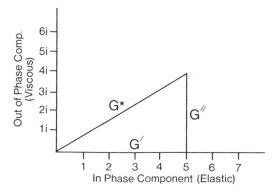

Fig. 21 Plot of complex modulus.

Note that G^*, G', and G'' are moduli, not viscosities; their units are units of stress not viscosity. Complex dynamic viscosity η^* is defined by Eq. (17):

$$\eta^* = \frac{G^*}{\omega} \tag{17}$$

where ω is the frequency of the sine wave in radians per second. The units of complex dynamic viscosity are the same as those of classic viscosity (i.e., dyne-s cm^{-2}, P, or Pa-s).

E. Mathematical Treatment of Viscoelastic Theory

In a dynamic experiment, the stress and strain are sine or cosine functions, and they can be treated as rotating vectors [17,18]. The magnitudes of the vectors are equivalent to the amplitudes of the maximum stress and maximum peak strain. One revolution of the vector is equal to a full cycle of oscillation.

The stress, strain, and rate of strain are complex variables (as previously discussed in Sec. III.D) that can be defined by the following equations:

$$\sigma^* = \sigma_0^{i(\omega t + \delta)} \tag{18}$$

$$\gamma^* = \gamma_0^{i\omega t} \tag{19}$$

where σ^* is the complex stress, γ^* is the complex strain, σ_0 is the maximum magnitude of the stress, γ_0 is the maximum magnitude of the strain, δ is the phase angle between strain and stress, t is time, ω is the angular frequency, and i equals $(-1)^{1/2}$. Differentiation of Eq. (19) is equivalent to a 90° counterclockwise rotation of the vector so that:

$$\frac{d\gamma^*}{dt} = i\omega\gamma_0^{i\omega t} = \omega\gamma_0^{i(\omega t + \pi/2)} \tag{20}$$

where $\omega\gamma_0$ is the magnitude of the rate of strain vector.

The complex shear modulus, G^*, is defined as the ratio of σ^* to γ^*.

$$G^* = \frac{\sigma^*}{\gamma^*} \tag{21}$$

By substituting Eqs. (18) and (19) into Eq. (21) we obtain

$$G^* = (\sigma_0/\gamma_0)^{i(\omega t + \delta)}\exp(-i\omega t) \tag{22}$$

or

$$G^* = (\sigma_0/\gamma_0)(i\delta) \tag{23}$$

From Euler's formula, one knows that

$$\exp(i\delta) = \cos \delta + i(\sin \delta) \tag{24}$$

Some special values of the complex exponential are $\exp(\omega i/2)$ equals i and $\exp (\pi i)$ equals -1. Equation (24) can be substituted into Eq. (23) to obtain:

$$G^* = (\sigma_0/\gamma_0) \cos \delta + i(\sigma_0/\gamma_0) \sin \delta \tag{25}$$

But:

$$G' = (\sigma_0/\gamma_0) \cos \delta \qquad \text{and} \qquad G'' = (\sigma_0/\gamma_0) \sin \delta \qquad \text{(26a and 26b)}$$

Consequently,

$$G^* = G' + iG'' \tag{13}$$

where G' is known as the elastic modulus, storage modulus, or the real modulus. The viscous modulus G'' is also known as the loss modulus, or the imaginary modulus.

The relationship between G' and G'' may be illustrated vectorically as two orthoganol vectors. The tangent between G'' and G' defines the phase angle δ as

$$\tan \delta = \frac{G''}{G'} \tag{27}$$

The physical significance of $\tan \delta$ becomes clearer when one considers the energy dissipated and stored per cycle of deformation for linearly viscoelastic materials. The energy dissipated per cycle is:

$$W = \int \sigma d\gamma = \int \sigma (d\gamma/dt) dt \tag{28}$$

So if it is assumed that the stress is the forcing function according to

$$\sigma(t) = \sigma_0 \sin (\omega t) \tag{29}$$

and the resultant strain can be represented by

$$\gamma(t) = \gamma_0 \sin (\omega t - \delta) \tag{30}$$

then Eq. (29) and (30), with the proper trigonometric identity, can be used to expand Eq. (28) to

$$\Delta W = \sigma_0 \gamma_0 \omega \int \sin(\omega t)[\cos(\omega t) \cos \delta + \sin(\omega t) \cos \delta] dt \tag{31}$$

The first term inside of the closed integral is an odd function and becomes zero after integration. The value of the integral of the second term is $(\pi/\omega) \sin \delta$, so that the energy dissipated per cycle of deformation is given as

$$\Delta W_{cycle} = \pi \sigma_0 \gamma_0 \sin \delta \tag{32}$$

The maximum energy stored per cycle, analogous to the potential energy of a spring at the maximum displacement is

$$W = \frac{1}{2} G(\gamma_o)^2 \tag{33}$$

where G' is the elastic modulus of the material, equivalent to the spring constant. Since $G' = G^* \cos \delta$ and $G^* \gamma_0 = \sigma_0$, then

$$W = \frac{1}{2} \sigma_0 \gamma_0 \cos \delta \tag{34}$$

Equations (32) and (34) can be combined to give the ratio of energy dissipated to maximum energy stored per cycle of deformation as

$$\frac{\Delta W}{W} = 2\pi \tan \delta = 2\pi \left(\frac{G''}{G'} \right) \qquad (35)$$

F. Temperature–Frequency Equivalence

The viscoelastic properties of pharmaceutical systems containing high molecular weight molecules, such as polymers, are extremely temperature-sensitive as well as shear frequency-dependent. Systems that typically contain high molecular weight molecules are semisolid dispersions, such as ointments or creams. Even though the effect of temperature on viscosity has been well documented for pharmaceutical systems, limited information is available on the effect of temperature on their viscoelastic properties. According to the theory of rubberlike elasticity, the elastic moduli of ideal elastomers are proportional to absolute temperature [18]. Since the deformation of a rubberlike material is an activated process in which molecular segments can move only by overcoming potential barriers, a direct relationship exists between the temperature and time-dependence of viscoelastic properties.

Modulus data taken over a range of shear frequencies (which is equivalent to reciprocal time) can be superposed in the same manner that time–temperature superposition is applied to creep and stress–relaxation data [19–22]. This phenomena is extremely useful because the limitations of instrumentation or time often do not allow the measurement of a complete modulus versus frequency spectrum. In spite of this limitation, a curve-shifting procedure can be used to construct a master curve (complete log modulus versus log frequency spectrum at a given temperature). A change in temperature shifts the distribution of modulus curves without changing the shape of the function. The shift of a modulus curve is quantitated in terms of a_T, the shift factor. Radebaugh and Simonelli applied the temperature–frequency relationship to the viscoelastic properties of anhydrous lanolin [23]. In these studies it was found that viscoelastic parameters, determined over a wide range of temperatures and shear frequencies, could be superposed. Elastic moduli (G') and viscous moduli (G'') obtained at low temperatures and frequencies were equivalent to moduli obtained at high temperatures and frequencies. Empirical shifts of modulus versus frequency data obtained at different temperatures were used to produce G' and G'' versus frequency master curves (Figs. 22 and 23). A method of reduced variables, in conjunction with an Arrhenius-type relation, proved useful in calculating the energy of activation for the structural processes involved in a major mechanical transition. The energy of activation was approximately 90 kcal/mol. This compares favorably with the magnitude of energies of activation of high molecular weight polymers undergoing a glass transition. This comparison is significant when one considers the generally low molecular weight composition of lanolin (99% of molecules have a molecular weight between 400 and 950). The magnitude of the energy of activation for lanolin suggests that the intra- and intermolecular forces are as great as those in high molecular weight polymers. Hence, the nature of the functional groups and the chain length of the molecules determine the strength of the structure of the system.

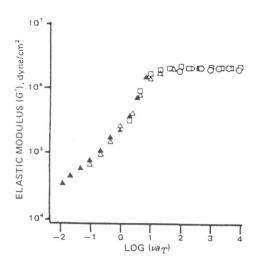

Fig. 22 Reduced frequency master curve of elastic modulus for anhydrous lanolin USP. Key: (○) 0°, (□) 5°, (Δ) 10°, and (▲) 15°.

At this point, it is necessary to examine the mathematical relationships behind temperature–frequency superposition. In general the concept can be expressed as

$$G(T_R, \nu) = G(T, \nu/a_T) \tag{36}$$

where G is either the elastic or viscous modulus, ν is the shear frequency, T_R is the reference temperature of superposition, T is the test temperature, and a_T is the shift factor. The effect of a change in temperature is the same as applying a multiplicative factor to the shear frequency scale. Ideally, there is often an inherent change in modulus brought about by changes in temperature. Each of these changes are compensated by vertical shifts during the construction of the log modulus versus log frequency curve.

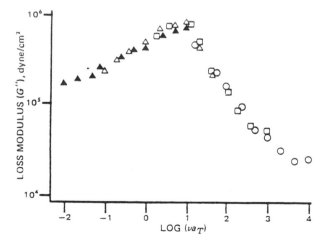

Fig. 23 Reduced frequency master curve of viscous modulus for anhydrous lanolin USP. Key: (○) 0°, (□) 5°, (Δ) 10°, and (▲) 15°.

Consequently, Eq. (36) can be modified to

$$\frac{G(T_R, v)}{T_R \rho(T_R)} = \frac{G(T, v/a_T)}{T\rho(T)} \tag{37}$$

where $\rho(T_R)$ and $\rho(T)$ are the densities of the test sample at the reference temperature and test temperature, respectively [20]. Division by the test temperature corrects for changes in modulus caused by the inherent dependence of modulus on temperature, whereas division by the density corrects for volume changes. To construct a master curve, a reference temperature is arbitrarily chosen, and moduli are measured at various frequencies and temperatures.

By rearranging Eq. (37), the modulus at any frequency relative to the reference temperature can be expressed as

$$G(T_R, v) = \frac{T_R \rho(T_R) G(T, v/a_T)}{T\rho(T)} \tag{38}$$

The shift factors are a function of temperature and are determined relative to the reference temperature. The values of the shift factors must be found empirically by matching the results of adjacent temperatures. Ferry was among the first to use this technique, so the procedure is often referred to as a Ferry reduction scheme [17,21,24]. Superposition, which is also referred to as the method of reduced variables, can reduce experimental work and extend the effective frequency range of results obtained with an instrument of limited frequency capabilities. When the temperature of testing is varied through an appropriate temperature range, a reduced frequency range of many more decades usually can be covered.

The power of this technique was demonstrated with the semisolid anhydrous lanolin [23]. It was demonstrated that one could predict the viscoelastic properties of anhydrous lanolin at shear frequences up to 100,000 s^{-1}, far greater than could be attained with any commercially available mechanical property tester. In reality, shear rates of this magnitude can occur in actual pharmaceutical use. Henderson et al. [25] established shear rates for a variety of situations: up to 120 s^{-1} for topical application of an ointment; 1,000–12,000 s^{-1} for a roller mill; and 5,000–100,000 s^{-1} for high-speed filling equipment.

It has also been theorized that the relationship between temperature and shift factors can be expressed as an Arrhenius-type equation:

$$a_T = A^{E_a RT} \tag{39}$$

where A is the preexponential term, R is the gas constant, T is temperature, and E_a is the energy of activation [17,26,27]. By taking the logarithm and then differentiating both sides of Eq. (39), it can be arranged to obtain

$$E_a = \frac{2.303\ R\ d(\log a_T)}{d(1/T)} \tag{40}$$

Therefore, the shift factors of superposition and be plotted as log a_T verus $1/T$, and the E_a for thermomechanical transitions (typically glass transitions for amorphous polymers) within the material can be calculated from the slope of the plot.

Another empirical relationship was developed by Williams, Landel, and Ferry [28] for amorphous polymers. It is known as the W-L-F equation, and is written as

$$\log a_T = \frac{-C_1(T - T_g)}{(C_2 + T - T_g)} \tag{41}$$

where C_1 and C_2 are constants and T_g is the glass transition temperature. The glass transition temperature is that temperature below which the configurational arrangements of the molecules essentially cease. The empirical constants C_1 and C_2, were originally thought to be universal, but have since shown slight variation from polymer to polymer [18]. The apparent energy of activation for a transition can also be calculated for data fit to the W-L-F equation. By taking the derivative of Eq. (41) relative to T, one obtains

$$\frac{d(\log a_T)}{dT} = \frac{-C_1 C_2}{(C_2 + T + T_g)^2} \tag{42}$$

Equation (42) can then be combined with Eq. (39) to obtain

$$E_a = \frac{2.303\, R C_1 C_2 T^2}{(C_2 + T + T_g)^2} \tag{43}$$

The magnitude of the energy of activation is an indication of the magnitude of the transition. Primary transitions usually have an energy of activation greater than 40 kcal. Their damping peaks will shift ≈ 7–$10°$ for every decade change in frequency. Minor or secondary transitions with much lower energies of activation are more sensitive to frequency and show greater movement on the temperature scale with changes in frequency.

The usefulness of Eqs. (40) and (43) was demonstrated by Radebaugh and Simonelli for anhydrous lanolin [23]. When the shift factors were plotted according to Eq. (40), E_a was approximately 90 kcal/mol. The significance of this value becomes more evident when the E_a is compared with values for polymeric systems. For main glass transitions in which T_R is taken as T_g, the E_a is of the order of 100 kcal/mol [29], secondary transitions at cryogenic temperatures are of the order of 1–10 kcal/mol. Comparisons of the E_a for anhydrous lanolin with experimentally obtained E_a values for polymers indicate that the structural transitions that occur in anhydrous lanolin rival those of a glass transition. This is not what one would expect, since the molecules are of low molecular weight, and the limiting value of the elastic modulus is not as large as one would expect for substances in the glassy state.

When the shift factors were plotted according to the W-L-F equation [Eq. (43)], it was found that anhydrous lanolin does not fit the "ideal" plot. The lack of fit to the W-L-F equation suggests that the transition in anhydrous lanolin is probably not a glass transition, because most polymers that undergo a glass transition obey the W-L-F equation. Even so, the magnitude of the E_a for anhydrous lanolin suggests that intra- and intermolecular force are as great as those in high molecular weight polymers. Hence, the nature of the functional groups and the chain length of the molecules determine the strength of the structure of the system.

IV. VISCOMETRY

There are several reasons for making rheological measurements:

1. To quantitate the effects of time, temperature, ingredients, and processing parameters on a formulation
2. To describe quantitatively the flow behavior of a material for the purpose of quality control
3. To measure the ease of product dispensation from a tube, bottle, or jar
4. To measure spreadability
5. To understand the fundamental nature of the system

The last of these is probably the most important for formulation

A. Fundamental Requirements

The prime objective of any rheological measurement is to determine the fnctional relationship between stress and strain or shear rate and, in the case of viscoelasticity, frequency. Some viscometers measure shear stress at only one shear rate (e.g., 1 kPa at 120 s^{-1}). Others measure stress continously over a wide range of shear rates: for example, the shear rate may vary from 1 to 1000 s^{-1}. No single viscometer is capable of all ranges of shear rates. A combination of viscometers may be used to generate shear rates over a range of 1×10^{-4}–1×10^4 s^{-1} or more.

No matter what instrumentation is used, the material being measured must have certain characteristics:

1. The fluid must be noncompressible. One should not attempt to assess rheological properties of materials that shrink in volume under stress. This type of error might occur in a heavily aerated emulsion. Pure shear involves no volume change.
2. No body forces can exist in the material: that is, the fluid is subjected to not only surface forces, but also to the force of gravity acting on each molecule. The force of gravity, or inertia, is a body force. Some body forces are always present, but they are usually small relative to the viscous forces and are ignored. Body forces can become important when high centrifugal forces are involved in the measurement or when a dispersed phase has an appreciably different density from that of the continuous phase.
3. The viscosity must be independent of pressure. Some rheometers can produce extremely high shear stresses (e.g., pressure-driven capillary rheometers). If the viscosity of the fluid is a function of pressure, the measured viscosity will depend on the pressure generated in the instrument and will not be consistent from instrument to instrument.
4. There must be no slipping at the shearing surfaces. In Fig. 3, the lower layer of fluid has a velocity of zero, the upper layer has a velocity of V_3. If either of these velocities changes owing to nonwetting of the shearing surface or other causes, the shear rate of the fluid will not be the same as the apparent shear rate being generated by the instrument, and the results will be meaningless. This problem can become critical in semisolids because of poor adhesion between the surface of the fluid and the shearing surface of the instrument. The problem also exists in tensile testing whenever the sample slips in the jaws of the tester, thereby creating an effective longer length.

5. Fully developed laminar flow must exist. Figure 3 illustrates laminar flow, each layer is flowing parallel to every other layer. The shear rate is defined in terms of the velocity gradient dv/dl, which assumes laminar flow.

6. The material must be at a constant temperature (isothermal) throughout the measurement. Viscosity is strongly dependent on temperature. This relationship can be expressed, in many cases, by an equation analogous to the Arrhenius equation, which is used in chemical kinetics:

$$\eta = A^{E_v/RT} \tag{44}$$

where E_v is the "activation energy" required to initiate flow between molecules, and A is a constant that is a function of molecular weight and molar volume of the fluid; R is the gas constant (1.987 cal mol^{-1}), and T is the absolute temperature (K). Note that e is raised to the positive E_v/RT not the negative value used in the Arrhenius equation and that E_v is also a function of temperature, since the bonds linking the molecules of the fluid are broken with increasing temperature. Thus, a plot of log η versus $1/T$ generally does not yield a straight line for large temperature differences.

B. Types of Rheological Instruments

Instrumentation used for rheological meaurements has been comprehensively covered by Whorlow [8] and also by Sherman and by Van Wazer [11,22]. The types of instruments can be divided into five categories: falling or rolling sphere, capillary or tube, steady rotation, dynamic, and miscellaneous.

1. Falling or Rolling Sphere Viscometer

A falling or rolling sphere viscometer consists of a cylindrical transparent tube having a graduated section near the middle of its length and, typically, a steel ball bearing that is allowed to fall through or roll along the tube. The tube is filled with the fluid of interest, and the time required for the ball to travel between the graduation marks is measured. The viscosity for newtonian fluids can be obtained directly from a relationship based on Stokes' law [30,31], as shown in Eq. (45):

$$\eta = \left(\frac{2}{9}\right)(\rho_1 - \rho_2)\frac{gr^2}{v} \tag{45}$$

where ρ_1 is the density of the ball, ρ_2 is the density of the fluid, g is the acceleration caused by gravity, r is the radius of the ball, and v is the velocity of the ball.

This equation assumes no wall effects; that is, an infinite value of fluid and a vertical tube. However, if the tube is calibrated against a fluid of known viscosity, Eq. (46) can be used:

$$\eta = K(\rho_2 - \rho_1)t \tag{46}$$

where K is an instrumental constant and t is the time required for the ball to travel between two marks on the cylinder. This method can be used for either falling or rolling balls. For the rolling ball, the tube would be at an angle other than 90°.

When the tube is at 90°, the shear rate is at the maximum and is defined as follows:

$$\dot{\gamma} = \frac{3v}{2r} \tag{47}*$$

where v is velocity of the sphere and r is radius of the sphere. At angles other than $0°$, at which the shear rate is zero (since the tube is horizontal and the ball cannot roll), the shear rate is difficult to quantitate owing to wall effects. The tube must be long enough for the ball to attain a constant velocity before reaching the first timing mark.

This method is not applicable to the complete characterization of nonnewtonian fluids, since the viscosity of nonnewtonian fluids varies with shear rate and since a falling ball generates only a single shear rate. However, the viscosity at a single shear rate can be determined for a nonnewtonian system.

The falling sphere viscometer can be used for a wide range of viscosiites (e.g., 10^{-4}–10^3 P), by varying the distance between the marks on the cylinder or by varying the density of the ball being used. It can also be used at high temperatures and high pressures.

2. *Capillary Viscometers*

Capillary viscometers span the range from simple glass tubes to very costly pressure-driven instruments. The capillary viscometer was invented in the mid-1800s by Hagen and Poiseuille, who also developed the law describing the viscosity of a fluid flowing through a capillary, Eq. (48) (for derivation see Ref. 8, p. 60):

$$\eta = \frac{\pi r^4 \Delta P}{8LQ} \tag{48}$$

where r is the radius, ΔP is the difference in pressure between the top of the capillary and the bottom, L is the length of the tube, and Q is the volume flowing through the tube *per second*. In CGS units, r and L are given in centimeters, ΔP in dynes per square centimeter, Q in cubic centimeters per second, and η in poise. The viscosity is measured by measuring the time for the liquid to flow between two points on the capillary.

The capillary viscometer can also be calibrated against a known fluid and then used for an unknown material, as shown in Eq. (49)

$$\frac{\eta_K/\rho_K}{\eta_u/\rho_u} = \frac{t_k}{t_u} \quad \text{or} \quad \eta_u = \frac{\eta_K \rho_u t_u}{\rho_K t_K} \tag{49}$$

where η_u is the unknown viscosity, η_K is the known viscosity, ρ_k and ρ_u are densities of the known and unknown fluids, respectively, and t_k and t_u are the flow times for the known and unknown fluids, respectively.

The measured viscosity of a liquid divided by its density [e.g., η_k/ρ_k in Eq. (49)] is known as the kinematic viscosity and is expressed in units of stokes. The stokes (St) has units of square centimeters per second.

The kinematic viscosity is important when a material is pumped through pipes. When a viscous fluid flows through a pipe, the flow may be laminar or turbulent. The

---

*This equation was derived by H. Lamb, Cambridge University Press, London, 1906), who showed that the maximum shear rate of a falling ball is $\dot{\gamma} = (\rho_1 - \rho_2) \, gr/3$. By substituting Eq. (45) for η into Lamb's equation, Eq. (47) is obtained.

conditions that describe whether the flow will be laminar or turbulent are expressed in a single value known as the Reynolds number. The Reynolds number is defined as

$$N_{Re} = \frac{\rho v D}{\eta}$$

where

N_{Re} = Reynolds number
ρ = density
v = velocity of the fluid
D = diameter of the pipe
η = the viscosity

and $\rho/\eta = 1$ over the kinematic viscosity; that is, as the kinematic viscosity increases, the Reynolds number decreases. When the Reynolds number is less than 2000, the flow in the pipe will be laminar, between 2000 and 3000 the flow is unstable, above 3000 the flow becomes turbulent. Turbulent flow requires more power to pump and may result in incorporation of air into a product.

The shear rate in a capillary viscometer is

$$\dot{\gamma}_{wall} = \frac{4Q}{\pi r^3}$$

$$\dot{\gamma}_{axis} = 0 \tag{50}$$

The shear rate at other positions between the axis of the tube depends on the profile of the flow. The viscosity is determined by the shear rate at the wall. For non-newtonian fluids the equation becomes much more complicated and will not be covered in this chapter. [Ref. 8 should be consulted for this information and the derivation of Eq. (50)].

a. Simple Capillary Viscometers

The simplest of capillary viscometers is a so-called Dudley pipette. The Dudley pipette consists of a standard transfer pipette with two timing marks. The time is measured for the pipette to empty the volume between the two timing marks. The time is compared with the time for a standard such as water. The viscosity is then determined from Eq. (49).

A number of U-tube capillary viscometers are available (Fig. 24). The simplest of these is the Ostwald viscometer (see Fig. 24a). The fluid is added to the bulb on the right side of the U and is pulled by suction to the upper mark on the bulk in the reservoir. The fluid is then allowed to flow back down through the capillary. The time for the liquid to pass between the two timing marks is measured, and the viscosity is calculated versus that of a standard liquid, as with the Dudley pipette.

Variations of the Ostwald (e.g., the Cannon-Fenske and the Ubbelohde viscometers) are designed to minimize errors caused by kinetic effects and head error. The pressure head in an Ostwald-type viscometer is always changing . Ideally, the backpressure should be kept constant. This is approximated in the Cannon-Fenske instrument by having a relatively small amount of fluid, with relatively low kinetic energy, flow into a relatively large reservoir such that the level of the reservoir changes very little. Glass capillary

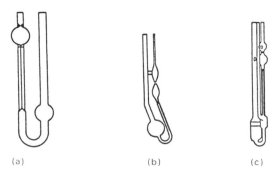

Fig. 24 Capillary viscometers: (a) Ostwald, (b) Cannon-Fenske, and (c) Ubbelohde. (From Ref. 15)

viscometers are available for kinematic viscosities between 0.6 and 10×10^4 cS. See "Rheological Measurements" in Kirk-Othmer, *Encyclopedia of Chemical Technology* [15].

b. Advantages and Disadvantages

There are some advantages to using capillary viscometers:

1. They are relatively inexpensive, except for pressure-driven viscometers.
2. High shear rates can be obtained
3. The flow is similar to processing flow.

The disadvantges are many:

1. Entrance and exit effects must be minimized by making the ratio of the length to the width of the capillary greater than 200. As this ratio increases, the relative contributions of entrance and exit effects become small. Also at larger ratios, laminar flow is assured.
2. The solids in dispersed systems sometimes tend to migrate toward the center of the capillary. This effect tends to lower the viscosity of the fluid in contact with the walls.
3. The shear rate is not constant. This makes data reduction difficult, particularly for nonnewtonian fluids.
4. The presure is not constant. This effect is closely tied to shear rate differences.
5. At high shear rates, laminar flow can become turbulent flow, which violates the initial assumptions for determining shear rates.
6. Disperse systems may yield different viscosities in capillary viscometers of widely different dimensions. If the dispersed particle is not several orders of magnitude smaller than the diameter of the capillary, the particles may interfere with basic assumptions for laminar flow, clog the capillary, or interact with each other. Capillary viscometers can supply answers for some types of systems, but one must be aware of their limitations and interpret the data with caution. They can be useful for emulsoins and suspensions containing a small percentage ($<1\%$) of suspended material. These fluids do not deviate too much from newtonian behavior.

3. *Rotational Viscometers*

The most frequently used rotational viscometers are the coaxial cylinder viscometer, the cone and plate type, and the rotating spindle type.

a. **Coaxial Cylinder Viscometers**

The coaxial cylinder viscometer consists of one cylinder inside another with a small gap between them (Fig. 25). The test material is placed between the two cylinders. Either cylinder may be driven at a constant angular velocity (ω). The stress generated on the other cylinder is measured as a torque (M).

The shear rate in a coaxial cylinder viscometer is different for newtonian and non-newtonian liquids when the cylinder is driven at the same angular velocity (ω). The shear rate at the outer wall for a newtonian fluid in a coaxial cylinder viscometer is

$$\dot{\gamma}_o = \frac{2\omega}{1 - (R_i/R_o)^2}$$

where ω is the angular velocity, and R_i and R_o are the inner and outer radii, respectively. Derivations for Eqs. (51a) and (51b) can be found in Reference 8. The shear rate at the inner wall is given in the following example.

The difference between R_i and R_o is typically 1–2 mm ($R_i/R_o \geq 0.98$). This small gap assures a relatively constant shear rate within the gap.

Example: Calculate the shear rates in a coaxial cylinder viscometers with ω 10 rad s^{-1} and R_i/R_o ratios of 0.98, 0.90, 0.50, and 0.10 at the inner and outer radii of the gap between the cylinders.

Solution:
$$\dot{\gamma}_o = \frac{2\omega}{1 - (R_i/R_o)^2} \qquad \dot{\gamma}_i = \frac{2\omega}{(R_o/R_i)^2 - 1}$$

$$= \frac{2 \times 10}{1 - (0.98)^2} \qquad = \frac{2 \times 20}{(1/0.98)^2 - 1}$$

$$= 505 \ s^{-1} \qquad = 485 \ s^{-1}$$

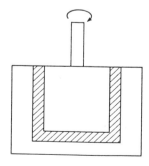

Fig. 25 Cross section of a coaxial cylinder viscometer.

R_i/R_o	$\dot{\gamma}_o$	$\dot{\gamma}_i$	$\Delta/\dot{\gamma}_o(\%)$
0.98	505	485	4.0
0.90	105.2	85.2	19
0.50	26.6	6.7	75.6
0.10	20.2	0.20	99

The shear rates $\dot{\gamma}_o$ given in the accompanying table are the shear rates of the driven (outer) cylinder. The corresponding shear rates at the inner cylinder $\dot{\gamma}_i$ are also shown, along with the percentage difference between the inner and outer cylinders. Ideally, the liquid in the instrument should experience a single shear rate. Since this is impossible in this type of instrument, the variation in shear rates should be held to a minimum. Therefore, an R_i/R_o ratio of 0.98 is the accepted minimum value.

For a nonnewtonian fluid (power law fluid) the shear rate is

$$\dot{\gamma} = \frac{2\omega}{N[1 - (R_i/R_o)]^{2/N}}$$

where N is defined as in Eq. (5), that is, $\dot{\gamma} = \psi \sigma^N$. Fluids of known viscosity can be used to calibrate the torque scale of the viscometer, which can then be used for non-newtonian fluids.

The shear rate for a Bingham material is even more complicated and will not be covered here: complete derivations are given in Whorlow [8].

The shear stress for all materials is given in Eq. (52):

$$\sigma = \frac{M}{2\pi R_o L} \tag{52}$$

where M is the measured torque, R_o is the outer radius, and L is the length of the inner cylinder.

The viscosity, therefore, is given by

$$\eta = \frac{\sigma}{\dot{\gamma}} = \frac{M}{2\pi R_o L \dot{\gamma}} \tag{53}$$

where $\dot{\gamma}$ is the appropriate shear rate, depending on the type of fluid being measured.

The concentric cylinder instrument has the advantages of being easy to use (at $\eta < 100$ P) and it can be made very sensitive.

Concentric cylinder viscometers exhibit a number of disadvantages: (a) if the value of R_i/R_o is less than 0.98, data reduction is difficult because the shear rate is not constant over the width of the gap—that is, the wider the gap, the greater the percentage change in the shear rates within the gap (see preceding example); (b) the instrument is hard to load with high viscosity liquids: (c) end effects can be a problem, particularly with nonnewtonian fluids; (d) dispersed systems may show slippage at the cylinder owing to phase separation; and (e) thixotropic materials will give varying viscosities as a function of time, as they do in all viscometers. This effect must be carefully monitored to avoid misinterpretation of the material's behavior. For example, a thixotropic material may be interpreted as being a simple thinning liquid.

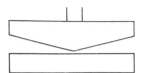

Fig. 26 Geometry of cone and plate viscometers.

Thixotropic characteristics of a material can be determined in this instrument by recording the torque readings as a function of time with the instrument rotating at a constant angular velocity.

b. The Cone and Plate Viscometer

The cone and plate viscometer (Fig. 26) consists of a cone, with an angle less than 5°, preferably 4–30°, and a flat plate. A small cone angle is required to generate a shear rate that is essentially constant throughout the gap. The shear rate of a cone and plate viscometer is

$$\dot{\gamma} = \frac{\omega}{\alpha} \tag{54}$$

where ω is the relative angular velocity between the cone and the plate (either the cone or the plate may be rotated while the nonrotating element is used to measure the stress generated), and α is the angle of the cone.

The viscosity measured by a cone and plate viscometer is given by

$$\eta = \frac{3M}{2\pi R^3 \dot{\gamma}} \tag{55}$$

where M is the measured torque and R is the radius of the cone or plate. A complete derivation of Eq. (55) may be found in Ref. 8 (p. 131).

Problem 7: Prove that the shear rate for a cone and plate viscometer is constant.

Solution: The shear rate is v/l, where v is the velocity and l is the thickness of the material. The velocity of the cone or disk at any radius r_i is $r_i\omega$. For small angles, $\tan\alpha = \alpha$ (radians). Therefore, the separation (l) between the cone and plate at any radius r_i is approximately $r_i\alpha$, since $\tan\alpha = l_i/r_i = \alpha$ (Fig. 27). Therefore, the shear rate is ($\omega r_i/\alpha r_i = \omega/\alpha$ for all values of r_i.

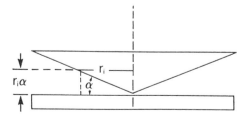

Fig. 27 Separation of cone and plate in terms of r_i and α.

That is, the shear rate is independent of the position within the gap. Therefore, the shear rate is constant throughout the gap.

The advantages of the cone and plate viscometer are:

1. The shear rate is constant. This simplifies data reduction.
2. Only a very small sample is necessary to fill the gap between the cone and plate.
3. Newtonian and nonnewtonian fluids can be measured over a wide range of viscosities.

The disadvantages are:

1. The temperature rise within the gap can be high at high shear rates.
2. High-viscosity materials can fail at the edge and be ejected from between the cone and plate.
3. Highly structured material may be destroyed while bringing the cone and plate together.
4. The cone and plate must be precisely aligned to obtain correct value.

A variation of the cone and plate viscometer is the parallel plate viscometer, which consists of two parallel plates instead of one plate and a cone. The shear rate in this case is

$$\dot{\gamma} = \frac{\omega r}{l} \tag{56}$$

where l is the separation between the plates. Most cone and plate viscometers can be converted to parallel plate viscometers by simply replacing the cone with another plate. For parallel plates, the shear rate is not constant throughout the gap, and the equations for nonnewtonian fluids become very complex.

c. The Rotating Spindle Viscometer

In all previously discussed methods of measuring viscosity, the sample is held between or within a structure that maintains a precisely defined geometry. For instance, in a coaxial viscometer the sample is placed between two cylindrical surfaces of precise radii; in a capillary viscometer the sample moves through a precisely defined capillary; only in the falling or rolling ball is it difficult to define the precise sample thickness; as a result, it is not suited for nonnewtonian fluids. The rotating spindle viscometer is another instrument in which the sample thickness is poorly defined.

Despite this problem, one brand of rotating spindle viscometer, or a variation thereof, is probably the most often used industrial pharmaceutical viscometer. It is manufactured by the Brookfield Engineering Laboratories, Inc., and is commonly called the Brookfield. The Brookfield consists of a motor (with four to eight fixed speeds), a scale to indicate torque, and a section of four to seven spindles. The full-scale torque range varies from approximately 675 to 57,500 dyn-cm for models LV and HB, respectively.

The shear rate and shear stress for cylindrical spindles are determined as follows:

$$\dot{\gamma} = \frac{2\omega R_c^2 R_b^2}{X(R_c^2 - R_b^2)} \tag{57}$$

$$\sigma = \frac{M}{2\pi R_b^2 L} \tag{58}$$

where

ω = angular velocity of spindle (rad s^{-1})
R_c = radius of container (cm)
R_b = radius of spindle (cm)
X = radius at which shear rate is being calculated
M = measured torque
L = effective length of spindle

The viscosity is defined in the usual way, $\sigma/\dot{\gamma}$.

The flow properties of nonnewtonian fluids, although given by the foregoing equations, do not always give consistent results between spindles. Therefore, a complete shear stress/shear rate diagram should be plotted using a single cylindrical spindle. The speed (rpm) of the cylinder is usually used instead of the actual shear rate, and the viscometer reads in scale units instead of the actual shear stress. A scale factor dependent on spindle size and speed is used to convert readings to viscosity.

The advantages of the Brookfield-type viscometer are

1. This type of viscometer is relatively inexpensive
2. The apparatus is rugged and easily used by inexperienced operators.
3. Samples are easily loaded (e.g., just placed in a beaker or pail).

The disadvantages are

1. The shear rate varies throughout the sample. The X in Eq. (57) determines the shear rate at a given point in the sample.
2. Operators may ignore the effects of container size and other variables associated with the measurement.
3. For nonnewtonian fluids the measured "viscosity" is dependent on spindle size.
4. Data reduction is difficult for nonnewtonian fluids.

4. Dynamic Measurements

The viscosity and shear rate–stress relationships of viscoelastic materials can be measured by any of the preceding methods. However, much of the information about viscoelastic materials is lost by making only steady-state shear measurements. Steady-state measurements do not establish that a material is viscoelastic, but only that it is nonnewtonian. As discussed in the section on viscoelasticity, viscoelastic materials exhibit both elastic and viscous characteristics. The measurement of the individual components gives much more information about the material than a single "viscosity" measurement.

The methods for evaluating viscoelastic characteristics are as varied as the ways to measure newtonian fluids and hookeian solids. There are two major techniques for measuring dynamic viscosity: (a) by applying a harmonic force to the material, and (b) by generating harmonic strains using a steady rotation.

a. Harmonic Strain

A harmonic strain may be applied in various ways. It may be applied through simple shear (Fig. 28a), tension–compression (see Fig. 28b), concentric cylinders (see Fgi. 28c), or oscillating fixtures (see Fig. 28d). There are several other variations of these meth-

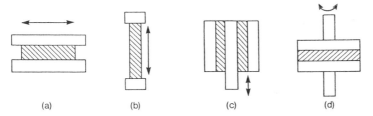

Fig. 28 Methods of applying harmonic strains: (a) simple shear, (b) tension–compression, (c) concentric cylinders, and (d) oscillating fixtures.

ods similar to that shown in Fig. 28d; for example, cone and plate or concentric cylinder configuration can be substituted for flat plates. Usually the harmonic strain is driven at a constant amplitude; that is, the maximum displacement is constant for the duration of the measurement (Fig. 29a). Some dynamic measurements use a free vibration instrument in which the oscillations are continually dampened by the fluid (see Fig. 29b). The latter will not be discussed in this chapter (a full discussion of this subject can be found in Ref. 8).

With the constant displacement instrument, the phase lag and the magnitude of the stress are measured. From these two values, the storage and loss moduli (G' and G'') can be calculated using Eqs. (16a) and (16b). The measurement is normally made by shearing the sample by a sinusoidal oscillation at one point and measuring the response at another point.

The complex modulus divided by the frequency of oscillation is the complex dynamic viscosity (η^*) (see the section on viscoelasticity for further discussion).

The advantages of this method are similar to those given for concentric cylinder, cone and plate, and parallel plate viscometers, since the geometry is essentially the same. This method also covers a wider time scale. For example, the range of oscillation frequencies can vary from 1×10^{-5} to 200 Hz. The information obtained by this method is unobtainable by most classic measurements. For instance, it can tell the investigator whether a prototype suppository base possesses enough elasticity to maintain its shape during insertion and still maintain a suitable viscosity to allow spreading in the bowel.

b. Eccentric, Rotating Disks

Figure 30 illustrates the test geometry of the eccentric, rotating disk (ERD). A sample is placed between two disks that rotate at the same anglular velocity ω, but around offset axes. The flow between the disks results in a shearing motion with material elements moving in circular paths relative to each other. The deformation is of a constant mag-

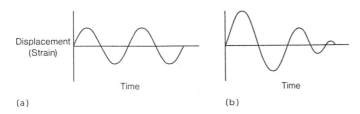

Fig. 29 (a) Constant and (b) attenuated harmonic oscillations.

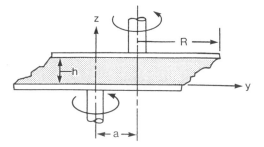

Fig. 30 Eccentric rotating disk geometry. (From Ref. 32.)

nitude, but changes direction continually. Any given element of material is sheared harmonically, but not in the same manner as in a conventional dynamic testing method. The stress experienced by all elements of the material is identical (i.e., independent of position).

The strain in an ERD is equal to the distance between the centers of the rotating disk α divided by the gap h between the disks (i.e., a/h). The elastic and viscous moduli are given by Eqs. (59a) and (59b).

$$G' = \frac{hF_Y}{\pi R^2 a} \tag{59a}$$

where

F_Y^u = force in the Y direction
R = radius of the disk
a = distance between the centers of the disks
h = separation between the disks

$$G'' = \frac{hF_X}{\pi R^2 a} \tag{59b}$$

Both F_Y and F_X are measured by sensors that monitor the two perpendicular forces on one of the disk shafts.

An example of the this type of instrument is the Mechanical Spectrometer of Rheometrics, Inc., which may be used either in the eccentric mode or as a conventional cone and plate or parallel plate rheometer.

The advantages of this type of instrumentation are

1. The equipment is easy to use.
2. The linearity of the instrumentation is good.
3. A wide range of strains may be obtained; especially very low strains.
4. A wide range of force amplitudes may be obtained: 1×10^{-4} to 1 N-m.

Many of the dynamic rheometers described here are found only in industrial research laboratories or well-funded universities. They are not typically used for quality control work or in routine formulation. However, the data generated by such instruments can provide information about the structure of the material that is not available from any other source.

5. *Miscellaneous Methods*

a. Penetrometer

A pentrometer typically consists of a weighted rod with a needle, cone, or sphere attached to the end. The penetrating element is allowed to drop vertically from a predetermined height into the sample. A graduated scale is used to measure the depth of penetration after a given time or until a given rate of penetration has been reached.

The yield value S_0 for a cone penetrometer is calculated from the depth of penetration p using the equation:

$$S_0 = \frac{K(wt)}{p^n} \tag{60}$$

where

S_0 = yield value

$K = \dfrac{1}{\pi} \cot 2\alpha \cot \alpha$ (K is an instrument constant and 2α is the cone angle)

wt = weight of the cone and attached parts that impinge on the sample

p = depth of penetration

n = a constant depending on the material, usually having a value near 2

A rod penetrometer consists of a metal rod with a platform for adding weight. The geometry is defined well enough to calculate shear stress (from the load) and velocity gradients. Pseudoplastic behavior can be defined as in Eq. (61)

$$v = \frac{1}{\psi} \sigma^n \tag{61}$$

where v is velocity gradient (i.e., shear rate), σ is shear stress, and ψ and n are constants characteristic of the material (ψ is sometimes called a pseudoviscosity).

Equation (61) is the "power law" as determined by a penetrometer (see Sec. III.B for other examples of power laws). Penetrometers are used to characterize waxes, greases, suppositories, and other semisolids.

b. Creep Measurement

The phenomenon of creep was introduced in connection with the modeling of rheological behavior. The present section is limited to a discussion of the instrumentation for creep measurements in dispersed systems. In a creep test, a sudden constant stress is applied to a system, and the strain is measured as a function of time. Creep measurements are useful for viscoelastic fluids, since nonviscoelastic fluids would release the stress instantaneously.

Creep measurements are probably the most inexpensive means of quantitating viscoelasticity. Barry [33] has pioneered the study of viscoelastic properties in pharmaceuticals and cosmetics. His work includes studies on the control of the consistency of emulsions of liquid paraffins in water through the formation of viscoelastic networks [34].

The creep of viscoelastic fluids can be measured in various ways: the double sandwich (Fig. 31a) or a variation thereof, the sliding coaxial cylinders (Fig. 31b), which can also be used in torsion (Fig. 31c). For semisolids, such as suppository bases, a mass placed on the upper surface of well-defined geometry (Fig. 31d) can be used for the con-

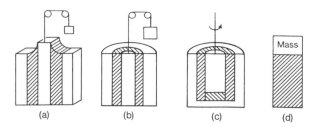

Fig. 31 Methods of measuring creep: (a) double sandwich, (b) sliding coaxial cylinders, (c) torsion, and (d) mass on upper surface.

stant load. (Note that a constant load is not the same as a constant stress. Stress is defined as a force/area; if the cross-sectional area is changing, the stress is no longer constant. The difference may not be important for small deformations.) The premise of linear viscoelasticity must be verified in all measurements of viscoelasticity. The strain must be directly proportional to the stress, or the material is not linearly viscoelastic, and the standard methods of analysis are not valid.

Analysis of creep curves.   Figure 32 illustrates a typical creep curve and its analysis. When a constant stress is rapidly applied to a viscoelastic material, the material responds with an instantaneous strain σ_0/G_0, where G_0 is the shear modulus at time 0. With time, the initial nonlinear response (A–B) typically becomes linear (B–C). The second region (A–B), for an ideal material, is known as retarded elasticity, described by G_r, the retardation shear modulus. Upon reaching linearity (B–C), the region of the curve is known as secondary creep, or viscous flow, which is observable in real materials [8]. After the load is removed (point C), there is an instantaneous recovery of a portion of the strain σ_0/G_0, followed by a slower recovery of the retarded elasticity σ_0/G_r , and finally a region of unrecoverable strain owing to viscous flow, $\sigma_0 t/\eta_N$, is reached.

Sherman [11] describes the creep curve in terms of molecular behavior as follows:
1.   The instantaneous strain region (origin–A) is due to the elasticity of the primary structure. If, at any point in this region, the stress is removed, the sample returns to its original dimensions. The instantaneous creep compliance J_0, of this portion is $1/G_0$ for shear or $1/E_0$ for tensile experiments. The curve in Fig. 32 is often plotted in terms of J, rather than σ_0/G. If J is used, the shape of the curve will be identical with that of Fig. 32; only the relative magnitude of the y axis will change.

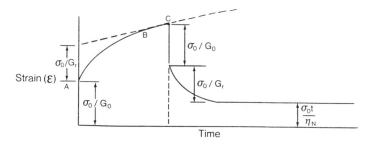

Fig. 32 Creep curve with major parameters.

2. In the retarded elasticity region (A–B), bonds break and re-form. However, not all bonds break and re-form at the same rate, since some are stronger than others. This concept is traditionally described mathematically by Eq. (62):

$$J_R = \sum_i J_i \left[1 - \exp\left(-\frac{t}{\tau_i} \right) \right] = \frac{\varepsilon_R(t)}{\sigma} \tag{62}$$

where J_R is the creep compliance for the retarded elastic region, $\sum_i$ indicates that all the elements from 0 to i are to be summed, J_i is the creep compliance for the ith element, exp indicates that e (the base of the natural logarithm) is raised to the $(-t/\tau_i)$ power, t is the time, and τ_i is the retardation time; that is, the time for the stress of that element to reach $1/e$ of its initial value. In addition, τ_i equals $J_i N_i$, which is often substituted into Eq. (62). The concept of τ is very important. The values of τ_i, where τ_i means that there are relaxation times $(\tau_1, \tau_2, \tau_3, \cdots)$, may vary from fractional seconds to literally days. These times are the length of time the strain in a given element of viscoelastic structure will decrease to $1/e$ (i.e., 36,8% of its initial value). Since each τ_i represents a different time, the total structure creeps at varying rates as time increases. This varying rate is expressed in Eq. (62) by the expression $\varepsilon_R(t)$. For example, in Fig. 32 the value of ε_R varies from A to C. Equation (62) states that the total shear compliance is made up of a number (i) of individual compliances (J). The individual compliances are the results of a range of bonding energies. Low bond energies yield elements with low shear compliances.

3. In the third region (B–C), newtonian flow takes place. The rupturing of all low-energy bonds has taken place, and the remaining structure can flow unimpeded in newtonian flow. The strain will increase as a function of time and viscosity:

$$\varepsilon_N(t) = \frac{\sigma t}{\eta_N} \tag{63}$$

where $\varepsilon_N(t)$ is newtonian strain as a function of time and η_N is newtonian viscosity.

Note: Liquids are not normally described in terms of strain; however, in the case of viscoelastic systems, this term can be appropriate. Equation (63) can be expressed as a strain rate $\eta_N(t)/t$, which is essentially a shear rate.

The total creep compliance–time plot is given by the sum of the three individual compliances, as shown in Eq. (64):

$$J(t) = J_0 + \sum_i J_i \left[1 - \exp \frac{-t}{\tau_i} \right] + \frac{t}{\eta_N} \tag{64}$$

where J_0 represents the instantaneous elasticity region, $\sum J_i[1 - \exp(-t/\tau_i)]$ represents the retarded elasticity region, and t/η_N represents the newtonian flow.

A graphic method was developed by Inokuchi [35] to determine the values of τ_i from experimental data. The experimental data points are plotted as creep compliance J as a function of time (Fig. 33a). The total curve is the sum of all the values for J_i (e.g., J_1 at 1 s. J_2 at 2 s, $\cdots$) or $J = \sum J_i$. The distance Q_1—that is, the distance at t_1, t_2, t_3, $\ldots$, between the extrapolated linear portion of the curve (B–D) and the retarded elastic portion of the curve (A–B)—is

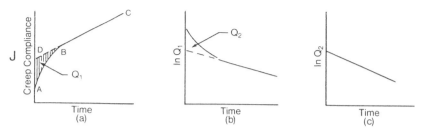

Fig. 33 Analysis of creep curves.

$$\sum_i J_i - \frac{\varepsilon_R(t)}{\sigma} = Q_1 \tag{65}$$

since

$$\frac{\varepsilon(t)}{\sigma} = \sum_i J_i - \sum_i J_i \exp\left(\frac{-t}{\tau_i}\right)$$

that is, the line (DBC) less the curve (AB) equals the retarded strain as a function of time divided by the stress. Therefore, we write

$$Q = \sum_i J_i \exp\left(\frac{-t}{\tau_i}\right)$$

A plot of $\ln Q_1$ versus time gives a straight line (if there is only one value of τ), with a slope of $1/\tau$, and an intercept of J_1 (see Fig. 33b). The process may be repeated (see Fig. 33c) for any curved portion of the line to determine the values for $\tau_2, \tau_3, \cdots$. Normally only three values of τ are meaningful, since τ becomes very small and beyond the precision of the measurement.

The values for τ can help the formulator determine whether a given system is able to maintain a long-term viscoelastic structure or will flow away rapidly.

Retardation spectrum.   Another way of analyzing a creep curve is by constructing a retardation spectrum. The retardation spectrum $L(\tau)$ is a continuum of relaxation times τ, rather than a series of discrete values. An approximation to the retardation spectrum is derived by first plotting $[J(t) - (t/\eta_N)]$ versus $\ln t$ and then plotting the slope of that curve as a function of time. Mathematically the approximate curve is

$$L(\tau) = \frac{d}{d \ln t}\left[J(t) - \frac{t}{\eta_N}\right] \tag{66}$$

The value of the newtonian viscosity η_N can be determined from the recovery curve by substituting the value of the initial stress σ_0 and the time of creep (after the curve becomes flat).

The procedure for graphically obtaining $L(\tau)$, sometimes called the compliance density, is shown in Fig. 34. Note that by using Fig. 34, the contribution of the retardation time τ of any element i may be determined by simply noting the relative value

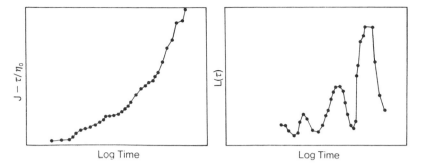

Fig. 34 Procedure for obtaining a retardation spectrum from a creep compliance curve. (From Ref. 33.)

of $L(\tau)$ for a given time (τ_i). The higher the value of $L(\tau)$, the greater the contribution for a given retardation time τ_i. It should be noted that L has dimensions of compliance (i.e., cm^2 dyn^{i-1}). The retardation spectrum is useful in examining long-time phenomena.

Relaxation spectrum. Stress relaxation was discussed under Section III.D in connection with modeling of rheological behavior. To review, in a stress relaxation experiment the material is held under a constant strain and the change in stress is followed as a function of time (Fig. 35a). The stress may be in tension, compression, shear, or bulk. A relaxation spectrum $H(t)$ may be obtained in a method analogous to that used for the retardation spectrum. The value of G or E, as determined from the relaxation curve (see Fig. 35a), is plotted (see Fig. 35b) versus the natural logarithm of time. The negative values of the instantaneous slopes of Fig. 35b (i.e., $-dG/dt$) are then plotted against the natural logarithm of the relaxation times (see Fig. 35c). Mathematically, $H(t)$ is approximated by

$$H(t) \text{ or } H(\tau) \approx \frac{-dG(t)}{d \ln \tau} \qquad (67)$$

Since $H(\tau)$ may span a very large range, the value of $\ln H(\tau)$ is often plotted versus $\ln \tau$. Unlike L, H has dimensions of modulus (i.e., dyne cm^{-2}). The relaxation spectrum is useful for short time phenomena. For those who wish to pursue this subject further. J. D. Ferry's book *Viscoelastic Properties of Polymers* [17] is an excellent resource.

c. Surface Rheometer

Surface rheometry is a technique that measures the surface rheological properties of molecules adsorbed at an interface. The techinque was successfully applied by Burgess et al. to measure the surface rheology of the proteins bovine serum albumin (BSA) and human immunoglobulin G (HIgG) adsorbed at the air–water interface [37]. It was also shown by the same researchers that the technique could be used to determine the stability of adsorbed protein layers [38]. The surface rheometer used consisted of a moving coil galvanometer; a platinum Du Noy ring, which is placed parallel to the interface and attached to the galvanometer; a control unit that varies the driving frequency and monitors the amplitude and motion of the ring; and a data-processing unit. The

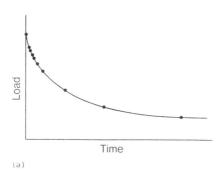

(a)

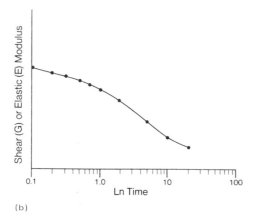

(b)

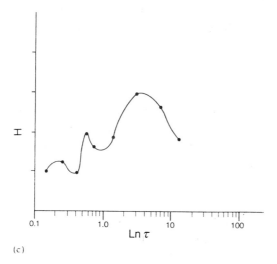

(c)

Fig. 35 (a) Relaxation curve, (b) G or E versus the natural logarithm of time, and (c) relaxation spectrum. (Adapted from Ref. 36.)

theory is explained by Sheriff and Warburton [39]. Values for the surface elasticity (G'_s) and surface viscosity (η'_s) are obtained as a function of time. G'_s and η'_s are defined as

$$G'_s = g_f \, I \, 4 \, \pi \, (f^2 - f_0^2) \tag{68}$$

and

$$\eta'_s = g_f \, I \, NC \, (1/X - X_0) \tag{69}$$

where I is the moment of inertia, f is the sample interfacial resonance frequence, f_0 is the reference interfacial resonance frequency, NC is the number of cycles of integration, X is the mean amplitude at the sample interface, X_0 is the mean amplitude at the reference interface, and g_f is the geometric factor.

d. Dynamic Light Scattering

In diffusion within polymer solutions, both macroviscosity and microviscosity affect hydrodynamics [40]. Microviscosity can be calculated from diffusion data by application of the Stokes–Einstein relation [41]:

$$D = \frac{KT}{6\pi\eta a} \tag{70}$$

where D is the diffusion coefficient, k represents Boltzmann's constant, T is the temperature, η denotes the (micro)viscosity of the diffusion media, and a is the radius of the diffusant. Diffusion, and consequently, diffusion coefficients can be measured by dynamic light scattering [42,43]. De Smidt and Crommelin used dynamic light scattering to measure the (micro)viscosity of aqueous polymer solutions [44]. They found that by measuring the diffusion coeffients of differently sized latex spheres in solutions of carboxymethylcellulose sodium, microviscosity effects could be observed.

e. Electron Paramagnetic Resonance

Kristl et al. developed an experimental technique whereby electron paramagnetic resonance (EPR) was used to study the motion of drug molecules in hydrocolloid suspensions [45]. The Li salt of the copolymer of methacrylic acid, and its methyl ester was dispersed in water to form gels of different concentrations. The model drug tempol, and the spin-labeled drugs lidocaine (sl-lid) and dexamethasone (sl-dex) where studied in the gels by EPR. Data suggested that the size and shape of the drug molecules strongly affect their motion, and there is a proportionality of the microviscosity of the hydrocolloids to the polymer concentration.

f. Electron Spin Resonance

An electron spin resonance (ESR) technique, essentially devoid of external mechanical stress force, was developed as an experimental technique to measure phase fluidity in semisolid petrolatum and polyethylene glycol systems [46]. Use of ESR is presented as a nondestructive technique that is capable of measuring the "rheological ground state" as discussed by Barry [33]. The ESR technique was adapted from the spin probe procedure for characterizing the transport properties of biological samples. It consists of dissolving a small concentration (approximately 10^{-4} *M*) of a stable free radical, di-*t*-butylnitroxide or DBNO, in about 0.5 ml of sample. Absorbance of microwave radiation by the DBNO probe is then obtained at its characteristic magnetic field in a suitable ESR spectrometer. The shape of the absorption band is a function of the rotational diffusion of the probe and, consequently, a measure for fluidity or viscosity. Hence, the shape of the ESR signal of the spin probe serves to measure fluidity or viscosity without the application of external mechanical stress.

V. RHEOLOGY OF DISPERSED SYSTEMS

A. Theory

Unfortunately, the rheological and mechanical properties of pharmaceutical dispered systems are not as well understood as the those of new newtonian systems. Dispersed systems include such diverse systems as liquid suspensions, liquid emulsions, semisolid powder-filled systems, semisolid liquid-filled systems, foams, and powder-filled solid polymeric systems. Powder-filled solid polymeric systems are typified by pharmaceutical film coatings. Evaluation of the rheological and mechanical properties of these systems is covered in an extensive review article [47]. Disperse systems also include those systems in which one continuous phase is dispersed within another. An example of this type of system would be a blend of two materials such as lanolin and polyethylene glycol. By definition, all of these systems can also be called composites [48]. The remainder of this chapter will concentrate on liquids, semisolids, and foams.

The rheological and mechanical properties of dispersed systems are not well understood, especially when the droplets or solid particles of the dispersed phase interact with one another, or interact with the surrounding bulk phase. The flow behavior of suspensions or droplets or particles in liquids is important because most theories of viscoelastic behavior also have their origin in the theory of the viscosity of suspensions. Einstein's equation for the viscosity of a suspension of spherical particles is fundamental to the theory [49,50].

$$\eta = \eta_1 (1 + k_e \phi_2) \tag{71}$$

The apparent viscosity η is a function of the viscosity of the suspending medium η_1, the Einstein coefficient k_e, and the volume fraction of the suspended phase ϕ_2. The volume fraction of the suspended phase is equal to the volume occupied by the suspended phase divided by the total volume of the dispersion. The equation holds only for dilute dispersions, where $\phi_2 \ll 1$, $k_e = 2.5$, and the spheres are noninteractive. In addition, the phases must be noncompressible; that is, Poisson's ratio equals 0.5. Attempts to extend the validity of Eq. (71) are numerous [51]. For example, as the volume fraction increases, the behavior can be modeled by a power series expansion:

$$\eta = \eta_2 (1 + 2.5 \phi + K\phi^2 + \cdots) \tag{72}$$

where the second-order coefficient K accounts for two-body interaction between particles in the dispersed phase.

One of the most useful extensions is the Mooney equation:

$$\ln\left(\frac{\eta}{\eta_1}\right) = k_e\phi_2\left[\frac{1}{(1-\phi_2)/\phi_m}\right] \tag{73}$$

where ϕ_m is the maximum volume fraction that the particles can attain when packed: ϕ_m is equal to the true volume of the dispersed phase divided by the apparent volume occupied by the dispersed phase [52]. Equation (73) is a constitutive equation that adequately describes the viscoisty of many kinds of suspensions, over a wide range of concentrations. Theoretically, ϕ_m is 0.74 for spheres in hexagonal packing, but generally the value is much less because of irregularities in particle shape and particle–particle interactions. Viscosity generally increases rapidly with concentration and state of aggregation. The Einstein coefficient has been estimated for shapes other than nonagglomerated spheres, including roughly spherically shaped agglomerates of rigid spheres [53]. Irregularities in shape generally increase k_e values.

When the concentration of the dispersed phase becomes high, suspensions become nonnewtonian and their viscosity becomes a function of shear rate $\dot{\gamma}$. For nonnewtonian suspensions that show a decrease η with an increase in shear rate, the Cross equation:

$$\eta = \eta_\infty + (\eta_0 - \eta_\infty)\left(\frac{1}{1 + \Omega\dot{\gamma}\,m}\right) \tag{74}$$

often holds [54,55]. The constants Ω and m depend on the system, and η_0 is the viscosity at zero shear rate, and η_∞ is the viscosity at high shear rates. It is generally assumed that the shear rate-dependence of viscosity seen in these systems is due to structural changes in the dispersion such as the breaking up of agglomerates by shearing forces. Other shear-dependent theories have been proposed by Krieger and Dougherty [56] and Gillespie [57,58].

For a given rheological test instrument, the theoretical equations for shear viscosity and shear modulus should be of the same form for a given instrument geometry [59,60]. Therefore, shear strain in the modulus equation replaces shear rate in the viscosity equation. For a dispersion of a rigid filler in a viscoelastic phase with a Poisson's ratio of 0.5, the relationship between relative viscosities an relative shear moduli can be expressed as:

$$\frac{\eta}{\eta_1} = \frac{G}{G_1} \tag{75}$$

where G is the shear modulus of the dispersion and G_1 is the shear modulus of the unfilled matrix phase. Consequently, the same theory that is used to determine the viscosity of the dispersion can be used to estimate its shear modulus. For example, G/G_1 can be substituted for η/η_1 in Eqs. (71) or (73) to yield corresponding equations for the relative shear modulus. The correlation between shear viscosity and shear modulus does not hold for systems in which Poisson's ratio is less than 0.5, but a theoretical equation has been developed that compensates for this condition [61]. In addition, if the rigidity of the dispersed phase is not much greater than that of the matrix, Eq. (75) is not applicable, as the modulus ratio will be substantially less than the viscosity ratio. Actual moduli, lower than predicted, can occur because of three reasons: (a) the Poisson's ratio of the matrix is less than 0.5, (b) thermal stresses reduce the apparent modulus, or (c) the modulus of the filler is not significantly greater than the modulus of the matrix. On the other hand, when the matrix is a rigid material, the Mooney equation [Eq. (73)] predicts shear moduli that are too high [62].

When the internal phase becomes deformable, such as in an emulsion, the viscosity is affected by the viscosities of the internal and the continuous phases as well as the shearing and interfacial forces. These conditions are expressed by two parameters, α' and β'.

$$\alpha' = \frac{\eta_0}{\eta_i} = \frac{\text{continuous phase viscosity}}{\text{internal phase viscosity}} \tag{76a}$$

and

$$\beta' = \frac{\eta_0 \dot{\gamma}}{u/a} = \frac{\text{shearing force}}{\text{interfacial force}} \tag{76b}$$

where $\dot{\gamma}$ is the shear rate, α is the radius of the internal phase, and u is the interfacial tension between phases. These parameters assume the absence of effects from buoyancy.

As the shearing force becomes larger, the interfacial tension is overcome, and the once spherical internal phase becomes elongated. The elongated particle rotates and traces out an effective volume larger than that of the spherical particle. As the shearing rate increases, the effect becomes more pronounced. This explains the reason for the non-newtonian behavior of emulsions of two newtonian fluids.

If the interfacial force is large compared with the shearing force, the internal phase remains spherical and behaves as a newtonian fluid, which follows, Eq. (77) [63]:

$$\eta = \eta_0 \left[1 + \frac{5}{2} \phi \left(\frac{1 + \frac{2}{5}\alpha'}{1 + \alpha'} \right) \right] \tag{77}$$

If the internal phase becomes very viscous compared with the continuous phase then $\alpha' \to 0$ and Eq. (77) reduces to the original Einstein equation, Eq. (71).

The viscosity of viscoelastic dispersions is dependent on the elastic properties of the internal phase, rather than the elasticity of the interfacial area. This elastic effect is independent of particle size, since the elasticity is dependent on only the shear modulus, which is an intrinsic property.

Finally, the effect of inertia of the internal phase is important. Batchelor [64] modified Einstein's equation to account for inertial effects; Eq. (78)

$$\eta = \eta_0 \left(1 + \frac{5}{2} \phi + 1.34 N_{Re}^{3/2} \right) \tag{78}$$

where N_{Re} is the shear Reynolds number; that is,

$$N_{Re} = \frac{a^2 \dot{\gamma}}{\nu} \tag{79}$$

where

a = radius of the particle
$\dot{\gamma}$ = shear rate
ν = kinematic viscosity of the continuous phase = viscosity/density

The unitless Reynolds number here characterizes the flow around the particle. This discussion touched only a few of the many factors contributing to and affecting the viscosity of disperse systems. Sherman's book [11 pp. 127–169] covers very thoroughly all factors that affect the viscosity of dispersed systems.

Another constitutive equation that can be used to predict the modulus of a dispersion of solid particles in the Kerner equation [65]. When the dispersed particles are more rigid than the matrix and deformation occurs by shear, the Kerner equation can be written as:

$$\frac{G}{G_1} = \frac{1 + 15(1 - \mu_1)}{(8 - 10\mu_1)(\phi_2/\phi_1)} \tag{80}$$

where μ_1 is Poisson's ratio of the matrix phase and ϕ_1, the volume fraction of the matrix phase, equals $(1 - \phi_2)$. This equation assumes the particles dispersed in the matrix phase are spherical and that there is good adhesion between the particles and the matrix phase. Good adhesion is assumed to exist if the externally applied stress does not exceed the frictional forces between the phases. In many cases where adhesion is poor, Eq. (80) holds because there is little, if any, relative motion across the dispersed particle–matrix interface. Viscoelastic response can vary dramatically from the case of perfect adhesion to that of no adhesion.

If Poisson's ratio equals 0.5, then the slope of the line predicted by a plot of [(G'/G'$_1$) –1] versus (ϕ_2/ϕ_1), from Eq. (80), is 2.5. Deviations from a slope of 2.5 suggest that one or more assumptions on which the equatoin is based do not hold. For example, slopes of >2.5 could be due to strong interactions between particles, which causes an increase in elastic structure. In contrast, slopes of <2.5 could be caused by slippage at the particle–bulk interface, which gives an apparent loss in elastic structure. Other deviations from a slope of 2.5 could be due to irregularities in the shapes of the particles of variations in Poisson's ratio.

The Kerner equation has been modified into other forms to account for deviations from the assumptions behind the original Kerner equation [62,66]. For example, constants have been incorporated to encompass the factors of filler geometry and packing fraction. These factors also account for the formation of strong aggregates between particles.

According to theory, the elastic modulus of a composite system is independent of the size of the filler (dispersed) particles, but experimental data indicates that there is an inverse proportionality between particle size and modulus [62]. When the dispersed phase volume fraction is held constant, an increase in the elastic modulus of the dispersion may be attributed to an increase in total particle surface area when particle size is reduced. As particle size decreases, the tendency for particle agglomeration increases, which causes a corresponding decrease in maximum packing volume and a resultant increase in the elastic modulus.

It has also been demonstrated that the distribution of particle sizes has an effect on the moduli and viscosity of suspensions [67–70]. Dispersions of various particle sizes can pack more closely than monosized particles. Consequently, there is a larger maximum packing fraction and, hence, a lower modulus at a given concentration of the dispersed phase.

Therefore, the modulus of the disperse system (or composite system) is dependent on the ratio of the moduli of the dispersed phase and the matrix phase. The larger the modulus ratio, the greater is the modulus of the disperse system. This is especially true for high concentrations of particles.

B. Energy Dissipation Considerations

Similar to the Kerner equation [Eq. (80)], the ratio of G'' to G', tan δ, is also an indicator of structural changes. In particular, tan δ is sensitive to the presence of fillers (solid, liquid, or gas). Changes in the dynamic mechanical properties of polymeric systems as a functional of ϕ_2 are often most evident in damping [71]. The change in tan δ of solid-filled polymers can be approximated by a volume averaging relationship [72,73]:

$$\frac{G''}{G'} = \left(\frac{G''}{G'}\right)_1 \phi_1 + \left(\frac{G''}{G'}\right)_2 \phi_2 \tag{81}$$

where $(G''/G') =$ tan δ, the damping of the filled polymer; $(G''/G')_1$ and $(G''/G')_2$ are the damping of the pure polymer and pure filler respectively; and ϕ_1 and ϕ_2 are the volume fractions of the pure polymer and pure filler, respectively. Since the damping of most rigid fillers (such as a powdered solid) is very small compared with that of the polymeric bulk phase, the term $(G''/G')_2 \phi_2$ is almost zero and can be neglected.

Experimentally, this equation was applied to powder-filled pharmaceutical semisolids by Radebaugh and Simonelli [74]. In general, Eq. (81) did not exactly predict the moduli of the filled systems. Even so, the equation did prove useful in postulating mechanisms of interaction between the filler and the bulk phase. For example, with starch-filled anhydrous lanolin, damping predicted by Eq. (81) was less than that determined experimentally over the entire shear frequency range tested. The increases in damping were postulated to be caused by newly introduced damping mechanisms that were not present in the anhydrous lanolin alone. The new damping mechanisms may have included (a) particle–particle friction, where particles touch each othre, as in weak agglomeration; (b) particle–bulk friction, where there is little or no adhesion at the interface; and (c) excess damping in anhydrous lanolin near the interface because of induced thermal stresses or changes in the bulk molecular configuration.

For these dispersions, it would be appropriate to modify Eq. (81) to the form

$$\frac{G''}{G'} = \left(\frac{G''}{G'}\right)_1 \phi_1 + \left(\frac{G''}{G'}\right)_2 \phi_2 + \text{interaction term} \tag{82}$$

where the interaction term accounts for deviations from idealized behavior. The interaction term will be negative when experimentally determined damping is lower than that predicted by Eq. (81). Conversely, the interaction term will be positive when experimentally observed damping is higher than that predicted by Eq. (81).

Radebaugh and Simonelli also studied the relationship between powder surface characteristics and damping of powder-filled semisolids [75]. The two powders studied were zinc oxide, with a hydrophilic surface, and colloidal sulfur, with a hydrophobic surface. Each were dispersed at multiple volume fractions in anhydrous lanolin. In each instance, experimentally determined damping was greater than predicted by Eq. (81). Even so, the damping achieved by zinc oxide dispersions was substantially greater than that achieved by colloidal sulfur dispersions. These studies demonstrated the importance of interactions between particles and between particles and the bulk.

C. Rheology of Dispersed Pharmaceutical Systems

There are many interactions that occur within dispersed systems. Cheng [76] suggested three primary types of interactions: hydrodynamic interaction between the continuous and internal phases, interparticle attraction, and particle–particle contact. These interactions, in turn, are affected by particle shape and size; particle concentration; viscosity or modulus of the suspending medium; rigidity or modulus of the suspended particles; surface properties of the suspended particles; and temperature.

1. Suspensions

The rheological properties of the continuous phase of a pharmaceutical suspension are primarily determined by a suspending agent, such as a soluble gum. It is not unusual for the rheological properties of the suspending agent to dominate the rheological properties of the entire suspension. An ideal suspending agent should be shear thinning. This means that it should have a high viscosity at low shear rates (such as sitting on a shelf) and low viscosity at high shear rates for easy dispensing (pouring) [16]. An example of such a material is the family of carboxyvinyl polymers marketed as Carbopol.

Sedimentation plays an important role in the physical stability of pharmaceutical products. The sedimentation rate v of spherical particles in a dilute suspension is given by a variation of Stokes' law, Eq. (83):

$$v = \frac{2r^2(\Delta\rho)g}{9\eta} \tag{83}$$

where: $\Delta\rho$ equals the density difference between the suspended phase and the continuous phase; g equals the acceleration owing to gravity; r is the radius of the particles; and η equals the viscosity of the continuous phase. For irregular particles, a modified form of Eq. (83) can be used:

$$v = \frac{Kr^2(\Delta\rho)}{\eta} \tag{84}$$

where K is an empirical constant that incorporates $2g$ and is determined experimentally. The limitation of Eq. (84) is that it has limited application to real pharmaceutical suspensions because the particles show hindered settling. This means that the faster-settling particles are held back by the slower-settling particles.

An excellent review by Hiestand [77] point out the importance of flocculation on the physical stability of coarse suspensions. In flocculated suspensions, particles are linked together into flocs, and they settle initially at a rate determined by the floc size and the porosity of the aggregated mass. *Subsidence* is a term often used to describe the settling of flocculated suspensions. The subsidence rate usually refers to the settling rate measured by following the boundary between the sediment and the clear medium overhead. There are many factors that affect flocculation, but one of them is the rheological properties of the suspending medium. The primary rate of disappearance of primary particles has been treated by von Smoluchowski [78,79] as a collision rate calculation that is diffusion controlled. The rate is given by

$$\left(\frac{dn}{dt}\right) = 4\pi DRn^2 \tag{85}$$

where n is the total number of particles, t is the time, D is the diffusion coefficient, and R is the collision radius, usually assumed to be equal to the particle diameter. If the diffusion coefficient is replaced by Einstein's equation, $D = kT/3\pi\eta R$, where k is the Boltzmann constant, η is the viscosity, and T is the absolute temperature, it may be shown that, $t_{1/2}$, required to reduce the total number of particles to one-half their original number, is

$$t_{1/2} = \frac{3\eta}{4kTn} \qquad (86)$$

Therefore, it can be readily seen that the collision rate can be reduced by increasing the viscosity of the suspending medium. In water (η = 0.01 cp) at 25°C for a 0.1% (by volume) suspension of spheres with r = 1.0 × 10^{-5} cm, one obtains $t_{1/2} \approx 1$ s.

The usual method for increasing the viscosity of the suspending medium is to incorporate a polymer into the suspending medium. In aqueous systems, a wide variety of hydrophilic polymers are available to increase viscosity. Even so, these polymers also stabilize suspensions by other mechanisms. For example, polymers can adsorb onto particle surfaces, thereby changing the nature of the interaction between the particles. Also, a given polymer chain can attach itself to more than one particle, thereby acting as a bridge between particles. These interactions are complex and have been thoroughly studied, but they are outside the realm of this chapter.

D. Rheology of Semisolids

Pharmaceutical semisolids include ointments, suppositories, pastes, and gels. In addition some raw materials, such as lanolin and petrolatum, are semisolids. Thus, not all semisolids are dispersed systems. However, some raw materials, which are commonly assumed to be nondispersed, may be mixtures of high- and low-melting triglycerides. The mixtures behaves like a newtonian fluid in the molten condition. Under use conditions, however, the high-melting triglyceride is dispersed in the low-melting material. The mixture then exhibits the properties of a Bingham solid: that is, it has a yield point and a plastic viscosity U.

Grant and Liversidge [81] demonstrated the importance of the rheological properties of the suppository base in the release and absorption of drugs. For instance, the yield point must be less than 300 N m^{-2}, which is the reported rectal pressure. Tukker et al. [82] found that levels of colloidal silica greater than 2% in suppositories inhibited the spreading of the molten suppository. This inhibition, no doubt, was due to the high yield value, above 300 N m^{-2}, of the resulting base. Up to 3% silica can be added to improve the flow characteristics of the suppository in the case of a cocoa butter and triglyceride base [83].

Barry [33] stresses the point that the true rheological nature of most semisolids cannot be obtained with a steady-state shear viscometer. Steady-state shearing measurements—that is, measurements in which the shear rates change only in direction—performed on viscoelastic materials, lose much of the information about the "rheological ground state" of the material. Typical rheological measurements destroy the structure of the material as it is being measured. Ideally, the measurement should be made in such a way that the structure is flexed, but not destroyed; that is, it is measured in its ground state. Creep, stress relaxation, and dynamic viscosity (sinusoidal oscillations) accomplish this. An examination of creep measurements on white, soft paraffin by Barry and Grace [84] demonstrates a practical application of the theory, instrumentation, and analysis of creep measraments (Fig. 36). Suzuki and Watanabe [85] showed that the sensory-perceived property of product "consistency" is closely related to Barry's rheological ground state.

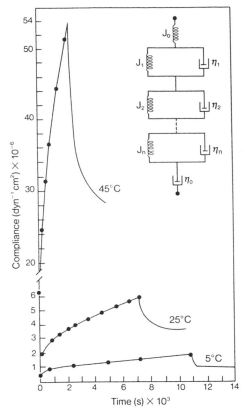

Fig. 36 Creep compliance curves for a sample of white soft paraffin BP, variation with temperature. The circles represent creep compliance values as calculated from the derived creep equation. Insert is a diagram of a mechanical model used to represent the viscoelastic properties of the material. (From Ref. 84.)

Modeling of the creep compliance for the curves at 25 and 5°C required five Voigt units and one Maxwell unit to completely describe the behavior of the material (see Fig. 17e and 17f). A Voigt unit is a hookeian element in parallel with a viscous element; a Maxwell unit is a hookeian element in series with a viscous element; a Maxwell unit is a hookeian element in series with a viscous element. The Maxwell unit in Fig. 36 consists of spring J_0 and dashpot η_0. At 45°C, the model consists of three Voigt units and one Maxwell unit. An explanation for the differences in the three curves in Fig. 36 is the melting of some crystal–crystal and crystal–amorphous areas in the paraffin. The individual points in Fig. 36 were calculated from the theoretical behavior of the corresponding series of Voigt and Maxwell units.

This type of analysis is useful for determining the buildup of structure with time and has been used to differentiate between paraffins [86] that show essentially the same steady-state viscosity, but an eightfold difference in creep compliance.

Dynamic mechanical testing of lanolin by Radebaugh and Simonelli showed that pharmaceutical semisolids have many of the rheological and mechanical properties of polymers [80]. In particular, they demonstrated that anhydrous lanolin can exist in a molecular state whereby the molecules are immobilized, similar to that of a glassy state [23]. These authors showed that temperature–frequency superposition could be used to predict a priori the viscoelastic properties of anhydrous lanolin at shear frequencies up to 100,000 s^{-1}, far greater than could be attained with any commercially available mechanical property tester. Predictions such as this are possible for pharmaceutical semisolids in general. The techniques that allow one to make these predictions are described in Section III.F. In addition, it was shown that mathematical models used to predict the mechanical properties of filled polymers are also useful to explain the molecular interactions in powder-filled pharmaceutical semisolids [74]. Of particular note was the development of models that were able to differentiate the mechanical properties of the filled semisolids based on the surface properties of the powdered filler [75]. Additional discussion on models for powder-filled semisolids was included in Sections V.A and V.B.

E. Rheology of Emulsions

Emulsions can show the whole gamut of rheological properties, from essentially newtonian to highly viscoelastic. The particle size of emulsions can vary from less than 0.05 μm to more than 100 μm. Some emulsions contain macroglobules; in this case, the two phases may be visibly distinguishable owing to the relatively large particle size.

Gums are frequently used to increase the viscosity and stability of emulsions. Gums or macromolecules can add long-range order to an emulsion. The long molecular chains of the gum can interact with each other by entanglement or electrostatic force to mechanically inhibit the coalescence of the internal phase and, thereby, stabilize the emulsion. A great deal of viscoelasticity can be induced into an emulsion system by using appropriate gums. The logical extreme of this type of formulation is a total gel which, after a small displacement, will recover its original size and shape. Montmorillonite clays (e.g., bentonite) are useful to impart this type of structure.

Pseudoplastic flow is also seen in emulsions containing macromolecules. Since macromolecules tend to show greater entanglement at rest than when subjected to shear, the viscosity is initially high and decreases, nonlinearly, as the shear rate increases. At high shear rates, the macromolecules align themselves and squeeze out water, thereby lowering the viscosity of the system.

When surfactant thickening agents are used in emulsions, thixotropy can be induced into the system. Thixotropic systems can also show a degree of viscoelasticity. Here, the gel nature of the gel–sol transformation is responsible. It is important to remember that some degree of gel nature exist throughout the thixotropic hysteresis loop.

Pseudoplasticity, thixotropy, and viscoelasticity are not mutually exclusive, all may occur simultaneously in a dispersed system. Emulsions normally do not show dilatancy, but they can exhibit shear thickening. Dilatant systems are normally suspensions containing a high concentration of deflocculated, fine particles.

Microemulsions [87] are at the lower limit of the particle size range for dispersed systems. At very low particle size (e.g., 0.04 μm), the dispersed phase tends to be very uniform—that is, spherical with a narrow size distribution. When a microemulsion aggregates, a characteristic viscoelastic gel stage is produced. A change in the rheological properties can accurately determine the occurrence of this intermediate stage in the inversion of a microemulsion. Rheologically, the yield point of an emulsion increases as its viscosity increases. Dynamic viscosity measurements are used to determine the exact nature of the gel stage by providing values for the elastic and viscous moduli.

Disperse systems show a wide range of rheological properties, depending on the nature of the dispersed particles they contain and on the composition of the dispersion media. The rheology of dispersed systems is among the most important of their physical properties, which influences not only the physical stability of the systems, but often also profoundly affects the performance features, their quality, and their utility. At least a working knowledge and understanding of rheology is essential, not only for those who design this class of production, but also for those responsible for their manufacture and evaluation.

REFERENCES

1. W. C. Brasie, *Ind. Eng. Chem. Fundam.*, 3:37 (1964).
2. M. M. Soci and E. L. Parrot, *J. Pharm. Sci.*, 69:403 (1980).
3. A. Ludwig and M. Van Ooteghen, *Drug Dev. Ind. Pharm.*, 14:2267 (1988).
4. A. K. Pennington, J. H. Ratcliffe, C. G., Wilson, and J. G. Hardy, *Int. J. Pharm.*, 43:221 (1988).
5. G. Dicolo, V. Carelli, B. Giannaccini, M. F. Serafini, and F. Bottari, *J. Pharm. Sci.*, 69:387 (1980).
6. G. W. Radebaugh, J. M. Murtha, J. Bondi, and T. Julian, *Int. J. Pharm.*, 45:39 (1988).
7. J. M. Dealy, *J. Rheol.*, 28:181 (1984).
8. R. W. Whorlow, *Rheological Techniques*. Halsted Press, New York, 1980.
9. H. B. Kostenbauder and A. N. Martin, *J. Am. Pharm. Assoc. Sci. Ed.*, 48:401 (1954).
10. B. Idson, *Costmet. Toiletries*, 93(7):23 (1978).
11. P. Sherman, *Industrial Rheology*. Academic Press, New York, 1970.
12. H. Green and R. N. Weltmann, *Ind. Eng. Chem.*, 15:201 (1943).
13. J. C. Boylan, *J. Pharm. Sci.*, 55:710 (1966).
14. S. S. Ober, H. C. Vincent, D. E. Simon, and K. J. Frederick, *J. Am. Pharm. Assoc. Sci. Ed.*, 47:667 (1958).
15. P. E. Pierce and C. K. Schoff, Rheological measurements, in *Kirk-Othmer Encyclopedia of Chemical Technology*, Vol. 20, 3rd ed. Wiley-Interscience, New York, 1982, pp. 259–319.
16. A. N. Martin, J. Swarbrick, and A. Cammarata, *Physical Pharmacy*, 3rd ed. Lea & Febiger, Philadelphia, 1983.
17. J. D. Ferry, *Viscoelastic Properties of Polymers*. 3rd ed. John Wiley & Sons, New York, 1980.
18. J. J.Aklonis, W. J. MacKnight, and M. Shen, *Introduction to Polymer Viscoelasticity*. Interscience, New York, 1972.
19. J. Bischoff, E. Catsiff, and A. V. Tobolsky, *J. Am. Chem. Soc.*, 74:3378 (1952).
20. A. V. Tobolsky and J. R. McLoughlin, *J. Polym. Sci.*, 8:543 (1952).
21. J. D. Ferry, *J. Colloid Sci.*, 10:474 (1955).
22. J. R. Van Wazer, J. W. Lyons, K. Y. Kim, and R. E. Colwell, *Viscosity and Flow Measurements—A Laboratory Handbook of Rheology*. Interscience, New York, 1963.
23. G. W. Radebaugh and A. P. Simonelli, *J. Pharm. Sci.*, 72:422 (1983).
24. J. D. Ferry, *J. Am. Chem. Soc.*, 72:3746 (1950).
25. N. L. Henderson, P. M. Meer, and H. L. Kostenbauder, *J. Pharm. Sci.*, 50:788 (1961).
26. R. C. Harper, H. Markovitz, and T. W. DeWitt, *J. Polym. Sci.*, 8:435 (1952).
27. E. Catsiff and A. V. Tobolsky, *J. Colloid Sci.*, 10:375 (1955).
28. M. L. Williams, R. F. Landel, and J. D. Ferry, *J. Am. Chem. Soc.*, 77:3701 (1955).
29. L. E. Nielsen, *Mechanical Properties of Polymers*, Vol. 1. Marcel Dekker, New York (1974).
30. R. B. Bird, R. C. Armstrong, and O. Hassager, *Dynamics of Polymeric Liquids*, Vol. 1. John Wiley & Sons, New York, 1977, p. 18.
31. F. Daniels and R. A. Alberty, *Physical Chemistry*, 2nd ed. John Wiley and Sons, New York, 1961, p. 351.

32. C. W. Macosko, *Rheol. Acta.*, 13:814 (1974).
33. B. W. Barry, *Adv. Pharm. Sci.*, 4:1 (1974).
34. B. W. Barry, *J. Colloid Interface Sci.*, 28:82 (1968).
35. K. Inokuchi, *Bull. Chem. Soc. (Jpn).*, 28:453 (1955).
36. G. M. Saunders, Ph.D. Thesis, Portsmouth Polytechnic, Portsmouth, England (1971).
37. D. J. Burgess, L. Longo, and J. K. Yoon, *J. Parenter. Sci.*, 45:xx (1991).
38. D. J. Burgess, J. K. Yoon, and N. O. Sakin, *J. Parenter. Sci.*, 46:150 (1992).
39. M. Sheriff and B. Warburton, *Polymer*, 15:253 (1974).
40. J. H. De Smidt, J. Offringa, and D. J. A. Crommelin, *Int. J. Pharm.*, *77:255 (1991)*.
41. W. Hess and R. Klein, *Prog. Colloid Polym. Sci.*, 69:174 (1984).
42. E. J. Derderian and T. B. Macrury, *J. Dispersion Sci. Technol.*, 2:345 (1981).
43. E. I. Al-Khamis, S. S. Davis, and J. Hadgraft, *Pharm. Res.*, 3:214 (1986).
44. J. H. De Smidt and D. J. A. Crommelin, *Int. J. Pharm.*, 77:261 (1991).
45. J. Kristl, S. Pecar, J. Smid-Korbar, and M. Schara, *Pharm. Res.*, 8:505 (1991).
46. J. N. Dalal, N. S. Dalal, and J. K. Lim, *J. Soc. Cosmet. Chem.*, 38:1 (1987).
47. G. W. Radebaugh, *Encyclopedia of Pharmaceutical Technology*, Vol. 6. Marcel Dekker, New York, 1992, pp. 1–27.
48. L. E. Nielsen, *Mechanical Properties of Polymers*, Vol. 2. Marcel Dekker, New York, 1974, p. 379.
49. A. Einstein, *Ann. Phys. (Paris)*, 19:289 (1906).
50. A. Einstein, *Ann. Phys. (Paris)*, 24:591 (1911).
51. I. R. Rutgers, *Rheol. Acta.*, 2:305 (1962).
52. M. Mooney, *J. Colloid Sci.*, 6:162 (1951).
53. T. B. Lewis and L. E. Nielsen, *Trans. Soc. Rheol.*, 12:421 (1968).
54. M. M. Cross, *J. Appl. Polym. Sci.*, 13:765 (1969).
55. M. M. Cross, *J. Colloid Interface Sci.*, 33:30 (1970).
56. I. M. Krieger and T. J. Dougherty, *Trans. Soc. Rheol.*, 3:137 (1959).
57. T. Gillespie, *J. Colloid Interface Sci.*, 22:554 (1966).
58. T. Gillespie, *J. Colloid Interface Sci.*, 22:563 (1966).
59. H. M. Smallwood, *J. Appl. Phys.*, 15:758 (1944).
60. E. Guth, *J. Appl. Phys.*, 16:20 (1945).
61. L. E. Nielsen, *Compos. Mater.*, 2:120 (1968).
62. T. B. Lewis and L. E. Nielsen, *J. Appl. Polym. Sci.*, 14:1449 (1970).
63. G. I. Taylor, *Proc. R. Soc. (Lond.)* A, 138:41 (1932).
64. G. K. Batchelor, *J. Fluid Mech.*, 41:545 (1970).
65. E. H. Kerner, *Proc. Phys. Soc., (Lond.)*, B69:808 (1956).
66. L. E. Nielsen, *J. Appl. Phys.*, 41:4626 (1970).
67. *United States Pharmacopiea,* 22nd Rev., U.S. Pharmacopeial Convention, Rockville, MD, (1970).
68. L. I. Conrad, *Am. Perfume Essent. Oil Rev.*, 6:177 (1954).
69. G. Barnett, *Drug Costmet. Ind.*, 80:610 (1957).
70. C. W. Macosko and J. Starita, *SPE J.*, 27:38 (1971).
71. F. R. Schwarzl, H. Bree, C. Nederveen, G. Schwippert, C. Struik, and C. van der Waal, *Rheol. Acta,* 5:270 (1966).
72. R. W. Gray and N. G. McCrum, *J. Polym. Sci.*, (Part A-2) 7:1329 (1969).
73. L. E. Nielsen, *Trans. Soc. Rheol.*, 13:141 (1969).
74. G. W. Radebaugh and A. P. Simonelli, *J. Pharm. Sci.*, 73:590 (1984).
75. G. W. Radebaugh and A. P. Simonelli, *J. Pharm. Sci.*, 74:3 (1985).
76. D. C-H. Cheng, *Chem. Ind. (Lond.),* 10:403 (1980).
77. E. N. Hiestand, *J. Pharm. Sci.*, 53:1 (1964).
78. M. von Smoluchowski, *Phys. Z.*, 17:757 (1917).
79. M. von Smoluchowski, *Z. Phys. Chem.*, 92:129 (1917).

80. G. W. Radebaugh and A. P. Simonelli, *J. Pharm. Sci.*, 72:415 (1983).
81. D.J. W. Grant and G. G. Liversidge, *Drug Dev. Ind. Pharm.*, 9:247 (1983).
82. J. T. Tukker, W. Van Vught, and C. J. DeBlaey, *Acta Pharm. Technol.*, 29:187 (1983).
83. J. Doucet, *Ann. Pharm. Fr.*, 33:253 (1975).
84. B. W. Barry and A. J. Grace, *J. Pharm. Sci.*, 60:1198 (1971).
85. K. Suzuki and T. Watanabe, *Am. Perfumume Cosmet.*, 85(9):115 (1970).
86. B. W. Barry and A. J. Grace, *Rheol. Acta*, 10:113 (1971).
87. L. M. Prince, in *Microemulsions: Theory and Practice* (L. M. Prince, ed.) Academic Press, New York, 1977, p. 12.

6

Surfactants

Martin M. Rieger

M. & A. Rieger Associates, Morris Plains, New Jersey

I. DEFINITIONS AND GENERAL PROPERTIES OF SURFACTANTS

The term *surfactant* is routinely used as shorthand for the more descriptive term *surface active agent*. Sometimes a surfactant is defined as any material that "lowers the surface tension of water." This definition of a surfactant is unsatisfactory, since the lowering of surface tension is a property of matter. Reduced surface tension is merely evidence for the adsorption of soluble or insoluble molecules at the interface of two phases (e.g., in the most common examples under discussion, at the border between air and water). Attempts to learn more about this phenomenon occupied some of the most creative scientists since Pliny the Elder's efforts to understand the calming effect of oil on turbulent seas [1].

To the theoretically inclined, the most satisfactory definition of a surfactant is based on the Gibbs adsorption equation. According to this thermodynamic equation, any material that makes a *surface contribution* to the free energy of the surface phase of a two-component system is a surfactant. A derivation of the Gibbs absorption equation, based on Gibbs' approach in 1876, can be found in most textbooks of physical chemistry and is based on ideal conditions. Some additional approaches are discussed by Adamson [2]. The best known form of the Gibbs equation:

$$\Gamma_2 = -\frac{a}{RT}\frac{d\gamma}{da} \tag{1}$$

where Γ_2 is the excess surface concentration of the solute (surfactant), γ is the surface tension, a is the activity of the solute, R is the gas constant, and T is the absolute temperature.

The Gibbs equation permits some concrete interpretation: If $d\gamma/da$, the change in surface tension with increase in activity (concentration), is negative, Γ_2 is positive. The practical result is that the concentration of the solute at or in the surface is greater than that in the bulk phase. Experimentally, this phenomenon has been demonstrated by comparing the composition of a bulk solution of a surfactant with that of a surface sample.

The Gibbs equation has universal applications. It can be applied directly to nonionic solutes; with ionizing solutes, the concentrations (activities) of both ions must be considered, and the resulting modification of the Gibbs equation becomes much more complex. The Gibbs equation (and its use in surface chemistry) is also applicable to both aqueous and nonaqueous systems. Since surfactants are customarily viewed as exhibiting their surface activity in aqueous systems, the subsequent discussion of surfactants will be concerned primarily with water-based systems.

The abstract concepts of the Gibbs equation can be clarified by a concrete explanation. Each molecule of solvent in the bulk solvent (water) is equally attracted in all directions to adjacent molecules by hydrogen bonding. On the other hand, the water molecules at the hypothetical surface [the air (vapor)–bulk interface] are experiencing attractive forces only laterally and into the bulk of the solvent. (The work required to enlarge this surface by 1 cm^2 against the opposing attractive forces is called the surface tension of water.) If a solute, such as ethanol, which is less hydrophilic than water, is now added to the water, the Gibbs equation demands that this solute, at equilibrium, be more concentrated on the surface than in the bulk. On the basis of molecular structures, Langmuir enunciated the "principle of independent surface action" some years ago. According to this concept, each segment of a molecule can act and interact independently from other portions of the same molecule. Thus, there is a strong attraction (hydrogen bonding) between the OH portion of ethanol and water. On the other hand, the hydrocarbon portion of the ethanol molecule bonds only weakly (by London dispersion forces) to water molecules. The result is that the ethanol molecules are not only squeezed to the surface, but are aligned on it such that the OH end faces (or is in) the aqueous medium, whereas the hydrocarbon end (CH_3–CH_2–) faces outward. The same principle, with minor modifications, applies to all systems containing surface-active agents.

Although quite hydrophilic, ethanol conforms to the Gibbs equation and lowers the surface tension of water. On the other hand, glycerol, which forms strong hydrogen bonds with water, does not concentrate at the surface and has almost no effect on the surface tension of water unless its concentration exceeds 50%.

The reduction of surface tension, as in an ethanol–water mixture or of more typical surfactants, results from the powerful (hydrogen bond) attraction of water molecules for each other. As a result, the less strongly hydrogen-bonded molecules of ethanol or of a surfactant are literally squeezed out of the bulk and find a "more comfortable home"—that is, concentrate—at the surface. As the hydrocarbon chain length of the alcohol increases, this tendency toward concentration at the surface also increases. If the concentration of the surfactant in solution is raised beyond the level at which the solute can be accommodated on the surface, an argument can be developed to explain the self-association of molecules to form micelles.

These thermodynamic considerations and their relation to molecular structure provide a meaningful definition of a surface-active agent. This definition fails, however, to satisfy the day-to-day needs of individuals who employ surfactants for various practical applications, because it includes molecules (e.g., ethanol) that do not function as surfactants. As a result, it is most useful to define a *functional surfactant* as a substance of fairly high molecular weight that possesses a polar and a nonpolar region on the same molecule. With this as a working definition, one can readily understand why such molecules will concentrate at or near the surface of the solvent. In the case of water, the polar end of such molecules will be in contact with "liquid" water, whereas the nonpolar portion will more likely be in contact with a second water-immiscible phase. In 1936, Hartley called such molecules "amphipathic" because one portion has sympathy and another antipathy for water. Today the term *amphiphilic* is used. The polar portion of an amphiphilic molecule is generally called the *head*, whereas the hydrocarbon chain of such a molecule is thought of as the *tail*. A very large number of organic molecules can exhibit the phenomenon of amphiphilicity, and molecules can be classified in accordance with their amphiphilic profile without much difficulty.

A realistic and up-to-date definition of a surfactant can now be given: a *surfactant* is an amphiphilic compound that (a) is soluble in at least one phase of the system, (b) forms oriented monolayers at phase interfaces, (c) exhibits equilibrium concentrations at phase interfaces higher than those in the bulk solution and forms micelles at specific concentrations, and (d) exhibits one or more of the following characteristics: detergency, foaming, wetting, emulsifying, solubilizing, and dispersing.

Surfactants, by virtue of their ability to adsorb at all types of interface, are used today in a multiplicity of industrial processes and personal (health) care products. Many of the products that are now taken for granted depend on the presence of surfactants for their usefulness or existence. Ore flotation, detergency, soap, mayonnaise, and emulsion polymers are just a few typical examples. Surfactants are critical for the formulation of disperse systems in drug and cosmetic products. They are required during the formulation and manufacturing processes and are essential for imparting physical stability to these systems.

II. PHYSICAL DESCRIPTION OF SURFACTANTS IN SOLUTION

In addition to the phenomenon of adsorption to the liquid–air interface (examined by Gibbs), surfactants exhibit two other key properties that account for a variety of surface phenomena. One of these is adsorption to surfaces other than the air–water interface, that is, adsorption to lipophilic or polar substrates; the other is self-association. The thermodynamic principle responsible for both phenomena is a balance between the removal of the hydrophobic portion of the surface-active molecule from its aqueous environment and the electrostatics of the system. As previously noted, the polar head group of an amphiphile at an air–water interface is dissolved in the aqueous medium, whereas the hydrophobic domain is in contact with the air. Similarly, the hydrophobic domains of amphiphiles at a hydrocarbon–water interface preferentially contact the hydrocarbon. This accounts, in part, for the ability of amphiphiles to effect emulsification.

In pharmaceutical practice, the use of surfactants is limited to dilute solutions. Only soap and detergent bars are distributed in concentrated forms by the pharmaceutical and personal care industries. As a result, the complex physical behavior of surfactants in concentrated solutions or in pure form needs to be discussed only briefly. The amphiphilic surfactant molecules tend to exhibit unusual solubilities and to form complex association structures in aqueous media in high concentration.

The temperature–solubility relationship of most anionic surfactants is not smooth. Instead, the solubility of most anionic surfactants, especially of carboxylates or soaps, increases at the so-called Krafft temperature. Concentrated solutions, once formed, exhibit complex phase behavior that has been extensively studied, especially by investigators in the soap industry [3]. Today, the unusual terminology of these phases persists in the description of phase changes of other anionic surfactants, which is based on X-ray diffraction patterns (neat, neat and nigre, middle). These phenomena and the formation of mesomorphic liquid crystals (smectic, nematic, and cholesteric) detected in polarized light are of limited interest to pharmaceutical product formulators. They are, however, critical in the development of the highly concentrated solid and liquid detergents marketed for household and industrial cleaning.

At temperatures below about 50°C and at concentrations below about 10–15%, surfactant solutions are still highly unusual. Early investigators of the physical and chemical properties of amphiphiles soon learned that aqueous solutions of surfactants were somewhat abnormal. For example, ionic surfactants in dilute solutions behave as true electrolytes in terms of conductivity; however, at higher concentrations the equivalent conductivity shows a sudden discontinuity. Other physical properties, including detergency, interfacial tension, and surface tension, also show sudden changes at or near a specific concentration (Fig. 1). The explanation of these phenomena on the basis of self-association (i.e., micelle formation) was highly controversial at the time [4]. For purely illustrative purposes, two early models of micelle structure are presented in Fig. 2, and discussion of other models is postponed (see Sec. II.C). The surfactant molecules are commonly viewed as stick figures, with a polar (round) head and a hydrocarbon (straight) tail. Today the concept that micelles are molecular aggregates formed in solutions of surface-active agents is universally accepted. Surfactants in very dilute aqueous solution can exist primarily as monomers; at higher concentrations several surfactant molecules may aggregate to form micelles, which are frequently (and probably erroneously) depicted as perfectly formed (Fig. 3).

In an aqueous medium, the polar groups of the micellized surfactant face outward, whereas the hydrocarbon tails form the core. The specific concentration at which the physical and chemical properties of a dilute aqueous solution of a surfactant undergo sudden discontinuities is referred to as the critical micelle concentration (CMC). Any

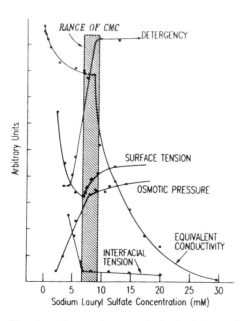

Fig. 1 Changes in several physical properties of aqueous sodium lauryl sulfate solutions as a function of concentration. (Modified from Ref. 138.)

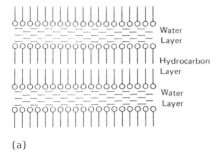

(a)

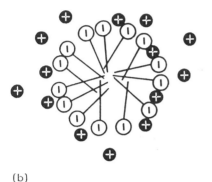

(b)

Fig. 2 Early models of micelles: (a) McBain lamellar micelle and (b) Hartley spherical micelle.

further increase in amphiphile concentration beyond the CMC usually has only a limited effect on most physical properties of the surfactant solution, as shown in Fig. 1. A more comprehensive pictorial description (Fig. 4) by Friberg and El-Nokaly [5] related the phenomena on the surface to those occurring in solution. The important point

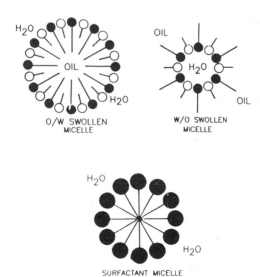

Fig. 3 Idealized cross-sectional designs of micelles of various types. (These micelles may be spherical or rod-shaped.)

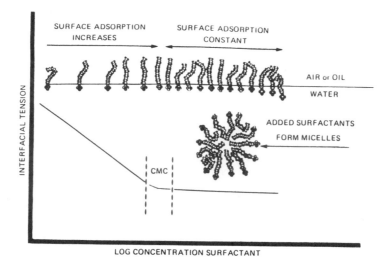

Fig. 4 Schematic showing surfactant adsorption. Surfactants adsorb strongly to a water–air interface or a water–oil interface owing to their amphiphilic nature (top). The accompanying reduction of interfacial tension [in accordance with Eq. (1), the Gibbs equation] ceases in a narrow concentraton range (the critical micellization concentration; CMC). At concentrations above this range, added surfactant will aggregate to form micelles. (From Ref. 5.)

to remember is that an increase of the concentration of the surfactant beyond the critical micelle concentration changes the numbers, the sizes, or the shapes of micelles, but does not provide an increase in the concentration of the monomeric species.

A. Micelle Formation

The events leading to the formation of micelles could be conceptualized as follows (see Fig. 4): In very dilute aqueous solution, amphiphiles tend to concentrate on the surface, in accordance with the precepts developed by Gibbs. As the concentration of the amphiphile is increased, the molecules of the amphiphile at the surface become more and more crowded until there is literally no more space in the surface layer. The amphiphilic molecules are then forced to remain in the aqueous solution, in which they cause significant disruption of the hydrogen-bonding between water molecules. To minimize this disruption, amphiphilic molecules tend to aggregate into multiple molecular structures. The dominant cause for this self-association is not the interaction between the hydrophobic tails of these surfactant molecules (i.e., hydrophobic bonding or London dispersion forces), but is found in the role of the self-attraction of water by virtue of (the energetically much larger) hydrogen bond formation. Tanford some years ago computed the free energy of attraction between water and a low molecular weight hydrocarbon to be about -40 ergs cm^{-2}. However, the attraction of water for itself is more than three times as high: -144 erg cm^{-2}. The unusual properties exhibited by aqueous solutions of amphiphiles are the result of disruption of water–water attractions. Thus, the driving force for micelle formation must be sought in the entropy gain resulting from the disruption of the water structure.

The CMC of anionic surfactants increases with increasing temperature, whereas that of nonionic surfactants decreases with increasing temperature. In aqueous solutions, the CMC of anionic surfactants is reached at about 0.2–0.3% (about 7.5 mM), depending on molecular weight and structure. Cationic surfactants tend to reach their CMC at about half that concentration, about 3 mM. Finally, the CMC of nonionic surfactants, especially those obtained by polyoxyethylation, is much lower (about 0.024 mM).

Amphiphiles also form micelles or association structures in nonaqueous systems. The driving force for this type of complex formation are dipole–dipole interactions of the polar head groups, which in this instance form the center of the "inverse" micelles, and dispersion forces between the nonpolar tails and the solvent. These complexes are believed to be responsible for the ability of amphiphiles to solubilize water in hydrocarbon solvents and form the basis for water-in-oil (W/O) emulsions, but neither their nature nor their structure is well understood. The existence of a CMC in these micellar systems is controversial.

In systems containing two or more surfactants, the micelles formed are likely to include more than one surfactant. Such mixed micelles (i.e., micellar aggregates of two or more surfactants) form readily, even if the surfactants are chemically different. Thus, anionic or quaternary surfactants can form mixed micelles with nonionic surfactants. In the micellization of cetyltrimethylammonium bromide (CTAB) and polyethylene glycol (PEG)-10 lauryl ether, the CMC varies as a function of the mole ratio (Fig. 5). Inves-

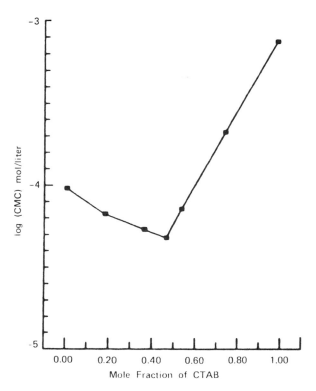

Fig. 5 Variation of the CMC of mixtures of cetyltrimethylammonium bromide and PEG-10 lauryl ether. [After Ref. 139.)

tigators actually believe that a secondary CMC exists in this system when the level of the surfactant mixture is raised at a constant mole ratio. Regardless of these complications, formulators must always remember that surfactants can interact, even in the absence of any chemical change. In the case at hand, the antimicrobial action of the quaternary is probably reduced by mixed micelle formation in the presence of the nonionic agent.

B. Thermodynamic Aspects of Micelle Formation

Several models have been developed to assist in the interpretation of micellar behavior, but only two of them will be discussed here. In the original one, the so-called mass action model, micelles are considered to be in equilibrium with the unassociated surfactant. Thus, for a nonionic surfactant, n (the aggregation number) molecules of the monomeric un-ionized surfactant(s) react in a single step to form a micelle, M:

$$nS \rightleftharpoons M \tag{2}$$

If the activity coefficient is ignored, the equilibrium constant for micelle formation K_m is then given as

$$K_m = \frac{[M]}{[S]^n} \tag{3}$$

In this and subsequent equations, the terms in brackets refer to the molar concentration of the species. Conventional thermodynamic arguments then show that—when n is large—the free energy of micellization at the critical micelle concentration is

$$\Delta G_m^0 = RT \ln[S]_{cmc} \tag{4}$$

where G_m^0 represents the standard free energy change for transferring 1 mol of S from the aqueous solution into its micellar form.

For an ionized surfactant, the ionic micelle derived from an anionic surfactant is formed by the association of n surfactant ions S^- and of $(n - p)$ firmly bound counterions (e.g., X^+) as follows:

$$nS^- + (n - p)X^+ \rightleftharpoons M^{-p} \tag{5}$$

Assuming ideality, the equilibrium constant for micelle formation is then given by

$$K_m^2 = \frac{[M^{-p}]}{[S^-]^n[X^+]^{n-p}} \tag{6}$$

As above, classic thermodynamics show that, when the aggregation number n is large, the free energy of micellization at or near the critical micelle concentration reduces to

$$\Delta G_m^0 = \left(2 - \frac{p}{n}\right) RT \ln[S^-]_{cmc} \tag{7}$$

If micellization of an ionic surfactant takes place in a system of high electrolyte content, Eq. (7) can be replaced by Eq. (6).

The second model, identified as the phase-separation model, considers micelles as a separate phase at the critical micelle concentration. Here μ_s and μ_m^0 are defined as the chemical potentials (per mole) of the free surfactant in the aqueous phase and of the associated surfactant in the micellar phase respectively. At equilibrium $\mu_s = \mu_{mt}^0$

If activity coefficients are ignored, μ_s is related to the surfactant's standard state μ_s^0 by

$$\mu_s = \mu_s^0 + RT \ln [S] \tag{8}$$

On the other hand, the micellar material is in its standard state, and $\mu_m = \mu_m^0$. The standard free energy of micellization is $\Delta G_m^0 = \mu_m^0 - \mu_s^0$. Upon combination with Eq. (8), this also yields Eq. (4) for ΔG_m^0. The analogous approach for an ionized surfactant yields.

$$\Delta G_m^0 = [1 + (n - p)]RT \ln [S^-]_{cmc} \tag{9}$$

where n and p are defined as previously.

The CMC of most surfactants is lowered by the presence of electrolytes. This phenomenon has been known for some time, and many have reported that CMC values may be in error owing to inadvertent contamination with neutral salts. Increasing levels of sodium chloride lower the CMC of alkyl sulfates (i.e., the CMC is reached at lower surfactant concentrations). Typical data are shown in Table 1, which demonstrate the sensitivity of the CMC of sodium lauryl sulfate to the presence of even small amounts of salt. The presence of electrolytes also affects the micellar aggregation number: Sodium dodecyl sulfate micelles in water may consists of about 60–80 molecules. This aggregation number is doubled in the presence of 0.5 M sodium chloride.

Relatively little attention has been paid to the mathematical treatment of mixed micelles. For the nonionic mixed micelles, the phase-separation model, assuming ideality, provides a satisfactory approach. On the other hand, mixed micelles of a nonionic and an ionized surfactant must take account of the counterions, and ideality is unlikely. Under these circumstances, the equations describing micelle formation become rather formidable. [Interested readers are referred to publications by D. G. Hall, e.g., *Colloids Surfaces*, 13:209–219 (1985).]

Micellization is exothermic and occurs more readily the colder the system. This is true for ionizing surfactants that show a CMC minimum [6,7] at approximately room temperature; the CMC rises sharply when the temperature is raised to about 50° or 60°C. For the nonionic micelles of the polyoxyethylene type, the CMC decreases with

Table 1 The CMC of Sodium Lauryl Sulfate in Water and NaCl Solutions at 25°C

NaCl (M)	CMC (mg/100 ml)
0	234
0.02	112
0.03	90
0.1	42
0.2	26
0.4	17

Source: Based on Ref. 135.

increasing temperature. Pressure also has an effect on CMC. As a rule, the CMC increases up to approximately 100 mPa and, then, decreases as the pressure is raised.

The rates at which micelles form and break and at which monomers enter and leave micelles are extremely rapid. Recent studies, briefly reviewed by Attwood and Florence, have shown that two processes are taking place [8]. One of these, the slow process, is related to the complete dissolution or dissociation of the micelle into monomers and, conversely, its re-formation. In addition, a fast process has been detected that is 100–1000 times faster and is believed to result from the exchange of monomers between micelles and the bulk solution but does not cause complete destruction of some micelles. In summary, micelles are not permanent structures. Instead, they constantly disintegrate and re-form. The average residence time of surfactant molecules in a micelle is only about 10^{-8} s.

Finally, nonmicellar association or, more specifically, premicellar aggregation should be considered. As a rule, dimers and trimers are formed in dilute solutions of molecules containing hydrophobic chains [9]. These aggregates form below the CMC. The evidence for the existence of these types of aggregations in ionic surfactants is highly controversial, since one would expect the electrostatic forces to repel these oligomeric complexes. Despite the controversial nature of this effect, its existence could be of great importance for surfactantlike drug molecules. Their in vivo diffusion and distribution could be seriously impeded by the formation of high molecular weight dimeric and trimeric structures. Thus, diphenhydramine HC1 has a micellar aggregation number of 3 [10] and tripelennamine HCL also has an aggregation number of 3 [11]. Much higher aggregation numbers have been reported for chlorpromazine, imipramine, and many other drugs. Micelle formation by "simple" drug molecules affects drug transport by virtue of an increase in "molecular" size. On the other hand, the drug's surface activity may alter the membrane's resistance to diffusion. Thus, estimates of a drug's activity based exclusively on the concentration of monomeric species generally underestimate the drug's efficacy [12].

C. Micelle Structure

Some principles of micelle formation have been discussed in the preceding section. McBain originally suggested that surfactant molecules form micellar structures by associating with each other in double leaflets to form lamellar micelles (see Fig. 2a). This concept was later modified by Hartley, who proposed the existence of loose spherical aggregates (see Fig. 2b). In Hartley's spherical micelles the molecules are *not* aligned radially, and the negatively charged heads and the positively charged counterions are not fitted to yield a perfect sphere.) [13].

Alternative shapes, such as oblate or prolate forms, have been suggested, especially for the polyoxyethylene derivatives (Fig. 6). Representations of micelles as perfect spheres or cylinders (see Fig. 3) should be identified as "idealized" models [14]. The idealized micelle shown in Fig. 6 also illustrates the uncertainties of the location of the counterions and differentiates between bound and unbound counterions. These problems are reflected in Eqs. (6) and (9), for the free energy of micelle formation.

Shape is related to size, and the latter is controlled predominantly by the aggregation number, n [cf. Eqs. (2) and (5)], that is, the number of molecules that associate to form a single micelle. Unfortunately, one cannot depend on reported aggregation numbers because they vary from author to author; more importantly, there is no assurance that all micelles in a given system have the same shape and aggregation number.

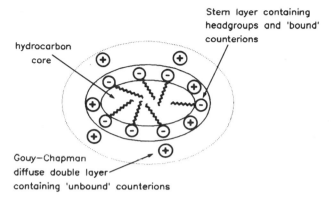

Fig. 6 Elliptical cross section through a (proloid spheroid) idealized anionic detergent micelle. (After Ref. 14.)

Studies of static light scattering with laser light suggest the following sequence of events in a cetyltrimethylammonium bromide (CTAB) solution in the presence of sodium bromide [15]. Aqueous solutions of CTAB above the CMC contain spherical micelles formed from 91 CTAB monomers. Rodlike and spherical micelles coexist at low sodium bromide concentrations. As the concentration of sodium bromide is raised, rodlike micelles become the preponderant species, and their association numbers can rise to about 9500. These huge, tortuous, threadlike structures are flexible and have a cross-sectional diameter of 4.5–6.0 nm. A few years ago, such structures, postulated on the basis of light-scattering studies, were actually observed by electronmicroscopy [16,17].

Interesting proposals for micelle structure include the pincushion model proposed by Menger [4,18] and the block model proposed by Fromherz [19]. Many published idealized micelle structural models (Figs. 3 and 7a) suggest that water does not contact the hydrophobic portion of the amphiphilic molecules in the micellar center and that the hydrophobic segments in the center are crowded. It can be safely concluded that the classic representation (see Fig. 7a) is unrealistic. Dill and Flory, therefore, proposed their so-called lattice model (see Fig. 7b) [20]. These authors were less concerned with the shape of the micelle than with the arrangement of alkyl chains in the micellar core. Their

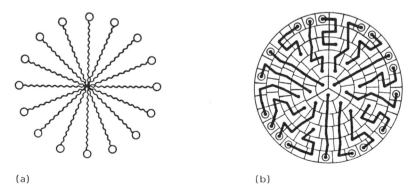

(a)   (b)

Fig. 7 Lattice model of micelle: (a) classical representation and (b) Dill–Flory lattice. (Courtesy of Prof. K. A. Dill.)

model allows chain bending to fill the limited space in the micellar core. Their construct also excludes water from the hydrocarbon core of micelles, but permits some contact between hydrophobic chains and the surrounding aqueous phase near the micelle's surface.

Imae and co-workers demonstrated that the geometric shape of micelles depends on the presence of electrolytes and on concentration [15]. In addition, Hoffman concluded that spherical micelles are preponderant in dilute surfactant solutions, whereas rodlike micelles are likely to form at somewhat higher concentrations [21]. Lamellar structures probably require still higher concentrations and represent a stage that precedes liquid crystals and microemulsion formation [22,23].

The discussion of micellar shape has so far neglected any contribution from the shape of the monomeric surfactant building blocks. This relation was formalized by Israelachvili [24]. A "critical packing parameter"—defined by the expression V/AL, where V is the volume of the hydrophobe of the amphiphile, L is the effective extended length of the hydrophobe (taking into account double bonds and other restrictions), and A is the *area* occupied by the hydrophilic head of the amphiphile—relates the expected aggregate structure to the surfactant's geometry (Table 2). This table also relates the surfactant's general nature to its critical packing parameter. Israelachvili's concepts can be applied directly to the selection of surfactants useful for emulsification, solubilization, and vesicle (liposome) formation. The concept of the critical packing parameter provides a scheme for predicting the shapes of the association complexes formed by surfactants and related substances. Not all association structures fit neatly into this scheme, but Israelachvili's generalizations help in understanding the geometry of most association complexes. More than 40 years ago the foresighted W. D. Harkins asserted that the number of molecules in a micelle is determined by their geometry. He asserted that the chains come together because of expulsion by the water and that the heads repel each other, thus increasing their spacing.

The principles of micellization are of great practical importance to the formulator, as discussed in Sections IV, V, and VI. In addition, micelles have an important and essentially unpredictable effect on the chemical stability of drug molecules. Also, they have the ability to solubilize active drug constituents by including them within their structure.

Micellization is an important mechanism of drug solubilization (see Sec. VI.B). The deliberate or inadvertent formation of so-called swollen micelles may affect the bioavailability of drugs in at least two ways: first, release of the drug for pharmacological action requires "destruction" of the micelle, and second, a micellized drug may not be able to diffuse to the target organ by virtue of its size.

D. Adsorption of Surfactants on Low-Energy Surfaces

The mechanism by which surfactants concentrate at an interface and form monolayers was previously described in connection with the derivation of the Gibbs adsorption isotherm for a surfactant solution in contact with air. For pharmaceuticals, aqueous solutions of surfactants are of primary interest. The interface between air and an aqueous surfactant solution is not ideal and cannot be precisely defined. The water at the interface exists partly as a liquid and partly as a vapor, and the latter is gradually diluted with air as a function of the distance from the true liquid. Thus, in fact, the interface is a region, and its precise nature is affected by the presence of solvents (e.g., propylene glycol) or of solutes (e.g., electrolytes), by temperature, and by pressure. Despite

Table 2 Relation of CPP[a] to Surfactants' Geometry

Surfactant features	Surfactant shape	Critical packing parameters[a]	Likely structure of aggregate	Nature of surfactant
Single alkyl chain, with large nonionic head or SDS[b] at low salt content	Cone	< 1/3	Spherical or ellipsoidal micelles (O/W)	Hydrophilic
Single alkyl chain, with small head or, e.g., SDS or CTAB[b] at high salt content	Truncated cone	1/3–1/2	Cylindrical or rod-shaped micelles (O/W)	Hydrophilic
Double alkyl chain, with large headgroup (lecithin, dialkyl dimethylammonium salts)	Truncated cone (close to cylinder)	1/2–1	Flexible bilayers or vesicle	Hydrophilic
Double alkyl chain with small headgroup	Cylinder	1	Planar bilayer	Hydrophilic/ hydrophobic
Double, bulky alkyl chain or multiple unsaturation with small headgroup	Inverted truncated	> 1	W/O micelles (inverted)	Hydrophobic

[a]The critical packing parameter of a surfactant is defined as

$$CPP = \frac{volume}{(area\ of\ hydrophilic\ head) \times (length\ of\ hydrophobe)}$$

[b]SDS, sodium dodecyl sulfate; CTAB, cetyltrimethylammonium bromide.

these complications, it is useful to examine surfactant solution adsorption phenomena at three interfaces: that with air, that with a liquid, and that with a solid.

1. *Surfactant Solution–Air Interface*

As defined by the Gibbs equation (Eq. 1) the presence of a water-soluble surfactant lowers the surface tension; for example, that of water from 72.8 mN/m to values as low as about 20–30 mN/m, as the surfactant's concentration approaches the CMC (see Fig. 1). Surface tension for the purposes at hand may be defined as a tangential force, on the surface of a liquid, that minimizes the interfacial area between the liquid and air. The lowering of the surface tension results from the coating of the air–solution interface by the alkyl chains of the surfactant.

The lowering of the surface tension of aqueous systems is also responsible for the generation of foam. Most foams are dispersions of a gas (air) in an aqueous solution of a surfactant. In foam, air bubbles are surrounded by a thin layer of the surfactant solution. The hydrophilic heads of the surfactant contact the aqueous phase, while the hydrophobic portions contact the gas phase. Once formed, the curved aqueous films tend to drain, producing a thinner film that ultimately collapses. The collapse is aided by gas diffusion, since the gas pressure inside the bubble (P) obeys the Young/Laplace equation, $P = 2\gamma/R$, where γ is the surface tension and R the bubble radius. As a result, the gas from smaller bubbles tends to diffuse into larger bubbles. The formation of stable foams in pharmaceutical products is generally undesirable, but foam is desirable in cosmetic products, such as shaving preparations and shampoos.

2. *The Surfactant Solution–Liquid Interface*

Monolayers similar to those between a gas and a surfactant solution are also formed when such a solution is in contact with an insoluble liquid. This phenomenon assists in the formation of emulsions. As a rule, an O/W emulsion will be formed if the surfactant has high water solubility [high hydrophilic–lipophilic balance (HLB); see Sec. III]. By analogy, oil-soluble surfactants (low HLB) also concentrate at an oil–water interface and yield W/O emulsions. The use of surfactants as emulsifiers in pharmaceutical dosage forms is discussed in detail in Chapter 3 and in Volume 2, Chapters 2 and 7.

The effect of surfactants on surface tension not only accounts for the spreading of insoluble liquids on surfactant solution (or the reverse phenomenon), but also for the spreading of liquids on solids, as described in the following.

3. *The Surfactant Solution–Solid Interface*

Several phenomena are involved in the interaction of a surfactant solution with a solid. One of these is the surfactant's ability to adhere to the solid, which is commonly called *adsorption*. It is a phenomenon that depends on characteristic interactions between a solid and a surfactant. The second phenomenon facilitates access of the surfactant's solute to the solid. This phenomenon, generally identified as *wetting*, is dominated by the interfacial energies of the (generally three-phase) system: solid, air, and solution. Both types of phenomena may occur simultaneously and require some additional comments.

Surfactant absorption onto solids is partly due to the amphiphilic nature of the surfactant and partly due to the surfactant's ionization. The adsorption of surfactants to solids (see Chap. 2, this volume, Vol. 2, Chap. 1) probably involves adsorption of single ions or molecules, rather than (mixed) micellar aggregates. Ionizing surfactants can be adsorbed to surfaces by ion-exchange or by ion-pairing mechanisms. The former involves the replacement of a counterion that is already adsorbed onto the substrate by an identically charged surfactant ion. In ion pairing, the surfactant ion is adsorbed directly onto an oppositely charged site on the substrate.

The third means of bonding is hydrogen bonding, in which hydrogen bonds are formed between the substrate and the adsorbed surfactant. A fourth adsorption mechanism involves dispersion forces in which there is some preferential interaction between the hydrophobic (water-repellent) portion of the surfactant molecule and a similar hydrophobic portion of the low-energy surface. Finally, it has been reported that bonding by polarization of π electrons between a strongly positively charged adsorbent and an electron-rich aromatic ring is possible.

In light of these various effects, the practical results of contact between a solid (powdered or continuous) and a surfactant solution can now be assessed in a more practical vein. The lowered surface tension of a surfactant solution facilitates wetting. Wetting of continuous solid surfaces is of critical importance in surface cleansing. The wetting of powdered substances facilitates removal of adsorbed or entrapped air and wetting-out of a powdered solid. This is vitally important for the creation of suspensions of insoluble solids in liquid media.

The wetting phenomenon is preferably viewed as a balancing of the free energies of the system's components; liquid, solid, and air (vapor). Details of these interactions and their description by Dupre and Young can be found in Chapter 2, this volume.

The presence of surfactants alters the surface characteristics of the solid and of the solution. Thus, all spreading and wetting phenomena encountered in pharmaceutical product development are critically dependent on surfactants. One of these is the so-called critical surface tension, which is determined by the relationship between a (wetting) liquid's surface tension and its contact angle on any solid. The critical surface tension of a solid is readily determined from a plot of the contact angle θ (see Chap. 2) versus the surface tension of various liquids and extrapolation to $\cos \theta = 0$. The critical surface tension of a solid is a characteristic property and is used to predict wetting of a solid by a liquid. Wetting occurs only if the surface tension of the liquid is equal to, or less than, the critical surface tension of the solid.

The critical surface tension plays a role in the incorporation of various pharmaceutical solids into finished dosage forms. Contact angles of water or aqueous systems on pharmaceutically important powders can be measured by compressing pharmaceutical powders or by preparing disks and the like by melting. Contact angles on finely divided solids can also be determined by packing the powder into a tube and measuring the penetration of liquids into the packing. Typical data have been developed by Lerk and co-workers [25,26], and some of their data are included in Table 3. The concepts that water-soluble materials exhibit a relatively low contact angle and that materials with high contact angles are classified as hydrophobic are clearly revealed by these data. For additional information on this topic see Chapters 2 and 3.

Mechanisms responsible for the adsorption of surfactants onto various substrates have already been mentioned. Regardless of the mechanism, surfactants are used to modify the surface properties of solids of all types, which may be either the substrate or a (drug) component of a finished pharmaceutical product. Such adsorption depends on pH, ionic strength, temperature, structure, charge density, and other properties of the adsorbent as well as the adsorbate. Initially, such adsorption is limited to a single layer of the surfactant (i.e., a Langmuir monolayer). Once the surfactant molecule is bound by electrostatic attraction to a solid, the surfactant's hydrophobic tail is exposed to the original aqueous medium, which was the solvent for the surfactant. This increases the interfacial tension between the liquid and the solid. Not unexpectedly, the remaining

Table 3 Contact Angles of Water with Various Substrates

Material	Angle (deg)
Glass	About 130
Paraffin	110
Human skin (not defatted)	75
Gold (a high-energy solid)	0
Lactose (powder)	30
Prednisolone (powder)	43
Prednisone (powder)	63
Aspirin (powder)	74
Magnesium stearate (powder)	121

Source: Based on data in Refs. 2 and 25.

surfactant in the aqueous phase may then begin to concentrate at this modified interface and form what may be called a bilayer on the surface of the solid. Such bilayers routinely result from hydrophobic bonding between two molecules of the surfactant. This type of sandwich adsorption reverses the polarity of the solid. For example, a negatively charged solid can be expected to adsorb a positively charged surfactant ion in the first step. In the second step, another layer of the surfactant is adsorbed hydrophobically. The resulting double layer now provides the solid with a positive charge. This can be extremely important for drug absorption in humans. Double-layer formation may also cause some rather undesirable effects during the use of antimicrobial agents based on cationic surfactants. For example, the adsorption of cationic surfactants onto dental enamel causes considerable staining. This has been explained on the basis of the formation of a bilayer of the cationic surfactant on the anionically charged enamel surface. As a result, the normally anionic enamel has now become a positively charged solid and is able to react with pigmented anionic constituents of ingested food.

An unusual example of adsorption was provided recently by El Falaha and co-workers [27]. These investigators demonstrated changes in the surface hydrophobicity of *Pseudomonas aeruginosa* strains that had been exposed to nonlethal concentrations of benzalkonium chloride or chlorhexidine. The effect on hydrophobicity occurred at about 1/20 of the minimal inhibitory concentration of the quaternary compound.

The tendency of amphiphiles to bind to proteins and polymers is of great practical and scientific importance. These topics are discussed later in Section IV.G.

III. CHEMICAL DESCRIPTION OF SURFACTANTS

The amphiphilic nature of surfactant molecules was used as the basis for describing their physical behavior in Section II. This description of assemblies of surfactant molecules and of their orientation at various interfaces depends on the presence of hydrophilic and hydrophobic segments in the same molecule. The molecule's hydrophilic portion can reasonably be expected to dissolve in, or at least attach itself to, the aqueous phase of the system, whereas the hydrophobic portion will dissolve in, or at least make contact with, the water-insoluble phase. All types of molecules, especially the amphiphiles, can provide links between two phases of markedly dissimilar polarities (e.g., water and oil). The balance between the hydrophilic and the hydrophobic properties of a surfactant has been codified by the hydrophile–lipophile balance (HLB) system, which is widely used in the formulation of emulsions with the aid of amphiphiles of all types (see Vol. 1, Chap. 3; Vol. 2, Chap. 2; Vol. 3, Chap. 2). Almost 40 years ago Griffin established an empirical scale of HLB values for a variety of nonionic surfactants [28]. Griffin's original concept defined HLB as the percentage (by weight) of the hydrophile, divided by 5 to yield more manageable values:

$$HLB = \frac{wt. \% \ hydrophile}{5}$$

Griffin studied primarily ethylene oxide (EO) adducts and routinely substituted "% EO" for "% hydrophile." Since that time, the HLB system has become so useful that it is applied today in the selection of emulsifiers. An abbreviated listing of HLB values is shown in Table 4. The HLB classification is not only useful in the formulation of emulsions and the like, but is also indicative of the solubility characteristics of surfactants in water. The practical usage of the HLB principle will be discussed on p. 267.

Davies and Rideal have provided a technique for calculating HLB values of surfactants of all types, and theoretical support for this concept was provided by the work of Lin in the early 1970s [see Ref. 29]. Although theoretically valid, these calculations for computing HLB values of surfactants from their structures (as described in Vol. 2, Chap. 2) frequently fail to yield correct HLB values. Evidently, the group numbers are not constant, but vary as a function of the number of repeating chemical groups. This system is of limited practical value but provides an important theoretical link to the concept of the critical micelle concentration (CMC). Becher related CMC to HLB to provide an important linkage between the utilitarian HLB concept and the more theoretical principles of CMC [6].

Griffin's HLB has been found particularly useful by emulsion technologists. It provides a practical and rational means for identifying combinations of emulsifiers and facilitates the formulation of stable emulsions. Details on the use of the HLB system will be found in other chapters in this book dealing with emulsification, especially Vol. 2. Chapter 2, and in Section VI.B.

The nature of the hydrophilic group (the head) provides the most useful means of chemically categorizing surfactants:

1. If the surfactant molecule is *not ionized*, the surfactant is classified as a *nonionic* surfactant. Of these, the polyoxyethylene (POE) derivatives are unquestionably the most important.

2. If the surfactant molecule carries a *negative* charge when it is dissolved or dispersed in water, the surfactant is classified as *anionic*. The most important groups of anionic surfactants include the alkylsulfates and the soaps.

3. If the surfactant can ionize to yield a *positive* ion, the surfactant is classified as *cationic*. The most important members in this class are the quaternary nitrogen compounds and amines, which can ionize to assume a positive charge. The quaternaries exhibit useful antimicrobial properties, as described in Section V.A.

4. Finally, the last group of surfactants includes those that carry both *positive and negative* charges. These are frequently referred to as *zwitterionic*, but this terminology should be applied to these surfactants only at those pH values at which a positive and negative charge reside on the same molecule (and are neutralizing each other). In all other circumstances, use of the term *amphoteric* surfactant is much more acceptable: this clearly indicates that at some pH conditions the molecule may carry a positive charge, whereas it might carry a negative charge at others.

The subdivision of surfactants into these four groups is universally accepted and will be used here for the discussion of the principal types of surfactant.

A. Nonionic Surfactants

Nonionic surfactants, as a group, find wide application in pharmaceutical and cosmetic products of all types. They are compatible with the other three classes of surfactants and retain this utility over a broad range of pH values. Their HLBs can range from about 2 up to about 18, depending on structure. Chemically, they include esters, ethers, amides and related compounds. As a rule, chemicals in this class act as surfactants only if they carry at least one free OH group or an ether grouping, normally derived from ethylene or propylene oxide.

Table 4 HLB Values of Selected Surfactants

Chemical name[a]	HLB	Characteristics in water	Function
Oleic acid	1.0	Immiscible; does not disperse	
Ethylene glycol distearate	1.5		
Sorbitan tristearate	2.1	Immiscible; does not disperse	Antifoam
Ethylene glycol monostearate	2.9		
Propylene glycol monostearate	3.4		
Glyceryl monostearate	3.8		
Glyceryl monooleate	3.8	Disperses with difficulty; separates on standing	W/O emulsifer
Propylene glycol monolaurate	4.5		
Sorbitan monostearate	4.7		
PEG-4 dilaurate	6.0		
Sorbitan monopalmitate	6.7		
N,N-Dimethyl stearamide	7.0	Forms milky dispersion that separates on standing	W/O emulsifier
Sucrose dipalmitate	7.4		
PEG-4 monoleate	8.0		
Sorbitan monolaurate	8.6		
Polyoxyethylene (4) lauryl ether	9.5		
PEG-4 monolaurate	9.8	Forms milky, stable dispersion	O/W emulsifier
Polysorbate 61	9.6		

	HLB		
Polysorbate 65	10.5		
Polysorbate 85	11.0		
PEG-8 monooleate	11.4		
PEG-8 monostearate	11.6	Forms translucent or clear dispersion	O/W emulsifier
Triethanolamine oleate	12.0		
Octoxynol-9	12.8		
Nonoxynol-9	13.0		
PEG-8 monolaurate	13.1		
Polysorbate 21	13.3		
PEG-32 dioleate	15.0		
Sucrose monolaurate	15.0		
Polyoxyethylene (20) oleyl ether	15.4	Yields clear solution	O/W emulsifier, detergent
Polysorbate 40	15.6		
PEG-40 monostearate	16.9		
Sodium oleate	18.0		
PEG-100 monostearate	18.8		
Potassium oleate	20.0		
Sodium lauryl sulfate	40.0		

Source: Comprehensive listings of commerical surfactants are included in the *CTFA International Cosmetic Ingredient Handbook*, 4th ed., 1992, The Cosmetic, Toiletry and Fragrance Association, Inc., Washington, DC, 1992; and the *Cosmetic Bench Reference*, Allured Publishing, Carol Stream, IL, 1992.

1. *Fatty Alcohols*

Fatty alcohols exhibit only marginal surfactant effects; they will form oriented films at interfaces and act as coemulsifiers in the presence of more hydrophilic amphiphiles. When fatty alcohols are included in drug or cosmetic compositions, they are frequently used as opacifiers and thickeners. Originally, fatty alcohols (C_8–C_{18}) were obtained by hydrogenation of fatty acids. Today, the Ziegler* and the Oxo† processes yield a range of synthetic fatty alcohols. By contrast, the branched-chain Guerbet‡ alcohols are almost never viewed as surfactants. A variety of these alcohols are used today to synthesize a wide range of surfactants.

2. *Nonionic Esters*

The nonionic esters (Table 5) are usually derived from fatty acids by esterification with polyhydric alcohols or polyethylene glycol. These fatty acid esters are relatively stable under neutral conditions, but can hydrolyze in acidic or alkaline media.

a. **Ethylene Glycol Ester**

The mono- and diesters of ethylene glycol (e.g., glycol stearate and glycol distearate) are rather poor emulsifiers. Even the more hydrophilic monoesters are used primarily for imparting opacity to liquid preparations and hardness to oil- or wax-based sticks and pastes.

b. **Propylene Glycol Esters**

Propylene glycol can form monoesters as well as diester with a variety of acids. Again, the monoesters of propylene glycol are relatively hydrophobic. For emulsification purposes, propylene glycol monostearate is, therefore, available in a pure form and in the form of a so-called self-emulsifying (SE) grade. This SE grade is prepared by adding a small amount of a soap to the pure ester. In this form, propylene glycol monostearate is an important emulsifier for creams and ointments of all types and has the added benefit of imparting viscosity to aqueous preparations.

c. **Glyceryl Esters**

Glyceryl esters are probably the most widely used surfactants in topical preparations of all types. Of particular importance is glyceryl stearate (or monostearate) which, like propylene glycol monostearate, is available in pure and self-emulsifying grades. Although glyceryl stearate is identified as a monoester, the commercial grades are mixtures of mono- and diglycerides, and most grades even contain some of the triester. Thus, the commercial grade of glyceryl stearate contains only about 40–45% of the monoester. However, purer grades (up to 90% of monoglyceride) are available and are more effective water-in-oil emulsifying agents than blends with higher diester content. Two major types of self-emulsifying grade are available: one contains a soap (potassium stearate) as the emulsifying agent; the other is based on nonionic water-soluble surfactants. In addition, grades containing a cationic surfactant to aid in emulsification have been manufactured.

---

*In the Ziegler process, metallic aluminum, hydrogen, and triethyl aluminum are reacted in the presence of ethylene to yield long-chain trialkyl aluminum derivatives, yielding alcohols on hydrolysis.

†In the Oxo process, carbon monoxide, hydrogen, and olefins are combined to yield aldehydes, which are then reduced to alcohols.

‡The Gourbet reaction yields branched-chain alcohols from the condensation of two straight-chain alcohols.

Table 5 Structures of Selected Nonionic Ester Surfactants

Formula	Names	Uses
$R-CO-OCH_2-CH_2OH$, where $R = CH_3(CH_2)_{16}-$	Ethylene glycol monostearate Ethylene glycol stearate	Opacifier; thickener
$R-CO-OCH_2-O-CO-R$, where $R = CH_3(CH_2)10-$	Ethylene glycol dilaurate	Opacifier
$R-CO-OCH_2-CHOH-CH_3$, where $R = CH_3(CH_2)_{14}-$	Propylene glycol myristate	Opacifier, emulsifier
$R-CO-OCH_2-CHOH-CH_2OH$, where $R = CH_3(CH_2)_{16}-$	Glyceryl monostearate Glyceryl stearate	Emulsifier
$CH_2OH-CHOH-CH_2-O(CH_2-CHOH-CH_2-O)_n-$ $-CH_2-CHOH-CH_2-O-COR$, where $R = CH_3(CH_2)_7CH =$ $=CH(CH_2)_7-$ and n averages 2	Tetraglyceryl monooleate Polyglyceryl-4 oleate	Emulsifier
RO, OR, CHOH-CH₂OR (sorbitan ring structure) where R = H or a fatty acid radical ($R'-CO-$)	Sorbitan (mono-, di-, tri-) acylate	Emulsifier

(continued)

Table 5 Continued

Formula	Names	Uses
	Sucrose (mono, di-, tri) acylate	Emulsifier
where R = H or a fatty acid radical (R'–CO–)		
$RCO-(OCH_2-CH_2)_n-O-COR$, where $R = CH_3(CH_2)_{16}-$ and n averages 150	PEG-150 distearate PEG-6000 distearate Polyoxyethylene-(150)-distearate	Solubilizer
$R-CO-(OCH_2-CH_2)_n-OH$, where $R = CH_3-(CH_2)_{10}-$ and n averages 8	PEG-8 laurate PEG-400 monolaurate Polyoxyethylene-(8)-monolaurate	Emulsifier
	Polysorbate 40 Sorbimacrogol palmitate 300 Polyoxyethylene-(20)-sorbitan monopalmitate	Emulsifier and solubilizer
where $R = CH_3(CH_2)_{14}-$ and $w + x + y + z$ averages 20		

The unesterified OH group(s) of monolgycerides can be esterified with low molecular weight carboxylic acids, such as tartaric or citric acid, to yield several groups of important food emulsifiers. Monoesters of fatty acids with glycerin have a long history of safe use in foods as well as in topical products, and this undoubtedly accounts for their wide use.

d. Polyglyceryl Esters

Polyglycerols are manufactured commercially by dehydration of glycerin. Even the lower members of this series possess rather complex structures, which may include cyclic compounds. The fatty acid esters of polyglycerol have recently become commercially available and are now finding application in pharmaceutical preparations as well as in foods. Depending on the length of the polyglyercyl chain and on the number of esterified hydroxyl groups, the resulting esters can be more or less hydrophobic.

e. Sorbitan Esters

Although esters of sorbitol with fatty acids can be prepared and have been used occasionally in the pharmaceutical industry, the derivatives of sorbitan are of much greater importance. 1,4-Sorbitan is obtained from sorbitol by dehydration or is formed during the acylation reaction. Although multiple esterification is possible, the monoesters are the most important and are widely used ingredients in pharmaceuticals, cosmetics, and foods.

f. Sucrose Esters

Sucrose, a polyhydric alcohol, can be esterified with a number of fatty acids and, depending on the degree of substitution, a variety of commercially important surfactants can be prepared. In light of their composition, these esters are particularly useful in foods as well as in a variety of pharmaceutical applications.

g. Ethoxylated Esters

When ethylene oxide is allowed to polymerize it forms a polyether, commonly referred to as polyethylene glycol (PEG) or polyoxyethylene (POE). The number following this name (e.g., 200) in the past referred to the average molecular weight of the ether. In modern usage, the (usually smaller) number refers to the average number of moles of ethylene oxide making up the polymer:

$$4CH_2\!\!-\!\!CH_2 \longrightarrow HOCH_2CH_2OCH_2CH_2OCH_2CH_2OCH_2CH_2OH$$
$$\backslash O /$$

Ethylene oxide

PEG 200 or PEG-4 or polyoxyethylene (4)

These ethers are mixtures, and it is preferable to indicate the chain length as follows:

$$H(OCH_2CH_2)_n\,OH$$

In the case of PEG-4, n would have an *average value* of 4. Derivatives of PEG are frequently identified as ethoxylated compounds or polyethoxylates.

The use of these ethers or of ethylene oxide for the manufacture of surface-active compounds has made it possible to create a wide range of surface-active agents with most unusual properties and stabilities. The fatty acid monoesters of PEG are normally prepared by the catalyzed polymerization of ethylene oxide in the presence of a fatty acid. They can also be made by esterifying fatty acids with preformed PEGs; however, this latter reaction can readily yield diesters. A host of surfactants can be synthesized in which the number of moles of ethylene oxide ranges from 2 to more than 100. Structurally, these compounds include a synthetic hydrophilic ether moiety and a fatty acid, which may or may not be of natural origin. The synthetic polyoxyethylene chain is a polyether; and, therefore it is widely assumed to be chemically stable under most conditions. On the other hand, the ester group is subject to hydrolysis whenever the pH conditions are adverse.

A very important group of ethoxylated esters is derived from sorbitan. These materials are obtained commonly be esterifying sorbitol or sorbitan with a fatty acid (cf. forgoing section: Sorbitan Esters) and then reacting this ester with ethylene oxide. The reverse, ethoxylation of sorbitan followed by esterification with a fatty acid, is evidently not commercially practiced. These materials are commonly referred to as polysorbates and have achieved wide use in pharmaceutical, cosmetic, and food preparations. One must always remember that these surfactants represent complex mixtures and that their method of synthesis is proprietary for each supplier.

3. *Nonionic Ethers*

Nonionic ethers (Table 6) are generally derived from polyethylene glycol or polypropylene glycol.

a. Fatty Alcohol Ethoxylates

The fatty alcohol ethoxylates, also known as polyoxyethylene ethers, are prepared from a (hydrophobic) fatty alcohol by reaction with ethylene oxide. Almost any fatty alcohol, including substituted phenols, can be reacted with ethylene oxide, and the levels of ethoxylation can range from 1 to 100 or even more. In light of these variables, an enormous range of ethers is available and to describe them all is impossible. The alcohols available for reaction with ethylene oxide range from lauryl alcohol to behenyl alcohol; the alcohols may be straight or branched-chain and derived from natural or synthetic sources (Oxo, Ziegler, or Guerbet); the alcohols may be sterols (cholesterol or lanolin derived) or alkyl phenols. All these ethers are considered to be chemically inert and can be used for emulsification and compounding at highly alkaline or strongly acid conditions.

b. Propoxylated Alcohols

Propylene oxide can be polymerized similarly to ethylene oxide; however, the polyoxypropylene derived from propylene oxide is not a hydrophilic material, but is, in fact, hydrophobic. Thus, if the reaction of propylene oxide is conducted in the presence of a fatty alcohol, a group of low HLB surface-active ethers results.

c. Ethoxylated/Propoxylated Block Polymers

A most interesting group of surfactants with particular usefulness for drugs and foods has been synthesized by preparing a hydrophobic polymer of propylene oxide, with a

Table 6 Structures of Selected Nonionic Ether and Nonionic Amide Surfactants

Formula	Names	Uses
C_8H_{17}–[phenyl]–$(OCH_2CH_2)_nOH$, where n has an average value of 9	Polyoxyethylene-(9)-octylphenylether PEG-9 octylphenylether Octoxynol-9	Solubilizer, spermicide
$CH_3(CH_2)_{14}CH_2$–$(OCH_2CH_2)_n$–OH, where n has an average value of 20	PEG-1000 cetyl ether PEG-20 cetyl ether Cetomacrogol 1000 Ceteth-20 Polyoxyethylene-(20)-cetyl ether	Emulsifier
$C_{13}H_{27}$–$(OCH_2CH_2)_n$–OH, where n has an average value of 3	Polyoxyethylene-(3)-tridecyl ether PEG-3 tridecyl ether	Emulsifier
C_4H_9–$(OCH-CH_2)_n$–OH, where n has an average value of 18 $\quad\quad\quad\;\; CH_3$	Trideceth-3 Polypropylene glycol-(18)-butyl ether Polyoxypropylene-(18)-butyl ether PPG-18 butyl	Emollient
$HO(CH_2CH_2O)_x$–$(CHCH_2O)_y$–$(CH_2CH_2O)_zH$, where $x = z$ $\quad\quad\quad\quad\quad\quad\quad CH_3$ and has the average value of 6 and y has the average value of 67	Poloxamer 401	Emulsifier
$CH_3(CH)_{10}$–CH_2–O–$(C_6H_{10}O_5)_xH$ where x may have a value of 1–3	Lauryl polyglucose	Foam booster Skin and hair
$CH_3(CH_2)_{16}CO$–NH–CH_2–CH–CH_3 $\quad\quad\quad\quad\quad\quad\quad\quad OH$	Stearoyl monoisopropanolamide Stearamide MIPA	Foam booster Emulsifier
RCO–NH–$(CH_2CH_2O)_nH$, where n has an average value of 5 and RCO represents the hydrogenated tallow fatty acid radicals	Polyoxyethylene-(5)-hydrogenated tallow amide PEG-5 tallow amide	Solubilizer Foam booster Skin conditioner

molecular weight of about 1200 or higher, and reacting the terminal hydroxyl groups of this polymer with ethylene oxide to add hydrophilic groupings. The resulting surfactants, known as poloxamers, are block polymers and possess a wide range of hydrophobic and hydrophilic properties, depending on the ratio of the building blocks. They are widely used for emulsification and solubilization in food, drug, and cosmetic products.

4. *Alkylpolyglycosides*

The alkylpolyglycosides represent a small, but growing, group of surfactants prepared by reacting a hydrophobic alcohol with glucose or a glucose oligomer. The average degree of polymerization of the carbohydrate portion is about 1.4. They are fully biodegradable. These surfactants are acetals and, thus, subject to degradation at low pHs. They can also undergo the Maillard reaction.

5. *Nonionic Amides: Alkanolamides*

The amides prepared from the reaction of a fatty acid or fatty acid ester with mono- or diethanolamine and other alkanolamines should be classified as nonionics (see Table 6). Most commercial products are, however, mixtures that include amine soaps, esters of the alkanolamines, and the like. Thus, commercial alkanolamides should not be viewed as truly nonionic surfactants. In addition, two broad classes exist, depending on the mole ratio of the fatty acid to the amine: the 1:1 condensates or superamides, and the 2:1 condensates or Kritchevsky types. The commercial amides prepared directly from alkanolamines yield derivatives containing only one or two hydroxyalkyl groups for each nitrogen atom. These compounds have found an important place in the preparation of water-based, surfactant-containing products intended for the cleansing of the skin and of the scalp.

Alkanolamides with long POE chains can be prepared by ethoxylation reactions of simple or complex fatty acid amides. Substances of this type find use as emulsifiers and solubilizers in the cosmetic industry. Finally, acyl amides can be alkylated directly. The most interesting surfactant in this group is *N*-lauryl pyrrolidone. This water-soluble amphiphile has found use as a cleansing agent in personal care products.

B. Anionic Surfactants

Anionic surfactants, as a group, are the most widely used surface-active agents in personal products and for industrial purposes. Their primary application is in products intended for cleansing and detergency.

1. *Carboxylates (Table 7)*

a. Soaps

The salts of long-chain fatty acids, commonly referred to as soaps, have been known for centuries and are used primarily for cleansing purposes, although most soaps are also good dispersing and emulsifying agents. Soaps have the general structure $RCOO^-M^+$, where R is usually a straight-chain saturated or unsaturated aliphatic group. The cation, M^+, most commonly found is sodium, although ammonium and potassium salts as well as other amine salts are occasionally employed. Short-chain fatty acid groups (i.e., those ranging from C_1 to about C_{10}) are not particularly useful as surfactants because they are too water-soluble, and their hydrophobic chains are too short. The upper limit on chain

Table 7 Structures of Selected Anionic Carboxylate-Type Surfactants

Formula	Names	Uses
$CH_3(CH_2)_{15}COONa$	Sodium palmitate	Cleanser Emulsifier
$[CH_3-(CH_2)_7COO]^-_2Al-OH^{2+}$	Aluminum distearate	Gelling agent
$[CH_3(CH_2)_7CO(-OCHCO)_n-O]_2\cdot Ca^+_2$, where n has the average value of 2 (branch: CH_3)	Calcium stearoyl-2-lactylate Calcium stearoyl lactylate	Emulsifier
$RCO-N-CH_2-COOH$, where RCO represents the mixed coconut fatty acid radicals (branch: CH_3)	N-Cocoyl-N-methyl glycine Cocoyl sarcosine	Skin cleanser
$CH_3(CH_2)_{10}CO-HN-C$ (COONa, CH_2CH_2COOH)	N-(1-Oxododecyl)glutamic acid, monosodium salt Sodium lauroyl glutamate	Skin cleanser; detergent bar
	$3\alpha,7\alpha,12\alpha$-Trihydroxy-5-β-cholan-24-oic acid Cholic acid	Natural constituent of intestinal tract

length is approximately C_{20}, because fatty acid salts containing only one carboxyl group and more than about 20 carbon atoms are quite insoluble in water. For use in pharmaceutical systems, sodium or potassium soaps are normally formed in situ by the addition of a melt of the fatty acid to an aqueous solution of the appropriate alkali. This technique is also used for the preparation of emulsions and suspensions. "Stearic acid" soaps are widely used emulsifiers, but commercial stearic acid normally consists of a mixture of 40% of stearic acid and 55% of palmitic acid, with an admixture of a wide variety of other fatty acids, including finite amounts of oleic acid, which is subject to oxidation. From a practical point of view, the use of mixed fatty acids is desirable because pure sodium stearate is quite insoluble in cold water and has a tendency to crystallize. This phenomenon is reduced by the use of mixed fatty acids, especially low molecular weight fatty acids, such as lauric and myristic. In recent years, soaps have been based on isostearic acid, which is a synthetically prepared fatty acid containing saturated branched-chain C_{18} fatty acid isomers. Salts of oleic acid are much more fluid than the soaps of stearic acid and are excellent emulsifiers. Unfortunately, the use of oleic acid is not advantageous; it can form malodorous peroxidation products, which may further decompose to form (sometimes irritating) derivatives, including aldehydes and acidic components that are undesirable in pharmaceutical preparations. Sodium stearate is readily soluble in hot water or hot ethanol; these solutions, at room temperature, can form gels, some of which are rigid enough to yield useful sticks for cosmetic or pharmaceutical applications.

The major disadvantage of soaps is that they can be used over only a limited pH range (i.e., above about 9). At pH values below about 9 the soap anion is converted to the free fatty acid, which is insoluble in water, but soluble in most organic solvents and lipids. A second disadvantage is that soaps form insoluble salts with polyvalent ions, such as calcium, magnesium, or aluminum and, therefore, cannot be used in hard water because "soap scum" (calcium stearate) is formed. Aluminum stearate, depending on the ratio of aluminum to stearic acid in the preparation, is a useful component for gelling hydrocarbons of all types. Aluminum tristearate, for example, can be dissolved in hot hydrocarbons and crystallizes on cooling to form a rigid network within the hydrocarbon. Finally, the very insoluble magnesium stearate crystallizes in plates and, therefore, finds use as a lubricant and glidant in pharmaceutical tableting processes.

b. Acyl Lactylates

Acyl lactylates are formed by the esterification of the hydroxy group of lactic acid with a fatty acid or fatty acid mixtures. During this esterification reaction, some self-esterification of lactic acid can occur and, as a result, the acyl lactylates normally comprise blends of two or more self-esterified lactic acid moieties, with one fatty acid substituent. These anionics may be viewed as soaps in which the hydrophilic head has been enlarged. Sodium and calcium salts are commercially available. They are metabolized on ingestion and are safe for food and pharmaceutical applications.

c. Ether Carboxylates

The ether carboxylate surfactants are commonly prepared by oxidation of the terminal OH group of fatty alcohol ethoxylates. Depending on the degree of ethoxylation, the resulting acids may not require neutralization to achieve solubility in aqueous systems. These surfactants can act as solubilizers and cleansing agents.

d. Acyl Amides of Anion Acids

This class of surfactants includes a variety of specialty amphiphiles. The acyl sarcosinates, the amides of *N*-methylglycine, are probably the most important representatives of this group. They are stronger acids than their parent fatty acids and are, at times, called "interrupted" soaps. Their alkali metal salts are useful in neutral and mildly acid pH solutions. The fatty acid amides of sarcosine are remarkably mild on contact with the skin and are preferred components in neutral skin-cleansing preparations. Other acyl derivatives of amino acids (e.g., those of glutamic acid) have limited application in specialty cosmetics and synthetic detergent bars.

The terminal amino groups of low molecular weight polypeptides can also be acylated, leading to the so-called fatty acid polypeptide condensates in which the peptide's remaining free carboxyl groups are commonly neutralized with either a potassium or an alkanolammonium ion. The polypeptides, generally derived from an animal collagen hydrolysate, have molecular weights of about 350–2000. These surfactants are used primarily for cleansing purpose in either skin or hair products, but only rarely as emulsifiers.

e. Natural Emulsifiers

Surface active materials found in the plant kingdom, such as the saponins, are glycosides of various steroids or triterpenoids and are of limited interest in drug products and topical preparations. The natural biological surfactants of primary interest include the bile salts and the phospholipids. Bile salts are derivatives of cholanoic acid and generally contain one to three hydroxyl groups. The most important of these is cholic acid; it is a half–moon-shaped molecule in which all hydroxyl groups are located in the concave portion, whereas the carboxyl group rotates freely along a series of singly bonded carbon atoms. This unique structure provides surface activity and helps micelle formation, which enables the body to absorb lipid materials from the intestinal tract. These micelles do not possess the classic palisadelike structure, but have been described as being composed of layers [30]. The presence of these compounds also influences intestinal drug absorption, because bile salts can form mixed micelles with a wide variety of synthetic and naturally occurring materials.

Bile salts increase the dissolution rates of insoluble drugs (e.g., griseofulvin) and alter membrane permeability. One of the most important functions of bile acids, especially sodium cholate, is the ability to solubilize cholesterol in the presence of the other naturally occurring group of surfactants, the phospholipids (see Amphoteric Surfactants). Finally, bile salts can react with certain cationic materials, making them or their micelles nonabsorbable, thereby reducing blood cholesterol levels.

2. *Esters of Sulfuric Acids*

Table 8 lists the esters of sulfuric acid, a group that comprises the alkyl sulfates and the so-called alkyl ether sulfates. Both types are widely used in cosmetic products as well

Table 8 Sulfur- and Phosphorus-Containing Anionic Surfactants

Formula	Names	Uses
$CH_3(CH_2)_{10}CH_2OSO_3Na$	Sodium lauryl sulfate Lauryl sulfate, sodium salt (SLS) Sodium dodecyl sulfate (SDS)	Cleanser Emulsifier
$CH_3(CH_2)_{10}CH_2(OCH_2CH_2)_nOSO_3NH_4$, where n has a value between 1 and 4	Ammonium lauryl ether sulfate Ammonium laureth sulfate Ethoxylated lauryl sulfate, ammonium salt	Cleanser Emulsifier
$CH_3(CH_2)_{10}-CH_2-\!\!\langle\bigcirc\rangle\!\!-SO_3H$	Dodecylbenzene sulfonic acid (DBS) LAS (common name for salts of DBS)	Hard surface cleanser
$CH_3(CH_2)_{10}\overset{O}{\overset{\|}{C}}-OCH_2CH_2SO_3Na$	Sodium lauroyl isethionate	Skin and hair cleansing; synthetic soap; bath products
$RC-\underset{CH_3}{\overset{O}{\overset{\|}{N}}}-CH_2SO_3Na$, where RCO— represents the coconut fatty acid radicals	Sodium N-cocoyl-N-methyl taurate Sodium methyl cocoyl taurate	Skin and hair cleansing; lime soap dispersant
$CH_3(CH_2)_{10}CH_2(OCH_2CH_2)_n-SO_3Na$, where n has an average value of 10	Sodium polyoxyethylene-(10)-laurylether sulfonate	Foaming agent Cleanser

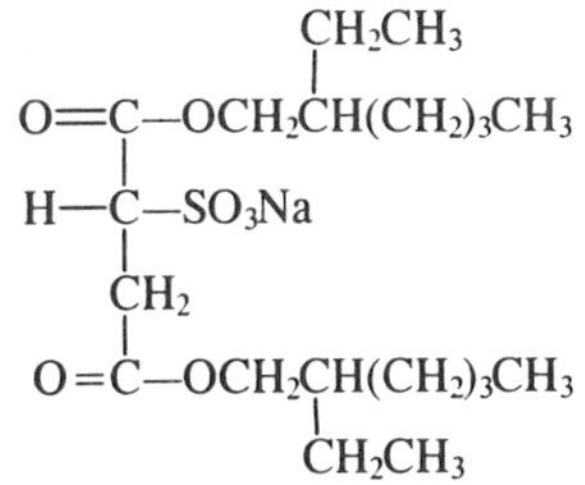

$$O=C-OCH_2CH(CH_2)_3CH_3$$
$$\quad\quad\quad\quad\quad\quad | $$
$$\quad\quad\quad\quad\quad\quad CH_2CH_3$$
$$H-C-SO_3Na$$
$$\quad | $$
$$\quad CH_2$$
$$O=C-OCH_2CH(CH_2)_3CH_3$$
$$\quad\quad\quad\quad\quad\quad | $$
$$\quad\quad\quad\quad\quad\quad CH_2CH_3$$

Dioctyl sodium sulfosuccinate
Di-(2-ethylhyexyl) sodium sulfosuccinate
Docusate sodium

Emulsifier
Suspending agent
Stool softener

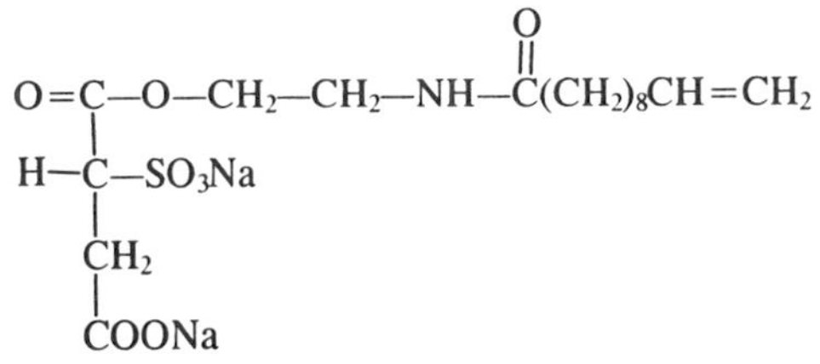

$$\quad\quad\quad\quad\quad\quad\quad\quad\quad\quad O$$
$$\quad\quad\quad\quad\quad\quad\quad\quad\quad\quad \|$$
$$O=C-O-CH_2-CH_2-NH-C(CH_2)_8CH=CH_2$$
$$H-C-SO_3Na$$
$$\quad | $$
$$\quad CH_2$$
$$\quad COONa$$

Disodium undecylenamideo-MEA-sulfosuccinate
Butanedioic acid, sulfo-, 4-[2-[(1-oxo-10-undecenyl)-aminoJethyl]ester, disodium salt

Foam booster
Antifungal surfactant

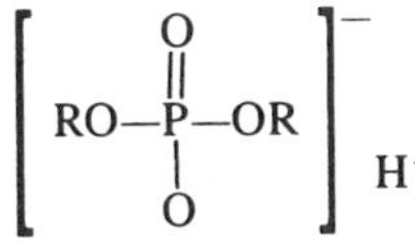

$$\left[\begin{array}{c} O \\ \| \\ RO-P-OR \\ | \\ O \end{array}\right]^{-} H_2^+N(CH_2CH_2OH)_2, \text{ where } R =$$

$$CH_3-(CH_2)_7-CH=CH-(CH_2)_7-CH_2-(OCH_2CH_2)_n-$$
or H where n has an average value of about 10

Diethanolammonium polyoxyethylene-(10)-oleylether phosphate

Emulsifier; thickener

as in pharmaceutical preparations. Chemically, these surfactants are monoesters of sulfuric acid in which the second hydrogen atom of the acid is replaced by a variety of cations. As esters, these derivatives are subject to hydrolysis in acidic or basic systems.

a. Alkyl Sulfates

The monoesters of sulfuric acid, commonly called alkyl sulfates, are formed by the reaction of a fatty alcohol with sulfuric acid. The neutralizing cations may include sodium, potassium, or alkanolamines. The alkyl sulfates of primary commercial interest are derived from lauryl alcohol, since the C_{12} moiety appears to produce optimum foaming. The source of the "lauryl" alcohol group can vary widely and includes reduction of fatty acids, Ziegler process alcohols, and oxoalcohols. Most of these alcohols are mixtures, and their properties may vary as a result of their chain length or branching. They foam in hard water, are unaffected by calcium or magnesium salts and, as a consequence, have become the key ingredients in shampoo compositions. They are also widely used as primary emulsifiers in oil-in-water preparations.

b. Ethoxylated Alkyl Sulfates

The ethoxylated alkyl sulfates are the monosulfuric acid esters of ethoxylated fatty alcohols in which the level of ethoxylation is generally less than 4. These so-called ether sulfates are prepared by reactions similar to those used for lauryl sulfate, and they exhibit essentially the same properties as the unethoxylated alkyl sulfates. The sodium salt of alkyl sulfate is relatively water-insoluble at low temperatures, but that of the ether sulfate exhibits higher solubility under these conditions. Thus, the ether sulfates are now slowly replacing the alkyl sulfates in commercial shampoos. Reports exist that suggest that the ether sulfates are somewhat less irritating than their unethoxylated counterparts.

3. *Sulfonates*

Various salts of sulfonic acids and sulfonic acid derivatives are widely used in surfactant applications because of their excellent stability in both alkaline and acidic conditions as a result of the chemical inertness of the carbon–sulfur bond. The most commercially important representatives of this group are the linear alkyl benzene sulfonates. Paraffinic sulfonates (i.e., alkane sulfonates) are produced in Europe, but are not widely used in the United States.

a. Linear Alkyl Benzene Sulfonates

The linear alkyl benzene sulfonates (commonly called LAS) are manufactured by the sulfation of alkyl benzenes in which the alkyl group is approximately 12–16 carbon atoms long. Branched-chain alkyl benzene sulfonates are no longer widely used because they are not biodegradable and, therefore, have been replaced by the linear alkyl group derivatives. In contrast with the alkyl sulfates or alkyl ether sulfates, these sulfonic acids can be supplied as free acids or as their salts, both generally in aqueous solution.

The LAS group includes the most widely produced surfactants in the world. They are the major ingredient in laundry and household detergents. They are prepared from the tetramer of propylene, which is condensed with benzene and finally (ring) sulfonated. The resulting compound, dodecyl benzene sulfonic acid, is a mixture that may contain

C_{12} and C_{15} chains. Other aliphatic hydrocarbons can be used, as well as naphthalene, to provide a wide range of compounds. These compounds are rarely used in pharmaceutical or cosmetic products.

The sulfonates of unsubstituted aromatics or of aromatics substituted with short alkyl chains include xylene and cumene sulfonates. These materials have the unusual property of thinning soap gels and detergent solutions and of increasing the solubility of phenols in aqueous products. These materials, commonly known as hydrotropes, are commercially important in light of their "solubilizing" characteristics.

b. α-Olefin Sulfonates

α-Olefin sulfonates are mixtures prepared by sulfonation of linear olefins and contain alkene and hydroxyalkane sulfonic acids as major components. They are useful detergents, especially in shampoos.

c. Alkyl Glyceryl Ether Sulfonates

Compounds of this type result from the reaction of a fatty alcohol with epichlorohydrin and subsequent conversion to the sulfonate. They have found use as detergents in dentifrices.

d. Alkylether Sulfonates

Alkylether sulfonates have recently been introduced into the market. These compounds can be described chemically as ethoxylates of a fatty alcohol in which the terminal OH group has been replaced by a sulfonic acid group. These substances foam well and reportedly can reduce the irritant properties of the alkyl sulfates.

e. Acyl Isethionates

The fatty acid esters of isethionic acid, called acyl isethionates, have characteristics more closely resembling those of the alkyl sulfates than those of the linear alkylaryl sulfonates. They are subject to hydrolysis, but are gentle to human skin and are used in synthetic detergent bars because they are relatively water-insoluble at room temperatures.

f. Acyl Taurates

The acyl taurates are interesting compounds produced by the reaction of *N*-methyltaurine (prepared from sodium isethionate plus methylamine) with an acid chloride. They can solubilize calcium soaps and exhibit surprising stability over a fairly broad pH range from about 4 to 10. *N*-Methylacyl taurates belong to the group of efficient anionic solubilizers for a variety of lipids. They are gentle to human skin and exhibit high water solubility.

g. Sulfosuccinates

A wide variety of sulfosuccinates can be prepared by the modification of one or two carboxyl groups of sulfosuccinic acid. Maleic anhydride is converted to mono- or disubstituted derivatives by esterification or amide formation; subsequent sulfonation of the double bond yields a broad range of sulfosuccinates. These compounds are widely used in agricultural emulsions. One sulfosuccinate, the bis(2-ethylhexyl) ester, commonly referred to as dioctylsulfosuccinate, has been used as a stool softener, and a complex undecylenic acid amide (see Table 8) has been reported to possess antifungal properties.

4. *Phosphoric Acid Esters*

Most of the phosphoric acid esters used in personal products are synthesized by esterification of a fatty alcohol or of a fatty alcohol ethoxylate with phosphoric anhydride or with polyphosphoric acid. The resulting mono- and diesters are typical anionic surfactants, whereas the triesters are nonionic. In cosmetic products, these esters are used as solubilizers, emulsifiers, or gelling agents for high–lipid-containing gels and sticks. Like the sulfates, the phosphates are subject to hydrolysis, especially under acidic conditions.

Another interesting group of derivatives results when a mono- or diglyceride of vegetable oil is converted to the phosphoric acid ester on the free OH group(s) of glycerin. A typical representative is the product that results from the reaction of glyceryl monooleate (which also contains some dioleate) with phosphorus oxychloride or pentachloride and subsequent neutralization with alkali. This complex mixture is called disodium oleoylglyceryl phosphate. Some of these mixtures have achieved food additive status in the United States.

C. Cationic Surfactants

Cationic surfactants (Table 9) are compatible with nonionic and amphoteric surfactants. As a rule, they cannot be used together with anionic surfactants because they interact to form water-insoluble salts (or complexes). Cationic surfactants are strongly adsorbed by negatively charged substrates, which include skin and hair, glass, ceramics, metallic oxides and clays, and most importantly, many types of microorganism.

Long-chain primary, secondary, and tertiary amine salts exhibit surface activity and find numerous industrial applications (ore flotation, corrosion inhibition in fuels and lubricants). On the other hand, quaternary ammonium salts are the major types of cationic surfactant used in cosmetics and toiletries.

1. *Quaternary Ammonium Salts*

Quaternary salts, normally in the form of their hydrochlorides or hydrobromides, are widely used in drugs and cosmetics in light of their antimicrobial properties and their substantivity to negatively charged surfaces. In contrast to primary, secondary, and tertiary amine nitrogens, the quaternary nitrogen atom retains its positive charge regardless of the pH of the medium. The most important members of this group are antimicrobials, which are characterized by possessing only one long-chain alkyl group; those that contain more than one fatty group are more useful as fabric- or hair-conditioning agents. The use of quaternaries as antimicrobial agents is discussed in greater detail in Section V.A.

2. *Betaines*

In the past it has been customary to classify the alkyl derivatives of *N*-trimethylglycine as amphoteric compounds. Since the nitrogen atom in these substances carries four substituents it is always positively charged, and these surfactants should be classified as quaternary compounds. They are used primarily in hair and skin preparations in light

Table 9 Cationic Surfactants

Structure	Name	Use
$[C_6H_5{-}CH_2{-}\overset{\overset{CH_3}{\mid}}{\underset{\underset{CH_3}{\mid}}{N}}{-}R]^+ \; Cl^-$ where R represents a mixture of alkyls, including all or some of the group beginning with capryl and extending through higher homologues, with lauryl, myristyl, and cetyl predominating	Benzalkonium chloride Alkylbenzyldimethylammonium chloride	Germicide; sanitizer
$(CH_3)_3CCH_2C(CH_3)_2{-}C_6H_4{-}OCH_2CH_2{-}O{-}CH_2CH_2{-}\overset{\overset{CH_3}{\mid}}{\underset{\underset{CH_2C_6H_5}{\mid}}{N}}{-}CH_3]^+ \; Cl^-$	Benzethonium chloride Diisobutylphenoxyethoxyethyl dimethylbenzyl ammonium chloride	Antiseptic; germicide
$[CH_3(CH_2)_{14}CH_2{-}\overset{\overset{CH_3}{\mid}}{\underset{\underset{CH_3}{\mid}}{N}}{-}CH_3]^+ \; Br^-$	Cetrimonium bromide Cetyltrimethyl ammonium bromide (CTAB)	Germicide; cationic surfactant
$[C_5H_5\overset{+}{N}{-}CH_2(CH_2)_{14}CH_3]^+ \; Cl^-$	Cetylpyridinium chloride 1-Hexadecylpyridinium chloride/CPC	Antiseptic; germicide

(continued)

Table 9 Continued

Structure	Name	Use
$$\left[\begin{array}{c} CH_3 \\ | \\ \bigcirc\!\!\!\!-CH_2-\overset{+}{N}-R \\ | \\ CH_3 \end{array} \right] Cl^-$$ where R represesnts a stearyl (C_{18}) alkyl chain	Stearyl dimethylbenzyl ammonium chloride Stearalkonium chloride	Hair conditioner
$$R-N \overset{(CH_2CH_2O)_xH}{\underset{(CH_2CH_2O)_yH}{}}$$ where R represents the coconut radical and $x + y$ has the average value of 15	PEG-15 cocamine Polyoxyethylene-(15)-coconut amine Polyethylen glycol-700 coconut amine	Emulsifying agent
$$CH_3(CH_2)_{10}CH_2-\overset{CH_3}{\underset{CH_3}{\overset{|}{\underset{|}{N^+}}}}-CH_2COO^-$$	Lauryl betaine N-Lauryl,N,N-dimethylglycine	Skin cleansers

of their substantivity. They are synthesized from a suitable tertiary amine by alkylation with chloroacetic acid.

3. *Ethoxylated Amines*

Ethoxylation of a primary amine increases its water solubility and provides nitrogen derivatives that, under certain pH conditions, can carry a positive charge. Alkylation of such ethoxylated amines with an alkyl halide leads to water-soluble quaternary compounds that have found application in the textile industry to reduce static charges and for dye leveling.

D. Amphoteric Surfactants

The amphoteric surfactant group (Table 10) is made up of a number of zwitterionic specialty materials. They are commonly used in skin and hair products as relatively mild detergents. They are not particularly useful as emulsifiers, but show pH-dependent substantivity to substrates. At high pH values they behave as anionics; at intermediate pH, they exhibit both anionic and cationic properties; finally, at low pH, they perform as cationics.

1. *Acrylic Acid Derivatives*

The acrylic acid derivatives include the so-called alkylaminopropionic acids as well as alkyliminodipropionic acids. The former are synthesized by the addition of one molecule of a fatty alkyl amine to acrylic acid. The resulting, relatively mild, water-soluble detergents can be used for skin-cleansing purposes and function as either cationic or anionic surfactants, depending on the pH of the medium. If the alkylaminopropionic acid is reacted with a second molecule of acrylic acid, the so-called iminodipropionic acids result. They exhibit essentially the same properties as the monosubstitution products. Both of these materials are available as free acids or as salts.

2. *Substituted Alkylamides*

When aminoethyl ethanolamine is reacted with a fatty acid, it forms a substituted imidazoline under anhydrous conditions. Under commercial conditions, this heterocyclic structure is unstable, and the secondary amide, $RCO-NH-C_2H_4-NH-C_2H_4OH$, becomes the major end product. Subsequent reaction of the reaction mixture with, for example, sodium monochloroacetate was, for many years, believed to yield an amphoteric imidazoline. Recent studies of these reactions indicate that the end products are mixtures of soap, the secondary amide, and of the mono- and di-β-carboxymethyl derivatives. These surfactants, nevertheless, find wide applications in shampoos, especially in shampoos that exhibit low eye irritation and cause minimal burning and stinging in the eyes.

3. *Phosphatides*

The natural emulsifiers, known generically as phosphatides, occur in both animals and plants. Their amphoteric characteristics are not significant when they are used industrially. The phospholipids play a particularly important role in living tissues in which their unique structural characteristics contribute to the (self)-assembly of membranes.

Phosphatides are the phosphoric acid esters of a diacylglyceride. These glycerophosphoric acids are further esterified with the hydroxyl group of amines (choline, ethanolamine, or serine) or of inositol. The choline esters are quaternaries, whereas the

Table 10 Amphoteric Surfactants

Structure	Name	Uses
$CH_3(CH_2)_{10}CH_2NH-CH_2CH_2COONa$	Sodium N-dodecyl-β-alanine Sodium lauraminopropionate	Skin and hair cleansers
$CH_3(CH_2)_{11}N\overset{CH_2CH_2COONa}{\underset{CH_2CH_2COOH}{\diagup}}$	Sodium N-lauryl-β-iminodipropionate Sodium lauriminodipropionate	Skin and hair cleansers
$CH_3-(CH_2)_{12}-\overset{O}{\overset{\|}{C}}-NH-CH_2CH_2-N\overset{CH_2CH_2OH}{\underset{}{-}}CH_2COONa$	Myristoamphoacetate	Hair cleansers
$\begin{array}{l}CH_2-O-COR\\ \| \\ CH-O-COR'\\ \| \\ CH_2-O-\underset{O}{\overset{O}{P}}-OCH_2-CH_2-N^+(CH_3)_3,\end{array}$	Lecithin 1,2-Diacyl-L-phosphatidylcholine	Edible surfactant Emulsifier Topical therapeutic agent

where RCO– and R′CO are naturally occurring acyl groupings

inositol derivatives must behave as anionics. Phospholipids in nature are derivatives of 1,2-diacyl-L-glycerol and display optical activity. The most important phosphatide is lecithin, which is identified chemically as diacylphosphatidylcholine. Commercial (egg or soybean) lecithins are mixtures of several phosphatidyl esters; in addition, the fatty acids may vary widely. Lecithin is water-dispersible in its pure form, but forms water-soluble lipoproteins in serum. These lipoproteins are good emulsifiers for lipids, including cholesterol. In the intestinal tract, natural phospholipids combine with sodium cholate and related bile salts to form mixed micelles, which are effective solubilizers for cholesterol.

Removal of the (normally unsaturated) acyl group from the second carbon atom of glycerin results in the formation of lysolecithin. Various grades of lecithin available from soybeans or eggs are widely used food emulsifiers and are employed in the preparation of parenteral nutritional systems. The choline esters of naturally occurring glycerophosphoric acids are the effective emulsifiers and solubilizers found in lecithins. The high degree of unsaturation in natural lecithin can lead to peroxide formation and unwanted degradation products.

Lecithins are used in the formation of liposomes, which are potentially useful drug delivery systems. Similar types of vesicles can also be prepared from certain nonionic ethers [31]. To ensure long-term stability, the use of synthetic (modified) phospholipids is widely practiced. Thus, dipalmitoyl phosphatidylcholine is commonly employed in the formation of liposomes intended for drug delivery.

Lecithins, as a group, possess two fatty acid chains, but only one amphoteric hydrophilic head. This accounts for their tendency to form micelles at low concentrations, which is vital for their biological (self-association) function. Phospholipids also play important roles in maintaining the health of living species; cephalins, lung surfactant, and plasmalogens are typical examples.

E. Additional Surfactants

Several other types of surfactant are available, in addition to the major group described in the foregoing. Only a few noteworthy examples will now be discussed briefly. Some of these surfactants, especially those based on higher molecular weight derivatives, may find increasing use in the pharmaceutical industry as the need for "nonabsorbable" surfactants increases.

1. *Amine Oxides*

Surfactants in the amine oxide group are derived from tertiary amines by oxidation, usually with hydrogen peroxide. As a result of the coordinate covalent bond between the nitrogen and the oxygen atom, these compounds, as a rule, behave as nonionic surfactants. Amine oxides (R'R"R'''NO) are good solubilizers for phospholipids in water and are useful in detergent compositions as well as in hair products.

2. *Perfluorinated Alkyl Derivatives*

Surfactants of various types in which the fatty alkyl group is replaced by a perfluorinated alkyl group have the property of lowering surface tension of water far below the normally achieved range of 25–30 dyn cm^{-1}. These materials find applications whenever low surface tension in water is desired. They are relatively expensive compounds and are used in low concentrations.

3. Starch-Derived Surfactants

As noted previously, low molecular weight polypeptides can be converted to useful surfactants by reaction with an acid chloride. Similarly, starch and cellulose, both highly polar polysaccharides, can be modified chemically by reaction with, for example, 2-chlorotriethylamine. The resulting tertiary amine can then be reacted with, for example, propanesultone, to yield a cationic sulfonic acid derivative analogous to the lauryl betaine shown in Table 9). If the starch is reacted with 3-chloro-2-hydroxypropyltrimethyl ammonium chloride, a quarternized starch is formed directly.

4. Polymeric Surfactants

An example of the polymeric-type surfactant results from the polymerization of an acrylate, such as 2-(acrylimidoamino)-2-methylpropanesulfonic acid, or its copolymerization with another vinyl derivative. This reaction leads to polyacrylates possessing varying degrees of substitution and functional groupings. Such polymers are now finding some uses in hair-conditioning systems.

5. Beeswax

Beeswax is a natural surfactant that contains high molecular weight alcohols, fatty acids, and their esters. It is commonly used in so-called cold creams in which the free fatty acids are neutralized with borax to create a soap.

6. Lanolin or Wool Fat

Lanolin is obtained during the purification of sheep wool. It is a complex mixture of esters of sterol alcohols and hydroxy acids. Lanolin is a component of so-called absorption bases, which are useful in emulsifiers because lanolin absorbs water directly by water-in-oil emulsification.

7. Ethoxylated Polysiloxane

These unusual emulsifiers have been particularly valuable for emulsifying polysiloxanes. They are prepared by proprietary procedures from dimethyl polysiloxanes end-capped with a silanol. Further reaction with ethylene oxide or propylene oxide provides an important series of chemically relatively inert emulsifiers.

IV. SPECIAL TOPICS

This section deals with diverse subjects that should be considered in the selection of surfactants for pharmaceutical applications and that may play important roles in the stability of finished formulations.

A. The Oxidative Stability of Polyoxyethylene Derivatives

As a rule, ethers are considered to be relatively inert because they do not readily undergo many of the classic chemical reactions. On the other hand, it is also well known that ethers can form peroxides which, if improperly handled, can decompose violently. Oxidative instability of polyoxyethylene has been recognized for about 30 years, but this phenomenon has sometimes been ignored by formulators. Stored polyoxyethylene derivatives may develop acrid odors that are unacceptable in pharmaceutical and cosmetic products. The instability of penicillins in the presence of polyethylene glycols was reduced materially by the addition of catalase, because it destroyed preformed peroxides. This finding demonstrates that peroxides can play a vital role in the stability of polyoxyethylene derivatives by themselves or in contact with other components of the preparation.

A systematic investigation of this phenomenon was conducted by Hamburger and co-workers, who examined the stability of PEG-20 ether (Cetomacrogol 1000, Ceteth-20) [32]. They established that the reaction was catalyzed by light and by heavy metals, especially copper, and resulted in a very rapid increase in the level of peroxide. These results have been confirmed by others, and today, nonionics are not used in biological work without careful purification because of their tendency to oxidize sulfhydryl groups.

The decompositions of polyoxyethylene ether peroxides not only cause oxidative and reductive problems, but also effect polyoxyethylene chain breakage. This rupture occurs subsequent to hydroperoxide formation on the carbon atom adjacent to the oxygen. After rupture, a variety of undesirable oxidation products are formed, including aldehydes and acids. Gradual ether peroxide decomposition can be responsible for lowering the pH of finished products. Peroxide decomposition products could be associated not only with adverse toxicological reactions, but also with chemical interactions between the newly formed species and a drug. In addition, the rupture (or shortening) of the polyoxyethylene chain alters the stability of the product because of accompanying changes in surface-active properties and in the CMC. The commonly observed reduction of the cloud point of oxidized polyoxyethylene derivatives demonstrates that, in the course of this oxidation, lower molecular weight surfactants are formed, and these may not be effective emulsion stabilizers [33]. The ether peroxides reportedly can react with amines to form hydroxylamines.

The oxidative attack on polyoxyethylene surfactants appears to proceed more rapidly in dilute solutions than in concentrated solutions and can be quantified in samples of nonionic surfactants by various chemical techniques. As a rule, polyoxyethylene derivatives should be stored in the dark, in the absence of heavy metal contaminants, and at relatively low temperatures.

Peroxide formation in polyethers may occur before use in pharmaceutical practice or in finished products. It is advisable, therefore, to avoid the use of nonionic surfactants that may have been subject to peroxide formation. The use of antioxidants in finished products may prove helpful.

B. Ester and Amide Hydrolysis

In Section III, devoted to the chemical description of surfactants, esters were identified as less stable to acid hydrolysis than amides. The modest stability of polyoxyethylene esters toward hydrolysis is complicated by the observation that monoesters of diethylene glycol or tetraethylene glycol, even at relatively low temperature—that is, 25°C in the absence of water—can rearrange (15% in the case of the monolaurate and 28% in the case of the monopelargonate) to form diesters and the corresponding unesterified polyoxyethylene glycols [34]. This type of internal transesterification must be taken into account whenever emulsion instability is observed in preparations containing these or similar esters. [The extent of this type of ester interchange is not assessable by the commonly used analytical assays (ester or saponification values) used for these ingredients.]

Transesterification reactions may also occur whenever drug molecules with free hydroxyl groups are incorporated into, or blended with, emollients or emulsifiers that are themselves ester-based.

Transesterification reactions of surfactants occur under surprisingly mild conditions and may cause not only instability, but also formation of unexpected products. The parabens have been reported to react with sorbitol to form esters of sorbitol with *p*-hydroxybenzoic acid. Entirely analogous reactions might occur between sorbitan esters and drugs carrying alcoholic or carboxylic acid functions.

Another form of ester hydrolysis has been reported for sodium di-2-ethylhexyl-sulfosuccinate. This frequently used drug ingredient has exhibited significant hydrolysis as early as 1 month after storage at 25°C in the presence of water and *n*-decane [35]. Whether the reported hydrolysis is in any way related to the presence of the hydrocarbon is not made clear. Nevertheless, these findings are another indication of the general instability of ester-type emulsifiers and a warning to the formulator to exercise care whenever esters are used in drug products.

The hydrolysis of sulfuric acid esters, the alkyl sulfates, and alkyl ether sulfates, has received attention from investigators [36,37]. The rate of acid hydrolysis of alkyl sulfate depends on the presence of other ionized species and the counterion. The controversy of whether alkyl sulfates are more or less stable than alkyl ether sulfates is of little practical value. These surfactants are unstable at pas below 4 and should not be used in such systems. They can, however, tolerate higher pHs and have been used in products exhibiting pHs above approximately 10.

If an alkyl or an alkyl ether sulfate is combined with a nonionic surfactant, the rate of hydrolysis increases, presumably because of mixed micelle formation. Micellar sodium lauryl sulfate evidently is more readily hydrolyzed than unassociated molecules in solution. The theory of micellar catalysis will be discussed later in Section IV.D. It is important to remember than kinetic rules, rates, and energetics established for chemicals in solution may not be valid whenever a surfactant is present, because of micellar catalysis.

Amide-derived surfactants (e.g., alkanolamides) are more tolerant of extreme pH conditions than esters. Amide-type surfactants are not widely used in pharmaceutical preparations, and no serious incompatibilities in personal products have been reported. It is noted here in passing that amide-type drugs can be protected against hydrolysis by incorporating them into surfactant micelles.

C. Phase Inversion Temperature

The *phase inversion temperature* (PIT) may be defined as the temperature at which an O/W emulsion changes to a W/O emulsion or vice versa. It is one of the most important concepts for formulating emulsions with nonionic emulsifiers, and its practical usefulness cannot be overemphasized. An emulsion's PIT is closely related to the surfactant's cloud point.

Aqueous solutions of nonionic surface agents become turbid and cloudy when heated, even in the absence of inorganic salts. The reproducible temperature at which this clouding occurs, the surfactant's PIT or cloud point, is concentration-dependent and generally increases as the concentration of the nonionic surfactant is raised. The clouding phenomenon is best described as representing insolubilization of the originally water-soluble surfactant or of a mixture of surfactants. The phase inversion phenomenon is limited to polyethylene glycol-derived, ether-type surfactants. Their solubility in water rests on the formation of hydrogen bonds between water and the ether oxygen atoms. When these hydrogen bonds are broken, or at least destabilized by heat or the presence of some electrolytes, the solubility of the surfactant is materially reduced. In this manner the PIT represents the temperature at which a phenomenon occurs, which is related to the HLB of the surfactant: when the originally water-soluble surfactant (possessing a high HLB) is heated in water, it becomes less and less soluble, until it finally is no longer soluble (reaches a point of low HLB). Thus, there is a distinct parallel between the HLB, as originally defined by Griffin, and the PIT, as characterized by Shinoda [38]. Consequently, the PIT of nonionic surfactants is also known as the HLB temperature. The PIT can also be viewed as that temperature at which a surfactant that is an oil-in-water emulsifier becomes a water-in-oil emulsifier.

Current understanding of the PIT has an important bearing on emulsification and solubilization. Nonionic emulsifiers and their mixtures exhibit temperature-dependent emulsification characteristics. As a rule, above the PIT, nonionic emulsions of lipids and water are of the W/O type, whereas below the PIT, such emulsions are of the O/W type. At the PIT (or in the range of the PIT) such systems invert, and this inversion generally results in the creation of small droplets that are required for long-term emulsion stability [39]. Optimum emulsion stability is achieved when the surfactant blend used is in equilibrium between the oil and water phases. Migration of a surfactant after completion of the emulsification process generally results in instability. Controversies exist on whether emulsification should be conducted above the PIT or just below (2–3°C) for optimal particle size reduction. No scientific publications dealing with optimization of complex pharmaceutical emulsions are available, but some practical rules for preparing and studying emulsions arise directly from the PIT concept.

1. Emulsification at the PIT (or at a temperature near it) and subsequent cooling optimizes particle size reduction and emulsion stability.
2. The PIT should be above the temperature at which an emulsion is stored.
3. Ambient climate and seasonal variations should be considered at all times.
4. Stability studies of emulsions should not be conducted above the PIT.

Förster and co-workers noted the relationships between temperature and emulsifier concentration which, in turn, impinged on interfacial tension, emulsification, and solubilization [39]. In their simple system of mineral oil, water, fatty alcohol, and fatty alcohol ethoxylate emulsifier, and at constant temperature (75°C), the minimum interfacial tension (10^{-5} mN/m) was reached at a mixed nonionic emulsifier concentration of 9%. A higher minimum interfacial tension (10^{-4} mN/m) at constant emulsifier concentration of 11% occurred at about 64°C. Both minima coincided with the range of microemulsion formation. Formulators will find much useful and practical information in the publication by Förster et al. [39].

The cloud point of nonionics is affected by the presence of ionized electrolytes. Some ionic species raise this temperature, whereas others lower it [40]. For example, the cloud point of a 2% aqueous solution of ethoxylated (10 mol) octyl phenol is lowered appreciably by 0.5 M ammonium sulfate, is raised moderately by 0.5 M zinc nitrate, and is essentially unaltered by 0.5 M ammonium bromide. The presence of organic constituents also affects the cloud point. The cloud point of polyoxyethylene (24) cetyl ether is lowered by benzoic acid to about 40–44°C and by cresols and phenols to room temperature [41].

D. Micellar Catalysis

During the discussion of the hydrolytic instability of alkyl sulfates, the important role played by micelle formation in the acid hydrolysis of these sulfuric acid esters was noted. A similar phenomenon, which influences the stability of other molecules, occurs when substances are solubilized or incorporated into surfactant micelles. One widely accepted principle of micellar catalysis is that the surfactant micelles have the ability to act as catalysts by bringing reactants together in a geometric arrangement that is conducive to, or interferes with, the reaction. Thus, in systems containing surfactants, one can expect, for example, that hydrolytic reactions will occur in the aqueous bulk as well as in or on the surfactant micelles. It is also feasible—and commonly observed—that incorporation of a reactive (drug) molecule into a micelle may actually protect it from hydrolysis; that is, the micelle exerts a negative catalytic or stabilizing effect.

The effect of micelles of common hydrolytic reactions involves both electrostatic and hydrophobic interactions. For example, a positively charged cationic micelle can increase the concentration of a nucleophilic reactant at the micelle–water interface, which presumably is close to the reactive site of the substrate. Hydrophobic aspects of micellar catalysis are exemplified by solubilizing the hydrophobic portion of a reactive compound in a micelle which, in turn, may make the reactive site more or less accessible to the attacking reagent. Reactions commonly subject to micellar catalysis include ester hydrolysis, as well as nucleophilic substitution reactions, and even photochemical reactions [42]. A typical pH-dependent phenomenon was reported by Yamada and Yamamoto, who determined that the rate of hydrolysis of aspirin in its un-ionized state was reduced by PEG-20 cetyl ether but that this surfactant did not stabilize the ionic form of this drug [43].

In 1974 Smith et al. [44,45] reported that the alkaline hydrolysis of benzocaine and of other *p*-aminobenzoates was retarded by the presence of PEG-24 cetyl ether. This effect was attributed by these authors to incorporation of the esters into the micelles which, in turn, provided protection against hydrolysis. About 10 years later, the hydrolysis of benzocaine in the presence of sodium dodecyl sulfate and small amounts of propylene glycol, between pH 10.5 and 12.5, was reexamined. The presence of sodium lauryl sulfate consistently increased the stability of benzocaine, and the optimum stability was found at a sodium dodecyl sulfate concentration of 5×10^{-2} M [44,45]. Indomethacin is a drug that is stabilized by high concentration of Poloxamer 407 [46] and generally by all surfactants [47]. Modern formulators often depend on micellar stabilization of drugs by formulating gelled solubilizates (see Sec. VI.B).

One final example demonstrates the unpredictable effect of micellar catalysis. Gani and co-workers studied the effect of cetyltrimethylammonium bromide on the base-catalyzed hydrolysis of 4-nitroacetanilide and reported both acceleration and retardation of the reaction rate, depending on pH and the presence of inert salts [48]. Additional examples and interpretive comments are included in the comprehensive review of De Oliveira and Chaimovich [49].

In summary, all available evidence suggests that inclusion of a drug species into a micelle can sometimes protect the drug against instability, or can facilitate degradation under other circumstances. In the absence of a predictive mechanism, long-term stability studies are required whenever reactive drugs are incorporated into formulations containing surfactants. Although hydrolysis reactions have received primary attention by investigators interested in micellar catalysis, other types of chemical reactions may also exhibit this type of catalysis.

E. Preservative Inactivation

It has been known for approximately 35 years that the presence of surfactants can "inactivate" the typical paraben preservatives used in pharmaceutical and cosmetic products. As reviewed some years ago, loss of preservative activity is now commonly explained on the basis of micellar binding of preservatives by surfactants [50].

Although several mechanisms have been suggested for a mathematical description of this phenomenon, the simplest one, based on the phase separation model, is entirely adequate for most needs. Here, the solubilized preservative is considered to be in a separate phase, and the condition is best described by a partition coefficient as follows:

$$K_m = \frac{P_b/V_m}{P_f/V_a}$$

where P_b is the amount of preservative (bound) in the micellar phase and P_f that (free) in the aqueous phase, V_m is the volume of the micellar phase, and V_a the volume of the aqueous phase. In this equation V_m is unknown, but is assumed to be proportional to be concentration of the surfactant S to yield:

$$K_m = \frac{(P_b/k')S}{P_f/V_a}$$

or

$$K_m k' = K'_m = \frac{[P_b] / [S]}{[P_f] / 100} \tag{10}$$

where K'_m is called the apparent partition coefficient, P_b in Eq. (10) is defined as the concentration (%) of micellized preservative; S is the concentration (%) of the surfactant, and P_f is the concentration (%) of the preservative in the aqueous phase. Now P_b is experimentally accessible from:

$$[P_b] = [P_t] - [P_f]\left(1 - \frac{[S]}{100}\right)$$

where P_t is the total preservative concentration (%) in the system.

These equations, based on the derivation of Shimamoto and Ogawa [51], are no different from those derived earlier by Kazmi and Mitchell [52], which define the binding capacity of the surfactant for the preservative. Various techniques have been used to determine the distribution of the preservative between the aqueous and the micellar phase or of the absolute value of P_b. Solubility, equilibrium dialysis, potentiometric techniques, titration techniques, and ultrafiltration as well as gel filtration have been employed.

The practical importance of the solubilization of preservatives by surfactant micelles cannot be overemphasized. Some of Shimamoto and co-workers' significant experimental results are shown in Table 11. In these experiments the fairly water-soluble methylparaben was included in a nonionic mineral oil-in-water emulsion (Formula 1). As a result of the preservative's inclusion into micelles, its presence in the aqueous phase and its antimicrobial activity were significantly reduced. Conditions for solubilization (micellization) are even more favorable for a water-insoluble preservative, such as propylparaben, as shown by the data of Blaug and Ahsan in Table 12 [53].

Table 11 Free Methylparaben (MP) Concentration
in Aqueous Phase of Formula 1

Total MP in emulsion (%)	Free MP in aqueous phase (%)[a]
0.0051	0.0010
0.0205	0.0043
0.0512	0.0116
0.102	0.0242
0.203	0.0566
0.307	0.0958
0.508	0.196

[a]Determined by an ultrafiltration technique [136].

Formula 1 Composition of Oil-in-Water Emulsions

Light mineral oil	30.0
Polyoxyethylene (2) palmityl ether	0.8
Polyoxyethylene (4) stearyl ether	0.9
Polyoxyethylene (6) stearyl ether	2.0
Polyoxyethylene (10) butyl ether	1.9
Methylparaben	0-0.5
Distilled water, qs ad	100.0%

Procedure
1. The emulsions were prepared by a phase-inversion process.
2. They were equilibrated for 7 days before chemical or microbiological study.

Solubilization of the parabens into micelles is no different from the solubilization of drugs into micelles. With preservatives, the practical effect is that microbial overgrowth can occur, even though "normal" concentrations of the preservatives have been added. For solubilized drugs, the pharmacological response may occasionally be less than that expected from the total concentration of the drug in solution.

Practicing formulators are familiar with the inability to predict preservative performance of a finished product containing surfactant. Models that attempt to correlate in vitro preservative availability with antimicrobial protection afforded to products become more and more complex and less reliable as the number of ingredients in the composition increases. Instead, formulators must depend on microbial challenge testing during product development, as reviewed by Haag and Loncrini [54].

F. Surfactant Interactions with Proteins and Polymers

Surfactant interactions with proteins and polymers may result from various adsorptive phenomena and complex formation. Recent investigations in the pharmaceutical field suggest that the number of potential interactions is high, since all major groups of surfactants (nonionics, anionics, cationics, and amphoterics) may react above and below

Table 12 Solubilization of Methylparabens and Propylparabens (PP) by Polysorbate 80

	Concentration (% w/v)	
Polysorbate 80	Total/free PP	Total/free MP
0	1	1
1	8	1.6
2	14	2.1
3	17	2.5
4	22	3.3
5	27	3.7

Source: Ref. 53.

their CMC with water-soluble or water-insoluble peptides and with all types of organic and inorganic polymers. Interest in this field is increasing as a result of the introduction of peptide and peptidelike drugs and the growing importance of nucleic acids in clinical medicine. Several mechanisms play a role in the phenomena described as "interactions" of surfactants with proteins and polymers.

Hydrophobic bonding to oleophilic sites is one process for removing an amphiphile from its aqueous environment. This process presumably competes with self-association (micellization) of the pure surfactant. Entirely different rules apply to interactions that depend on ionic interactions, which are particularly important for binding between so-called conditioning surfactants and the human integument and between certain clays and cationic surfactants.

1. Water-Insoluble Proteins

Water-insoluble proteins, such as keratin or zein, can adsorb amphiphiles by electrostatic attraction or hydrophobic bonding and the like. The phenomenon of substantivity of surfactants is one of the results of adsorption [55]. Surfactant substantivity, especially of quaternary ammonium compounds, is widely used in the treatment of skin, hair, and fabrics. The hoped for result is monolayer adsorption to provide these substrates with a hydrophobic surface to reduce static electricity during friction. Although substantivity to the human integument is generally desirable, some surfactant–protein interactions can cause unwanted effects on skin or hair due to excessive buildup and bilayer formation.

Aqueous alkyl sulfates bond to stratum corneum proteins primarily hydrophobically and effect extensive swelling. Nonionic or cationic amphiphiles cause no swelling of corneal proteins because their bonding, if any, generates no new hydrophilic sites for water swelling. Cationics presumably react primarily with negative sites in skin, converting hydrophilic sites in stratum corneum to hydrophobic sites [56]. The effect of surfactant binding per se on transdermal permeation of drugs remains obscure. For example, Zatz's recent review [57] and Ashton et al.'s publications [58,59] attribute the changes in drug penetration in the presence of surfactants to effects on the solubility and solubilization of drugs or to effects on the barrier properties of skin lipids.

2. Water-Soluble Proteins

The interactions of water-soluble proteins and surfactant result from cooperative binding and protein conformational changes. These interactions depend on specific characteristics of the protein and of the surfactant. Reactions of this type are commonly called protein denaturation. As with surface adsorption, the surfactant molecules participating in this process must be monomeric, and detergent-induced denaturation can take place below the CMC. Sometimes the interaction itself is referred to as micellization, especially when the soluble protein and surfactant molecules form aggregates. These interactions play an important role in the use of sodium dodecyl sulfate in polyacrylamide gel electrophoresis. The interested reader is referred to Reynold's review of the subject of interactions between proteins and amphiphiles [60].

The enzymes, a second group of water-soluble proteins, are subject to deactivation by surfactants. These types of enzyme inhibitions have been used to rate the relative safety of surfactants. Saccharase inhibition evidently has been used to confirm the mildness of sulfosuccinates in comparison with an alkylether sulfate [61]. Examples of enzyme denaturation by surfactants have been reported. For example, polyoxyethylene-(9)-octylphenyl ether and polyoxyethylene-(23)-lauryl ether inhibit the hydrolysis of triglyercides by pancreatic lipase, even below the CMC [62]. Another example is the totally unexplainable effects of surfactants on L-glutamic acid deydrogenase: Polysorbate 20 and 40 enhanced reactivity, and polysorbate 60 inhibited activity; the enzyme was not soluble in polysorbate 80, which had no effect on activity [63].

3. Water-Insoluble Polymers

The water-insoluble polymers that interact with surfactants may be inorganic or organic. All water-swelling–layer silicates tend to sorb cationic surfactants. Sodium and calcium bentonites, montmorillonite, and hectorite exchange water-soluble cations with quaternaries, such as cetyltrimethylammonium chloride. The amount of quaternary held is quite high owing to double-layer formation and is a function of the clay's tendency to swell in water [64]. The resulting "quaternized" clays are widely employed today as suspending and deflocculating agents.

Organic water-insoluble polymers have only a limited tendency to interact with surfactants by hydrophobic bonding.

4. Water-Soluble Polymers

The water-soluble polymers that interact with surfactants include nonionic polymers as well as polyelectrolytes. Binding studies between substances, such as polyoxyethylene, PVP, polyvinylacetates, and cellulosic ethers, and especially, sodium dodecyl sulfate, suggest that the interaction is controlled by a hydrophobic-binding mechanism and that the polymer's chain conformation is modified by surfactant sorption. Usually, the hydrophobic binding of a charged surfactant causes expansion of the polymer coil in water. An alternative concept views the mechanism as one in which the polymer chain surrounds the surface of a micelle. Cationic surfactants seem to produce comparable effects in the presence of nonionic polymers. As expected, interactions between nonionic surfactants and nonionic polymers are of limited interest.

Polyelectrolyte polymers react with surfactants similarly to proteins. Depending on the charges of the interacting species, neutralization or salt formation by a surfactant tends to collapse the polyelectrolyte's expanded coil. Polyelectrolyte–surfactant interactions are important in pharmaceutical systems because the polymers are widely used as thickening agents, dispersing aids, and binders. The interaction processes are highly pH-dependent and may result in the formation of micellelike structures at reactive sites on the polyelectrolyte polymer. The interactions of a charged polymer and an oppositely charged surfactant may also result in insolubilization or in unusual viscosity phenomena at or near the stoichiometric equivalence point [65].

V. BIOLOGICAL EFFECTS OF SURFACTANTS

Surfactants exhibit a variety of biological effects by themselves and additional effects through modfication of the activity of other substances present in the system. In this section, one highly desirable effect, antimicrobial action, and one clearly unwanted effect, toxicity, will be briefly reviewed.

A. The Antimicrobial Action of Surfactants

Signficant antimicrobial effects of surface active agents have generally been associated only with quaternary compounds. Depending on their structure, quaternaries exhibit antimicrobial activity at relatively low concentration. By contrast, almost all surfactants, regardless of their chemical classification, resist attack by microbial organisms whenever their concentrations are high enough (about 30%) by virtue of osmotic effects.

Only a few selected surface-active materials exhibit broad-spectrum antimicrobial activity in dilute solutions. Quaternary ammonium and some phosphonium compounds find application as topical disinfectants, and these materials are employed in commercial dermatological and pediatric products [66]. Quaternary compounds are also used in preoperative scrubs and in the irrigation of skin wounds. The most commonly used quaternary agents for this purpose are benzethonium chloride, cetylpyridinium chloride, cetyltrimethylammonium bromide, and benzalkonium chloride (see Table 9).

The antibacterial activity of commercially available benzalkonium chlorides varies as a result of the alkyl chain distribution [67]. The antibacterially most effective (against *Staphylococcus aureus*, *Escherichia coli*, and *Pseudomonas aeruginosa*) was a preparation showing the following alkyl composition: 3.5% C_{10}, 67.5% C_{12}, 24.0%, C_{14}, and 5.0% C_{16}. The importance of alkyl chain distribution in this type of compound is also recognized compendially (*USP XXI*). As a rule, quaternary surfactants with more than one long-chain aliphatic group are less active than those carrying only one hydrophobic chain, and the optimal chain length for germicides is C_{12} and C_{14}.

Most commercially used germicidal quaternary surfactants exhibit broad-spectrum activity at relatively high dilution in vitro. Their antimicrobial activity is adversely af-

Table 13 Phenol Coefficients of Quaternary Antiseptic Surfactants (at 37°C)

Compound	*Staphylococcus aureus*	*Salmonella typhosa*
Benzalkonium chloride	150–360	175–275
Benzethonium chloride	320	200
Cetylpyridinium chloride	350	130
Cetyltrimethylammonium bromide		
pH 5.0	300	—
pH 6.7	500	—

Source: After Ref. 66.

fected by the presence of proteinaceous impurities. Typical data (Table 13) on the activity of quaternary detergents against bacteria, fungi, bacterial spores, and protozoa have been reviewed by Lawrence [66]. The antimicrobial action may depend on protein denaturation, enzyme inhibition, or disruption of the cell membrane, with subsequent cell lysis.

Surfactants that contain more than one quaternary (or positively ionizable) group are among the most active substances known in terms of antimicrobial performance. This group includes compounds such as dequalinium acetate and chlorhexidine gluconate. These substances are frequently not considered as surfactants, but they exhibit many surfactantlike properties. Quaternary compounds, as a group, are substantive to the skin or other negatively charged surfaces, including dental enamel. Therefore, they provide residual activity after they have been rinsed from the substrate. Quaternary-based antimicrobial mouthwashes are believed to exert their long-term activity as a result of substantivity to the oral mucosa as well as to the teeth.

Lysis of cells can also occur in the presence of anionic surfactants, even though anionic agents are believed to exhibit only weak antimicrobial effects. For example, Kabara showed that fatty acids, especially dodecanoic acid and unsaturated acids, inhibit the growth of gram-positive bacteria [68]. A Lever Brothers Co. patent (U. S. patent 4,150,151, see the Appendix) discloses that sodium dodecyl sulfate (0.3%) effects the kill of a mixed oral bacterial population in less than 15 s.

The antimicrobial action of individual surfactants, described in the foregoing, is readily modified by the presence of other surface active agents, which may alter the nonmicellar concentration available for antimicrobial action. The effect of the CMC on antimicrobial activity is difficult to demonstrate, but efforts have been made in the self-association of benzalkonium chloride [69]. Similar conditions should prevail for mixed micelles and other combinations that may affect the CMC.

Another interesting group of antimicrobial agents based on surfactants are the "solutions" of iodine in surfactants, also known as iodophors. Although surfactants of all types can be used to solubilize iodine, the most interesting ones are phenolic derivatives of polyoxyethylene, which can dissolve more than 20 or 30% of iodine by weight. Most of the iodine is available for antimicrobial action, and the ability to provide high concentrations of iodine in essentially aqueous solution makes iodophors useful antimicrobial systems.

B. The Toxicology of Surface Active Agents

It is accepted wisdom that "the toxicological evaluation of a chemical material always requires knowledge of a specific amount which, under the conditions of test, can penetrate into the human body" [70]. This fundamental precept of toxicology is not an absolute criterion for assessing the toxicological potential of surfactants. Surfactants that have not been absorbed into the human body can, nevertheless, be responsible for adverse responses. For example, the presence of a completely unabsorbed surfactant in the intestinal tract can affect digestive processes, or may enhance, or interfere with, the penetration of ingredients present in the chyme. Similar reasoning is pertinent to surfactants applied to the epidermal surface. Here, the surfactant may alter the so-called barrier properties of the epidermis and, as a result, allow normally excluded materials to penetrate into the skin. The assessment of a surfactant's safeness, therefore, should not be exclusively based on the surfactant's toxicological profile.

An extensive review of the toxicology of topically applied surfactants was published a few years ago [71]. A more recent review of topically applied surfactants addresses the problem of irritation and swelling of stratum corneum [72]. Particularly noteworthy is the absence of irritation during human patch testing of polysorbate 20, in contrast with severe irritation from sodium lauryl sulfate. Reference 71 includes a brief survey of the toxicity of systemically administered surfactants. Today formulators generally rely on surfactants with established safety records for use in ingested or parenteral products or whenever systemic absorption is suspected.

A realistic appraisal of the toxicity of surfactants, as a group, is complicated because as a rule, surfactants applied to the external surface of the body can penetrate or cause toxicological effects only in nonmicellar form (i.e., as monomers). Size restrictions inhibit the permeation of complete micelles. On the other hand, ingested surfactants can be adsorbed from the intestinal tract by endocytosis, which does not require that the molecules of the surfactants be present in unassociated form.

In the past, complete evaluations of potential systemic effects of surfactants included determination of carcinogenic, mutagenic, teratogenic, and reproductive effects, in addition to the usual parameters of chronic toxicity. Such studies have been conducted for only few surfactants. At times, studies are carried out only as a result of some unexpected adverse effects elicited by a commercial product.

McNamara reviewed the gross toxicity of several important surfactants some years ago, and Table 14 shows that certain surfactants are significantly more toxic than others [73]. Black's comprehensive up-to-date review includes a wealth of information on the safety of anionic surfactants [74]. Since surfactants are frequently used in food products, much safety information has been submitted to various governmental agencies to support the regulatory status of ingested surfactants. A listing of surfactants permitted in food distributed in the United States, based on the Code of Federal Regulations (CFR), is provided in Table 15 [75]. It is generally assumed that surfactants accepted as food additives may be safely used in oral drug products. In addition, hundreds of surfactants, not listed as food additives, are used in drugs or topical preparations.

After gastrointestinal absorption, surfactants are fairly rapidly metabolized, and the metabolites are excreted in the urine and feces. Most of the metabolic activity takes place in the liver; however, other organs of the body show presence of surfactants after administration of radioactively labeled surfactants. Not unexpectedly, gastrointestinal absorption of ingested surfactants is dose-dependent, which is especially significant for cationic substances in light of their extremely high substantivity for the usually anionically charged proteins of the body.

The potential for harmful effects from ingested surfactants is best illustrated by some examples from the literature. Tagesson and Edling demonstrated that food additive types of surfactants (polysorbate 60 or 80) affect the integrity of intestinal mucosa by examining their effects on various enzymes leached from rat intestinal cells [76]. The polysorbates have essentially no effect on alkaline phosphatase or 5'-nucleotidase, but increase the level of N-acetyl-β-glucosaminidase in the extracellular fluid. Octoxynol-9 also materially increases the activity of N-acetyl-β-glucosaminidase. The surfactants, as a group, reduce phospholipase A_2 activity.

Gut permeability is increased by surfactants, as demonstrated by passage of sodium fluorescein into the animal's blood. Thus, ingested surfactants may facilitate penetration or absorption of potentially toxic or pathogenic compounds. This, in turn, may result in adverse effects on other organs.

Table 14 Selected Data of Subchronic and Chronic Oral 24-Month Toxicity Studies on Surfactants

Compound	Species	NOEL[a]	MOEL[b]	Response
Sodium lauryl sulfate	Rat	1.0 g kg^{-1}d^{-1}	4.0 g kg^{-1}d^{-1}	Retarded growth
Dioctyl sodium sulfosuccinate	Rat	0.5% (diet)	1.0% (diet)	Retarded growth
Benzalkonium chloride	Rat	0.063% (diet)	0.125% (diet)	Retarded growth
Nonoxynol-4	Rat	1.9% (diet)		
	Dog	0.12% (diet)	Emesis	
Nonoxynol-9	Rat	0.27% (diet)		
	Dog	0.09% (diet)	0.27% (diet)	Liver weight
Polysorbate 60	Rat	2.0% (diet)	10.0% (diet)	Diarrhea
PEG-8 stearate	Rat	10.0% (diet)	25.0% (diet)	Weight retardation
	Dog	1.0 g kg^{-1}d^{-1}		
PEG-40 stearate	Rat	10.0% (diet)	25.0% (diet)	Retarded growth
Sorbitan stearate	Rat	10.0% (diet)	25.0% (diet)	Retarded growth
	Dog	5.0% (diet)		

[a]No-observed-effect level.
[b]Minimum-observed-effect level.
Source: After Ref. 73.

Table 15 Surfactants with Food Additive Status in the United States

Name	Classification[a]	CFR Ref.
Glyceryl monostearate	GRAS F.S.	182.1324
Diacetyl tartaric acid esters of mono- and diglycyerides of edible fats or oils, or edible fat-forming fatty acids	GRAS E.	182.4101
Mono- and diglycerides of edible fats or oils, or edible fat-forming acids	GRAS E.	182.4505
Monosodium phosphate derivatives of mono- and diglycerides of edible fats or oils, or edible fat-forming fatty acids	GRAS E.	182.4521
Glycerol ester of wood rosin		172.735
Stearyl monoglyceridyl citrate	H.F.	172.755
Succistearin (stearoyl propylene glycol hydrogen succinate)	H.F.	172.765
Dioctyl sodium sulfosuccinate	H.F.	172.810
Hydroxylated lecithin	H.F.	172.814
Methyl glucoside–coconut oil ester	H.F.	172.816
Sodium lauryl sulfate	H.F.	172.822
Sodium mono- and dimethyl naphthalene sulfonates	H.F.	172.824
Sodium stearyl fumarate	H.F.	172.826
Acetylated monoglycerides	H.F.	172.828
Succinylated monoglycerides	H.F.	172.830
Monoglyceride citrate	H.F.	172.832
Ethoxylated mono- and diglycerides	H.F.	172.834
Polysorbate 60	H.F.	172.836
Polysorbate 65	H.F.	172.838
Polysorbate 80	H.F.	172.840
Sorbitan monostearate	H.F.	172.842
Calcium stearoyl-2-lactylate	H.F.	172.844
Sodium stearoyl-2-lactylate	H.F.	172.846
Lactylic esters of fatty acids	H.F.	172.848
Lactylated fatty acid esters of glycerol and propylene glycol	H.F.	172.850
Glyceryl-lacto esters of fatty acids	H.F.	172.852
Polyglycerol esters of fatty acids	H.F.	172.854
Propylene glycol mono- and diesters of fats and fatty acids	H.F.	172.856
Sucrose fatty acid esters	H.F.	172.859
Fatty acids	H.F.	172.860
Oleic acid derived from tall oil fatty acids	H.F.	172.862
Salts of fatty acids	H.F.	172.863
Synthetic fatty alcohols	H.F.	172.864

[a]GRAS F.S., generally recognized as safe food substance; GRAS E., generally recognized as safe emulsifier; and H.F., permitted for direct addition to human food.
Source: After Ref. 75.

A most important issue is the tumor-promoting action of surfactants. A recent comprehensive genotoxicity study indicated that more than 50 tested surfactants had negligible potential for causing genetic damage by themselves [77]. On the other hand, surface-active agents can act as tumor promoters. Some years ago polysorbate 85 was shown to exhibit some tumorigenic properties when applied to rabbit skin [78].

The topical toxicity of surfactants must be discussed separately from their toxicity after ingestion. Topical application of surfactants may result in irritation or allergic responses, including additional adverse effects owing to exposure to light (photodermatoses). Surfactants not only defat the epidermis, they remain in or on the stratum corneum, causing irritation or enhancing their own skin penetration. Their nonspecific binding depends not only on the site of application and electrostatic interactions, but also on the chain length of the hydrophobe. The C_{12} alkyl chain is particularly prone to cause adverse side effects on skin [see Refs. 72 and 79 for possible mechanisms].

Topically applied surfactants in emulsions or solubilizers remain on the skin surface and will be concentrated by evaporative water loss or skin penetration. As a result, lipids, emulsifers, and other nonvolatiles are concentrated on the skin, and this affects skin penetration [80]. The interaction of surfactants with skin membrane lipids was recognized many years ago and may play a role in penetration enhancement (see Sec. VII.A).

About 30 years ago, Bettley (who had been studying the interaction of soaps with the skin surface) asserted that the barrier zone—as expected at that time—is not permeable to soap [reviewed in Ref. 79]. Instead, soap acts on the barrier to make it permeable to water, to other solutes in the water, and ultimately, to the soap. The concept that surfactants increase permeability as a result of lipid or lipoprotein solubilization has been questioned, because the penetration-enhancing effect of surfactants is readily reversed, at least partially, by removal of the surfactant. Thus, alternative mechanisms for these phenomena were sought.

In their review, Cooper and Berner pointed out that surfactants may have specific denaturing (uncoiling) effects on proteins [79], whereas Rhein and Simion sought the explanation in keratin binding [72]. Regardless of the mechanism, enhanced penetration can be the result of a surfactant's effect on the protein pathway. The basic concept that surfactants can facilitate their own entry and that of other materials into the body must be kept in mind whenever the toxicological properties of surfactants are discussed. Once the surfactant has breached the skin barrier, it and accompanying ingredients can enter the systemic circulation without any alteration by the digestive system. A similar rationale can be applied to surfactant absorption by mucosal membranes.

By contrast, ingested surfactants are subject to digestive hydrolysis, and it is noted that most of the surfactants listed in Table 14 are modified by digestive processes before they can enter into the systemic circulation. Toxicologists have consistently observed that surfactants can affect bodily performance, enzymatic activity, metabolism, and other important functions required by mammalian species, depending on concentration and frequency of administration.

In summary, regardless of the route of administration, there are no surfactant molecules that are 100% safe under all conditions of use unless they undergo significant chemical modification before they reach potential target organs. Rapidly hydrolyzed surfactants that yield innocuous substances (e.g., sucrose monoleate) probably produce only minor adverse effects. Some surfactants used in the industry are natural constituents of the food chain, and their toxic side effects are probably also insignificant. The occasional administration of low levels of surfactants required for drug formulation is probably safe. However, the selection of a surfactant for use in a drug or a cosmetic must be made with care.

VI. USE OF SURFACTANTS IN DRUG PRODUCTS

Relatively few surfactants exhibit pharmacological effects that have been exploited for therapeutic purposes. As a result, the major use of surfactants in drugs arises from their utility as adjuvants. This use of surfactants is based on their ability to emulsify, suspend, or solubilize drugs and, finally, on their tendency to increase drug absorption. This last effect of surfactants is dependent not only on a surfactant's ability to interact with the drug, but to an equal degree on its ability to alter the barrier properties of membranes through which the drug must diffuse. The ability of surfactants to enhance membrane diffusion is critical to sound pharmaceutical development: on one hand, this effect can be highly beneficial; on the other, membrane damage accounts for most of the toxicological phenomena associated with the use of surfactants. The desired pharmacological actions of a surfactant, as well as the occasional adverse side effects resulting from its use, depend on the surfactant's ability to solubilize lipids, remove lipids from biomembranes and, in general, react with proteins of all types. This unique attribute accounts for the ability of surfactants to effect fusion of mammalian cell membranes, destruction of viruses, lysis of bacterial cells, and various phenomena of biological importance.

Many investigators are reported to have studied the surfactantlike properties of numerous drug molecules [8]. These properties may contribute to drug distribution and efficacy in the body. By contrast, relatively few surfactant molecules that meet the surfactant characteristics mentioned earlier (detergency, foaming, wetting, emulsifying, solubilizing, and dispersing) find any use as drugs.

A. Surfactants as Active Drugs

The fact that many surfactants possess antimicrobial activity and that the quaternary nitrogen derivatives are particularly useful germicides has already been noted (see Sec. V.A). Use of quaternary antimicrobial antiseptics in the oral cavity is widespread. Some additional applications have been mentioned in Section V.A. An interesting example was provided by Vitzthum and Rupprecht, who showed that adsorption of cationic surfactants on various silicas and on *E. coli* enhanced sorption of disodium EDTA and suggested that this finding explains the synergistic effect of EDTA–cationic surfactant mixtures [81].

Numerous experiments have established that cationic molecules are adsorbed onto a variety of proteinaceous substrates, such as hair and skin, from which they are not removed by simple rinsing with water. This substantivity (sorption), which occurs below the CMC, probably results from cation reaction with negative protein sites, and it is generally of the monolayer type. Cation exchange can also occur above the CMC, but, in addition and quite commonly, ion pair absorption occurs simultaneously, leading to bilayer formation. The adsorption of cationic materials by proteins, especially keratin, is clearly pH-dependent, and more is adsorbed at higher than at lower pH values. Keratins are also known to absorb anionic surfactants; in this latter case, adsorption is increased by the presence of acid.

The microbicidal action on microorganisms after sorption depends on their release from the substrate. This slow elution of the quaternary from the substrate can provide an environment of continuing antimicrobial action sometime after the initial application of the surfactant. An antimicrobial agent that is so tightly bound (substantitive) to a substrate that none of the germicidal material is released may still provide a bactericidal surface that may kill microorganisms on contact. Such complexities caused by substantivity play a role in the antimicrobial testing of quaternaries by the classic zone of inhibition technique.

During the discussion of disodium octylsulfosuccinate, the long-term use of this material as as laxative was mentioned. The mechanisms of this action have not been fully explained. Certain nonionic ethers of nonyl- and octylphenol are widely used as spermicides in concentrations ranging as high as about 5%. The spermicidal action of these nonionic ethers might be attributed to their ability to disrupt viable membranes or at least to dissociate lipids from lipoproteins.

B. Use of Surfactants as Drug Adjuvants

The major use of surfactants in drug and cosmetic products is as adjuvants. When used for this particular purpose, surfactants can perform various important tasks. The use of surfactants makes it possible to dilute a particular drug with an inert constituent to provide an acceptable dosage form. For example, oil-soluble drugs can be diluted with an aqueous system either by emulsifying the drug directly in water or by diluting the drug first with a solvent and then emulsifying the resultant mixture. Examples of these uses of surfactants in drugs are provided in the appendix (West German patent 1,667,911 and U. S. patent 4,496,556). Surfactants assist in the dispersion of insoluble substances, which facilitates their oral or parenteral administration. Surfactants provide a means of achieving fine dispersion of drug particles to accelerate their rate of absorption. Surfactants are also useful to increase patient acceptance of drugs (topical and oral) by modifying their texture, taste, or other characteristics. Patient acceptance is particularly critical in topically applied products, whether they be drugs or cosmetics. Surfactants play an important role in providing a suitable texture or skin finish to the consumer. It comes as no surprise, therefore, that almost all drug forms can, and frequently do, contain surfactants.

The rate of dissolution of drugs in a solvent is generally increased in the presence of a nonreacting surfactant. This feature is dependent primarily on increased wetting. Conceivably, micellization can play a secondary role in this rate process. More importantly, dissolution accompanied by micellization can be expected to raise the amount of a drug "dissolved" in the medium from that normally achievable from the solvent and the solute in the absence of other influences.

1. *Use of Surfactants in Emulsions*

Emulsions are widely used in cosmetics as well as in pharmaceutical preparations. They can be applied to the skin (topical), they can be ingested (drugs, nutrients, and such), and they can be injected by the usual parenteral techniques. Emulsions are difficult to prepare and have questionable stability; nevertheless, they are the preferred dosage form for many drugs and toiletry products. The theoretical aspects of emulsions are described in Chapter 3, and details for preparing pharmaceutical emulsions can be found in Volumes 2 and 3. As a result, this review of emulsions will be concerned primarily with the choice of surfactants for emulsification.

The principles of the HLB system for the sake of characterizing surfactants have already been described (see Sec. III). It will be recalled that some surfactants are oil-in-water (O/W) emulsifiers, whereas others are water-in-oil (W/O) emulsifiers, a feature directly attributable to the emulsifier's HLB (see Table 4). In addition, many lipids and lipidlike ingredients require a specific HLB (of a surfactant or surfactant mixture) to emulsify them in water, or vice versa. An abbreviated list of these HLB values is given in Table 16. This listing clearly demonstrates that O/W emulsification of the different lipids used in cosmetics and pharmaceuticals requires approximately the same HLB. Thus, one could argue that only a single emulsifier is required to emulsify all types of oils. Nothing could be further from the truth. Formulators have learned through trial and error that the effects of emulsifiers on a particular lipid blend are quite unpredictable. They have learned that mixtures of emulsifiers are more useful than single emulsifiers. The HLB of a blend of emulsifiers can normally be evaluated by allegation (see Vol. 2, Chap. 2). For example, an HLB of 9.5 could be reached by merely using polyoxyethylene-(4)-lauryl ether alone but can also be obtained by using a mixture of polyoxyethylene-(40)-stearate (HLB 16.9; 32 parts) and propylene glycol monolaurate (HLB 4.5; 68 parts) $[0.32 \times 16.9 + 0.68 \times 4.5]$.

Commercially available polyoxyethylene ethers and esters are not pure compounds and may contain a wide range of ethoxylates. For example, polyoxyethylene-(7)-myristyl ether (HLB about 10.5) contains about 2% free alcohol and about 1–2% of the 14-mol ethyleneoxide adduct [82]. All the other adducts are present in a gaussian distribution, with a peak at the 7-mol ethyleneoxide adduct. The sum of the 5-, 6-, 7-, 8-, and 9-mol adducts accounts for about 62% of the total. Thus, the commercially available ethyleneoxide-based emulsifiers are mixtures and, depending on source, could be used singly. Practitioners prefer mixed emulsifiers to a single emulsifier to form a mixed disperse phase. Any surfactant blend is adsorbed to this interface in accordance with basic physicochemical principles. The ability of this adsorbed film to resist deformation, to tolerate changes in temperature, and to maintain its mechanical strength may depend on liquid crystal formation by mixed emulsifier systems (see Vol. 1, Chap. 3). Therefore, the HLB system is essentially a useful preliminary guide to the development of a stable emulsion. As a rule, ester-type surfactants behave differently from ether-type surfactants, regardless of pH, and chemical features of the fatty alkyl chain enter into the problem

Table 16 HLB Values Required for Emulsification of Various Lipids

Lipid	Emulsion	
	O/W	W/O
Cetyl alcohol	15	—
Stearyl alcohol	14	—
Stearic acid	15	—
Lanolin, anhydrous	10	8
Mineral oil	12	—
Cottonseed oil	10	5
Petrolatum	12	5
Beeswax	12	4
Paraffin wax	11	4

of emulsification. Typical examples utilizing a number of emulsifiers are included in Formula 1 (p. 256) and in the Appendix (European Patent 072,462, p. 279).

The choice of emulsifiers exerts important effects on the stability of an emulsoin. The most significant side effect of surfactants affecting emulsion stability is the recently discovered phenomenon of liquid crystalline gel phase formation in emulsion systems. About 15 years ago, Barry and his co-workers studied the rheological properties of various emulsions that had been stabilized by mixed emulsifiers and fatty alcohols [83–86]. They concluded that the increase in the viscosity of these emulsions with increased levels of the emulsifying system could be explained only by postulating the formation of a gelled network structure of liquid crystalline phase in the system. A few years ago, Friberg asserted that the traditional concept of an emulsion as a two-phase system should be replaced with one that views emulsions as three-phase systems [5,87]. In addition to the oil phase and the water phase, he distinguishes a multimolecular-layer phase, comprising emulsifier, oil, and water. The existence of these liquid crystalline association structures has been confirmed by freeze-fracture micrography and other techniques. The modern definition of an emulsion recognizes the presence of several phases (including lamellar liquid crystals) in emulsions (International Union of Pure and Applied Chemistry).

Drugs in emulsified form have become popular since it was reported that they exhibit better topical or mucosal bioavailability than unemulsified drugs [88,89]. Emulsions intended for internal use can be prepared only with systemically nontoxic emulsifiers (see Table 15). The use of such nontoxic emulsifiers is also preferred for emulsions intended for external use, because absorption of emulsifiers through the skin can occur.

Selection of emulsifiers for parenteral emulsions requires still more rigid control of the emulsifying agent. Particularly well-suited for this purpose are the polyethylene oxide–polypropylene oxide block polymer types of emulsifier, as well as phosphatides derived from soybeans or eggs. Side effects are materially reduced by purification of the emulsifiers. Other useful emulsifiers include polyethylene glycol palmitate and the tartaric acid ester of cotton seed oil fatty acid monoglycerides [90].

2. *Use of Surfactants in Suspensions*

Theoretical and practical aspects of the formation of stable suspensions are discussed in Volume 1, Chapter 2, and in several chapters in Volume 2. Some phenomena discussed in this chapter impinge on the formulation of suspensions. The ability of surfactants to wet various types of solids was discussed in Section II.D. Similarly, the effects arising from the absorption of ionic surface-active agents on solid particles and the resulting changes of the charge on the particle have also been described. As a rule, the presence of wetting agents in suspensions not only helps the wetting of the particles, but also affects particle–particle interactions, which are critical for maintaining the dispersion in a stable state or for facilitating redispersion if the suspension flocculates. A few practical examples demonstrating the unpredictable effects of surfactant–solid drug interactions follow.

A dispersion of a drug, such as sulfamerazine, in the presence of a low level of an alkyl ether sulfate forms a resuspendable flocculated system. Higher levels of the surfactant yield a less-flocculated system, which is suspended with increased difficulty. Particularly striking is the effect of sodium chloride on this system: it causes a tightly packed sediment to appear, but when the concentration of sodium chloride is raised further, a more-flocculated precipitate is formed [91].

Nonionic ethers that are adsorbed onto drug particles by hydrophobic bonding also exert an important effect on the redispersibility of pharmaceutical suspensions [8]. Surfactants can alter the viscosity of aqueous suspensions, as demonstrated by Moriyama [92].

Wetting agents can also alter the dissolution and bioavailability of drugs from tablets. Thus, El-Sabbagh and co-workers studied sulfadiazine tablets granulated with a 10% solution of gelatin, with and without polysorbates 20, 60, or 80 [93]. Tablet dissolution times decreased with an increase in surfactant concentration. In addition, significantly increased drug bioavailability was observed in the presence of the surfactants in human tests. On the other hand, Heng and Wan reported that low concentrations of polysorbate 80 reduced the dissolution rate of sulfanilamide granulates [94]. They noted that starch also retarded the disintegration or dissolution rate, but that, in this case, the addition of the surfactant accelerated dissolution.

3. *Use of Surfactants in Solubilization*

For the purpose of this discussion, *solubilization* is defined as the process of preparing a visually clear solution of a substance that is only slightly soluble in the "solvent." The resulting system is expected to remain clear to the naked eye within a reasonably narrow temperature range. Solubilization excludes any system in which chemicals react with each other to become clear (e.g., the hydrolysis of a triglyceride in alkali and water); nor does solubilization imply dissolution of a solid below its limit of solubility in the solute. Finally, cosolvency—that is, the use of a nonsolvent and a solvent to provide a clear solution of the solute—does not constitute solubilization. Two concepts to the formation of solubilizates within the foregoing definition exist: one of these is formation of a microemulsion; the other is formation of a swollen micelle. Although the approaches to creating a microemulsion or a solubilizate by forming a swollen micelle may be different, modern practitioners do not always make this rigid distinction. Microemulsions are thermodynamically stable isotropic solutions; this differentiates them from macroemulsions, which are thermodynamically unstable. Microemulsions, like macroemulsions, may be O/W or W/O.

The formation of a microemulsion depends on the creation of extremely low interfacial tensions between the components. The adsorption of a single surfactant at an interface follows the Gibbs equation (see Eq. 1). The Γ_2, the excess surface concentration of the single surfactant, is insufficient to achieve the required lowering of the interfacial tension because of limitations owing to the CMC or the geometry of the system. The use of a properly selected cosurfactant changes not only the geometry at the interface, but also increases the CMC (to make more monomolecular surfactant available for adsorption). This principle was employed in the preparation of microemulsions of hexadecane in water in the presence of 1–3% soy lecithin and about 10–15% *i*-propanol [95].

In the early development of microemulsions a coarse O/W emulsion of a hydrophobic oil was clarified with the aid of a cosolubilizer. The resulting clear microemulsions were believed to contain droplets of the internal phase surrounded by the surfactant molecule and the cosolvent (e.g., hexanol), which is intercalated into the surface film of the surfactant. This concept is frequently referred to as the mixed film theory. The more modern view of microemulsions includes not only the spherical droplets postulated by earlier investigators, but also lamellar phases and other association structures, in addition to swollen micelles. This is defined as the micellar solution theory. The debate about these concepts and the mechanism of solubilization continues, and no resolution is in sight [96,97].

For the practitioner, solubilization is a useful tool, regardless of the theoretical aspects. To form a micellar solution, the polyoxyethylated surfactant is dissolved in water. After addition of the oil at an appropriate (low) temperature, it may be solubilized into the interior of the micelle, producing a swollen micelle "dissolved" in the aqueous phase. Clarity is lost at or above the PIT, and additional phases may be formed [98]. For practical applications, microemulsions are best prepared from mixtures of nonionic emulsifiers. There is an optimum temperature for solubilization by nonionics. Ionizing surfactants are too hydrophilic to act singly as solubilizers; instead, a somewhat lipophilic cosurfactant or cosolubilizer must be added. It is not at all unusual to use the concepts of solubilization and cosolvency simultaneously. Typical examples include modern mouthwash preparations, which contain alcohol or glycols, or both, in addition to solubilizers to provide clarity at low temperatures by solubilization and at higher temperatures by cosolvency.

Once a swollen micelle (or microemulsion) has been formed, the solubilized substance is shielded from adverse influences of the environment [see micellar catalysis and Refs. 40–49]. Transparent solubilizates exhibiting gel-like viscosities currently receive much interest from formulators. A typical transparent oil–water gel (15% polyoxyethylene-(7)-glyceryl monococoate, 15% polyoxythylene-(30)-cetyl/stearyl ether, 5% isopropyl palmitate, and 65% water) for drug (indomethacin) solubilization was recently described [99].

The solubilization of flavor oils is commonly believed to have no effect on perceived intensity, although a lowering of odor intensity of solubilized fragrances has been carefully documented by several investigators. Since flavor intensity of volatile oils is judged in the turbinate area of the nares, any material that lowers volatility of flavor oils (including solubilization) can be expected to reduce the perceived flavor level. The subject of the effect of solubilization on fragrance intensity was recently reviewed by Bell [100], who included a number of earlier references. Headspace analysis has been used to demonstrate that water-soluble flavor cosolvents alter not only the CMC of the surfactant, but also the amount of flavorant (menthone) found in the headspace [101]. By analogy, the solubilization of hydrocarbons in aqueous surfactant systems lowers their vapor pressure [102]. The solubility of a variety of gases is enhanced significantly by the presence of surfactants. Some typical recently published data are included in Table 17.

Further information on microemulsion will be found in Volume 2, Chapter 2.

4. *Use of Surfactants in Liposomes*

Liposomes have been examined for their ability to act as drug carriers since their discovery some years ago. Multilamellar liposomes are onionlike structures in which water layers alternate with lipid bilayer membranes. Multilamellar vesicles form spontaneously when phospholipids are allowed to hydrate [103]. Water-soluble drugs can be included in the aqueous phase, and oil-soluble drugs may be added to the membrane-forming phospholipid. Unilamellar vesicles are generally formed from multilamellar vesicles by ultrasonification and may be thought of as "bags" of water in a bilayer lipid membrane.

When prepared by the classic technique, liposomes have been compared with cells; however, such structure can evidently also be formed from synthetic surfactants, such as alkyl polyglyceryl ether [104] and by specialized ultrasound equipment [105]. Lipo-

Table 17 Solubility of Gases in Surfactant Solutions: Moles of Gas per Atmosphere per 1000 g H_2O at 26°C

Surfactant	Surfactant concentration (*M*)	Gas solubility (mol $\times$ 10^3)		
		O_2	C_3H_8	CF_4
Decyltrimethyl-ammonium	0	1.41	1.42	0.27
bromide	0.10	1.41	2.07	0.28
	0.30	1.41	3.70	0.41
	0.50	1.66	10.40	0.45
Cetyltrimethyl-ammonium	0.10	1.52	6.20	0.42
bromide	0.30	1.72	11.44	0.42
	0.50	1.79	15.66	0.56
Sodium dodecyl sulfate	0.10	—	—	0.37
	0.30	—	—	0.48
	0.50	—	—	0.58

Source: Ref. 137.

somes assume the surface charges of the surfactants used in their preparations. Even antigenically active components can be included, and their presence makes liposomes targetable drug delivery systems, since liposomes reportedly do not release entrapped drugs in the body until they are absorbed intracellularly by endocytosis or fusion.

Efforts to use liposomal therapy topically, orally, or parenterally have been in progress for about 20 years. A comprehensive review of liposomes will be found in Volume 3, Chapter 2.

VII. EFFECT OF SURFACTANTS ON DRUG EFFICACY

The preceding sections have shown that surfactants may be used to produce solutions or dispersions of drugs in solvents in which they are normally insoluble. Alternatively, surfactants can be used to stabilize drugs physically to facilitate their application. The principle remains that, regardless of the drug form or the presence of surfactants, the drug must ultimately penetrate a body membrane to perform its pharmacological function. Large drug particles are not readily absorbed by the skin or, with the exception of the gastrointestinal tract, by mucous membranes, nor would one expect them to diffuse readily from a depot injection. As a result, insoluble drugs are customarily administered in the form of emulsions or solubilizers (i.e., in relatively finely divided form).

Wagner, in his 1961 review article on drug absorption, questioned much of the information found in the literature [106], and a few years thereafter, Levy et al. [107] asserted: "Numerous studies of the effects of surfactants on drug absorption have shown that these agents can either increase, decrease, or exert no apparent effect on the transfer of drugs across biological membranes." In Levy's study of the effect of various concentrations of polysorbate 80 on the absorption of ethanol or sodium secobarbital by goldfish, low concentration of the surfactant increased the absorption of the barbiturates, whereas higher concentration actually decreased the absorption. On the other hand, the absorption of ethanol was unaffected by the presence of the surfactant. The authors of this classic paper demonstrated (a) that the surfactants did not affect the membrane of the fish, because alcohol penetration was not altered by the presence of the surfactant; (b) that low concentrations of polysorbate 80 provided some enhancement of penetration, conceivably by virtue of complexation between a few molecules of the polysorbate and the drug; and (c) that a significant increase of the concentration of polysorbate decreased absorption, presumably as a result of incorporation of the drug into a polysorbate micelle. In fact, not much more scientific knowledge has been added to the understanding of the absorption phenomenon, except for the key observation, probably first reported by Bettley, that the barrier itself may be affected by the presence of a surfactant (in his particular study, soap). This inherent characteristic of surfactants, in turn, can increase penetration of materials, not only through the epidermis, but also through other membranes.

The use of high levels of surfactants in oral dosage forms is rarely practical in modern pharmaceutical products. As a result, the levels of surfactants in the gastrointestinal tract are low and have only limited influence on drug absorption. On the other hand, the inclusion of surfactants in solid or liquid (clear and suspension) dosage forms can be expected to increase the rate of drug dissolution as a result of the lowering of surface tension [108]. The bioavailability of a solubilized drug can be affected by a variety of in vivo modifications; these include micellar life times and, especially, micellar stability in contact with body fluids and body surfaces. For example, emulsified or solubilized drugs are not likely to persist in the digestive tract because of dilution effects and the hydrolysis of surfactants in the gastrointestinal environment. Thus, the practical effect of surfactants on drug availability is expected to be limited unless the surfactant has a direct effect on the residence time at the absorption site.

A. Percutaneous Absorption

Percutaneous absorption is of increasing importance in modern pharmaceutical technology because of the great interest in the transdermal administration of drugs. Therefore, an understanding of the kinetics of the penetration mechanism and how these kinetics are affected by the presence of surfactants is important. Absorption of a topically applied drug is a function of the activity—not the concentration—of the drug in the product. Since drugs can be incorporated into micelles, form complexes, or undergo other modifications in a finished formula, drug activity in the presence of surfactants is best related to the concentration of the nonmicellized drug. Polano and Ponce studied the penetration of radiolabeled hydrocortisone-17-butyrate through cadaver skin from solutions in ethanol or various vehicles containing propylene glycol [109]. They found that the in vitro penetration from an oil-in-water cream or from a petrolatum–polyethylene base without propylene glycol was slower than that from the alcohol–propylene glycol blend. The addition of PEG-2 cetyl ether to the petrolatum–polyethylene base enhanced in vitro penetration, and this effect was also observed in their in vivo testing on psoriatic patients. No effort was made to explore this phenomenon further, except to note that the surfactant enhanced the solubility and improved the penetration rate. A more comprehensive interpretation of the penetration phenomenon was provided by Lippold and Schneemann in 1984 [110]. They found in their study of β-methasone-17-benzoate on human volunteers that the penetration rate, as determined by blanching, depended primarily on the tendency of the drug to remain in the vehicle; in other words, the high solubility of the drug in the vehicle resulted in its low bioavailability. The distribution coefficient of the drug between the vehicle and the epidermis is critical for drug efficacy. As a rule, water-soluble drugs, such as urea, penetrate more effectively from an oil-in-water emulsion than from a water-in-oil emulsion, as shown by Wohlrab [111].

Percutaneous adsorption is significantly influenced by the ability of a surfactant to "delipidize the epidermal tissue." This effect was reported by Vinson and Choman, as early as 1960, in their study of the penetration of nickel ion through guinea pig skin in the presence of sodium lauryl sulfate or sodium dodecylbenzenesulfonate [112]. Nonionic surfactants have been reported to have similar effects [113]. Modern investigations suggest that lipid loss from skin during surfactant contact is minimal [114].

The issue of the "size" that can penetrate mammalian skin has not been entirely clarified. Thus, Komatsu reported that some micellar drug penetration may occur through male guinea pig skin in vitro in the presence of polysorbate 80 or of PEG-8 dodecylether [115]. On the other hand, Dalvi and Zatz reported that percutaneous absorption of benzocaine from nonionic micellar solutions was proportional to the concentration of the "free" drug [116]. They showed that the steady-state flux of the drug through hairless mouse skin was proportional to the concentration of the free drug. An increase of the saturation concentration of benzocaine in water by various nonionic surfactants did not affect the average flux, which remained the same (within statistical variations) as that from a saturated aqueous solution (Table 18).

Modification by surfactants of a drug's skin permeation depends on a balance of several vehicle-related factors:

1. If the vehicle is occlusive (i.e., reduces water evaporation from the skin), permeation is enhanced. The presence of surfactants in an occlusive vehicle normally reduces occlusivity.
2. Micellization of a drug lowers its thermodynamic activity in solution and should reduce its permeation.
3. The permeation of emulsified drugs may depend on two drug transfers: migration of the drug into the continuous phase of the emulsion and subsequent transfer of the drug into the stratum corneum. Similar considerations apply to suspend drugs. The specific effect of surfactants on these transfers is uncertain.
4. Emulsions applied to the skin may lose solvent. In addition, the emulsions's components diffuse as separate entities through the skin. In practice, the loss

Table 18 Effect of Polyoxyethylene Nonylphenols on Benzocaine Penetration Through Hairless Mouse Skin

Polyoxyethylene chain length, n	Surfactant concentration		Total benzocaine concentration (mg/ml^{-1})	Average flux (mg hr^{-1} cm^{-2} $\times$ 10^3 $\pm$ SD)
	% w/v	M		
—	—	—	1.262	60.0 $\pm$ 3.9
9	1.4	0.0227	—	59.1 $\pm$ 3.2
15	0.2	0.00227	1.265	51.8 $\pm$ 3.2
15	1.0	0.01135	2.168	67.5 $\pm$ 8.3
15	2.0	0.0277	3.308	58.7 $\pm$ 3.5
30	3.5	0.0227	—	63.6 $\pm$ 1.0
50	5.5	0.0227	4.275	58.5 $\pm$ 7.0

of water increases the concentration of nonvolatile constituents of the emulsion, including surfactants. As a result, the drug distribution coefficients (emulsion–continuous phase and emulsion–skin) can be expected to change.

5. Many emulsifying surfactants (including fatty acids) may act as penetration enhancers by virtue of some interaction with skin.
6. The presence of both a solvent (e.g., propylene glycol) and a surfactant affects the micellization of the surfactant, alters the solubility of the drug, and influences the skin's lipid barrier.
7. Some surfactants may enhance drug permeation in vivo as a result of irritative effects.

Additional factors may influence skin permeation, but the variety of available surfactants exhibiting diverse effects makes broad generalizations impossible.

B. Mucosal Absorption

As a rule, surfactants of all types increase the permeability, at least in vitro, of a variety of epithelial tissues. These effects are normally studied by treating the tissue with the surfactant and *then* determining the permeability to a given ion or molecule before and after exposure. The tissues so studied include the cornea of the eye, the jejunum, the epidermis (as already noted), the gastrointestinal mucosa, and the oral mucosa. These effects are unrelated to the presence of any drug and are merely evidence that the mucosal tissue has been modified by the surfactant.

The basic objective of much of this work is unrelated to drug administration from disperse systems. Instead, the effort is directed to the enhancement of absorbance of an administered drug, regardless of its solubility state. Mucosal drug absorption may occur from oral, nasal, vaginal, or gastrointestinal tissues. As a general rule, mucosal drug absorption is increased by the presence of surfactants that are identified as penetration enhancers [117]. In practice, this generalization may be confounded by (a) the differences that can be expected from the polarity and the molecular weight of the drug; (b) the presence of extraneous materials in the oral cavity, in the stomach, or in the intestines; (c) the survival of micellized drugs after administration; and (d) any micellization or complexation by other chemicals that may occur before the absorptive process. In addition, the system drug–surfactant–mucosa can often be quite specific. For example, a surfactant useful in a suppository may not be appropriate for use as a permeation enhancer in the mouth because mucosal membranes differ in their physical characteristics [118]. A specific example is Siegel and Gordon's demonstration that surfactants can increase the in vivo permeability of the ventral tongue mucosa of adult male rats to a variety of substances having different chemical and physical properties [119]. Included in these studies were butyric acid, butanol, urea, sucrose, and inulin. Today, most investigators agree that the presence of surfactants increases mucosal absorption of drugs. Included are such diverse drugs as vitamin B_{12}, insulin, iron, dicumarol, and griseofulvin.

Particularly critical to the absorption of drugs is the presence of bile salts, which are involved in the absorption of lipids from the intestines and can increase the absorption of a variety of drugs. Much of the earlier work dealing with this use of bile salts was performed by Gibaldi in 1970, and his work and more recent studies were summarized by Attwood and Florence [Ref. 8, p. 425].

Current interest in orally or mucosally administration of macromolecular (protein) drugs centers on

1. Preventing acid-catalyzed degradation in the stomach

2. Proteolysis in the gastrointestinal tract
3. Enhancing permeability across the mucosa
4. Inhibiting first-pass metabolism

As a result, any oral vehicle for protein drug administration should be stable in the gastrointestinal tract, protect the protein drug against degradation, and exhibit safety.

Drug absorption through mucosal tissues may be achieved from a variety of emulsions or suspensions. Both drug toxicity and drug bioavailability may be modified by the presence of the presumably safe excipients of these dosage forms. The influence of surfactants or emulsions on drug toxicity is most critical in parenterally administered drugs. As noted earlier, however, these effects are specific, and no generalizations can be made.

A unexpected effect of emulsification was reported by Engel and Fahrenbach, who observed that heparin, which is not absorbed gastrointestinally from aqueous solutions, is absorbed by rodents when administered orally in emulsion form [120]. Rectally administered heparin is also more readily absorbed in the presence of a glyceryl mono-oleate–sodium taurocholate emulsion (mixed micelle), as reported by Taniguchi et al. [121]. The number of studies dealing with intestinal absorption of emulsified drugs in animals is large. Relatively few in vivo human bioavailability studies have been conducted. In one of these, vitamin A was found to be particularly well absorbed by cystic fibrosis patients from an orally administered O/W emulsion [122].

According to De Greef, "The oral use of emulsion systems offers the advantage of improving the biological availability of different drugs, for example, griseofulvin, sulfonamides, vitamin A, and macromolecules" [123]. No specific reasons for this phenomenon are given.

Rettig reviewed the bioavailability and rate of absorption of orally administered emulsified or suspended drugs and provided a most instructive scheme of the various factors influencing bioavailability from disperse systems (Fig. 8) [124]. He also discussed some of the factors involved in drug absorption and identified various rate-controlling steps.

There has been much interest recently in the nasal administration of systemically active drugs. Since there is only limited commercial use and to conserve space, some typical studies dealing with surfactant-assisted mucosal drug administration are listed in Table 19.

C. Parenteral Administration

The intramuscular injection of solubilizing drugs can result in precipitation of a poorly soluble drug as the micellizing surfactant is diluted, resulting in delayed release. Relatively few studies have been conducted to establish the effects of surfactants on intravenously injected drugs. Evidently, a polyoxyethylene derivative of castor oil facilitated the intravenous injection of diazepam and provided better anesthetic effects than solutions in propylene glycol [131]. Similarly, the intramuscular injection of diazepam in the presence of the surfactant provided more rapid high blood levels than administration in a propylene glycol vehicle. In other studies of diazepam in emulsion form, it was also observed that the toxicity of the drug was clearly related to the composition and nature of the emulsion vehicle. Thus, the presence of surfactants in injectables can have some unexpected and, sometimes, adverse effects.

The toxicity of solubilized injectable drugs can also be altered by instability of the

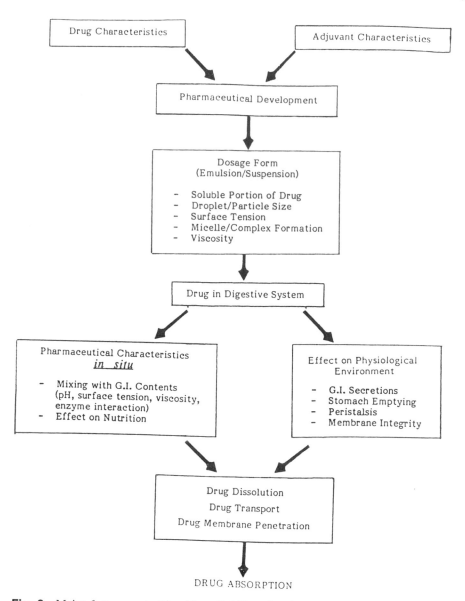

Fig. 8 Major factors controlling bioavailability of oral suspensions and emulsions.

solubilizing system. Teelmann and co-workers concluded that a mixed micellar systems of lecithin and glycocholic acid was well tolerated at reasonable dosages by various species [132]. They did, however, observe adverse effects when the solubilizing system was deliberately degraded at elevated temperatures to yield high levels of lysolecithin.

The choice of surfactant (nonionics or phospholipids) can influence absorption and transport [133]. Intravenously administered O/W emulsions are normally formulated with excess surfactant. As a result, emulsions of this type may include idealized emulsion droplets (i.e., a core coated by a single emulsifying layer), droplets with bi- and oligo-layered structures, and large unilamellar vesicles [134]. In the studied model emulsion

Table 19 Surfactant-Assisted Mucosal Penetration

Surfactant	Drug	Species	Ref.
Sodium cholate	Insulin	Rat	125, 126
PEG-(24) cholesterol ether	Ergot peptide alkaloid	Rat	127
PEG-(22) tocopheryl ether	Cyclosporine	Man	128
Sodium deoxycholate	Cholecystekinin octapeptide	Dog/rabbit	129
Sodium glycocholate plus linoleic acid	Tyrosylarginine (Kyotorphin)	Rat	130

(based on 25% soybean oil, 1.8% egg phospholipids, 2.24% glycerol, and water) the emulsifier can evidently disperse the internal phase into several forms.

As with percutaneous or mucosal drug efficacy, the performance of a parenterally administered drug in the presence of surfactants is unpredictable. Each combination of drug and amphiphile, therefore, must be studied for unexpected effects.

APPENDIX: PRACTICAL EXAMPLES

U. S. Patent 4,150,151 of April 17, 1979 (to Lever Brothers Co.)

This patent describes the formulation of a clear mouthwash that exhibits antimicrobial activity in the absence of a quaternary germicidal agent.

Preferred Composition and Preparation

Ethanol, 190 proof	12.50%
Flavor oil mixture	0.25%
Nonionic surfactant	0.25%
Sodium alkyl sulfate blend	0.30%
Sorbitol	12.00%
Buffers, sweeteners, salts	0.17%
Water, qs ad	100.00%

The flavors are dissolved in the ethanol. The aqueous phase, which comprises all the remaining components, is then added with stirring to the alcoholic mixture.

Comments

The inventors report that, in the absence of the nonionic surfactant, pure sodium dodecyl sulfate did not produce a clear product at room temperature. A clear product resulted if the mixed alkyl sulfate included the following alkyl chain percentages: C_{12}, 97.5%; C_{14}, 1.3%; C_{10} and C_{18}, 1.2%. Even this clear solution became cloudy on cooling at 35°C. Clarity was maintained at low temperatures only when polysorbate 20 or 60, PEG-20 isohexadecyl ether, or PEG-100 stearate, or PEG-10 stearyl ethers and mixtures thereof were added. Clarity was not achievable unless the alkyl sulfate blend was used at a level of about 0.3% or higher. This system is a demonstration of the criticality of the blend of chemicals required to maintain clarity in a solubilizing system (surfactants) in the presence of a cosolvent (ethanol). This patent also includes the following data on the antimicrobial activity of specific alkyl sulfates.

Gradient Plate Evaluation

Ingredient	Activity	PPM required to inhibit[a]				
		Rich	Ca	Ssal	Anti	Lepto
Sodium decyl sulfate	100%	1,800	1,000	1,900	2,100	1,800
Sodium dodecyl sulfate	100%	190	250	250	470	2,500
Sodium tetradecyl sulfate	100%	140	130	150	180	710,000
Sodium hexadecyl sulfate	100%	10,000	170	190	240	2,900

[a]Rich, Richberg's oral *Staphylococcus*, a mouth isolate; Ca, *Candida albicans*, a yeast registered with the American Type Culture Collection (ATCC No. 10231); Ssal, *Streptomyces salivarius*, a mouth isolate, ATCC No. 9756; Anti, antibiotic-resistant *Streptococcus*, a mouth isolate; and Lepto, *Leptotrichia*, an antibiotic-resistant mouth isolate.

These data are an indication that alkyl chain length has an important effect on biological activity not only for quaternaries (see Sec. V.A), but also for anionics.

West German Patent 1,667,911 of June 16, 1971 (to Richardson-Merrell)

This older patent describes a clear, stable pharmaceutical gel that contains about 15% of mixed essential oils, two nonionic emulsifiers, and water. The transparent gel requires high-melting emulsifiers, since the high level of essential oils (menthol, camphor, eucalyptus oil, methyl salicylate, and others) makes production of a firm paste difficult. The product reportedly maintains its gel-like nature and clarity at temperatures up to 40°C.

Typical Composition and Preparation

PEG-14 cetearyl ether	17.7 parts
PEG-20 oleyl ether	4.2 parts
Mineral oil	3.0 parts
Aromatic oils (mixed)	16.0 parts
Water	51.6 parts
1,2,6-Hexanetriol	4.7 parts
Poloxamer (70% ethylene oxide)	2.8 parts

The essential oils are dissolved in the emulsifiers in the presence of the mineral oil. The remaining ingredients are dissolved in the water, and the oil–emulsifier blend is added to the water. Stirring at 55–60°C is continued until the mass is poured into suitable containers, in which it gels at or near room temperature.

Comment

A mixture of emulsifiers is employed for optimal solubilization. The ratio is not unusual for solubilizates of the swollen micelle type. The triol and the poloxamer contribute to clarity at low temperature. The gel formation in this system must be attributed to the presence of association structures (liquid crystals).

U.S. Patent 4,496,556 of January 29, 1985 (to Orentreich)

This formulation shows how emulsification can provide a potent steroid (dehydroepian-drosterone)-containing cream for reducing age-related dry skin—in a diluted and patient-acceptable form.

Composition of Cream and Preparation

Dehydroepiandrosterone (alcohol)	1.0%
Preservatives	0.2%
Squalane	2.0%
Stearyl alcohol, NF	2.8%
Cetyl alcohol, NF	4.2%
PEG-20 cetyl ether	5.0%
Mineral oil, NF	5.0%
Petrolatum, USP	5.0%
Water	74.8%

The method of preparation is not provided. Presumably, all components–except any water-soluble preservative are blended at about 60–70°C and then added with agitation to the water (plus preservative).

Comment

This is a simple emulsion, using a single emulsifier and fatty alcohols as gelling agents and coemulsifiers. The oily components (mineral oil and petrolatum) probably provide a somewhat greasy finish to the product. In this cream form a low concentration of a drug can be administered readily to a large area of the body.

European Patent 072,462 of February 23, 1983 (to Toko Yakuhin Ind. Co.)

This patent describes a topical anti-inflammatory cream based on a mixed emulsifier system.

Typical Composition and Preparation

Flurbiprofen	1.0% w/w
Peppermint oil	3.0% w/w
Stearic acid	5.0% w/w
Cetyl alcohol	5.0% w/w
Liquid paraffin	15.0% w/w
White vaseline	3.0% w/w
Polysorbate 60	2.0% w/w
Sorbitan monostearate	0.6% w/w
Preservatives	0.1% w/w
Triethanolamine (10% aqueous)	3.5% w/w
Sodium lauryl sulfate	0.1% w/w
Purified water	61.7% w/w

The drug is dissolved in the peppermint oil at 70–80°C. The stearic acid, cetyl alco-hol, paraffin, vaseline, and any oil-soluble preservative are added, maintaining the temperature at 70–80°C. The water-soluble preservative, the triethanolamine, and lauryl sulfate are dissolved in the water at 70–80°C and added to the oil phase with stirring. The emulsion is then cooled.

Comments

This preparation demonstrates the use of a diluent to dissolve a drug. The product is a complex emulsion using four emulsifiers. The mole ratio of stearic acid to triethanolamine is about 0.02:0.002. This emulsion, thus, contains little if any soap, since 0.004 mol of the acidic nonsteroidal anti-inflammatory is present. The presence of the free stearic acid probably raises the viscosity of the product and provides a pearly appearance. The use of the small amount of the alkyl sulfate is interesting in light of its tendency to cause irritation (and enhance skin penetration) during continuous use.

British Patent 2,143,433 of February 13, 1985 (to Patel, H. M.)

This patent describes the preparation of liposomally entrapped methotrexate (MTX) and its efficacy in psoriasis therapy.

Composition and Preparation

	Neutral liposome	Negatively charged liposome
Cholesterol	2 parts	2
Phosphatidylcholine	10 parts	10 parts
Dicetylphosphate	—	1 part
MTX (50 mg/5 ml of saline per gram of lipid)	+	+

The lipids are dissolved in a suitable volatile solvent and dried. The MTX in saline is added, and the mixture is allowed to stand with occasional shaking. The suspensions are then sonicated under nitrogen for about 10 min. The resulting unilamellar liposomes are allowed to stand for 1 h. Unentrapped MTX is then removed by extensive dialysis against saline.

Five milliliters of liposomes (1000 mg lipid and 3–5 mg entrapped MTX) is mixed with white soft paraffin or an amphiphilic cream before administration to patients. Both preparations reduced or eliminated psoriatic lesions.

Animal testing with tagged MTX shows increased cutaneous absorption of lipsomally entrapped MTX over comparable dosing with a normal MTX containing product.

Comments

The data show that this type of "emulsion" provides good therapeutic efficacy. Interestingly, multilamellar (unsonicated) liposomes appear to effect better penetration than unilamellar preparations in animals; nevertheless, unilamellar preparations were used in human therapeutic trials.

The author provides no data on the long-term stability of this dosage form. Nevertheless, liposomes may provide the formulator with highly effective drug delivery, even in the absence of the desirable long shelf life.

REFERENCES

1. R. H. Tregold, Organic monolayer imaged, *Nature*, 313:348 (1985).
2. A. W. Adamson, *Physical Chemistry of Surfaces*, 4th ed. John Wiley & Sons, New York, 1982.
3. F. B. Rosevear, Liquid crystals: The mesomorphic phases of surfactant compositions, *J. Soc. Cosmet. Chem.*, 19:581–594 (1968).
4. F. M. Menger, On the structure of micelles, *Acc. Chem. Res.*, 12:111 (1979).
5. S. E. Friberg and M. A. El-Nokaly, Surfactant association structures of relevance to cosmetic preparations. In *Surfactants in Cosmetics* (M. M. Rieger, ed.) Marcel Dekker, New York, 1985.
6. P. Becher, Hydrophile–lipophile balance: History and recent developments, *J. Dispersion Sci. Technol.*, 5:81 (1984).
7. J. J. H. Nusselder and J. B. F. N. Engberts, Toward a better understanding of the driving force for micelle formation and micellar growth, *J. Colloid Interface Sci.*, 148:353–361 (1992).
8. D. Attwood and A. T. Florence, *Surfactant Systems*, Chapman & Hall, London, 1983, p. 108.
9. P. Somasundaran et al., Dimerization of oleate in aqueous solutions, *J. Colloid Interface Sci.*, 99:128 (1984).
10. D. Attwood and O. K. Udeala, Aggregation of antihistamines in aqueous solution. The effect of electrolyte on the micellar properties of some diphenylmethane derivatives, *J. Pharm. Pharmacol.*, 27:395 (1975).
11. D. Attwood and O. K. Udeala, Aggregation of antihistamines in aqueous solution: Effect of counterions on self-association of pyridine derivatives, *J. Pharm. Sci.*, 65: 1053 (1976).
12. G. E. Amidon, Ph.D. thesis, University of Michigan, 1980, cited in Ref. 8, p. 180.
13. K. Shinoda, *Colloidal Surfactants*, Academic Press, New York, 1962.
14. L. R. Fisher and D. G. Oakenfull, Micelles in aqueous solution, *Chem. Soc. Rev.*, 6:25 (1977).
15. T. Imae et al., Formation of spherical and rod-like micelles of cetyltrimethylammonium bromide in aqueous NaBr solutions, *J. Colloid Interface Sci.*, 108:215 (1985).
16. J. N. Ness and D. K. Moth, Direct electron microscopial observation of rod-like micelles of cetyltrimethylammonium bromide in aqueous sodium bromide solution, *J. Colloid Interface Sci.*, 123:46 (1988).
17. J. R. Bellare et al., Seeing micelles, *Langmuir*, 4:1066 (1988).
18. F. W. Menger et al., The water content of a micelle interior. The fjord vs. reef models, *J. Am. Chem. Soc.*, 100:4676 (1978).
19. P. Fromherz, The nature of the surfactant-block model of micelle structure. In *Surfactants in Solution*, Vol. 1 (K. L. Mittal and B. Lindman, eds.), Plenum Publishing Corporation, New York, 1984.
20. K. A. Dill and P. J. Flory, Molecular organization in micelles and vesicles, *Proc. Natl. Acad. Sci. USA*, 78:676 (1981).
21. H. Hoffman et al., Rheology of surfactant solutions, *Tenside Detergents*, 22: 290 (1985).
22. J. Tabony, Occurrence of liquid-crystalline mesophases in microemulsion dispersions, *Nature*, 319: 400 (1985).
23. J. Tabony, Formation of cubic structures in microemulsions containing equal volumes of oil and water, *Nature*, 320:338 (1986).
24. J. N. Israelachvili, *Intermolecular and Surface Forces*, Academic Press, New York, 1985.
25. C. F. Lerk et al., Contact angles and wetting of pharmaceutical powders, *J. Pharm. Sci.*, 65:843 (1976).
26. C. F. Lerk et al., Contact angles of pharmaceutical powders, *J. Appl. Pharm. Sci.*, 66: 1480 (1977).

27. B.M.A. El-Falaha et al., Surface changes in *Pseudomonas aeruginosa* exposed to chlorhexidine diacetate and benzalkonium chloride, *Int. J. Pharm.*, 23:239 (1985).
28. W. C. Griffin, Classification of surface-active agents by "HLB," *J. Soc. Cosmet. Chem.*, 1:311 (1949).
29. C. Fox, Cosmetic emulsion. In *Emulsions and Emulsion Technology* (K. J. Lissant, ed.), Marcel Dekker, New York, 1974.
30. D. G. Oakenfull and R. L. Fisher, Study of the properties of oxidized wood charcoals, *J. Phys. Chem.*, 81:1838 (1977).
31. M. N. Azmin et al., The effect of non-ionic surfactant vesicle (niosome) entrapment on the absorption and distribution of methotrexate in mice, *J. Pharm. Pharmacol.*, 37:237 (1985).
32. M. Donbrow, Stability of the polyoxyethylene chain. In *Nonionic Surfactants* (M. J. Schick, ed.), Marcel Dekker, New York, 1987.
33. T. Sato et al., Changes in physico-chemical properties during decomposition of nonionic surfactant solutions. *J. Am. Oil Chem. Soc.*, 63:695 (1986).
34. N. Parris and J. K. Weil, Determination of diester formation in diethylene glycol and tetraethylene glycol monoesters, *J. Am. Oil Chem. Soc.*, 56:775 (1979).
35. P. Delord and F. C. Larche, Hydrolysis of aerosol-OT and phase diagram, *J. Colloid Interface Sci.*, 98:277 (1984).
36. C. J. Garnett et al., Kinetics of the acid-catalysed hydrolysis of dodecylsulphate and dodecyldiethoxysulphate surfactants in concentrated micellar solutions, *J. Chem. Soc. Faraday Trans. I*, 79:953, 965 (1983).
37. C. J. Garnett et al., Kinetics of the acid-catalysed hydrolysis of dodecylsulphate and dodecyldiethoxysulphate surfactants in concentrated micellar solutions, *J. Chem. Soc. Faraday Trans. I*, 79:953 (1983).
38. L. Marszall, HLB of nonionic surfactants: PIT and EIP methods, In *Nonionic Surfactants* (M. J. Schick, ed.), Marcel Dekker, New York, 1987, Chap. 9.
39. T. Förster, F. Schambil, and W. von Rybinski, Production of fine disperse and long-term stable oil-in-water emulsions by the phase inversion temperature method, *J. Dispersion Sci. Technol.*, 13:183–193 (1992).
40. H. Schott et al., Effect of inorganic additives on solutions of nonionic surfactants *J. Colloid Interface Sci.*, 98:196 (1984).
41. M. Donbrow and E. Azaz, Solubilization of phenolic compounds in nonionic surface-active agents, *J. Colloid Interface Sci.*, 57:20 (1976).
42. N. J. Turro et al., Photophysical and photochemical processes in micellar systems, *Angew. Chem.*, 92:712 (1980).
43. H. Yamada and R. Yamamoto, Biopharmaceutical studies on factors affecting rate of absorption of drugs. I. Absorption of salicylamide in micellar solution, *Chem. Pharm. Bull.*, 13:1279 (1965).
44. G. G. Smith et al, Hydrolysis kinetics of benzocaine and homologs in the presence of a nonionic surfactant, *J. Pharm. Sci.*, 63:712 (1974).
45. R. A. S. Bhuri et al., *J. Pharm. Univ. Karachi*, 2:25 (1983) (from *Chem. Abstr.*, 101: 157598c, 1984).
46. H. Tomida et al., Hydrolysis of indomethacin in Pluronic F-127 gels, *Acta Pharm. Suec.*, 25:87 (1988).
47. M. S. Suleiman et al., Kinetics of alkaline hydrolysis of indomethacin in the presence of surfactants and cosolvents, *Drug Dev. Ind. Pharm.*, 16:695–706 (1990).
48. V. Gani and P. Viout, Effets de micelles cationiques sur l'hydrolyse alcaline d'acetanilides a groupe acyle active par des substituants electro-attracteurs, *Tetrahedron Lett.*, 34:1337 (1978).
49. A. G. DeOliveira and H. Chaimovich, Effect of detergents and other amphiphiles on the stability of pharmaceutical drugs, *J. Pharm. Pharmacol.*, 45:850 (1993).
50. M. M. Rieger, Current aspects of cosmetic science I. The inactivation of phenolic preservatives in emulsions, *Cosmet. Toiletries*, 96(5):39 (1981).

51. T. Shimamoto and Y. Ogawa, Interaction of methyl *p*-hydroxybenzoate with polyoxyethylene dodecyl ethers, *Chem. Pharm. Bull.,* 23:3088 (1975).

52. S. J. A. Kazmi and A. G. Mitchell, Dialysis method for determining preservative distribution in emulsions, *J. Pharm. Sci.,* 60:1422 (1971).

53. S. M. Blaug and S. S. Ahsan, *J. Pharm. Sci.,* 50:138–141; 441–443 (1961).

54. T. E. Haag and D. F. Loncrini, Esters of parahydroxybenzoic acid. In *Cosmetic and Drug Preservation* (J. J. Kabara, ed.), Marcel Dekker, New York, 1984, p. 63.

55. J. A. Faucher and E. D. Goddard, Interaction of keratinous substrates with sodium lauryl sulfate: I. Sorption, *J. Soc. Cosmet. Chem.,* 29:323 (1978).

56. L. D. Rhein et al., Surfactant structure effects on swelling of isolated human stratum corneum, *J. Soc. Cosmet. Chem.,* 37:125 (1986).

57. J. L. Zatz, Modification of skin permeation by surface-active agents. In *Skin Permeation* (J. L. Zatz, ed.), Allured Publishing, Carol Stream IL, 1993.

58. P. Ashton et al., Surfactant effect in percutaneous absorption. I. Effects on the transdermal flux of methyl nicotinate, *Int. J. Pharm.,* 87:261 (1992).

59. P. Ashton et al., Surfactant effects in percutaneous absorption. II. Effects on protein and lipid structure of the stratum corneum, *Int. J. Pharm.,* 265 (1992).

60. J. A. Reynolds, Interactions between proteins and amphiphiles. In *Lipid–Protein Interactions,* Vol. 2 (P. C. Jost and O. H. Griffith, eds.), John Wiley & Sons, New York, 1982.

61. P. Thau, Surfactants for skin cleansers. In *Surfactants in Cosmetics* (M. M. Rieger, ed.) Marcel Dekker, New York, 1985.

62. P. Canioni et al., Interaction of porcine pancreatic colipase with a nonionic detergent, *Lipids,* 15:6 (1980).

63. T. S. Seibles, Interaction of dodecyl sulfate with native and modified β-lactoglobulin, *Biochemistry,* 8:2949 (1969).

64. W. Röhl et al., Adsorption von Tensiden an niedrig geladenen Schichtsilikaten Teil 1: Adsorption kationischer Tenside, Prog. Colloid Polym. Sci., 84:206 (1991).

65. E. D. Goddard et al., Novel gelling structures based on polymer/surfactant systems, *J. Soc. Cosmet. Chem.,* 42:19 (1991).

66. C. A. Lawrence, Germicidal properties of cationic surfactants. In *Cationic Surfactants* (E. Jungermann, ed.), Marcel Dekker, New York, 1970, p. 491.

67. R. M. E. Richards and L. M. Mizrahi, Differences in antibacterial activity of benzalkonium chloride, *J. Pharm. Sci.,* 67:380 (1978).

68. J. J. Kabara, Fatty acids and derivatives as antimicrobial agents—a review. In *The Pharmacological Effect of Lipids* (J. J. Kabara, ed.), American Oil Chemists Society, Champaign, IL, 1978, Chap. 1.

69. E. Tomlinson et al., Effect of colloidal association on the measured activity of alkylbenzyl-dimethylammonium chlorides against *Pseudomonas aeruginose,* J. Med. Chem., 20:1277 (1977).

70. F. Wingen et al., Screening-untersuchgen zur Frage der Hautresorption Kosmetikfarbstoffen: Parts I and II, *J. Soc. Cosmet. Chem.,* 34:47 (1983).

71. E. J. Singer and E. P. Pittz, Interactions of surfactants with epidermal tissues: Biochemical and toxicological aspects. In *Surfactants in Cosmetics* (M. M. Rieger, ed.) Marcel Dekker, New York, 1985, Chap. 6.

72. L. D. Rhein and F. A. Simion, Surfactant interaction with skin. In *Interfacial Phenomena in Biological Systems* (M. Bender, ed.), Marcel Dekker, New York, 1991, Chap. 2.

73. B. P. McNamara, Concepts in health evaluations of commercial and industrial chemicals. In *New Concepts in Safety Evaluation* (M. A. Mehlman et al., eds.), Hemisphere Publishing, Washington, DC, 1976, Chap. 4.

74. J. G. Black, Interaction between anionic surfactants and skin. In *Pharmaceutical Skin Penetration Enhancement* (K. A. Walters and J. Hadgraft, eds.), Marcel Dekker, New York, 1993, Chap. 3.

75. Code of Federal Regulations, Title 21, Part 172, Subparts H and I, as of April 1, 1992.

76. C. Tagesson and C. Edling, Influence of surface-active food additives on the integrity and permeability of rat intestinal mucosa, *Food Chem. Toxicol.,* 22:861 (1984).

77. J. Yam et al., Surfactants: A survey of short-term genotoxicity testing, *Food Chem. Toxicol.,* 22:761 (1984).

78. M. Mezei and A. K. Y. Lee, Dermatitic effect of nonionic surfactants, IV. Phospholipid composition of normal and surfactant-treated rabbit skin, *J. Pharm. Sci.,* 59:858 (1970).

79. E. R. Cooper and B. Berner, Interaction of surfactants with epidermal tissues: Physicochemical aspects. In *Surfactants in Cosmetics* (M. M. Rieger, ed.), Marcel Dekkere, New York, 1985.

80. S. E. Friberg and B. Langlois, Evaporation from emulsions, *J. Dispersion Sci. Technol.,* 13:223 (1992).

81. J. Vitzthurn and H. Rupprecht, Coadsorption of cationic surfactants and sodium ethylene diamine tetraacetate on silica surfaces and *Escherichia coli,* Acta Pharm. Technol., 36:67 (1990).

82. K. L. Matheson et al., Peaked distribution ethoxylates—their preparation, characterization and performance evaluation, *J. Am. Oil Chem. Soc.,* 63:365 (1986).

83. B. W. Barry, Rheology of emulsions stabilized by sodium dodecyl sulfate/long-chain alcohols, *J. Colloid Interface Sci.,* 32:551 (1970).

84. B. W. Barry and G. M. Saunders, The self-bodying action of the mixed emulsifier cetrimide/cetostearyl alcohol, *J. Colloid Interface Sci.,* 34:300 (1970).

85. B. W. Barry and G. M. Saunders, Rheology of systems containing cetomacrogol 1000-cetostearyl alcohol: I. Self-bodying action, *J. Colloid Interface Sci.,* 38:616 (1970).

86. B. W. Barry and G. M. Saunders, Rheology of systems containing cetomacrogol 1000-cetostearyl alcohol: II. Variation with temperature, *J. Colloid Interface Sci.,* 38:626 (1972).

87. S. Friberg, Three-phase emulsions, *J. Soc. Cosmet. Chem.,* 30:309 (1979).

88. A. Takamura et al., Physicopharmaceutical characteristics of an oil-in-water emulsion-type ointment containing diclofenac sodium, *J. Pharm. Sci.,* 73:676 (1984).

89. T. T. Kararli et al, Enhancement of nasal delivery of a renin inhibitor in the rat using emulsion formulations, *Pharm. Res.,* 9:1024 (1992).

90. B. A. Mulley, Medicinal emulsions. In *Emulsions and Emulsion Technology* (K. J. Lissant, ed.), Marcel Dekker, New York, 1974, p. 292.

91. J. V. Bondi et al., Effect of adsorbed surfactant on particle–particle interactions in hydrophobic suspensions, *J. Pharm. Sci.,* 62:1731 (1973).

92. N. Moriyama, Effects of surfactants and inorganic phosphates upon apparent viscosities of pigment–water (50–50) suspensions, *J. Am. Oil Chem. Soc.,* 52:198 (1975).

93. H. M. El-Sabbagh et al., Effect of surfactant treated binder on the physical properties and bioavailability of sulfadiazine tablets, *Acta Pharm. Technol.,* 30:243 (1984).

94. P. W. S. Heng and L. S. C. Wan, Surfactant effect on the dissolution of sulfanilamide granules, *J. Pharm. Sci.,* 74:269 (1985).

95. K. Shinoda et al., Lecithin-based microemulsions: Phase behavior and microstructure, *J. Phys. Chem.,* 95:989 (1991).

96. L. M. Prince, The mixed film theory, Chapter 5; and S. Friberg, Microemulsions and micellar solutions, Chapter 6. In *Microemulsions, Theory and Practice* (L. M. Prince, ed.) Academic Press, New York, 1977, pp. 91; 133.

97. K. Shinoda and S. Friberg, Microemulsions: Colloidal aspects, *Adv. Colloid Interface Sci.,* 4:281 (1975).

98. S. J. Holland and J. K. Warrack, Low-temperature scanning electron microscopy of the phase inversion process in a cream formulation, *Int. J. Pharm.,* 56:225 (1990).

99. A. DeVos, L. Vervort, and R. Kinget, Solubilization and stability of indomethacin in a transparent oil–water gel, *Int. J. Pharm.,* 92:191 (1993).

100. M. Bell, The solubilization of perfumery materials by surface active agents, *Soap Perfum. Cosmet.,* 58:263 (1985).

101. J. N. Labows, Surfactant solubilization behavior via headspace analysis, *J. Am. Oil Chem. Soc.,* 69:34 (1992).

102. G. A. Smit et al., Solubilization of hydrocarbons by surfactant micelles and mixed micelles, *J. Colloid Interface Sci.,* 130:254 (1989).

103. M. Ostro, *Liposomes,* Marcel Dekker, New York, 1983; see also G. Gregoriades in additional reading.

104. U. S. patent 4,217,344 to L'Oreal (Aug. 12, 1980).

105. A. A. Siciliano, Topical liposomes—an update and review of uses and production methods, *Cosmet Toiletries,* 100(5):43 (1985).

106. J. G. Wagner, Biopharmaceutics: Absorption aspects, *J. Pharm. Sci.,* 50:359 (1961).

107. G. Levy et al., Effect of complex formation on drug absorption III, *J. Pharm. Sci.,* 55:394 (1966).

108. P. Finholt and S. Solvay, Dissolution kinetics of drugs in human gastric juice—the role of surface tension, *J. Pharm. Sci.,* 57:1322 (1968).

109. M. K. Polano and M. Ponce, *Arch. Dermatol.,* 112:675 (1976).

110. B. C. Lippold and H. Schneemann, The influence of vehicles on the local bioavailability of betamethasone-17-benzoate from solution- and suspension-type ointments, *Int. J. Pharm.,* 22:31 (1984).

111. W. Wohlrad, Vehikelabhängigkeit der Harnstoffpenetration in die menschliche Haut, *Dermatologica,* 169:53 (1984).

112. J. Vinson and B. R. Choman, Percutaneous absorption and surface active agents, *J. Soc. Cosmet. Chem.,* 11:127 (1960).

113. M. Mezei and K. J. Ryan, Effect of surfactants on epidermal permeability in rabbits, *J. Pharm. Sci.,* 61:1329 (1972).

114. J. L. Lévêque, J. deRigel, D. Saint Léger, and D. Billy, How does sodium lauryl sulfate alter the skin barrier function in man? A multiparametric approach, *Skin Pharmacol.,* 6:111 (1993).

115. H. Komatsu, Percutaneous absorption of butylparaben in vitro. II. Effects of micellar trapping of the drug and percutaneous absorption of nonionic surfactants, *Chem. Pharm. Bull.,* 32:3739 (1972).

116. U. G. Dalvi and J. L. Zatz, Effect of nonionic surfactants on penetration of dissolved benzocaine through hairless mouse skin, *J. Soc. Cosmet. Chem.,* 32:87 (1981).

117. D. Harris and J. R. Robinson, Drug delivery via the mucous membranes of the oral cavity, *J. Pharm. Sci.,* 81:1 (1992).

118. D. C. Corbo et al., Characterization of the barrier properties of mucosal membranes, *J. Pharm. Sci.,* 79:202 (1991).

119. I. A. Siegel and H. P. Goron, Surfactant-induced increases of permeability of rat oral mucosa to nonelectrolytes in vivo, *Arch. Oral Biol.,* 30:43 (1985).

120. R. H. Engel and M. J. Fahrenbach, Intestinal absorption of heparin in the rat and gerbil, *Proc. Soc. Exp. Biol. Med.,* 129:772 (1968).

121. K. Taniguchi et al., Enhanced intestinal permeability to macromolecules II. Improvement of the large intestinal absorption of heparin by lipid–surfactant mixed micelles in rat, *Int. J. Pharm.,* 4:219 (1980).

122. W. J. Warwick et al., Absorption of vitamin A in patients with cystic fibrosis, *Clin. Pediatr.,* 15:807 (1976).

123. H. H. DeGreef, Emulsies als orale doseringsvorm, *Pharm. Weekbl.,* 118:252 (1983).

124. H. Rettig, Aspects of [drug] bioavailability from oral suspensions and emulsions, *Acta Pharm. Technol.,* 24:143 (1978).

125. E. Zis et al., Bile salts promote the absorption of insulin from the rat colon, *Life Sci.,* 29:803 (1981).

126. S. Hirai et al., Mechanism for the enhancement of the nasal absorption of insulin by surfactants, *Int. J. Pharm.,* 9:173 (1981).

127. J. Urbancic-Smerkolj et al., Enhancement of the bioavailability of some ergot peptide al-kaloids in the rat, *Yugosl. Physiol. Pharmacol. Acta*, 23:127 (1987).

128. R. J. Sokol et al., Improvement of cyclosporin absorption in children after liver transplan-tation by means of water-soluble vitamin E, *Lancet*, 338:212 (1991).

129. S. J. Hersey and R. T. Jackson, Effect of bile salts on nasal permeability, *J. Pharm. Sci.*, 76:876 (1987).

130. P. Tengamnuay and A. K. Mitra, Bile salt–fatty acid mixed micelles as nasal absorption promoters of peptides. I. Effects of ionic strength, adjuvant composition, and lipid struc-ture on the nasal absorption of [D-Arg^2]Kyotorphin, *Pharm. Res.*, 7:127 (1990).

131. M. A. K. Mattila et al., Prevention of diazepam-induced thrombophlebitis with cremophor as a solvent, *Br. J. Anaesthiol.*, 51:891 (1979).

132. K. Teelmann, et al., Preclinical safety evaluation of intravenously administered mixed mi-celles, *Arzneimillelforschung*, 34:1517 (1984).

133. S. Davis and P. Hansvani, The influence of emulsifying agents on the phagocytosis of lipid emulsions by macrophages, *Int. J. Pharm.*, 23:69 (1985).

134. K. Westersen and T. Wehler, Physicochemical characterization of a model intravenous oil-in-water emulsion, *J. Pharm. Sci.*, 81:777 (1992).

135. R. J. Williams et al., *Trans. Faraday Soc.*, 51:728–737 (1955).

136. T. Shimamoto et al., *Chem. Pharm. Bull.*, 21:316–311 (1973).

137. W. Prapaitrakul and A. D. King, Jr., *J. Colloid Surface Sci.*, 106:186 (1985).

138. W. C. Preston, *J. Phys. Colloid Chem.*, 52:84 (1978).

139. M. Olteanu and I. Mandru, *J. Colloid Interface Sci.*, 106:247 (1985).

ADDITIONAL READING

Adamson, A. W., Physical Chemistry of Surfaces, 4th ed., John Wiley & Sons, New York, 1982.

Attwood, D. and A. T. Florence, *Surfactant Systems*, Chapman & Hall, London, 1983.

Becher, P., *Dispersion Sci. Technol.*, 5:81–96, 1984. [HLB]

Eccleston, G. M., *Crit. Rep. Appl. Chem.*, 6:124–156, 1984. [Nonionic emulsifiers]

Gloxhuber, C., *Anionic Surfactants*, Marcel Dekker, New York, 1980.

Gregoriades, G., *Liposome Technology*, 2nd ed., CRC Press, Boca Raton, 1992.

Jungermann, E., *Cationic Surfactants*, Marcel Dekker, New York, 1970.

Linfield, W. M., *Anionic Surfactants*, Parts 1 and 2, Marcel Dekker, New York, 1981.

Lucassen-Reynders, E. H., *Anionic Surfactants*, Marcel Dekker, New York, 1981. [Physical chemistry]

Myers, D., Surfactant Science and Technology, 2nd ed., VCH Publishers, New York, 1992.

Mulley, B. A., Medicinal emulsions. In *Emulsions and Emulsion Technology*, Part I (K. J. Lissant, ed.), Marcel Dekker, New York, 1974.

Rieger, M. M., *Surfactants in Cosmetics*, Marcel Dekker, New York, 1985.

Tanford, C., *The Hydrophobic Effect*, 2nd ed., Wiley-Interscience, New York, 1980.

Tomlinson, E. et al., in *The Interation of Phenothiazines with Alkyl Sulfates in Solution Chem-istry of Surfactants* (K. L. Mittal, ed.), Plenum Press, New York, 1979, pp. 889–902.

van Olphen, H. and K. J. Mysels, *Physical Chemistry: Enriching Topics from Colloids and Sur-face Science,* Theorex, La Jolla, CA, 1975.

7

Viscosity-Imparting Agents in Disperse Systems

Joel L. Zatz

Rutgers—The State University of New Jersey, Piscataway, New Jersey

Joseph J. Berry

Bristol-Myers Squibb Company, New Brunswick, New Jersey

Daniel A. Alderman

The Dow Chemical Company, Midland, Michigan

I. INTRODUCTION

Polymers are used in suspensions, emulsions, and other dispersions, primarily to minimize or control sedimentation. The rheological character given to disperse systems also plays a role in maintaining pharmaceutical preparations at their application site. For example, highly fluid skin lotions may run, whereas viscous preparations tend to remain in place for longer time periods. A related application is in ophthalmic preparations, for which polymers are used to enhance drug retention.

In addition to their effect on dispersion rheology, polymers may also play a role in determining the flocculation state of suspended particles. By virtue of their surface activity, some polymers can directly improve emulsion stability; the ability of acacia to function as an emulsifier is well known.

Various substances have been used over the years to build viscosity in aqueous drug systems. Included are such familiar compounds as sucrose and other sugars, and polyols such as glycerin. These materials suffer from two major disadvantages. They are needed in high concentration to product significant viscosity changes, and their aqueous solutions are newtonian in nature (see Chap. 5).

On the other hand, only small amounts of many polymers (depending on chemistry and molecular weight) are needed to bring the viscosity of an aqueous preparation to almost any desired value. Furthermore, most polymer solutions or dispersions are nonnewtonian; in addition to being pseudoplastic, they may exhibit a yield point or thixotropy. These properties are advantageous in combining sedimentation resistance with processing ease. This point is explained further in Section III.

The nonnewtonian nature of polymer solutions makes it difficult to compare the properties of different polymers. Viscosity is a function of shear rate and, quite often, shear history, so that the numerical value of viscosity that is measured is a function of the method and conditions of measurement. Typically, manufacturers quote viscosity figures obtained from a single measurement at relatively high shear; this is insufficient to characterize a nonnewtonian material, particularly since its application to sedimentation control will take place under quiescent (low-shear) conditions.

As a consequence, the viscosity data provided by raw material suppliers is useful in only a very general way. Such data can show, for example, that certain polymer grades yield more viscous solutions than other grades made by the same manufacturer. However, it is extremely difficult to compare data on different polymers supplied by different manufacturers. It is not uncommon to find that two polymers, the solutions of which have nearly the same quoted viscosity value, affect a disperse system in markedly different ways.

Within a polymer family, an increase in molecular weight results in an increase in molecular asymmetry; hence, in viscosity. Different viscosity grades, based on a difference in average molecular weight, are described in several ways. With methylcellulose, the viscosity of a 2% aqueous solution measured in a standard manner is provided. Polyethylene glycols are described in terms of average molecular weight, whereas designations, such as low, medium, and high, are used in connection with viscosity grades of carboxymethylcellulose. All aqueous systems containing polymers require a preservative. Many polymers of natural origin are attacked directly by microorganisms. Cellulose derivatives are degraded by cellulases, enzymes that may be produced by microbial agents. Even if the polymer chosen is totally resistant to bacteria and molds, the aqueous medium may allow growth, and a preservative is still necessary.

Certain inorganic agents are also used as viscosity builders. Examples are colloidal magnesium aluminum silicate (Veegum) and microcrystalline silica. These substances do not support bacterial or mold growth and are relatively inert from a physiological standpoint.

II. POLYMER SOLUTION RHEOLOGY

Typically, polymer solutions are nonnewtonian. The three most commonly observed behaviors for polymer solutions are plastic, pseudoplastic, and thixotropic. Plastic systems flow only after a critical shear stress is exceeded (yield value). In pseudoplastic or shear-thinning systems, the viscosity decreases with increasing rates of shear. Thixotropy is the case in which a plastic or pseudoplastic system exhibits a time-dependent recovery, resulting in a hysteresis loop if shear stress is alternatively increased and decreased.

The type of rheological behavior, as well as the magnitude of the viscosity, is a critical factor determining the usefulness of a particular polymer for each potential application. For example, pseudoplasticity, the existence of a yield point, and some degree of thixotropy are useful characteristics for a polymer used as a suspending agent. Thus, xanthan gum, which has a yield value and is highly pseudoplastic, was a more effective retardant of creaming in mineral oil-in-water emulsions than either methylcellulose or carboxymethylcellulose [1], despite that comparisons were made at concentrations yielding the same range of measured viscosity values. Thus, it is not possible to evaluate polymer usefulness on the basis of a single viscosity value measured under arbitrary conditions.

The situation is complicated because rheological characteristics of polymer solutions may vary, depending on the concentration and degree of substitution. For example, solutions of medium- and high-viscosity grades of carboxymethylcellulose that are not highly substituted tend to exhibit thixotropic behavior, whereas more highly substituted grades are pseudoplastic.

It is sometimes advantageous to combine viscosity builders with different properties. The addition of xanthan gum to dispersions of magnesium aluminum silicate reduced the extent to which the viscosity of the latter increased over time [2]. Magnesium aluminum silicate is highly thixotropic in dispersions by itself; this was reduced by the gum. In addition, steady-shear measurements suggested synergy between the two materials in both viscosity and yield value.

Viscoelastic properties of the same materials were investigated by oscillatory shear [3]. The storage modulus G' was essentially independent of frequency for 1 and 3% clay dispersions containing no gum. The addition of gum shifted the behavior, and the data for the combined materials contained some of the rheological characteristics of each of the pure substances. The results were interpreted in terms of a reduction in structural rigidity of the clay and an increase in flexibility.

A recent study evaluated combinations of magnesium aluminum silicate with three carbomers [4]. The data suggested enhancement of the structure (yield value) in comparison with the properties of the two substances taken separately.

Specialized applications require specific rheological characteristics. For example, viscoelastic substances are used in eye surgery to prevent mechanical damage to sensitive tissues and avoid adhesions [5]. Polymer solutions are used in cataract, corneal, and glaucoma surgery. Among the agents employed are sodium hyaluronate, hydroxypropyl methylcellulose and chondroitin sulfate.

Power law relations are frequently used to describe the behavior of pseudoplastic polymer solutions. As part of a research program on natural polymer properties, the effects of concentration and temperature on the behavior of guar gum dispersions were evaluated [6]. A plot of the logarithm of shear rate was a linear function of the logarithm of shear stress and the following equation was applied to each flow curve:

$$v = a\sigma^b$$

where

v = shear rate
σ = shear stress
a and b are constants

The power constant b was directly proportional to gum concentration and inversely related to temperature. From the data, the authors were able to formulate a single empirical equation that permitted calculation of shear rate from shear stress, concentration, and temperature over a relatively wide range of values.

III. SEDIMENTATION CONTROL IN DISPERSE SYSTEMS

The control of sedimentation is of primary importance in maintaining the integrity of a disperse system. Stokes' law [7] defines the sedimentation rate of a sphere in a fluid as

$$V = \frac{2r^2(d_s - d_L)g}{9\eta}$$

where

V = sedimentation rate
r = particle size
d_S = density of sphere
d_L = density of liquid
g = gravitational constant
η = viscosity of continuous phase

Although most drugs in suspension are not perfect spheres and the suspensions are not dilute enough to follow Stokes' law, the equation is still useful. From the equation, three methods of controlling sedimentation present themselves: (a) particle size reduction, (b) density matching, and (c) viscosity building.

Since particle radius is raised to the second power, a modest change in this parameter translates into a much larger change in sedimentation rate. In practice, it is difficult to achieve particle reduction into the submicron range.

If the densities of the medium and the suspended particle are the same, no sedimentation will occur. An exact match is usually difficult to obtain, but it is occasionally possible to add ingredients that will bring the density of the continuous phase closer to that of the dispersed phase. Salts, if appropriate to the formulation, sugar, and other polyols may be used in aqueous suspensions for this purpose. Often the amount of density-increasing agents required to make the densities of the two phases equal would be too great to be practical.

A common method of controlling sedimentation is through use of viscosity-building agents, alone or in combination with one or both of the aforementioned approaches. The rheological characteristics of the polymer solutions used to stabilize disperse systems are very important. Systems that exhibit shear thinning are useful. They allow the dispersion to have a high "resting" viscosity and also enable redispersion of any settled material. Furthermore, it is possible to pour material from the container, even though the viscosity of the dispersion at rest may be considerable. It is not always feasible, or even necessary, to completely arrest the sedimentation of suspended particles. However, for suspensions that do settle, it is important that they be easily resuspendible (see Sec. V).

Zatz [8] has reviewed the merits of several thickeners, as well as how rheological behavior affects sedimentation stability of disperse systems. Relatively small increases in the concentration of xanthan gum dramatically reduced the sedimentation rate of sulfamerazine suspensions. The logarithm of the initial settling rate was a linear function of gum concentration.

IV. VISCOSITY CHANGES DURING PRODUCT AGING

The shelf-life of a dispersion depends on the chemical stability of its ingredients, as well as the physical stability of the system as a whole. Because of the importance of viscosity in terms of stability and certain use characteristics, major changes in viscosity over a time period are cause for concern.

Several factors may be responsible for changes in dispersion viscosity over time. Some are obviously due to alterations in the viscosity-building agent or its interaction with the rest of the system. Other factors, such as particle growth, may be independent of polymer content, although the polymers present may reduce the rate of change of particle size.

Depolymerization results in a decrease in average molecular weight; hence, a decrease in viscosity. Although processing under high shear may result in depolymerization, further viscosity changes would not be expected after manufacture unless chemical degradation of the polymer were to take place. Degradation of cellulosic derivatives by cellulase is an example of such a process. Cellulases may be introduced by microorganisms, or may be present as contaminants in other raw materials. Other chemical changes, such as hydrolysis of polymers at low pH values, are also possible.

Chemical changes in the system over time, producing a drift in pH or generating ionic products, may alter viscosity by virtue of the effect of these environmental alterations. Polymers may introduce a second-order effect on viscosity by acting as either flocculating or deflocculating agents in certain instances (see following section).

Time-dependent hydration of polymers or other viscosity-building agents can also result in a change in measured viscosity over time. In contrast with many of the other influences, continuing hydration results in an increase in viscosity after manufacture. Typically, viscosity reaches a plateau value after 1 or 2 weeks.

Because of the variety of factors that can alter viscosity over time, some of which increase viscosity, whereas others have the opposite effect, it is often difficult to pinpoint the exact cause in a particular situation. Small drifts in apparent viscosity are often encountered and are usually considered acceptable. However, substantial changes are cause for concern because of changes in the resistance to sedimentation and, also, because they suggest that chemical or physical changes of some kind are taking place. In other words, they are a sign that chemical or physical stability are not all that they should be.

In a study of polymer stabilization of 10% mineral oil emulsions, the apparent viscosity at 25°C was measured over time [1]. In emulsions containing 1% emulsifier and 1% carbxoymethylcellulose (CMC), high-viscosity grade, the apparent viscosity dropped from about 780 mPa s 1 week after manufacture to about one-tenth that value after 448 days. Apparent viscosity of emulsions containing other CMC concentrations also decreased over time. The effect of storage on apparent viscosity of another anionic polymer, xanthan gum, depended on gum concentration. Apparent viscosity decreased when the gum concentration was 0.1%, remained essentially constant at a 0.2% gum level, and increased over time at higher concentrations. Although several factors may be involved in these changes, the patterns observed suggest that small amounts of ionic products were produced during storage [1,9].

Elevated storage temperature can have an adverse effect on polymer stability that will result in a viscosity change over time. In a study of methylhydroxyethylcellulose, single-point measurements were used to track stability of several polymer grades at different temperatures over time [10]. There was little change in viscosity following storage for 2 months at room or refrigerator temperature. Storage at 40°C, however, usually caused losses of 15% or more. Storage temperatures of this magnitude may be encountered in tropical areas. Another concern is that high temperatures produced during manufacture, even for a short period., may adversely affect viscosity.

V. FLOCCULATION AND DEFLOCCULATION PHENOMENA

Flocculation is a process in which particles are allowed to come together and form loose agglomerates. Unlike coalescence, the total surface area is not reduced during the flocculation process. Deflocculation is the opposite, that is, breakdown of clusters into individual particles. Table 1 lists the properties of both types of suspensions.

Table 1 Properties of Flocculated and Deflocculated Suspensions

Property	Flocculated	Deflocculated
Sedimentation rate	Rapid	Slow
Supernatant	Clear	Cloudy
Sediment	Voluminous	Compact
Redispersibility	Easy	Difficult

It can be seen from the table that the chief advantage of a flocculated suspension is its redispersibility. Deflocculated suspensions settle more slowly and look more elegant while settling, but typically the sediment is close-packed and cannot be redispersed by shaking the container. The goal of controlled flocculation is to produce reasonably sized aggregates or flocs. In this way redispersibility is maintained while sedimentation rate is kept within reasonable bounds.

The difference in sediment density can be used as a means for characterizing the flocculation state. After allowing a group of suspensions containing the same active solid at the same concentration to settle completely, it is possible to compare the volume of sediment to identify those that are flocculated. In practice, the parameter measured is the sedimentation volume, the ratio of the volume of sediment to total suspension volume, often abbreviated as F [7]. In a series of suspensions, those that are deflocculated have the smallest values of F. Flocculated suspensions generally have F values at least twice as large as those for the deflocculated systems. The extent of flocculation is sometimes assumed to be proportional to the F value of a flocculated system.

Flocculation can be achieved by various means. The use of a polymeric agent is one common method. Polymers that contain chemical groups that interact with the suspended particles can be added to the continuous phase. In such a case, polymer segments can then attach to individual particles to form a polymer–particle complex. As a polymer links two or more particles, a floc can be formed. This flocculation process is called polymer bridging and is often concentration-dependent. When the concentration of polymer is high, particles can be completely surrounded by polymer and, thus, little floc formation can occur. Felmeister et al. [11] observed this concentration-dependent behavior in sulfaguanidine suspensions that were flocculated with an ionic polysaccharide. An increase in sedimentation volume was noted as polymer concentration was increased, but as concentration was increased still further, sedimentation volume decreased.

Law and Keyes [12] have shown that multilayer absorption of certain water-soluble cellulose derivatives can lead to deflocculation. The authors examined various concentrations of polymers. At high polymer concentrations deflocculation was usually observed. This effect was believed to be caused by steric repulsion.

A second method of flocculation is based on electrical charge. Suspended particles often have an associated charge. These charged particles will repel each other and, thereby, resist forming flocs. Reduction of surface charge may be accomplished by added electrolytes or surfactants of opposite charge. Reduction of particle repulsion permits the particles to become close enough to allow the attractive van der Waals forces to dominate. The complex nature of these particle interactions are explained by DLVO theory, which is covered by Hiemenz [13].

Components other than the suspended drug can influence flocculation by polymers. In a study of sulfamerazine suspensions, two surfactants, one anionic and the other nonionic, were employed as wetting agents [14]. Primafloc C3, a cationic polymer used in water purification, was added at different concentrations that spanned a wide range. Some of the results for suspensions containing the anionic wetting agent, docusate sodium, are shown in Fig. 1, in which sedimentation volume F is plotted as a function of the logarithm of polymer concentration. At very low concentrations, the suspensions were deflocculated and settled to form a nondispersible cake; variations in polymer concentration had no significant effect. But, at a concentration of about 0.1% polymer in suspensions containing 0.2% surfactant, the suspension volume was increased significantly, signaling a change from a deflocculated to a flocculated state (see curve 1, Fig. 1). The addition of more polymer had little effect until its concentration reached 1%, at which point the suspension was once again deflocculated.

A similar pattern was observed in suspensions containing 1% docusate sodium but flocculation occurred at higher polymer concentration (see curve 2, Fig. 1). The choice of wetting agent influenced the results obtained. When a nonionic surfactant, polysorbate 40, was used in place of docusate sodium, addition of the polymer resulted in a minimal increase in sedimentation volume. Combinations of the two surfactants at the same total concentration were employed in some experiments. The polymer concentration at the flocculation peak was a function of the weight fraction of docusate sodium in the surfactant mixture.

Figure 2 contains diagrams that suggest the mechanisms involved in determining flocculation state of the suspensions. In the absence of polymer, or at low polymer concentrations (see Fig. 2a), the negatively charged particles repel each other, preventing flocculation. At higher polymer concentrations (see Fig. 2b), electrostatic attraction results in simultaneous polymer adsorption to more than one particle, leading to flocculation. At much higher concentrations, the ratio of polymer to particle area is such that adsorption tends to cover each particle with a positively charged polymer layer, once again producing a deflocculated system (see Fig. 2c).

The same surfactants were employed in a study of flocculation of magnesium carbonate suspensions by xanthan gum [15]. The gum carries a negative charge, whereas the particle surfaces are positively charged in aqueous dispersion. Aqueous magnesium carbonate dispersions were flocculated in the absence of additives. The addition of the gum increased the sedimentation volume (enhanced flocculation), whereas the opposite effect resulted from incorporation of docusate sodium, an anionic surfactant. When both

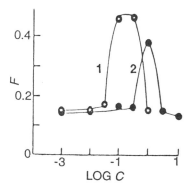

Fig. 1 Sedimentation volume (F) of sulfamerazine suspensions containing docusate sodium as a function of polymer concentration (C). Curve 1, 0.2% docusate sodium; curve 2, 1.0% docusate sodium. (From Ref. 11.)

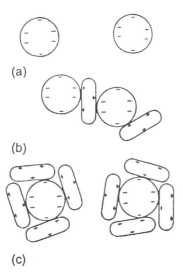

(a)

(b)

(c)

Fig. 2 Schematic representation of sulfamerazine particles in suspension. Spheres are particles; rods are polymer molecules. (a) Deflocculation at low polymer concentration; (b) flocculation by bridging; (c) deflocculation at high polymer concentration. (From Ref. 11.)

the gum and docusate sodium were present, the net result in terms of flocculation state depended on the relative concentrations of the two materials. This was rationalized in terms of competitive adsorption between the surfactant and polymer on the particle surface. A bridging mechanism implies adsorption of the polymer; if this is blocked by surfactant adsorption, flocculation enhancement by the polymer is reduced or does not occur. On the other hand, the nonionic surfactant polysorbate 40 did not itself influence flocculation of the particles or block the effect of the gum. Apparently, the lack of charge on this surfactant reduced its adsorption, thereby, allowing molecules of the gum to attach to the particle surface.

VI. EXCIPIENT COMPATIBILITY

Suspension dosage forms and other disperse systems may contain a large number of additives. Among them typically are surfactants, polymers, electrolytes, and polyols. There are many possibilities for complex interactions among these agents and between them and the drug [16].

As a general guide, precipitation reactions can be anticipated when charged polymers are mixed with other polymers or surfactants of opposite chemical type. Thus, anionic polymers tend to be compatible with other anionic polymers or nonionic polymers, or with nonionic or anionic surfactants, but not with cationic polymers or surfactants. Occasionally, precipitation can be avoided if one of the interacting species is present in much larger concentration than the other. Added salts sometimes block the reaction.

A troublesome interaction, although it does not usually lead to precipitation, is the binding (complexation) of phenolic and carboxylic preservatives by nonionic polymers and surfactants. Complexation may result in a shortage of sufficient free preservative to effectively protect against microorganisms. If it is not possible to substitute another, less interactive, preservative, or to remove the offending adjuvant, one must resort to an increase in preservative concentration.

Some caution should be exercised when charged polymers are combined with oppositely charged particles. The adsorption that results may lead to flocculation, which can be desirable (see previous section). However, excessive flocculation should be avoided, or the suspensions may turn into an inelegant, yogurtlike mass.

VII. POLYMER SELECTION

A number of decisions have to be made in selecting a viscosity-building agent for a formulation. General rheological behavior and possible interactions with the particles and other components of the dispersion are major factors. The following considerations help provide general guidance, but the selection process may not always follow a step-by-step procedure. After eliminating those materials that are obviously not suitable and selecting likely candidates from those that remain, empirical testing is necessary to identify the best candidates.

A. Biological Compatibility

It is obvious that certain polymeric agents will be removed from consideration, depending on the route of administration or application. With the possible exception of novel polymers with truly unique properties, only those that have been approved for a particular use should be tested.

B. Physicochemical Compatibility

In general, the chemical type of the polymers and surfactants in a disperse system must be mutually compatible. A knowledge of the charge on the particle surface is helpful in anticipating changes in flocculation character. These considerations were discussed more fully in the section on flocculation–deflocculation phenomena.

C. Natural Versus Synthetic

To obtain a polymer derived from a natural source, it is necessary to go to that source. If the desired material is obtained from a plant exudate, consider the site where the plant grows. Political changes, climatic changes, or local disasters of one kind or another can influence availability of a natural raw material as well as the quality of what is available. Thus, given recent events in Iran and Afghanistan, traditional sources for gum tragacanth, it is not surprising that the price of this substance has skyrocketed and that high-grade material is currently difficult to obtain. Natural products produced domestically by fermentation, such as xanthan gum, do not suffer from the same limitation.

Another consideration is the degree of chemical uniformity. In general, synthetic polymers and modified natural polymers (such as cellulose and chitin derivatives) might be expected to have more reproducible characteristics than plant exudates, provided that suitable care is taken in raw material selection and manufacture. Certainly, the ability to procure pharmaceutical dispersion adjuvants with predictable, consistent rheological properties is an important factor in selection.

The vulnerability of materials of natural origin to microbiological attack is often cited; however, natural raw materials do differ in susceptibility. Furthermore, many synthetic and semisynthetic polymers may also undergo degradation. Consequently, preservatives are required in all aqueous systems.

D. Viscosity Type and Concentration

Major considerations that come into play here involve effectiveness in retarding sedimentation (low-shear rheology), patient handling (medium-shear rheology), and processing during manufacture (high-shear rheology). A complete rheological description at various concentrations, therefore, is of great help, but empirical testing is likely to be necessary in fine-tuning the selection process.

VIII. VISCOSITY-BUILDING SUBSTANCES

In this section, the most frequently employed viscosity-building agents are reviewed, and specific information useful to the formulator is provided. Water-soluble polymers are emphasized, but thickeners for nonaqueous and partially aqueous systems are also available. Many of the same substances can be used to produce gels. Many polymer properties are summarized in Table 2. Additional information on substances useful in topical formulations is also available [17].

Synthetic and semisynthetic polymers are generally available in several grades, varying in chemistry and molecular weight and, therefore, in rheological properties. Most of the cellulose derivatives, for example, can be obtained in a variety of grades that have different degrees of substitution and molecular weight. In the natural polymers, functional differences are introduced by a process of selection or by chemical treatment. Thus, several alginates, differing in molecular weight and calcium content (and, consequently, viscosity) are offered commercially.

Most of the specific agents, the descriptions of which follow, are generally recognized as safe (GRAS) for use in foods. Many are listed in the *United States Pharamcopeia/National Formulatory* (USP/NF). In some instances, specific grades have been approved for use in foods and pharmaceuticals, whereas others have not. Before using any of these substances, its current status should be verified.

A. Natural Polymers

Water-soluble polymers are widely found in nature; they are derived from plant exudates, seaweed extracts, seed extracts, and fermentation processes of certain microorganisms. These polymers may be either nonionic or anionic. Different structures, branching, and molecular weight are responsible for the various properties of each polymer [18–20].

1. *Alginates*

Algin [21] is an anionic seaweed polysaccharide made up of linear groupings of mannosyluronic and gulosyluronic acids (Fig. 3). Monovalent salts and some salts of divalent ions (notably magnesium) are water-soluble. A firm gel is produced if a hydrated alginate is brought into contact with calcium or certain other polyvalent ions. The rate of gel formation may be controlled, or its onset delayed, by the use of slightly soluble calcium salts or sequestrants. Sodium alginate gels below a pH of 3–4 because of the protonation of carboxyl groups (see Chap. 10 on gels in Volume 2 for further details).

Table 2 Summary of Properties of Selected Viscosity-Imparting Agents

Agent	Derivation	Structure	Regulatory status	Ionic charge	pH factors	Temperature factors	Rheology	Yield point	Relative viscosity	Important features
Alginates, NF	Kelp extract	Polysaccharide	Alginate salts and alginic acid are GRAS	Anionic	Stable at pH 3–10	Poor temperature stability	Pseudoplastic	No	Medium to high	Polyvalant ions will crosslink polymer to form gels
Propylene glycol alginate, FCC	Modified kelp extract	Polysaccharide	PGA approved as a direct food additive	Anionic	Stable at pH 3–6,7	Poor temperature stability	Pseudoplastic	No	Medium to high	
Gum arabic (acacia, NF)	Plant exudate	Polysaccharide	GRAS as a direct food additive	Anionic	Viscosity is affected by pH	Reversible viscosity loss at elevated temperature	Newtonian at <40% conc.; pseudoplastic at >40% conc.	No	Very low	Low viscosity; ability to be made at high concentration; excellent sugar compatability
Carrageenan, FCC	Seaweed extract	Polysaccharide	GRAS	Anionic	Stable at pH 3–10	Reversible viscosity loss at elevated temperature	Thixotropic	No	Moderate	Will complex with casein in milk; strong gel formation possible
Guar gum NF	Seed extract	Polysaccharide	GRAS	Anionic	Stable at pH 4–10	Viscosity degradation at elevated temperatures and time	Pseudoplastic	No	High	High viscosity for natural gums
Gum karaya FCC	Plant exudate	Polysaccharide	GRAS	Anionic	Becomes ropey above pH 7.0	Very poor, viscosity drops irreversibly at elevated temperatures	Thixotropic water;	No	High	Insoluble, but swells in degrades at low pH; limited dry shelf life; used as a bulk laxative
Locust bean gum	Seed extract	Polysaccharide	GRAS	Nonionic		Viscosity will degrade at elevated temperatures with time	Pseudoplastic	No	High	Subject to shear de-polymerization; viscosity affected by temp. history
Gum tragacanth	Plant exudate	Polysaccharide	GRAS	Anionic	Stable at pH 1.9–8.5; excellent low pH stability	Good temperature stability; reversible viscosity loss at elevated temperatures	Pseudoplastic	No	High	Surface active; good low pH stability; composed of soluble and insoluble portions
Xanthan gum NF	Biosynthetic polymer	Polysaccharide	Approved as a direct food additive 21 CFR 172.695	Anionic	Good stability at pH 1–12	Good temperature stability; viscosity not affected by temperature changes	Pseudoplastic	Yes	High	Good enzyme resistance; yield point, viscosity unaffected by pH; high viscosity at low conc. (efficient)

Table 2 Continued

Agent	Derivation	Structure	Regulatory status	Ionic charge	pH factors	Temperature factors	Rheology	Yield point	Relative viscosity	Important features
Carboxy methyl-cellulose USP	Cellulose	Cellulose ether	GRAS 21 CFR 182, 1745	Anionic	Stable at pH 4–10	Good temperature stability; reversible loss of viscosity at elevated temperatures	Thixotropic at $DS^a = 0.4$ Pseudoplastic at $DS^a = 0.7$; 0.9, 1.2	Yes	Low to high	Not stable with some salts
Ethyl-cellulose NF	Cellulose	Cellulose ether	Approved for human consumption in 21 CFR 121.230	Nonionic	Stable at pH 4–10	Irreversible loss at viscosity at elevated temperature over extended time	Not reported	No	Low to medium in organic solvent	Hot water-soluble; soluble in many organic solvents; can be used to thicken alcohol
Hydroxy ethylcellu lose, NF	Cellulose	Cellulose ether	Approved for direct *food contact* only, 176.170, 176.180, 177.20 175.300, 173.103	Nonionic	Stable at pH 4–10	Good temperature stability	Pseudoplastic	No	Low to high	Not approved for human consumption; efficient thickener
Hydroxy propyl cellulose, NF	Cellulose	Cellulose ether	Approved as a direct food additive 21 CFR 172.870	Nonionic	Stable at pH 4–10	Precipitates at elevated temperature (reversible)	Pseudoplastic	No	Low to high	Good organic solvent solubility; good micro-biological resistance
Hydroxy propyl methyl cellulose 2906 USP 2910 USP 2208 USP 1818 USP	Cellulose	Cellulose ether	USP grades 2906, 2910, and 2208 approved as direct food additive 21 CFR 172.814	Nonionic	Stable at pH 4–11	Good temperature stability; viscosity reduces reversibly with increasing temperature until a reversible thermal gel is formed.	Pseudoplastic	No	Low to very high	Reversible thermal gelation; wide range of viscosities available; good microbial resist-ance; food additive status
Methyl cellulose USP	Cellulose	Cellulose ether	GRAS as a direct food additive 21 CFR 1892.1400	Nonionic	Stable at pH 4–11	Good temperature stability; viscosity reduces reversibly with increasing temperature, until a reversible thermal gel occurs	Pseudoplastic	No	Low to high	Thermal gelation; food additive status, variety of viscosities available

Material	Source	Description	Regulatory status	Ionic character	pH stability	Temperature stability	Rheology		Viscosity	Comments
Microcrystalline cellulose blends (MCC + CMC)	Cellulose	Crystalline cellulose and cellulose ether	Individual components approved as food additives	Anionic	Stable at pH 4–10	Good stability; viscosity unaffected by temperature	Thixotropic	Yes	Low	Yield point gives good suspension properties; dispersions opaque
Chitosan	Shells of crustaceans	Deacetylated chitin		Cationic	Soluble only at pH < 6.0	Good	Not reported	Not reported	Moderate to low	Cationic; poor tolerance to anions; low pH stability
Carbomer, USP	Acrylic acid	Crosslinked polyacrylate	Cleared for food contact only	Anionic	Soluble at pH > 4.0	Good temperature stability	Pseudoplastic	Yes	Very high	Very efficient thickener; poor salt tolerance reduces viscosity rapidly; good suspending agent organic agent solubility; excellent rheology for topical medications
Polyvinyl pyrrolidone (PVP) povidone USP	n-vinyl-2-pyrrolidone	Polyvinyl pyrrolidone	Used in medicine; not approved as food additive; substantial toxicological information available	Nonionic	pH does not affect viscosity	Good temperature stability	Not reported	No	Very low	Extremely low viscosity; can complex with some drugs
Polyvinyl alcohol USP	Polyvinyl acetate	Linear polyhydroxy polymer	Cleared for food contact only	Nonionic	5–7	Good temperature stability	Not reported	Not reported	Low	Not approved for human consumption; used in some eye preparations
Sodium hyaluronate	Rooster combs, fermentation	Polysaccharide	Solution approved for intraocular lens implantation	Anionic	4–8	Unstable at elevated temperature	Pseudoplastic	No	High	
Magnesium aluminum silicate, USP/NF	Mineral deposits	Complex silicate	GRAS	Anionic	3.5–11	Good temperature stability	Thixotropic	Yes	Low-medium	White; synergistic in presence of polymers; rheology sensitive to cations; many grades available for specific applications
Bentonite	Mineral deposits	Montmorillonite clay	GRAS	Anionic	Dispersions best at neutral pH or above	Good temperature stability	Thixotropic	Yes	Low-medium	Buff colored

[a]DS, degree of substitution on the cellulose backbone.

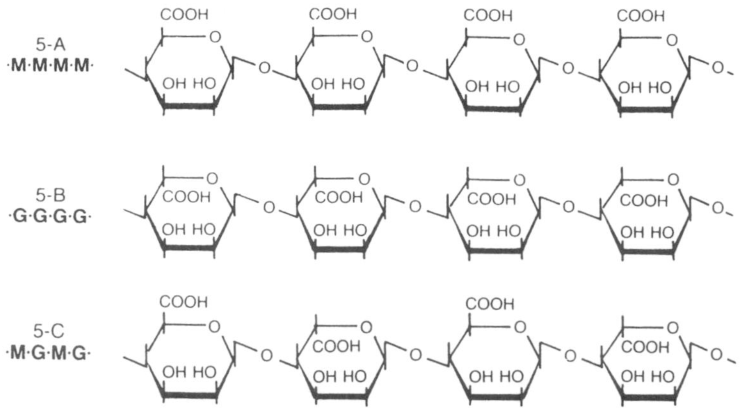

Fig. 3 Structure of polymers segments contained in alginic acid. (From Ref. 18.)

Propylene glycol alginate is a nongelling form that is useful over a pH range of 3–7. Alginate solutions exhibit pseudoplastic flow properties.

2. Gum Arabic

Gum arabic (acacia gum) is the dried exudate of trees of the genus *Acacia* [22]. Gum arabic results from an infection of the tree and is produced only by unhealthy trees. The tree bark is cut to accelerate exudation and formation of the gum exudate. Acacia gum may be defined as an anionic exudate polysaccharide that is a highly branched complex of arabic acid. Its molecular weight is on the order of 240,000.

Gum arabic is soluble in hot or cold water, with almost no solubility in organic solvents. Addition of ethanol to aqueous solutions of gum arabic rapidly decrease viscosity, and finally causes precipitation at a 60% ethanol concentration. Unlike most natural gums, acacia exhibits very low solution viscosities; concentrations of 40–50% polymer in water are possible. At concentrations under 40%, solutions exhibit newtonian flow; higher concentrations behave in a pseudoplastic manner. The solution viscosity of nonsterile gum arabic declines with time because it is very susceptible to bacterial contamination and growth, but this effect can be slowed with proper use of preservatives.

Gum arabic is most often used in emulsification and colloid stabilization. The gum is surface-active, and this helps to form and stabilize emulsions.

The low viscosity characteristic is also useful in obtaining minimum particle size in emulsification. It has been especially useful in the emulsification of flavor oils for beverages or baking. Gum arabic is listed in the *USP/NF*.

3. Carrageenan

Carrageenan is an anionic polysaccharide derived from seaweed [23]. Different types of carrageenan can be identified by the structure of the basic repeating units. The possible structures are identified by the Greek letters μ, ν, λ, ξ, κ, ι, and θ, as pictured in Fig. 4. Commercial products are usually mixtures of the κ-, ι-, and λ- carrageenans.

Properties such as water-solubility and gelation are greatly affected by the composition of carrageenan. For example, although all the forms of carrageenan are soluble

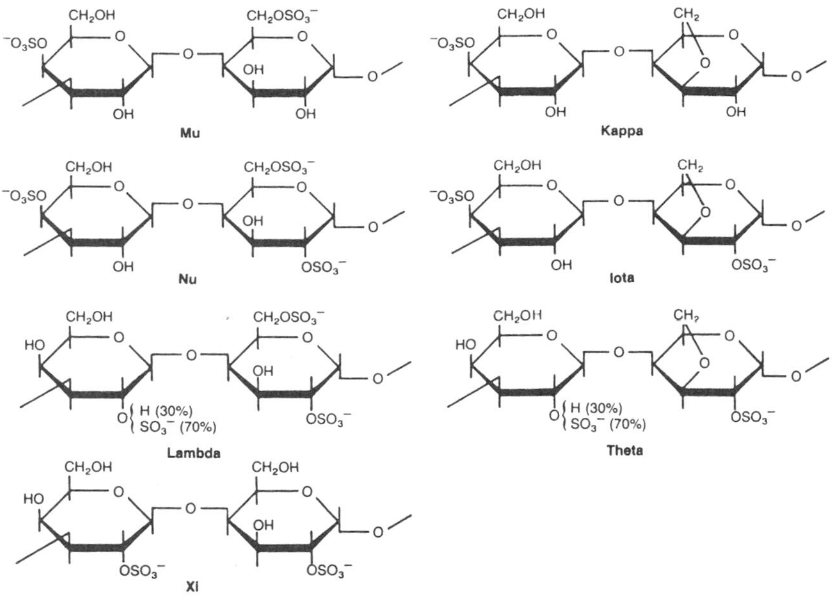

Fig. 4 Idealized structure of carrageenan repeating units. (From Ref. 18.)

in hot water, only the λ salt forms are soluble in cold water. The λ form is also the only nongelling form. After heating and cooling in the presence of certain ions, such as calcium and potassium, gels from that can exhibit great strength and have definite melting temperatures, depending on composition. Carrageenan is not soluble in organic solvents, but may tolerate the presence of some water-miscible organic solvents in solutions or gels.

Solutions of carrageenan have a yield point when used in sufficient concentration, and they are also thixotropic. Carrageenan solutions generally have a pH of 6–10, but exhibit increasing hydrolysis rates at a pH of less than 6. They are least stable under strongly alkaline conditions, and strong oxidizing agents can cause depolymerization. Gel formation exhibits a well-known completing reaction with the casein in milk. At low levels, carrageenan stabilizes milk emulsions and alters mouth feel; consequently, its polymers are often used in milk products.

4. *Guar Gum*

Guar gum, listed in the *National Formulary*, is a nonionic seed polysaccharide made up of a straight-chain mannose backbone, with regular branching of a galactose unit on every second mannose (Fig. 5) [22]. Guar gum is soluble in water. Solutions may exhibit turbidity, owing to the presence of insoluble endosperm components. It takes at least 3 h at room temperature for guar to reach its maximum viscosity in water, but hydration time can be shortened at elevated temperatures. Since guar gum retains some of its particulate characteristics in solution, the use of a fine–particle-sized product to ensure a smooth, homogeneous dispersion is important. Guar gum is not soluble in organic solvents, and viscosity will rapidly decrease with the addition of miscible solvents to aqueous polymer solutions.

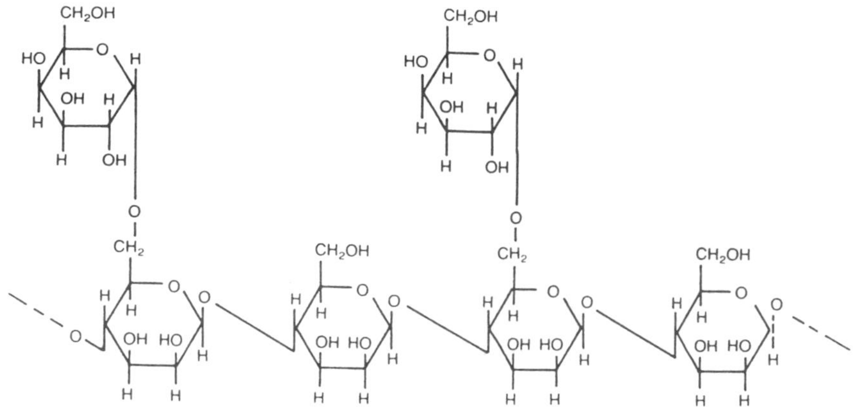

Fig. 5 Idealized structure of guar gum. (From Ref. 18.)

The rheology of an aqueous guar gum solution is pseudoplastic and exhibits no yield point. Guar gum may exhibit shear depolymerization when subjected to high shear rates for even a brief period. Maximum viscosity is obtained at a pH close to 6, with a loss of viscosity above pH 10. Guar solutions then reversibly with increasing temperature and may degrade irreversibly with time at elevated temperature.

5. Karaya Gum

Karaya gum is an anionic exudate polysaccharide complex of galactose, rhamnose, and glucuronic acid, partially acetylated [18,22]. Gum karaya is the least soluble of the exudate polymers. It does not form a true solution, but its particles swell in water to form a colloidal dispersion. The viscosity of gum karaya in water increases rapidly with concentration so that a dispersion with a concentration of 2–3% acts as a gel. Higher concentrations can be made, as in bulk laxative applications, by cooking karaya in steam. This reduced dispersion viscosity so that 20–25% dispersions can be made. Karaya gum dispersions in water have a pH between 4 and 5. Viscosity increases with pH, but solutions become stringy above pH 8. Gum karaya is not soluble in organic solvents and does not tolerate water-miscible organic solvents. The major pharmaceutical applications for gum karaya are bulk laxatives and denture adhesives.

6. Locust Bean Gum

Locust bean gum, a nonionic seed polysaccharide, with a straight-chain mannose backbone, has limited solubility in cold water [24]. Complete hydration requires heating to 82.2°C (180°F). The method of solution preparation dramatically affects the final solution viscosity. Locust bean gum is not soluble in organic solvents. It is one of the more efficient thickening natural polymers, along with guar, tragacanth, and karaya gums. Solutions of locust bean gum are pseudoplastic and have no yield point. Solutions of locust bean gum tend to react with inorganic salts, especially divalent ions, which may cause insolubilization, precipitation, or gelation. Combinations with other gums, such as xanthan, form gels.

7. Tragacanth Gum

Gum tragacanth NF is an anionic polysaccharide made up of a soluble portion, tragacanthin, and an insoluble portion, bassorin [25]. Tragacanth swells in cold water to produce a highly viscous, colloidal dispersion. It is insoluble in alcohol or organic solvents. Gum tragacanth is one of the most efficient natural polymer thickeners. The highest viscosities are obtained when solutions are made in cold water. The use of heat in solution preparation causes a certain amount of degradation and, owing to chain scission, a loss of at least 1/3 the viscosity achievable at lower temperatures. Tragacanth is graded by its viscosity in water. Ribbon grade tragacanth exhibits the highest viscosity, and flake grade is slightly lower. Solutions of gum tragacanth exhibit pseudoplastic flow.

Tragacanth solutions are stable over a wide pH range. In fact, these solutions exhibit good stability at low pH. For this reason, it is often chosen as the thickener for low pH food products, such as salad dressings and sauces. Divalent and trivalent cations, as well as storage at elevated temperatures, may cause a reduction in viscosity.

8. Xanthan Gum

Xanthan gum NF is a natural anionic biopolysaccharide made up of different monosaccharides, mannose, glucose, and glucuronic acids (Fig. 6) [26]. Soluble in water, but not in organic solvents, this gum can tolerate up to 50% of water-miscible organic solvents. Xanthan gum exhibits pronounced pseudoplastic rheology, with a definite yield point.

Enzymes that would commonly degrade other natural polymers, such as cellulose, do not affect xanthan. This has been attributed to the uniform polymer structure and shielding of the backbone by side chains. Xanthan solutions will tolerate divalent and trivalent ions, particularly at acidic pH values. Solutions are stable at relatively low pH; thus, xanthan is often used in low-pH food products. Xanthan exhibits a unique tem-

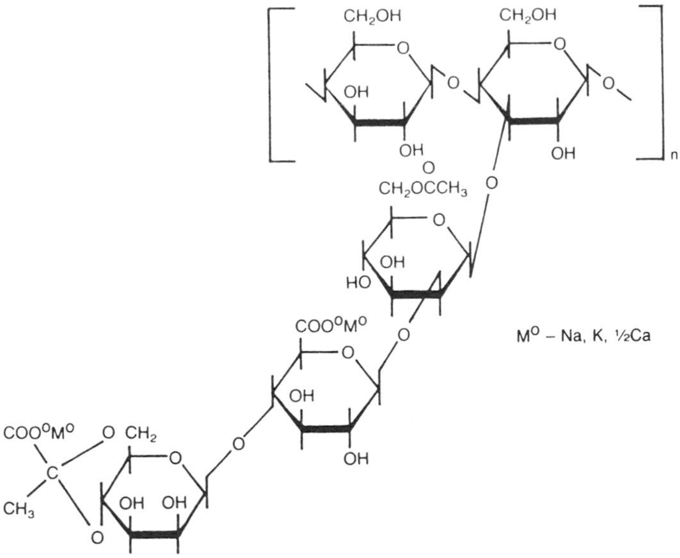

Fig. 6 Idealized structure of xanthan gum. (From Ref. 26.)

perature–viscosity relationship. Rather than thinning with heat, xanthan solutions (of at least 1% concentration) exhibit relatively constant viscosity. This polymer is resistant to shear depolymerization.

B. Cellulose Derivatives

Cellulose is one of the most widely used starting materials for the manufacture of modified natural polymers. It is common to use highly purified cotton or wood cellulose in the manufacture of food- or pharmaceutical-grade cellulose ethers. The cellulose molecule depicted in Fig. 7 shows the basic building block, the anhydroglucose unit, with its three possible sites for substitution. The degree of substitution of cellulose is defined in terms of the average number of hydroxyl groups substituted per unit (up to a maximum of 3.0). Steric hindrance makes complete substitution unlikely.

The Properties of cellulose derivatives depend on the nature of the substituent, the degree of substitution, and the uniformity of substitution. Native cellulose is not water-soluble even though each monomeric unit contains hydroxyl substituent groups, which are rather polar. This apparent contradiction may be attributed to extensive hydrogen bonding and associations that tightly bind polymer chains to one another in "crystalline" regions, thereby preventing hydration and dissolution. Substitution with bulkier moieties interferes with this self-association of polymer chains and allows water to interact more easily with the remaining hydroxyl groups.

Even the addition of hydrophobic substituents, such as methyl groups, can impart solubility in water by reducing internal hydrogen bonding and intermolecular association. The number of substituted groups per monomer unit necessary to produce water solubility varies with substituent type. A degree of substitution (DS) of hydroxypropyl as low as 0.1, for example, can impart water swelling properties. A DS of 0.4 of the hydroxyethyl substituent makes this cellulose polymer water-soluble. As substitution is increased, the cellulose ether begins to swell in organic solvents. At a DS of 2.3–2.5, it is soluble in polar organic solvents.

The uniformity of substitution is important to many polymer properties, including aqueous and organic solubility, and enzyme resistance. Uniform substitution results in the highest solubility at a given degree of substitution. When the degree of substitution is high (greater than 2.0) and the substitution is uniform, enzymes are blocked from breaking the cellulose backbone. Thus, highly substituted cellulose derivatives are more resistant to enzymatic and microbial attack.

Polymers for which the chains are not uniformly substituted, especially at lower DS values, may not uniformly solvate. The result may be solutions containing undissolved polymer chains that appear as turbidity or specks of "dust" in what would otherwise be a clear solution.

All of the cellulose ethers are generally quite stable in aqueous solution. They are relatively unaffected by pH within the range of 3–11; acid degradation occurs at pH

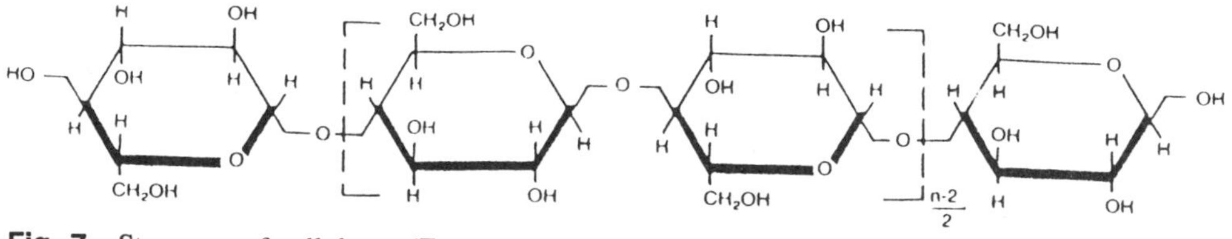

Fig. 7 Structure of cellulose. (From Ref. 30.)

values below 3. The viscosity stability of solutions exposed to long-term elevated temperatures is very good. Cellulose ethers with methyl substitution generally form a gel at elevated temperatures. Gel formation is reversed when the temperature is reduced. Nonionic cellulose ethers show good tolerance to most salts, although at higher levels increased competition for the available water can salt out the cellulose ether. The level at which this salting out phenomenon occurs depends on the ability of the polymer to compete for available water. Cellulose derivatives with more hydrophilic substituents, such as hydroxyethyl groups, can tolerate greater levels of salts (Table 3).

1. Carboxymethylcellulose

Sodium carboxymethylcellulose (CMC), an anionic polymer, is available in three grades: food, pharmaceutical, and technical [27]. It is also available with a variety of molecular weights and degrees of substitution. Carboxymethylcellulose is soluble in hot or cold water, but not in organic solvents. It is offered in several degrees of substitution: 0.4, 0.7, 0.9, and 1.2. Higher substitution leads to greater water solubility and better tolerance to other solution components, such as salts. The sodium content of the polymer increases with increasing substitution.

Carboxymethylcellulose is more resistant to microbial attack than most natural gums, but still must be preserved in aqueous systems. Heat sterilization and chemical preservation of solutions is recommended. As with most hydrocolloids derivatives, long-term exposure to extremes in temperature, pH, or oxidizers will result in chain scission and consequent viscosity loss. The viscosity of carboxymethylcellulose solution decreases reversibly with increasing temperature. Permanent viscosity loss is seen only after extended times at elevated temperature or in combination with low pH. Salts containing the polyvalent cations (e.g., Al) cause precipitation or gelation of cellulose gum. The rheology of aqueous carboxymethylcellulose solution depends on the degree of substitution. Low-substituted carboxymethylcellulose products exhibit thixotropy; higher substitution leads to pseudoplastic behavior.

2. Ethylcellulose

Ethylcellulose (EC) is available in several grades and types, but there are only two types of "premium" food or pharmaceutical grades [28]. The commercial forms of ethylcellulose are water-insoluble because of the high degree of hydrophobicity of the ethyl substituent on the cellulose backbone. The average DS (degree of substitution) for ethylcellulose NF is 2.3–2.5. Lower levels of ethyl substitution, not commercially available in the United States, exhibit water solubility. Ethylcellulose has been used to thicken alcoholic systems and to provide film formation for water-resistant sun screens. Organic solutions of ethylcellulose will tolerate very little water before precipitation occurs. The

Table 3 Chemistry of Some Cellulose Derivatives

Substituent	Polymer name
$O-CH_2-COONa$	Carboxymethylcellulose, cellulose gum
$-OCH_3$	Methylcellulose
$-O-C_2H_5$	Ethylcellulose
$-O-C_2H_4-OH$	Hydroxyethylcellulose
$-O-CH(CH_3)-CH_2OH$	Hydroxypropylcellulose

use of ethylcellulose in typical liquid dispersion systems is very limited because of these solubility properties.

3. *Hydroxyethylcellulose*

Hydroxycellulose (HEC) is a nonionic ether derivative of cellulose. Additional hydroxy groups are available to create long side chains [29]. An idealized structure of hydro-xyethylcellulose is shown in Fig. 8.

Hydroxyethylcellulose is soluble in water over a broad temperature range, to form clear, homogeneous solutions that do not gel at elevated temperures. It is not soluble in organic solvents, but can tolerate addition of some water-miscible organic solvents to aqueous polymer solutions. Solutions of hydroxyethylcellulose exhibit pseudoplastic flow and have no yield point.

4. *Methylcellulose*

Methylcellulose (MC) is a nonionic cellulose ether made by reacting methyl chloride with alkali cellulose [30]. The degree of substitution specified in the *USP* monograph for methylcellulose is in the range of 1.7–1.9.

Methylcellulose is soluble in cold water, but not in hot water. Once in solution and heated, methylcellulose solutions form an opaque, rigid gel that reversibly "melts" on cooling to the original viscosity. The gelation temperature depends on polymer concentration as well as the concentration of soluble additives. Figure 9 shows the effect of concentration on gel temperature. Methylcellulose is not soluble in organic solvents except for solvent blends, such as methylene chloride–ethyl alcohol. The rheology of aqueous methylcellulose solutions is pseudoplastic, and there is no yield point.

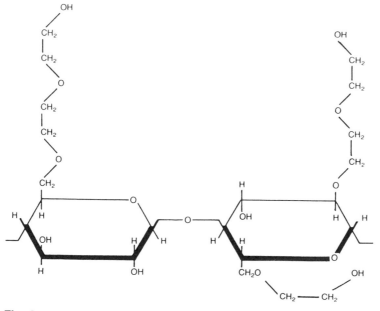

Fig. 8   Idealized structure of hydroxyethylcellulose. (From Ref. 29.)

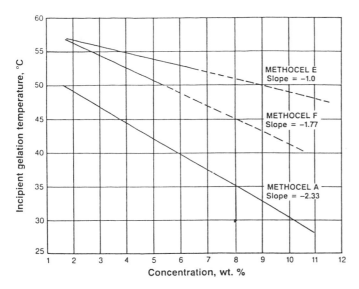

Fig. 9 Incipient gelation temperature of different Methocel products as a function of concentration. (From Ref. 30.)

5. *Hydroxypropyl Methylcellulose*

Hydroxypropyl methylcellulose (HPMC) is a nonionic cellulose ether available in a variety of types and viscosities [30]. There are four distinct USP grades of hydroxypropyl methylcellulose, with varying levels of methyl and hydroxypropyl substitution.

The methyl substitution imparts to HPMC one of its unique features, thermal gelation. The strength of the gel and the temperature at which it forms (60–90°C) depends on the polymer substitution and concentration in water. Figure 9 shows the effect of product type and concentration on gel temperature. Solutions of hydroxypropyl methylcellulose may be sterilized by autoclaving, without loss of viscosity.

Hydroxypropyl methylcellulose is a surface-active agent and reduces surface tension and interfacial tension. Solutions of HPMC exhibit pseudoplastic rheology, and there is no yield point.

C. Microcrystalline Cellulose

Dispersions of microcrystalline cellulose do not have viscosities that are significantly greater than that of water. However, combinations with carboxymethylcellulose are used to thicken aqueous solutions [31]. Cellulose in nature is made up of polymer chains arranged in amorphouse and crystalline regions. In the manufacture of microcrystalline cellulose, the amorphous segments are hydrolyzed and removed. To prevent aggregation after drying, the microcrystals are coprocessed with sodium carboxymethylcellulose and spray-dried (Avicel RC-591 and CL 611 grades) or bulk-dried (Avicel RC-501, RC-581 grades).

These four grades may be dispersed in water to form colloidal dispersions. Approximately 93% of the product is the insoluble, but swellable, microcrystalline cellulose. The spray-dried versions may be dispersed in water, with high shear. The bulk-dried versions required even higher shear, such as homogenization, to fully disperse the micro-crystalline particles. Viscosity continues to increase up to 24 h after the dispersion is formed.

The colloidal dispersions of microcrystalline cellulose blends exhibit thixotropic rheology. Viscosity is not affected by temperature. The dispersions also exhibit a yield point. Therefore, colloidal microcrystalline cellulose can be an effective suspension aid, although it is a relatively inefficient thickener. Care must be taken to obtain a proper colloidal dispersion. The microcrystalline cellulose should be fully dispersed in water before the addition of other ingredients. Cations in the dispersion may cause product flocculation, but protective colloids, such as cellulose gum or methylcellulose, can minimize the problem. A pH of less than 4.0 may be expected to lead to flocculation.

D. Chitosan

Chitosan is a derivative of chitin, the important organic component in the skeletal material of invertebrates. The major available commercial source of chitin is the exoskeletons of crustaceans. Chitin is produced by first removing the protein and calcium carbonate found in crustacean shell. Deacetylation to form chitosan is carried out in strong alkaline solutions at elevated temperature. The molecular structure is shown in Fig. 10. Chitosan is soluble in water only under acidic conditions. The pH of a chitosan solution must be kept below 6.0 to prevent precipitation or gelation. Chitosan may best be formulated at the pH 2–3 region. The acid solutions of chitosan are compatible with nonionic polymers, but are incompatible with sulfates and most anionic water-soluble polymers.

E. Synthetic Polymers

1. *Carbomer (Polyacrylic Acid)*

The acid form of this polymer (Carbopal, Goodrich) can be dispersed in water to give a pH of 2.8–3.2, but it does not dissolve [32]. Neutralization of the acid functionality with a base, such as sodium, potassium, or ammonium hydroxide, produces negatively charged carboxylate groups. This causes the polymer to uncoil and allows it to thicken aqueous systems. Carbomer also has solubility in a wide variety of polar organic solvents. Carbomer is an extremely efficient thickener in the neutralized state. The viscosity of a carbomer solution drops rapidly in the presence of a monovalent salt, and even more rapidly with salts containing di- and trivalent cations. Below a pH of 10, carbomer solutions are subject to viscosity loss under prolonged ultraviolet light exposure.

Solutions of carbomer are very pseudoplastic. They exhibit a yield value. Because of the extreme shear-thinning, thick gels may be pumped easily. This shear-thinning has made it an excellent choice as a thickener in creams and lotions.

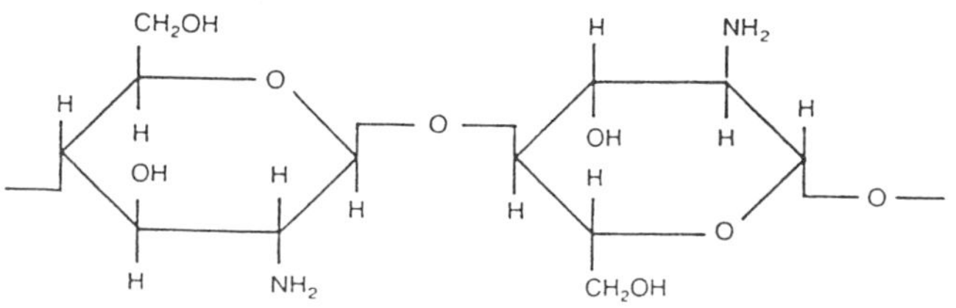

Fig. 10 Section of a deacetylated chitin molecule. (From Ref. 19.)

2. *Polyvinylpyrrolidone*

Polyvinylpyrrolidone (PVP) is formed by polymerization of *N*-vinyl-2-pyrrolidone [33]. It is soluble in cold water and many organic solvents, such as alcohols and some chlorinated compounds. Solutions of PVP in water exhibit a very low solution viscosity. Polyvinylpyrrolidone acts as a protective colloid; it can also form complexes with many substances. This property has been used effectively to increase solubility or, conversely, to cause precipitation. Complex formation with PVP has been used to modify the toxicity of certain drugs or to enhance or prolong the action of others.

Solutions of polyvinylpyrrolidone are stable for extended time periods if protected from molds. Solutions are stable at elevated temperature, but viscosity drops reversibly with increasing temperature. The pH of polymer solutions will not appreciably affect viscosity, but a precipitate will form in strong caustic.

3. *Polyvinylalcohol*

Polyvinylalcohol (PVA) is manufactured through the hydrolysis of polyvinylacetate. Manufacturers create different products by altering the chain length and degree of hydrolysis of polyvinylacetate [34]. Polymers with 99% hydrolysis are considered completely hydrolyzed, and varieties of partially hydrolyzed versions also are available. Completely hydrolyzed polyvinylalcohol is soluble in water, but not in organic solvents, it will tolerate up to 30% alcohol in an aqueous solution. Tolerance to higher levels of alcohol in water solutions of PVA is gained with a lower degree of hydrolysis. The viscosity of aqueous solutions tends to be quite low; solution viscosities are little affected by temperature.

4. *Magnesium Aluminum Silicate*

Magnesium aluminum silicate is a complex silicate that is refined to a white product. The manufacturer states that stable aqueous dispersions may be prepared within a pH range of 3.5–11 [35]. Specialized grades permit this range to be extended. A new product, Veegum Plus, provides increased viscosity and a higher yield value when compared with the standard material [36].

IX. SAMPLE FORMULATIONS

A. Trisulfapyrimidines Oral Suspensions

Veegum (magnesium aluminum silicate)	1.00 g
Syrup USP	90.60 g
Sodium citrate	0.78 g
Sulfadizaine	2.54 g
Sulfamerazine	2.54 g
Sulfamethazine	2.54 g

Directions: Add Veegum slowly and with continuous stirring, to the syrup. Incorporate the sodium citrate into the Veegum–syrup mixture. Premix the sulfa drugs and add to the syrup. Stir and homogenize. Add sufficient 5% citric acid to adjust the pH of the product to 5.6 (from *Remington's Pharmaceutical Sciences*, 18th ed., Mack Publishing Company, Easton, PA, 1990, p. 1542). This suspension is buffered to minimize dissolution of the sulfa drugs. The platelike Veegum clay particles are structured through the interaction of the positively charged ends with negatively charged edges. This serves to support and separate the drug particles. Veegum is partially flocculated by electrolytes. Although the suspension eventually sediments, it can be redispersed without difficulty.

B. Kaolin Mixture With Pectin

Veegum	0.88 g
Sodium CMC	0.22 g
Purified water	79.12 g
Kaolin	17.50 g
Pectin	0.44 g
Saccharin	0.09 g
Glycerin	1.85 g

Directions: Add Veegum and sodium CMC to water with continuous stirring. Add the kaolin with mixing. Add the pectin, saccharin, and glycerin to the suspension with continuous mixing (from *Remington's Pharmaceutical Sciences*, 18th ed., Mack Publishing Company, Easton, PA, 1990, p. 1542).

Sedimentation is retarded by Veegum, CMC, and pectin, the latter acting as a stabilizer as well as an active ingredient. The combination of Veegum and CMC results in augmented viscosity (greater than the sum of the viscosities of the two ingredients measured separately) and an increase in yield value, which tends to keep the finely divided solids in suspension. Another polymer that works well in combination with Veegum is xanthan gum.

C. Antacid Suspension

A: Al–Mg Fluid Gel (Reheis Chemical)	36.20 g
B: Sorbitol solution 70%	7.00 g
C: Antifoam AF emulsion (Dow Chemical)	1.70 g
D: Methylparaben	0.22 g
E: Propylparaben	0.04 g
F: Flavor	0.30 g
G: Methocel K4M (Dow Chemical)	0.60 g
H: Deionized water	53.94 g

Directions: (1) combine C and H, using an Epenbach Homomixer; (2) add A, mix 10 min; (3) transfer to overhead stirrer; (4) combine B and F mix thoroughly and add to formula while mixing; and (5) combine D, E, and F upon solution, add to rest of formula and mix 5 min (from *Drug and Cosmet. Ind.,* (May): 48, 1985).

The sorbitol helps to avoid caking in antacid suspensions. The concentration of Methocel K4M (hydroxypropyl methylcellulose) in this formation is relatively low, so that viscosity-building probably plays a minor role in stabilization. It may function here as a protective colloid. The properties of this nonionic polymer are not affected very much by electrolytes. There is also little effect of this polymer on the flocculation state of the particles. Aluminum hydroxide particles are often positively charged, and many anionic polymers will interact with them to produce a yogurtlike mass, because of excessive flocculation. Polyphosphates and other deflocculants may serve to avoid this incompatibility [37].

D. Glycerin (Glycerol) and Rose Water Lotion

Glycerin (glycerol)	48.8 g
Water	48.8 g
Carbopol 941 resin (Goodrich)	0.2 g
Triethanolamine	0.2 g
Glyceryl monostearate (self-emulsifying opacifier)	2 g
Perfume	qs

Directions: (1) Slowly add the Carbopol 941 resin to the water using good agitation and stir until the Carbopol 941 resin is fully dispersed; (2) add the glycerin; (3) add the glyceryl monostearate; (4) mix in the perfume; and (5) lastly add the triethanolamine (from *Personal Care Products Formulary* GC - 68, Carbopol Resin, B. F. Goodrich).

Triethanolamine is used to neutralize the Carbopol resin (carbomer). The resulting product is a viscous liquid; at higher carbomer concentrations (about 0.5%), a gel would result. The viscosity of preparations containing carbomer is reduced in the presence of salts. Polar organic liquids can be thickened by neutralizing carbomer with an organic base, such as an amine.

E. Cream Lotion Shampoo

Water	68.85%
Stepanol WAT (Stepan)	35.00%
Keltrol, xanthan gum (Kelco)	0.80%
Timica pearl white (Mearl)	0.20%
Methylparaben	0.15%

Directions: (1) Add the Keltrol to the water slowly and with good agitation. Mix thoroughly. (2) Add the Stepanol WAT. (3) Add the other ingredients (including color as desired) and mix completely. (4) Package (from *Kelco Product Formulation* SS-4636, Kelco Div., Merck and Co., 2/81).

Xanthan gum is responsible for the texture of this dispersion. Solutions of this gum are highly pseudoplastic, and they exhibit a yield value. Viscosity of solutions of xanthan are relatively insensitive to variations in temperature, pH, and ionic content. It is one of the few anionic thickeners that function well in acid media. It may be used in combination with other stabilizers, such as Veegum and microcrystalline cellulose.

F. Lubricant Jelly

Water, deionized	403.5 g
Propylene glycol	90.0 g
Kelcosol sodium alginate	5.5 g
Keltrol T xanthan gum	1.0 g
Preservative and fragrane	*to suit*
	500.0 g

Directions: (1) Slurry Kelcosol and Keltrol T in propylene glycol. (2) With good agitation, add gum slurry to water. (3) After gums are fully hydrated, add preservative add fragrance (from *Kelco Product Formulation* SS-5262, Kelco Div., Merck and Co., 3/86).

Jellies of the type exemplified by this formulation are sometimes characterized as "soft gels." They are very viscous solutions, with a small yield value. The gums (sodium alginate and xanthan gum) provide the viscosity. They also contribute to the lubricity of the product.

G. Tetracycline Suspension

Tetracycline	2.50 g
Avicel RC-591 microcrystalline cellulose	0.75 g
Sodium carboxymethylcellulose (CMC), medium viscosity	0.15 g
Dibasic sodium phosphate	1.40 g
Citric acid	1.00 g
Sorbitol solution (70)	35.00 ml
Glycerin (glycerol)	5.00 ml
Methyl *p*-hydroxy benzoate	0.18 g
Propyl *p*-hydroxy benzoate	0.02 g
Distilled water	q.s. to make 100 ml

Procedure

1. To 50 ml distilled water, slowly add the Avicel RC-591, while mixing with an efficient agitator. Mix for at least 30 min or until the Avicel is completely dispersed.
2. Add the preservatives and mix until dissolved.
3. Slowly add the CMC and mix well until dissolved.
4. Add the sorbitol solution and glycerin (glycerol) while mixing.
5. Dissolve the dibasic sodium phosphate and citric acid in 5 ml distilled or deionized water, add to the bulk and mix.
6. Disperse the tetracycline until homogeneous.
7. Adjust to volume with distilled water. Mix well.
8. Homogenize and remix (from FMC Corporation).

Avicel RC-591 contains CMC, in addition to cellulose microcrystals. These microcrystals form asymmetric aggregates (in the presence of low electrolyte concentrations) that link to produce a three-dimensional network throughout the suspension. The network provides bulk and retards drug sedimentation. Because of the small particle size, relatively low Avicel concentrations are required. High electrolyte concentrations reduce interparticle repulsion, making it difficult to disperse Avicel. Sequestrants may be of value in such situations.

The CMC acts as a protective colloid, facilitating dispersion of the microcrystalline cellulose. Xanthan gum also functions well for this purpose.

REFERENCES

1. J. L. Zatz and B. K. Ip, *J. Soc. Cosmet. Chem.*, 37:329–350 (1986).
2. P. A. Ciullo, *J. Soc. Cosmet. Chem.*, 32:275–285 (1981).
3. C. R. Chen and J. L. Zatz, *J. Soc. Cosmet. Chem.*, 43:1–12 (1992).
4. P. A. Ciullo, *Cosmet. Toiletries*, 106:89–95 (1991).
5. T. J. Liesegang, *Surv. Ophthalmol.*, 34:268–293 (1990).
6. L. Ben-Kerrour, D. Duchene, F. Puisieux, and J. T. Carstensen, *Int. J. Pharm.* 5:59–65 (1980).

7. A. R. Gennaro, ed., *Remington's Pharmaceutical Sciences*, 18th ed., Mack, Easton, PA, 1990, pp. 294–298.
8. J. L. Zatz, *J. Soc. Cosmet. Chem.,* 36: 393–411 (1985).
9. J. L. Zatz, and K. Knapp, *J. Pharm. Sci.,* 73:468–471 (1984).
10. A. Huikari, and A. Karlsson, *Acta Pharm. Fenn.,* 98:231–238 (1989).
11. A. Felmeister, et al., *J. Pharm. Sci.,* 62:2026–2027 (1973).
12. S. L. Law and J. B. Keyes, *Drug Dev. Ind. Pharm.,* 10:1049–1069 (1984).
13. P. C. Hiemenz, *Principles of Colloid and Surface Chemistry*, Marcel Dekker, New York, 1986, pp. 677–731.
14. J. L. Zatz, L. Schnitzer, and P. Sarpotdar, *J. Pharm. Sci.,* 68, 1491–1494 (1979).
15. J. L. Zatz, P. Sarpotdar, G. Gergich, and A. Wong, *Int. J. Pharm.,* 9:315–319 (1981).
16. J. L. Zatz and R. Y. Lue, *J. Pharm. Sci.,* 76:157–160 (1987).
17. R. Y. Lochhead and W. R. Fron, *Cosmet. Toiletries*, 108 (5):95–135 (1993).
18. R. L. Davidson, *Handbook of Water-Soluble Gums and Resins*, McGraw-Hill, New York, 1980.
19. R. I. Whistler and J. N. BeMiller, *Industrial Gums*, Academic Press, Orlando, FL, 1959.
20. E. Ott, H. M. Spurlin, and M. W. Grafflin, *High Polymers*, Vol. 5(1–3), Interscience, New York, 1955.
21. *Kelco Algin* 2nd ed., Kelco Technical Brochure.
22. Meer Technical Support System, *Meer Technical Bulletins on Natural Gums.*
23. *General Carrageenin Application Technology* (G-31), FMC Corp., Marine Colloids Div. (1988).
24. *Locust Bean Gum*, Celanese Polymer Product Data Bulletins.
25. *Supercol Gums*, Henkel Gum Tragacanth Technical Brochure.
26. *Xanthan Gum, A Natural Biopolysaccharide for Scientific Water Control*, Kelco Technical Bulletin.
27. *Cellulose Gum*, Hercules Technical Bulletin.
28. *ETHOCEL Ethylcellulose* Resins, Dow Chemical Company, Technical Brochure, #192–818–1284.
29. *NATROSOL Hydroxyethylcellulose*, Hercules Technical Brochure.
30. *METHOCEL Handbook*, Dow Chemical Company.
31. *AVICEL Microcrystalline Cellulose Product Description*, FMC Technical Bulletin G-34.
32. *CARBOPOL Water Soluble Resins*, B. F. Goodrich Technical Brochure.
33. *PVP, Polyvinylpyrrolidone*, GAF Technical Brochure.
34. *Elvanol Polyvinyl Alcohol*, DuPont Technical Brochure.
35. *Veegum*, R. T. Vanderbilt Company Technical Brochure.
36. D. B. Braun, and P. A. Ciullo, Presented at the 11th Congress of Latin American and Iberian Cosmetic Chemists, Montivideo, Uruguay, November 1993.
37. J. L. Zatz, D. Figler, and K. Livero, *Drug Dev. Ind. Pharm.,* 12: 561–568 (1986).

8

Bioavailability of Disperse Dosage Forms

Maureen D. Donovan and Douglas R. Flanagan

University of Iowa, Iowa City, Iowa

I. INTRODUCTION

Disperse systems have been broadly classified as systems in which one substance, the dispersed phase, is distributed throughout another substance, the continuous phase or vehicle. They are important to pharmacy because of their widespread use. Pharmaceutical dosage forms that can be classified as disperse systems are suspensions, emulsions, creams, ointments, pastes, foams, suppositories, and aerosols. These dosage forms are used for many routes of administration (e.g., oral, dermatological, ophthalmic, parenteral, respiratory, and rectal). Depending on the route of administration, the disperse phase may vary in particle size from less than 1 μm for inhalation and ophthalmic use, to about 10–100 μm for dermatological use, and up to 200 μm for oral use. A small particle size will hasten dissolution and also reduce the chance of abrasion to susceptible tissues.

Although disperse pharmaceutical dosage forms are relatively complex to formulate and prepare, bulky, and prone to various routes of physical degradation (i.e., segregation, aggregation, coalescence, and caking), which lead to inaccurate dosing, there are certain advantages to their use. If the drug is easily oxidized or hydrolyzed, a disperse system, when compared with a solution, may provide adequate shelf life for the product. Also, for the very young and the elderly, an oral fluid, disperse formulation is easier to administer than a tablet or capsule. For drugs that are poorly soluble, disperse dosage forms are smaller in volume than a solution of the same dose and, therefore, more convenient for patient use. Finally, a disperse system is advantageous in masking the taste of drugs.

Although a disperse pharmaceutical dosage form can be considered readily available for absorption, the correlation of absorption to formulation variables is often unclear. Frequently, the drug must first dissolve in the vehicle before it can be absorbed. Here, the dissolution rate of the drug, first in the vehicle, then into the environment in which the dosage form resides, can limit the bioavailability. The dosage form may also be present at the site of administration or absorption for a relatively short time. This may limit the bioavailability or therapeutic effectiveness by limiting the amount of drug present at its active site. Because of the relative instability of disperse systems when they come into contact with the body fluids present at the absorption site, correlations between in vitro dosage form performance and in vivo behavior can be difficult to ascertain. As a result, physiological and anatomical constraints at various sites of administration significantly influence the bioavailability of a drug when formulated in disperse systems as much as do the formulation factors. Consequently, the formulator must have a fundamental understanding of the environment in which the drug resides before the absorption of drug, or a poorly bioavailable product may result.

II. FORMULATION FACTORS AFFECTING DRUG RELEASE FROM DISPERSE SYSTEMS

A. Wetting

The initial dispersion of particles in a suspension requires wetting by the dispersion medium. If the material from which a suspension is prepared exhibits hydrophobic characteristics, it is difficult to remove air from the particle surface. Entrapped air often promotes particles that rise to the top of the dispersion medium, particle deaggregation, or in other ways the generation of an unstable suspension. Poor wetting of individual drug particles gives rise to disperse formulations with poor physical stability and poor dissolution properties. Entrained air decreases the effective surface area for dissolution, thereby decreasing bioavailability.

B. Particle Size

Dissolution rate is a direct function of total surface area for a dispersed phase. The surface area increases inversely with the particle size according to the expression, $S_v = 6/d$, where S_v is the specific surface area and d is the average particle diameter. The *United States Pharmacopeia* (*USP*) requires that griseofulvin, for example, have a specific surface area between 1.3 and 1.7 m²/g. This area corresponds to an average particle size between 3 and 4 μm. Such a particle size is important to achieve adequate absorption of a poorly soluble drug such as griseofulvin. Insulin suspensions also have particle size requirements that affect their onset and duration of action. Extended action zinc insulin suspensions are crystalline and have a particle size of 10–40 μm, which delays onset of action for 4–6 h and prolongs action to 36 h. On the other hand, prompt zinc insulin suspensions are composed of amorphous particles, with a particle size smaller than 2 μm, which gives a prompt onset of action in 1–3 h and a duration of action of 12–16 h.

C. Viscosity

The overall viscosity of a dispersion arises from two sources—the intrinsic viscosity of the dispersion medium and interaction of the particles of dispersed phase. The intrinsic viscosity of the medium affects the dissolution rate of particles through its effect on the diffusion coefficient D. The Stokes–Einstein equation, $D = kT/6\pi\eta r$, shows the relationship between viscosity (η) and diffusion coefficient, where k is Boltzmann's constant, T is absolute temperature, and r is molecular radius. As viscosity increases, the diffusion coefficient decreases which also gives rise to a proportionate decrease in rate of dissolution.

III. PRINCIPLES OF DRUG RELEASE FROM DISPERSE SYSTEMS

A. Particulate Dissolution Models

1. *Diffusion-Controlled Dissolution*

To evaluate the dissolution characteristics of solid particles, one must consider two aspects of such systems. The first aspect concerns the most appropriate basic models for single particle or monosized multiparticulate systems. The second aspect is: How does the size distribution affects the dissolution profiles for polydisperse systems, and how are these effects included in the basic dissolution models? First, dissolution models without size distribution effects will be considered, then various approaches to account for polydispersity will be reviewed.

The basic diffusion-controlled model for solid dissolution was developed by Noyes and Whitney [1,2] and was later modified by Nernst [3]. This model is represented by the following equation:

$$\frac{dQ}{dt} = \frac{DA[C_s - C_b]}{h} \tag{1}$$

where

dQ/dt = dissolution rate
D = diffusion coefficient
h = diffusion layer thickness
C_s = solubility
C_b = bulk solution concentration
A = surface area of particle

This model assumes that a rapid equilibrium is achieved at the solid–liquid interface, producing a saturated solution that diffuses into the bulk solution across a thin layer of solution, called the diffusion layer. This diffusion process across the diffusion layer is rate-controlling, which effectively converts the heterogeneous process of dissolution to one governed by the homogeneous process of liquid-phase diffusion. Even though the concept of a stagnant or unstirred layer of liquid adhering to the solid surface is somewhat naive, models using this concept have been useful and have been the basis for modeling more complex dissolution systems.

For spherical particles with a changing surface area, Hixson and Crowell [4] derived the well-known cube-root relationship shown below:

$$W_t^{1/3} = W_0^{1/3} - K_{1/3}t \tag{2}$$

where

W_t = particle weight at time, t
W_0 = initial particle weight
$K_{1/3}$ = dissolution rate constant

Under sink conditions (i.e., where $C_s \gg C_b$), the dissolution rate constant $K_{1/3}$ is given by the expression, $(4\pi/3\rho^2)^{1/3} . DC_s/h$, where ρ is the solid density and other symbols are as defined previously. The Hixson–Crowell cube-root relationship is most useful for the dissolution of macroscopic solid spheres [5] in which the diffusion layer is considered constant and small compared with the size of the sphere.

For multiparticulate systems, the Hixson–Crowell cube-root relationship has shown some utility [6]. In such systems Eq. (2) can be applied with W_t and W_0 representing the total mass of monosized spherical particles, and the rate constant, $K_{1/3}$, would include a factor, $N^{1/3}$ (number of particles). Not all such dissolution data can be explained by the cube-root relationship which led Niebergall and Goyan [7] to derive the square-root relationship shown below:

$$W_t^{1/2} = W_0^{1/2} - K_{1/2}t \tag{3}$$

Under sink conditions, the dissolution rate constant $K_{1/2}$ is given by the expression, $(3\pi/2\rho)^{1/2} \cdot DC_s/k$, where k is the proportionality constant between diffusion layer thickness and particle size. In this model, Niebergall and Goyan assumed that the diffusion layer exhibits a square-root dependency on particle size. This conclusion was reached empirically, based on the observation that a square-root dependency on weight gave a constant dissolution rate constant for different particle size fractions of a particular solid. The cube-root constant varied under these conditions.

Neither the cube-root nor the square-root models were intended to describe particle dissolution down to very small sizes. Higuchi and Hiestand [8] attempted to deal with particulate dissolution systems in which the size was much smaller than the diffusion layer thickness. With such an assumption, they derived the following relationship:

$$W_t^{2/3} = W_0^{2/3} - K_{2/3}t \tag{4}$$

Under sink conditions, the dissolution rate constant $K_{2/3}$ is given by the expression, $2\sqrt{2}/3\sqrt{\rho})^{2/3}DC_s$. They showed that this model correlated well with data for the dissolution of micronized methylprednisolone in water [9].

Under nonsink conditions more complex mathematical models have been derived to describe the time course of particulate dissolution [10,11]. These models are mathematically cumbersome and of limited use for general application to particulate dissolution systems.

Other conditions for describing the dissolution behavior of particulate systems have come from the work of Mauger and Howard [12,13]. They have applied Nielsen's model [14] for the hydrodynamics around a falling sphere to modify the Higuchi–Hiestand model to explicitly include a factor for the effect of hydrodynamics on diffusion layer thickness. They have applied their approach to the dissolution behavior of suspensions.

To account for the size distribution effects in most real particulate dissolution systems has been a more challenging problem than the development of the basic single or monosized particulate models. In general, the initial size distribution can be described by

$$N = \int_{a_{os}}^{a_{ol}} n_i \cdot da_{oi} \tag{5}$$

where
  a_{os} = smallest initial size
  a_{ol} = largest initial size
  n_i = number of particles of size a_{oi}
  N = total number of particles

The total particle mass is

$$W = \int_{a_{os}}^{a_{ol}} w_i n_i \, da_{oi} = \int_{a_{os}}^{a_{ol}} \left(\frac{\pi\rho}{6}\right) a_i^3 n_i \, da_{oi} \tag{6}$$

where

w_i = weight of particles of size a_i

To properly account for distribution effects, two time periods during the dissolution process must be considered: one period before any particles completely dissolve and a second after the first (i.e., smallest) particles have dissolved. The time at which the first changes to the second is called the critical time, t_c. The t_c for a particular system can be calculated, if the initial particle size distribution is known, by applying one of the previous models [see Eqs. (2–4)] to the smallest-sized particles in the system. After t_c, the lower limit for the distribution integrals [see Eq. (5) or (6)] becomes the smallest particle from the original distribution that still exists at time, t.

Higuchi and Hiestand [7] considered that many drug powders exhibit log-normal size distributions, which could be approximated by $n_i = K/(a_{oi})^4$. Later they observed that the distribution of micronized methylprednisolone could be approximated by $n_i = K/(a_{oi})^2$ [8]. Carstensen and Musa [15] dealt more directly with a log-normal particulate system, which led to the following expression:

$$W = \int_{\log a_{os}}^{\log a_{ol}} \left(\frac{N\pi\rho}{6}\right)\left[a_{oi} - \frac{2DC_s t}{h}\right]^3 \cdot \left(\frac{1}{\sqrt{2\pi}\,\log\sigma_{geo}}\right) \cdot$$
$$\exp[-1/2(\log a_{geo} - \log a_{oi}/\log\sigma_{geo})]^2 \, d\log a_{oi} \tag{7}$$

where

σ_{geo} = log-normal standard deviation
a_{geo} = geometric mean size

They claimed that truncated distributions can be employed if the distribution is truncated at $3\log\sigma_{geo}$. Computer simulations of Eq. (7) for various log-normal powder distributions were presented by these authors to show how their equations would work in practice. Their approach has been criticized as having some deficiencies [16].

Brooke has also dealt with log-normal size distributions [17]. His equation for the weight undissolved (W_t) is given below:

$$W_t = r[\exp 3(\mu+3\sigma^2/2)] \, (1-F[\ln\tau-(\mu+3\sigma^2)/\sigma])$$
$$- \; 3r\tau[\exp 2(\mu+\sigma^2/2) \, [\, (1-F[\ln\tau-(\mu+2\sigma^2)/\sigma])$$
$$+ \; 3r\tau^2 \, [\exp (\mu+\sigma^2/2] \, (1-F[\ln\tau-(\mu+\sigma^2)/\sigma])$$
$$- \; r\tau^3 \, (1-F[\ln\tau-\mu\sigma]) \tag{8}$$

where

r = $\pi\rho N/6$
τ = Hixson–Crowell particle size at time t
   ($t = 2DC_s t/\rho$)
μ = log-normal mean size

σ = log-normal standard deviation
$F[\ ]$ = standard normal distribution variable

Even though this equation is complex, it is claimed that no integrations are required, and the expression can be evaluated with a calculator and standard mathematical tables. Brooke points out potential problems with using truncated distributions versus the exact log-normal distribution. One must know whether a truncated distribution or the exact distribution better represents the actual drug powder employed. If one or the other is used incorrectly, the effect can be to omit or add a significant mass of large particles, which could give poor fit between the dissolution model and experimental data.

Veng-Pedersen and Brown have represented a series of papers attempting to deal with size distribution and nonspherical particle shape problems in a comprehensive fashion [18–23]. They have proposed an approach requiring dissolution data normalization and time scaling that deals with the aforementioned size distribution problems in a unified fashion. Figure 1 shows general normalized dissolution profiles of powders, initially log-normally distributed, dissolving according to the three aforementioned particle models [23]. By normalizing and scaling the time axis c, where c is the fraction of time required for complete dissolution, the effect of size distribution on each model can be easily observed and compared. The Higuchi–Hiestand model ($m = 3/2$) appears most sensitive to size distribution effects and the Hixson–Crowell model ($m = 3$) the least sensitive. Such a plot also shows that initial dissolution data appears quite linear for each model, but the initial slopes deviate markedly from the theoretical slope of –1 for an ideal monodisperse system (dashed line). Thus, good linearity in such plots is not sufficient to demonstrate the powder is monodispersed nor that size distribution effects are negligible. The approach of Veng-Pedersen and Brown is supported by only limited experimental dissolution data (i.e., on tolbutamide [20] and glyburide [21] powders). There needs to be further experimental evaluation of this approach to determine its robustness and ease of use.

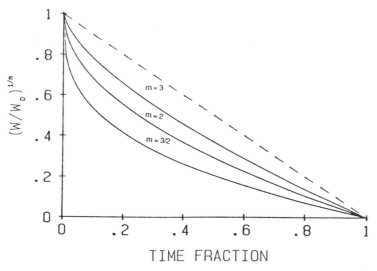

Fig. 1 Normalized dissolution profiles of powders initially log-normal: $m = 3/2$, Higuchi–Hiestand model; $m = 2$, Niebergall–Goyan model; $m = 3$, Hixson–Crowell model; dashed line represents a monodisperse powder.

Matsuura [24,25] has recently evaluated the dissolution behavior of monodisperse and polydisperse powders of alkylparabens. He has shown good correlation of expressions derived on the basis of the cube-root relationship [see Eq. (2)] with multiparticulate dissolution data. He was also able to show that powdered mixtures prepared from two different particle sizes followed predicted dissolution profiles.

2. Surface-Controlled Dissolution

Even though diffusion-controlled dissolution processes appear to predominate, there are instances for which the surface processes of molecular or ionic solvation and detachment appear to be rate-controlling. Wurster and Taylor, in their review [26], refer to examples for which diffusion-controlled dissolution does not completely account for the observed behavior. They have suggested that surface control may be operative in the dissolution of prednisolone polymorphs [27] as well as conditions under which adsorbed surfactants alter the surface properties of the dissolving solid [28]. Wurster and Kildsig [29] also have attributed the dissolution behavior of *m*-aminobenzoic acid to surface control when high concentrations of caffeine as a complexing agent have been employed.

Piccolo and Tawashi [30–32] studied the effect of adsorbed dyes on particle dissolution and demonstrated a significant saturable dissolution inhibition phenomenon with low levels of several dyes on diethylstilbestrol and other drugs. They demonstrated that both anionic and cationic dyes can produce dissolution inhibition of diethylstilbestrol at concentrations as low as 0.1 mg/ml [32]. Figure 2 shows the relative dissolution rate for diethylstilbestrol with various dyes as a function of concentration. As can be seen, dissolution could be inhibited almost tenfold with the typical maximal inhibition being three- to fivefold. Further support for surface inhibition of drug dissolution by dyes or other formulation additives is lacking.

Work on the dissolution mechanism of cholesterol into complex bile salt–lecithin systems has also been clearly shown to be surface-controlled in some systems [33–36].

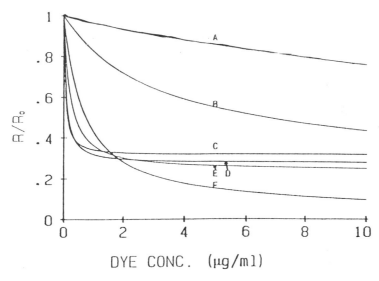

Fig. 2 Relative dissolution rates of diethylstilbestrol as a function of dye concentration. Key: A, D&C Green No. 5; B, FD&C Red No. 3; C, Malachite Green; D, Ext. D&C Blue No. 1; E, FD&C Blue No. 1; F, FD&C Violet No. 1.

This phenomenon has been well studied and represents on of the few well-established surface-controlled dissolution processes. Surface control has often been invoked to account for unusual dissolution behavior, but on more detailed study of several such claims, no clear evidence of surface control has been found [36].

3. *Experimental Methods*

Experimental test systems for measuring the dissolution characteristics of multiparticulate solids or suspensions have been quite varied. A simple method has been reported to obtain the dissolution profiles of powders that correlates well with the particle size of the powders [37]. For nitrofurantoin formulations, dissolution profiles have been obtained for both tablets and suspensions by the *USP* method for tablets [38]. More recently, Mauger and Howard [39,40] have studied the dissolution characteristics of prednisolone acetate suspensions. They have employed the spin-filter system of Shah [41], which is particularly useful for suspensions and disintegrating dosage forms, since the rotating cylindrical filter is nonclogging and, thus, permits efficient intermittent or continuous sampling. Both particle size and suspending agent gave rise to significant differences in dissolution profiles for three commercial ophthalmic suspensions. These same authors have subsequently used this same method to evaluate dissolution profiles for various-sized fractions of prednisolone acetate [40].

B. Factors Affecting Release From Emulsion Systems

The study of drug release from or through emulsion systems has received considerable treatment, both theoretically and experimentally, in the past 40 years. There have been models for drug penetration through viscous emulsion systems, typified by topical formulations, as well as models for less viscous systems, typified by oral emulsions. Interfacial transport mechanisms in such systems have been of interest as models for biological transport into and through lipoidal membranes.

The earliest emulsion release or permeation models in the pharmaceutical literature were proposed by Higuchi and Higuchi [42]. They drew an analogy between the dielectric behavior of heterogeneous systems and their permeability coefficients (P). They found that the Clausius–Mosotti [see Eq. (9)] and Bruggeman [see Eq. (10)] equations shown below correlate well with release data for a water–oil (W/O) emulsion:

$$\frac{(P_\varepsilon - P_1)}{(P_\varepsilon + 2P_1)} = \frac{(P_2 - P_1)}{(P_2 + 2P_1)}\Phi_2 \tag{9}$$

$$\left(\frac{P_1}{P_\varepsilon}\right)^{1/3} = (1 - \Phi_2)\left(\frac{P_1 - P_2}{P_\varepsilon - P_2}\right) \tag{10}$$

where
  P_ε = effective permeability coefficient
  P_1 = external phase permeability coefficient
  P_2 = internal phase permeability coefficient
  Φ_2 = internal phase volume fraction

In this equation, the permeability coefficients (P_i) are defined as D_iK_i (D = diffusion coefficient; K = partition coefficient). Equation (9) can be rearranged to explicitly give P_ε as a function of P_1, P_2, and Φ_2:

$$P_\varepsilon = \frac{P_1[P_2(1 + \Phi_2) + 2P_1(1 - \Phi_2)]}{P_2(1 - \Phi_2) + P_1(2 + \Phi_2)} \tag{11}$$

A similar simplification of Eq. (10) is not possible. Both expressions [Eqs. (9) and (10)] are reasonable representations for the permeation characteristic of such disperse systems [42]. For the amount released (Q) as a function of time, the assumption of a quasi-infinite reservoir gave adequate fit to the data up to at least 30% released. Such an assumption leads to a concentration profile [$C(x,t)$] for this system described by the following error function (erf) expression:

$$C(x,t) = C_\varepsilon \text{erf} \frac{x}{2\sqrt{D_\varepsilon t}} \tag{12}$$

where

C_ε = effective initial concentration
x = distance
D_ε = effective diffusion coefficient

Applying Fick's first law of diffusion ($J = -D\partial C/\partial x$) to Eq. (12) and integrating over time gives

$$Q = 2C_\varepsilon A\sqrt{\frac{D_\varepsilon t}{\pi}} \tag{13}$$

where

Q = amount released as a function of time
A = release area

Such equations ignore specific details, such as emulsion droplet size or distribution, the possible presence of oil–water interfacial barriers, and the effect of micelles in the external phase. Models have been derived for uptake of drug into the internal phase of an O/W emulsion, assuming that external (aqueous) phase diffusion of micellar-solubilized drug is rate-limiting [42] as shown in the following:

$$\ln\left(\frac{\alpha}{\alpha - \beta C_{do}}\right) = \frac{\beta A}{\Phi_2}\left(\frac{D_d}{KC_{sa}} + D_{dm}\right)t \tag{14}$$

where

K = micellar partition coefficient
C_{do} = drug concentration in oil
C_{sa} = surfactant concentration
D_d = free drug diffusion coefficient
D_{dm} = drug–micelle diffusion coefficient
α, β = precalculated functions of K, C_{sa}, D, true oil/water partition coefficient, and total initial drug content.

All parameters for Eq. (14) can be independently determined except C_{do}, which is measured during an emulsion transport study. The log-linear behavior with time predicted by Eq. (14) can be compared with experimental data. Modifications to Eq. (14) have also been presented to include the effect of electrical charges on emulsion droplets and micelles [44]:

$$\ln\left(\frac{\delta}{\delta - \varepsilon C_{do}}\right) = \left(\frac{4\pi\varepsilon}{\gamma\Phi_2}\right)t \tag{15}$$

where δ, ε, and γ are complex constants of experimental parameters (C_{sa}, C_{dm}, K, electrical surface potential, and so forth), which can be independently determined. Again, the functional relationship for C_{do} is log-linear with time which can be easily compared with experimental results.

More complex models have been proposed that include droplet size distribution and interfacial barrier contributions [44]. The rate of change of drug concentration (dC_{wi}/dt) caused by an emulsion droplet of particular size (a_i) is:

$$-\frac{dC_{wi}}{dt} = \frac{3D_a P(C_{wi} - C_a)}{Ka_i(D_a + a_i P)} \tag{16}$$

where

$\quad D_a$ = aqueous diffusion coefficient
$\quad P$ = permeability coefficient of an interface
$\quad C_a$ = aqueous drug concentration
$\quad C_{wi}$ = aqueous drug concentration at the surface of droplet of size a_i
$\quad K$ = oil–water partition coefficient

For an emulsion of known size distribution, a series of equations based on Eq. (16) can be written for each droplet size, and the results summed over all the droplets to yield release profiles from such emulsions. It is apparent that emulsifier effects arise in the interfacial permeability term P, which will vary with emulsifier type and concentration.

IV.   IN VITRO–IN VIVO CORRELATIONS

For over 30 years, studies have been conducted to correlate in vitro dissolution test results with in vivo parameters. Since Levy and Procknal [45] showed a linear correlation between the percentage of aspirin absorbed in vivo with the percentage dissolved in vitro for tablet dosage forms, improvements in methods and correlations with in vivo data have been sought. Excellent reviews [46–48] were written about in vitro–in vivo correlations.

Cabana [48], in his 1973 review, revealed that 80–90% of documented nonbioequivalence resulted from poor dissolution. By the late 1960s and early 1970s, assay technology had also developed to the point that plasma concentrations of most drugs could be adequately detected. Consequently, studies were conducted on many generic and standard products to determine the extent of nonbioequivalence.

The results of these studies indicated that a significant number of generic and standard products were nonbioequivalent. Therefore, the Food and Drug Administration (FDA) in 1977, initiated regulations that required manufacturers of generic products to show bioequivalence before receiving approval to market a new generic product. The bioavailability regulations published by FDA [49] specified the types of studies that could satisfy a bioequivalence requirement for a particular product. In addition to well-controlled human studies, FDA stipulated that an in vitro test that had been correlated with human in vivo bioavailability data could be used to satisfy a bioequivalence requirement.

Studies involving in vitro–in vivo correlations often included suspensions as a reference standard for comparison with tablets and capsules. For example, Bates et al. [50] successfully correlated the percentage of salicylamide dissolved in 15 and 20 min with the amount of drug excreted in 1 h. In a similar study, a suspension of micronized oxazepam was compared with four tablet formulations [51]. Peak serum concentration was used as a measure of absorption rate, which correlated linearly with the percentage dissolved in vitro in 5 min using a 3-L–flask apparatus.

Although suspensions are often assumed to dissolve rapidly, a potential exists for bioavailability differences. The following example illustrates that correlations and, hence, dissolution standards are necessary for oral suspensions to ensure bioequivalence. Colaizzi and co-workers [52,53] established a suitable dissolution test method for correlation of in vivo data of seven different commercially available oral trisulfapyrimidine suspensions. The in vivo measurement of peak serum levels of sulfadiazine was linearly correlated with the percentage of drug dissolved in 30 min. The FDA's paddle method was used at 37°C and 25 rpm in 900 ml of pH 3.4 aqueous medium. The range of percentage dissolved was 20–100%, with an observed range of peak serum levels of 6–12 mg/ml for the commercial suspensions. An equally good correlation was obtained for sulfamerazine, but not for sulfamethazine. Their results demonstrate the potentially large differences that can exist for suspension dosage forms containing sulfonamide drugs.

V. PHYSIOLOGICAL FACTORS AFFECTING BIOAVAILABILITY

Disperse dosage forms are usually administered parenterally, orally, and topically. Figure 3 shows a simple cross-sectional view of several of the administration sites of disperse systems. The absorption barrier for each route of administration is the layer that is most resistant to drug penetration. Frequently, this barrier is the layer that is in contact with the external environment (skin, cornea, gastrointestinal epithelium). For parenteral delivery, the rate-limiting barrier can be muscle or adipose tissue, or it may be the capillary endothelium. Although it is important to identify the rate-limiting barrier to absorption, other physiological characteristics, such as pH, blood flow patterns, and clearance properties, can also have significant effects on bioavailability. The formulator's knowledge of both the physicochemical properties of the dosage form, along with the physiological properties of the administration site can have a significant effect on the development of an optimally bioavailable disperse dosage form.

A. Skin

For all but very hydrophobic compounds transferring across the skin, the rate-limiting barrier is the stratum corneum—a layer that consists of several layers of keratinized, metabolically inactive cells. The cells are flattened and hexagonal and represent the remains of the living epidermis, which is the layer directly below the stratum corneum. The stratum corneum is 8- to 16-layers thick and varies with body region, but over most of the body the thickness is about 10 μm. The hydration level of the stratum corneum is about 10–25%. Several possible pathways for percutaneous absorption exist across the stratum corneum. One, the transcellular route, represents drug movement through the

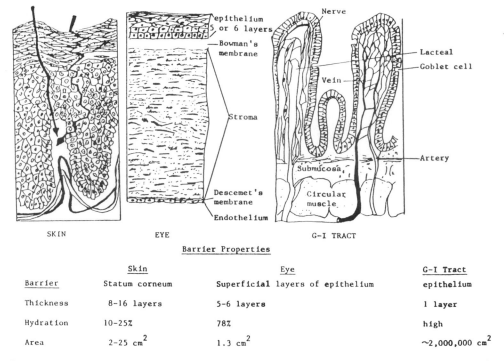

Barrier Properties

	Skin	Eye	G-I Tract
Barrier	Statum corneum	Superficial layers of epithelium	epithelium
Thickness	8-16 layers	5-6 layers	1 layer
Hydration	10-25%	78%	high
Area	2-25 cm^2	1.3 cm^2	~2,000,000 cm^2

Fig. 3 A comparison of the superficial layers of the skin, eye, and gastrointestinal tract pertinent to drug absorption.

cells themselves. Most of this movement takes place through the hydrated keratin layers and is frequently referred to as the "polar" route. Another, the intercellular route, follows a pathway between the cells where compounds interact with a liquid crystalline phase of lipids. Hydrophobic drugs dissolve in this lipid phase and diffuse across the stratum corneum by passing through the spaces between the cells. The epidermis and the dermis are situated just below the stratum corneum. They frequently provide much less resistance to drug penetration than does the stratum corneum, yet they can provide a formidable barrier to hydrophobic compounds for which the solubilities in the lipoidal stratum corneum are much greater than their affinities for the more aqueous environment of the epidermal and dermal tissues. The third pathway, the transfollicular route, follows along the hair shafts to reach the systemic circulation through the capillaries and venules that supply the hair follicle.

B. Eye

The epithelium of the cornea provides the greatest diffusional resistance for most ophthalmic drugs. It contains five to six layers and is about 50 μm thick. Bowman's membrane, the stroma, Descemet's membrane, and the endothelium are adjacent layers, but only with lipophilic drugs do these layers provide significant resistance to penetration. The hydration level of the cornea is 78%, which is significantly greater than that of the skin. The surface area of the corneal absorption site is about 1.2 cm^2, compared with typical application site areas for the skin that are 2–25 cm^2. Although the transcorneal route is considered to be the primary pathway to the internal eye tissues, scleral permeation as well as access through conjunctival blood vessels are possible alternatives. Drug solutions instilled into the cul-de-sac of the eye also have the potential for systemic bioavailability owing to the clearance of the solution by the lacrimal duct. Depending on the volume instilled, the cleared volume may contain sufficient drug for absorption by the nasal membranes, resulting in systemic drug effects.

C. Gastrointestinal Tract

1. *Stomach*

The gastric mucosa is composed of a simple columnar epithelium, with numerous interspersed specialized cells (parietal, chief) and glands that contain cells that secrete substances such as mucus, gastrin, intrinsic factor, and pepsin. Drug permeability through this tissue is generally limited to nonionized forms of drug compounds. Because of the relatively low pH value of the stomach [typical pH range is 1 (fasted) to 5 (fed)], there is a preferential absorption of weakly acidic compounds from the stomach region. Because of the relatively short residence time and low surface area in comparison with the small intestine, the fraction of total drug absorbed from the stomach is often quite small.

2. *Small Intestine*

The epithelial cells of the small intestine are columnar, 1 μm in length, and have a rapid renewal rate of 2 days. The total length is approximately 300 cm, and the total surface area is about 2 million cm^2, owing to the many folds (villi) on the mucosal surface. Approximately one-half of the total absorptive surface area of the small intestine exists within the first 25% of its length (duodenum and proximal jejunum). The mucosal cells in the small intestine are capable of absorbing both nonionized and ionized compounds. The absorption of nonionized compounds generally occurs by passive diffusion across the lipoidal cell membrane, whereas the absorption of ionized compounds frequently requires the presence of a specific carrier on the cell surface, or a specialized pathway accessible to small electrolytes. The pH within the small intestine varies along its length. Generally, the pH ranges within each segment are as follows: duodenum, 4.5–6.5; jejunum, 5–7; and ileum, 6.5–7.5. The pH changes are mediated by the secretions present within the small intestine, some of which contain bicarbonate, bile salts, water, and many digestive enzymes. Because of the rather harsh environment within the intestinal lumen, drug instability within the small intestine can be a limitation to good oral bioavailability.

Gastrointestinal absorption is not complete until drug reaches the systemic circulation. Therefore, the drug must cross the hepatoportal system intact and enter the inferior vena cava before being systemically bioavailable. Consequently, permeability across the epithelial cell layer, although rate-determining, is only the initial step in the process constituting gastrointestinal absorption.

3. *Large Intestine (Colon)*

The large intestine is approximately one-half the length of the small intestine (150 cm) and possesses a significantly reduced surface area owing to the lack of villi on the mucosal surface. The pH of the colon is generally in the range of 5.5–7, and the lumenal fluids contain significantly lower concentrations of degradative enzymes than are present in the small intestine. The colon does possess a substantial bacterial population, however, which can be responsible for the metabolism of drug agents before their absorption. Significant water is reabsorbed within the colon, and some charged species are also capable of being absorbed across the epithelia.

4. *Rectum*

The distal 12 cm of the large intestine is classified as the rectum. The epithelium in this region is considerably thicker than that of the rest of the large intestine, and the rectal tissue is more highly vascularized. Approximately one-third of the rectal blood supply drains into the rectal plexus, which then drains into the systemic venous system. This blood flow pattern enables some fraction of drug compound absorbed from the rectum to bypass the hepatoportal system and to enter the systemic circulation without undergoing hepatic metabolism.

D. Oral Cavity

The mucosae within the oral cavity are characterized by regions of both keratinized and nonkeratinized stratified squamous epithelium. The regions of keratinization include most of the hard palate, the gingiva, and the dorsum of the tongue. The tissues of the soft palate, the floor of the mouth, the lips, and the cheek (buccal region), all are non-keratinized. As with other mucosal tissues, the oral mucosa is most permeable to lipophilic, nonionized compounds. The total surface area of the oral mucosa is in the range of 200 cm^2, and the mucosa ranges in thickness from 100 to 600 μm. The keratinized tissues appear to be a barrier to some, but not all, permeants [54]. Similar to the skin, the intercellular space also represents a significant permeability barrier. Although the blood supply to and from the oral mucosa allows drugs absorbed from this site to bypass hepatic metabolism, the tissues themselves are quite metabolically active, and a significant fraction of applied drug may be lost to local metabolism before absorption. In general, the permeability of the buccal mucosa appears to be intermediate between that of the cornea and the skin.

E. Vaginal Mucosa

Although drug delivery to the vaginal mucosa is frequently limited to treatment of local infection or inflammation, systemic absorption from this site is also a possibility. The vaginal mucosa is an approximately 150- to 200-μm–thick layer of stratified squamous epithelium, which overlies a connective tissue layer (lamina propria), and layers of circular and longitudinal muscles fibers. The mucosa does not contain glands, rather the surface is bathed by cervical secretions. These secretions are generally acidic (pH 4–6), as a result of the metabolism of glycogen, present in high concentration in the epithelial cells, to lactic acid. This metabolic transformation is performed by the normal vaginal bacterial flora; therefore, it is important that vaginal dosage forms neither affect the bacterial populations present, nor significantly alter the pH at the mucosal surface.

VI. METHODS OF ASSESSING DRUG BIOAVAILABILITY

Bioavailability can be simply defined as the measurement of the rate and extent of drug absorption. Both the rate and extent of absorption are assessed separately from profiles of the concentration of drug in systemic fluids (usually blood or plasma) over time following administration of the drug at a particular site of absorption.

Figure 4 illustrates a typical plasma concentration–time curve following drug absorption in which the maximum drug concentration (C_{max}) is reached at t_{max}. Plots of drug concentration–time curves, such as shown in Fig. 4, can be characterized well by the following equation:

$$C = \frac{FDk_a}{V(k_a - K)} (e^{-k_a t} - e^{-Kt})$$ (17)

where

$\quad C$ = plasma concentration
$\quad F$ = fraction of the dose D absorbed
$\quad k_a$ = first-order absorption rate constant
$\quad K$ = first-order elimination rate constant
$\quad V$ = the apparent volume of distribution

Although Eq. (17) theoretically represents a drug that follows one-compartment model pharmacokinetics, it is often correct empirically to represent the plasma profile of a drug that may also follow multicompartmental pharmacokinetics.

Equation (17) accurately predicts changes in the plasma concentration of a drug whenever the extent of absorption, or the rate of absorption, is influenced by the release from the dosage form. The extent of absorption is measured by F, whereas the rate of absorption is proportional to k_a. Figures 5 and 6 show the expected changes in the drug concentration–time profile if either k_a or F change.

These two parameters are theoretically ideal for measuring the rate and extent of absorption, but difficulties arise that discourage their use in bioavailability assessment. F is determined by Eq. (18), in which AUC represents the area under the plasma con-

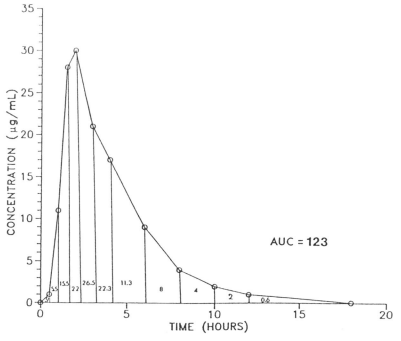

Fig. 4 A summation of trapezoids to yield the area under the concentration–time curve (AUC).

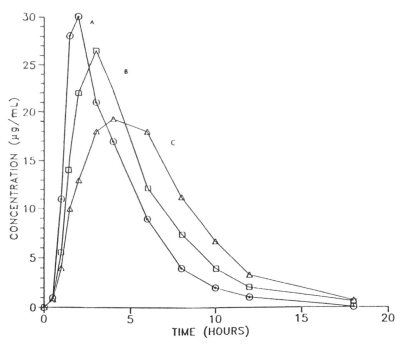

Fig. 5 A comparison of concentration–time curves in which k_a decreases from curves A to C. All other pharmacokinetic parameters are constant.

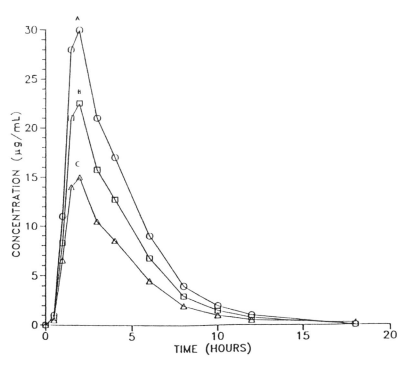

Fig. 6 A comparison of concentration–time curves in which F decreases from 1, to 0.75, to 0.5 for curves A to C. All other pharmacokinetic parameters are constant.

centration–time curve, and the subscripts o and iv represent the oral and intravenous routes of administration:

$$F = \frac{AUC_o}{AUC_{iv}} \tag{18}$$

Although AUC can be easily determined by summing trapezoids (Fig. 4), many drugs cannot be administered by rapid intravenous injection without submitting the subject to the risk of toxicity from a high dose of drug. The parameter k_a can be determined by the method of residuals, or by established deconvolution methods [55]. Either way, temporal variations in plasma level or the need to accurately assess F before determining k_a results in unreliable estimates of k_a [56–58].

Consequently, parameters with less error associated with their estimation have replaced F and k_a. C_{max}, t_{max}, and AUC_o, although less than ideal theoretically, have proved adequate for measuring bioavailability. Equations (19)–(21) show the relationship between k_a or F and C_{max}, t_{max}, and AUC_o.

$$C_{max} = \frac{FDk_a}{V(k_a - K)} \left(e^{-k_a t_{max}} - e^{-K t_{max}} \right) \tag{19}$$

$$t_{max} = \frac{\ln(k_a/K)}{V(k_a - K)} \tag{20}$$

$$AUC_o = \frac{FD}{VK} \tag{21}$$

In Eq. (19), C_{max} is a function of both k_a and F, such that changes in either rate or extent of absorption also result in changes of C_{max}. However, as long as the same subjects are crossed over in a comparative study and K remains constant, t_{max} changes only with changes in k_a.

Observed (C_{max}, t_{max}, and AUC) and pharmacokinetic parameters (k_a and F) can be used to measure the bioavailability of oral products. However, observed parameters are commonly used because of the ease with which they can be measured and their independence from modelistic assumptions. A statistical analysis is applied to the rate or extent, or both, measurements to determine if a difference exists between two generic products. Statistical differences in C_{max} and t_{max} indicate a difference in the rate of absorption for two or more products, whereas, a difference in the extent of absorption occurs if C_{max} and AUC_o are statistically different. Standard deviations associated with the measurement of t_{max} are often relatively high; therefore, t_{max} associated with two different products may not show statistically significant differences with this parameter. This occurs because t_{max} is a discrete measurement, not necessarily associated with the theoretically correct value represented by Eq. (20). Values of t_{max} for individual subjects will be associated with the sampling times, which may not be chosen over small enough intervals, resulting in large differences in the observed t_{max} values for individuals.

Whereas F measures the absolute bioavailability of a drug product, a ratio of the AUC for the test (or generic) product to a reference standard of the same drug is a measure of the relative bioavailability. This relationship is shown in Eq. (22):

$$\text{Relative bioavailability} = \frac{AUC_{test}}{AUC_{stnd}} \tag{22}$$

It is important to distinguish between absolute and relative bioavailability. For example, a generic and standard product may yield an average AUC of 55 and 65% of the AUC of an equally high intravenous dose and, therefore, show poor absolute bioavailability. However, when the relative bioavailability is determined (55/65 = 0.85), the generic product may be acceptable, provided the parameter differences for rate and extent are statistically equivalent. Under these conditions, the products would be considered bioequivalent and, therefore, therapeutically equivalent. Consequently, oral products may be acceptable for clinical use, yet possess poor absolute bioavailability because of gastrointestinal or first-pass effects, which are beyond the control of the formulator. On the other hand, if the reduction in bioavailability is due to formulation variables, the formulator should consider correcting the problem. A reduction in bioavailability is almost always accompanied by variable absorption between or within the patient population, often resulting in variable therapeutic efficacy as well.

The FDA considers drug products to be therapeutically equivalent if they are bioequivalent. Bioequivalence applies to drug products that contain the same therapeutic moiety. The products should also be identical in strength, dosage form, and route of administration. Before approval by the FDA, many generic drug products are tested for bioequivalence to an appropriate standard. However, not all generic drug products must undergo a comparison of blood or plasma levels in a properly conducted crossover study. Some drugs do not present a known or potential bioequivalence problem. Each year the *USP* publishes a list of drugs, identifying currently marketed drug products, relative to their bioequivalence status. The publication, *USP DI Volume III: Approved Drug Products and Legal Requirements* is available from the United States Pharmacopeial Convention.

A. Dermatological Bioavailability

It is generally accepted that the transdermal permeation of drugs from various topical delivery systems is governed by one of two factors: (a) penetration rate of drug through the skin and, in particular, penetration through the stratum corneum which, in most cases, is the rate-limiting barrier; (b) release of drug from the delivery system (i.e., solution, ointment, gel, polymer, or device).

The skin is a living dynamic organ that has permeability characteristics that depend upon various factors that can be summarized as

1. Thickness of stratum corneum
2. Integrity of stratum corneum
3. Hydration level of skin
4. Partition coefficient
5. Application of permeability enhancers

Factors 1 and 2 are manifested in age, sex, race, and body region effects on skin permeability. Factors 3 and 5 are manifested when formulation or treatment conditions are altered that affect the skin's overall permeability characteristics. Factor 4 is manifested in the lipophilicity of the drug or the relative solubilities of drug in stratum corneum versus donor vehicle.

Since skin is a heterogeneous, laminated substance, its permeability characteristics can be viewed as a series of barriers. The total diffusional flux through these barriers may be represented by:

$$J = \left[\frac{1}{\sum_{i=1}^{n} 1/P_i} \right] \Delta C \tag{23}$$

where

J = membrane flux
P_i = permeability coefficient of a particular barrier
ΔC = concentration difference

Total mass flow can be obtained from Eq. (23) by multiplying by the area A of coverage. Each of the barriers of the skin may, in turn, be complex barriers containing parallel diffusional paths. The flux across such barriers is given by

$$J = \left(\sum_{i=1}^{n} f_i P_i \right) \Delta C \tag{24}$$

where

f_i = fractional area of a particular pathway

Even though Eqs. (23) and (24) present a complicated diffusional picture for skin permeation, they can be reduced to simpler models involving only two or three barriers in series [see Eq. (23), $n = 2$–3] or two parallel routes [see Eq. (24), $n = 2$] for a particular barrier. These models can be further simplified by assuming that most of the diffusional resistance, R, resides in the stratum corneum. When such is the case, the series-barrier model reduces to a one-barrier system. The stratum corneum may also be considered to have two possible parallel pathways, one being lipophilic and one being hydrophilic.

More complex models have been proposed for predicting intrinsic skin permeability. These have been reviewed by various authors [59–62]. All such models incorporate varying contributions of polar versus nonpolar permeation routes, partition coefficient dependency, interfacial resistance factors, and aqueous solubility, combined with the series- and parallel-barrier concepts.

The permeability characteristics of a barrier or parallel path is, thus, described by its permeability coefficient P or its diffusional resistance R, which is the reciprocal of the permeability coefficient. These are represented by

$$P = \frac{DK}{h} \tag{25}$$

and

$$R = \frac{h}{DK} \tag{26}$$

where

D = diffusion coefficient
K = partition coefficient
h = barrier or pathway thickness

From Eqs. (25) and (26) it is apparent that differences in drug permeation rates arise from differences in diffusion coefficient, partition coefficient into the skin, and variations in skin thickness between individuals and within the same individual from site-to-site. Since the stratum corneum is the usual rate-limiting barrier for drug permeation through skin, these physicochemical parameters can be more closely identified with this layer than other anatomical layers of the skin.

In general, skin permeability rises proportionately with the oil/water partition coefficient K, except at extremes in the partition coefficient [63]. At intermediate partition coefficients, the proportionality arises from increases in affinity or solubility of the drug in stratum corneum versus a reference solvent (usually water). At low partition coefficients, permeation is often higher than expected from the partition coefficient because hydrophilic pathways through the stratum corenum become the preponderant route of transport. At high partition coefficients, the permeation rate is often lower than expected because there is a change in the rate-limiting barrier from the stratum corneum to other more hydrophilic layers of the skin. These generalities are based on the observation that it is primarily the nonionized form of a compound that diffuses across the stratum corneum. There have been several reports of the permeation of ionic species across excised skin samples, however. Kushla and Zatz [64] studied the penetration of lidocaine across excised human and mouse skin. After thoroughly characterizing the degree of ionization in the propylene glycol/water suspensions at various pHs, it was found that both the ionized and nonionized forms of lidocaine diffuse across human and mouse skin. Interestingly, the permeation of the ionized form was far greater in the mouse skin than in that of humans. Alternatively, the observed lower permeation rate can be accounted for by release from the vehicle becoming rate-limiting.

Diffusion coefficients of molecules vary with the cube-root of their molecular volumes in solution. The diffusion coefficients of most drug molecules do not vary greatly because of this low dependency on molecular size or molecular weight. When there are apparent changes in diffusivity with molecular structure, these are often due to specific interactions that occur between the diffusing species and the barrier.

The third factor affecting permeability coefficients is the thickness term h in Eqs. (25) and (26). The thickness of importance is that of the stratum corneum, which varies across the body, between individuals, and with hydration levels. Stratum corneum varies from 10 to 30 μm across various body regions. Hydration caused by occlusion of the skin or in some way altering moisture loss often exhibits variable effects on skin permeability. Even though the thickness of the stratum corneum increases with hydration, its permeability often increases as well. The classic work of Wurster and Kramer [65] showed that hydrated skin demonstrated higher permeability for a series of salicylate esters. The degree of permeability enhancement was proportional to the ester's aqueous solubility and inversely related to its partition coefficient. Similar hydration effects on permeation were observed for methyl ethyl ketone [66], alkylacetates from the vapor phase [67] and sarin [68].

A later study has shown that the rate of permeation of polar compounds, such as methanol and ethanol, are unaffected by hydration, whereas less polar compounds, such as butanol, hexanol, and heptanol, exhibit twofold permeability increases in hydrated hairless mouse skin [69]. A different permeability picture was obtained for these same alcohols when Swiss mouse or rat skins were employed under conditions that caused hydration levels to increase [70,71]. One must be cautious in attempting to generalize how skin hydration affects permeability for molecules of widely differing polarity and size, since diffusion coefficient, partition coefficient, and thickness, each are altered and may have opposing effects on permeation [72-74].

1. *Vehicle Effects*

In addition to the intrinsic permeability of the skin, drug release from the vehicle may be rate-limiting for skin permeation. Higuchi proposed mathematical expressions describing the rate of release of solid drugs suspended in ointment bases [75,76]. One expression he proposed is given below:

$$Q = \sqrt{C_s(2A - C_s)Dt} \tag{27}$$

where

Q = amount released per unit area
C_s = solubility in external phase of vehicle
A = total drug concentration (suspended and dissolved) in vehicle
D = effective diffusion coefficient

If the drug is completely dissolved in the vehicle, models have been presented that assume fickian diffusion from the base [77]. Equation (28) is based on a Fourier series solution to Fick's law:

$$Q = hC_0\left[1 - \frac{8}{\pi^2}\sum_{m=0}^{\infty}\frac{1}{(2m+1)^2}\exp\left(\frac{-(2m+1)^2\pi^2 Dt}{4h^2}\right)\right] \tag{28}$$

where

Q = amount of drug released per unit area
h = thickness of vehicle
C_0 = initial drug concentration in vehicle
D = effective diffusion coefficient
m = Fourier series index
t = time

Such an expression is somewhat unwieldy for simulation of release profiles. A simplified expression [Eq. (29)] has been proposed that approximates Eq. (28) up to a 30% release [77]:

$$Q = 2C_0\left[\frac{Dt}{\pi}\right]^{1/2} \tag{29}$$

The foregoing expression was obtained by considering the layer of vehicle as being of infinite thickness and using the appropriate error function solution. Even though the author predicted accuracy only up to 30% release, it can be shown that Eq. (29) is reasonably accurate up to about 60% release.

Extensions of these models have been recently reviewed [78]. Equations (27) and (28) can be modified to include diffusional boundary layers or the diffusional contribution of the skin in series with the vehicle. Comparisons of diffusion profiles can then be made for solution systems versus suspension systems. The general approach can be applied to any topical delivery formulation, including those systems that include rate-controlling polymeric membranes.

2. Experimental Techniques

Whenever drug penetration across the skin is dependent on the release rate of drug from the vehicle, optimal penetration can be attained by maximizing this rate. Besides the basic need for understanding those formulation variables that can optimize release, a product should be selected that has the best chance of success in the clinic. For these reasons it is useful to study in vitro drug release rates to predict and, therefore, optimize in vivo efficacy.

In vitro release can be studied by placing a semisolid preparation in one half of a diffusion cell and measuring the appearance of drug in the other half. The receiving half of the cell usually contains a well-stirred liquid that provides a large reservoir for the released drug and is mechanically separated from the semisolid by a semipermeable membrane, usually cellophane. This simple in vitro apparatus has been used to study the effect of formulation variables on the release of drug, with subsequent correlation to the vasoconstrictor response of steroids [79,80].

Ostrenga et al. [79] used an in vitro apparatus similar to the one described earlier and found a rank order correlation between release, percentage drug solubilized, and vasoconstrictor response for a series of creams containing 0.05% (w/w) fluocinonide. A similar correlation existed between percentage drug solubilized and the vasoconstrictor response for five different ointment formulations.

Another in vitro apparatus, which has been used routinely for correlation purposes, is the "skin cell" [81], which consists of excised skin mounted between two halves of a diffusion cell. Semisolid preparations containing drug can be placed on the epidermal side of the excised skin. A saline reservoir is placed on the receiving, or dermal, side of the skin into which drug penetrates with time. Excised skin is difficult to maintain in viable condition; therefore, more variability occurs with the skin cell method than with the in vitro release apparatus just described. However, results associated with the skin cell method correlate more closely with results obtained clinically [80,82].

Ostrenga et al. [82] used the skin cell method to correlate penetration across normal human abdominal skin for a series of topical gels containing fluocinolone acetonide or fluocinonide. The composition of the gels varied by the inclusion of 0–100% propylene glycol. Figure 7 shows the relationship between the amount penetrated and percentage glycol for the two steroids. The maximum penetration rate for each drug corresponds to the minimum glycol concentration necessary to solubilize each steroid. Under these conditions the thermodynamic activity of the drug in the vehicle is at its maximum. The results in Fig. 8, relating the vasoconstrictor response at 24 h for both drugs to percentage composition of propylene glycol, correspond very well with the in vitro results shown in Fig. 7. The investigators [82] concluded that the similarity in results in Figs. 7 and 8 indicated that the rate-determining step for absorption was in the skin. They also concluded that efficacy was optimal when the drug was near saturation in the vehicle. This occurred at a propylene glycol concentration of 30%, which just solubilized the 0.025% fluocinolone acetonide. At 5% glycol most of the drug was in suspension; however, penetration and vasoconstrictor response was equally high. The similarity in results at 5 and 30% glycol was attributed to a very high partition coefficient of the 5% glycol gel offsetting the decrease in concentration of the drug in solution.

B. Ophthalmic Bioavailability

Because of the difficulties in directly measuring drug concentrations in the aqueous humor, C_{max} and particularly t_{max} are not reliable parameters to assess ophthalmic bio-

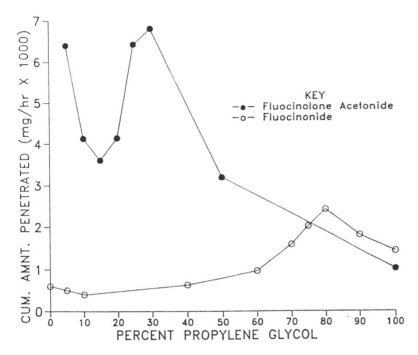

Fig. 7 Cumulative amount of steroid penetrating human abdominal skin as a function of propylene glycol content.

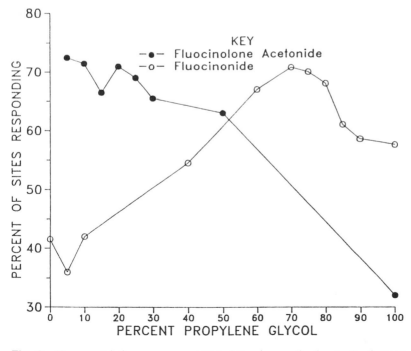

Fig. 8 Vasoconstriction response at 24 h following application to the forearm of subjects ($n =$ 40) as a function of propylene glycol content.

availability differences. Also, animal data must be used to determine bioequivalence; however, other problems in interpreting results further complicate the issue. In particular, the onset of activity, as measured by the rate of absorption, is of much less importance than an overall improvement in therapy, which is primarily dependent on the extent, and not the rate, of absorption. Therefore, AUC should be the primary determinant of ophthalmic bioequivalence, since AUC is less affected by aqueous humor concentration-time curves, which are not necessarily smooth throughout. The AUC comparisons should provide a reasonably accurate assessment of ophthalmic bioequivalence.

VII. IN VIVO BIOAVAILABILITY ASSESSMENT

A. Parenteral Bioavailability

Administration by the "alternative" parenteral routes: subcutaneous, intrademal, intramuscular, intra-articular, and intraperitoneal, frequently cannot match the bioavailability of an equivalent intravenous (IV) dose. Toxicity following IV administration or the desire for an extended-release parenteral dosage form are two common reasons for the development of such dosage forms. The bioavailability of parenteral dosage forms is covered in detail elsewhere in these volumes, yet a brief review of the bioavailability characteristics of disperse parenteral dosage forms also seems appropriate in this chapter.

1. *Suspensions*

Suspensions for subcutaneous or intramuscular administration can use either water, a limited number of nontoxic oils (sesame, peanut, or olive), or an equally limited number of organic solvents (propylene glycol, polyethylene glycol, or glycerin) as suitable vehicles. Typically, if an aqueous vehicle is used, the water and dissolved drug rapidly diffuse into the body tissues, leaving a depot of undissolved drug at the injection site. The dissolution characteristics of the drug at the injection site then control the rate at which drug is absorbed into the systemic circulation and its resulting bioavailability.

The various types of insulin available for subcutaneous administration are excellent examples of the usefulness of parenteral suspension dosage forms. Insulin can be administered subcutaneously in an aqueous solution, yet its absorption is so rapid that it requires dosing every 4–6 h. Various insulin complexes (zinc or protamine zinc insulin) are delivered as suspensions that have hypoglycemic activities for periods of 12–36 h. The extent of duration is determined by the crystal structure of the complex along with the size of the crystalline or amorphous particles. Intramuscular administration of aqueous drug suspensions can also provide sustained blood levels for several days. Procaine penicillin G, an insoluble salt of penicillin G, is administered intramuscularly as a suspension and frequently results in measurable blood levels of penicillin G for longer than 48 h. Penicillin G potassium solution, in comparison, is absorbed rapidly following intramuscular administration, yet is frequently administered twice daily, rather than once daily, as for the suspension dosage form.

Nonaqueous suspensions are also frequently used for parenteral therapy, especially for drugs that have limited aqueous solubility or stability. Su et al. [83] reported on the development of a nonaqueous suspension of cefazolin sodium, a drug that has insufficient stability in water for formulation in an aqueous vehicle. An acceptable formulation was developed using ethyl oleate as the vehicle. The performance of the suspension was compared with that of both an intravenous or intramuscular aqueous solution. There were no differences in the plasma AUCs for any of the dosage forms. There were also no differences seen in the C_{max} and t_{max} values between the aqueous solution and the nonaqueous suspension. In this case, a nonaqueous formulation was developed that mimicked the behavior of an aqueous intravenous or intramuscular dose, yet showed improved stability characteristics.

In an attempt to develop an extended-release formulation of another cephalosporin antibiotic, cefotaxime, Guerrini and colleagues studied the absorption of the drug from aqueous solution or arachis oil suspension following either subcutaneous or intramuscular administration to sheep [84]. The C_{max} was somewhat lower and the t_{max} somewhat longer for the oil formulation given intramuscularly, yet the bioavailabilities from the two formulations were statistically equal. From the subcutaneous route, the oil solution gave continuous low and prolonged plasma levels of cefotaxime, whereas the aqueous solution behaved similarly to both the arachis oil and aqueous suspension following intramuscular administration.

Toutain and co-workers reported an interesting phenomenon following the intra-articular administration of methylprednisolone acetate [85]. While investigating the mechanisms of prolonged anti-inflammatory activity in the joints of cows that had been given intra-articular injections of methylprednisolone acetate suspension, these investigators found that methylprednisolone levels were measurable in the synovial fluid for longer than 100 days. Plasma levels of methylprednisolone were not detectable for this period, yet significant adrenal suppression could be detected for at least 6 weeks after dosing. On necropsy, the investigators found that there were many fibrin-encapsulated deposits of methylprednisolone within the joint cavity itself. These results indicate that because of its slow dissolution and poor solubility, much of the administered dose remained as solid drug within the joint itself for prolonged periods. The slow diffusion of methylprednisolone acetate from the fibrin-encapsulated depots resulted in sustained levels of drug in the synovial fluid for extended periods. These results indicate that when determining the bioavailability of a parenteral suspension dosage form, plasma levels may not always reflect the total amount of drug available, owing to an extended slow dissolution of the dosage form or entrapment of drug within an isolated physiological compartment.

2. *Parenteral Emulsions*

In an attempt to prolong the activity of physostigmine while limiting its toxicity, Benita et al. [86] developed an emulsion dosage form that doubled the typical 1- to 2-h activity of an aqueous solution. The oil–water emulsion consisted of a mixture of soybean oil, purified phospholipids, Pluronic F68, water, and mannitol to adjust the osmotic pressure. The bioavailability in rabbits of an intramuscular dose of physostigmine in normal saline was approximately 25%. The bioavailability from the physostigmine emulsion system was approximately 50% as was the bioavailability from a solution of drug and the Pluronic emulsifier. Further investigation into the disposition of physostigmine from a micellar Pluronic vehicle indicated that Pluronic gave high initial plasma concentrations, yet they were not measurable for periods any longer than those from an aqueous intramuscular injection. The emulsion dosage form was the only formulation to give both therapeutically effective and prolonged plasma concentrations of physostigmine.

3. Colloidal Dispersions

Injectable dosage forms of vitamin E (α-tocopherol acetate) have been scrutinized owing to reports of toxicity and questionable efficacy. An intravenous formulation was associated with the deaths of 38 infants (all of whom received extremely high doses) [87]. Intramuscular injectable formulations using oily vehicles (olive oil, glycerol, cottonseed oil, sesame oil, polyethylene glycol), all have had extremely poor bioavailabilities in neonates [87–89]. In comparison, an aqueous colloidal dispersion of α-tocopherol acetate administered intramuscularly resulted in a bioavailability (of α-tocopherol) of approximately 26%. There is evidence that the absorption of α-tocopherol acetate from the injection site is the rate-limiting step in the availability from this dosage form, yet competing hydrolysis to form the parent compound complicates the data analysis, and further studies are necessary to confirm this observation.

4. Liposomes

The disposition of liposomes following parenteral delivery has been studied by several investigators [90,91]. Following intravenous delivery, most of the liposomes are trapped within the tissues of the reticuloendothelial system. Therefore, depending on liposomal size and charge, high concentrations are found within the liver, spleen, lungs, or bone marrow.

Following subcutaneous administration, liposomes are cleared from the injection site by the lymphatics and, frequently, are concentrated in the regional lymph nodes, where they can provide slow and prolonged release of entrapped drug [90]. Technetium ^{99m}Tc-labeled liposomes of various sizes, charge, and lipid composition were injected into the foot pad of rats by Osborne et al. [91]. The distribution of ^{99m}Tc was followed by scanning the animals with a γ-camera. After 5 h, ^{99m}Tc showed localization in the primary and other regional lymph nodes. Sonicated, neutral or positively charged liposomes were taken up by regional lymph nodes more efficiently than negatively charged ones at 5 and 30 h. Larger unsonicated liposomes were not taken up by the lymph nodes and disappeared slowly from the site of injection.

Sasaki et al. compared the absorption of mitomycin (MMC) and its more lipophilic prodrug, nonyloxycarbonyl mitomycin (n-MMC), following intramuscular administration to rats in liposomes and in an oil-water emulsion system [92]. Mitomycin, a relatively polar compound, was rather poorly incorporated into either the liposomes or the emulsion system, whereas the more lipophilic n-MMC showed complete incorporation into the liposomes, as well as good emulsion stability. Following intramuscular administration, MMC was rapidly (< 1 h) removed from the injection site, regardless of dosage form. Both liposomal and emulsified n-MMC were retained at the injection site for significantly longer periods (>> 2 h), as were the lipids in both of the formulations (> 24 h). The n-MMC concentrations were measurable in the regional lymph nodes almost immediately following injection, and remained at reasonably high levels over the next 2 h. Although this study shows little difference between the liposomal and emlusion formulations, further studies need to be conducted to select the optimal dosage form for n-MMC.

The use of liposomally encapsulated insulin for prolonged hypoglycemic response has also been studied. When injected subcutaneously, most of the liposomes remained at the injection site. The duration of hypoglycemia in diabetic dogs was significantly longer with insulin entrapped in large, negatively charged liposomes than with free insulin [93,94]. When 10 units of liposomally entrapped insulin were injected subcutaneously, plasma insulin levels of 18 μU/ml were maintained for up to 7 h, with detectable levels remaining at 24 h. The plasma glucose concentration fell from 16 mM to 3.3 mM and remained low for 9 h. Insulin in neutral liposomes gave a much smaller biological effect. Free insulin gave a high 1-h plasma level of 480 μU/ml, which fell rapidly to control levels in 3 h, with the plasma glucose showing similar rapid decline with a fast return to preinjection levels. Thus, liposomally entrapped insulin seems to have a more prolonged time course of activity, compared with unentrapped insulin when given in large negative liposomes.

B. Gastrointestinal Bioavailability

The bioavailability of an oral dosage form is determined by the extent of absorption of the drug throughout the entire gastrointestinal (GI) tract. Gastric contents move along the GI tract at various rates, depending on the physiological status of the individual and the physical size of the dosage form or its subunits. Under normal conditions, gastric contents are moved down the GI tract as a result of the contractions of the smooth muscles underlying the intestinal mucosa. The coordinated contractions are the result of both electrophysiological and hormonal control mechanisms. The presence or absence of food or liquids in the stomach controls the type and frequency of the contractions. When food is present, increased contractile activity in the stomach assists in the early stages of food digestion by performing particle size reduction and mixing of the stomach contents. The pylorus controls the emptying of the stomach contents into the duodenum. In general, particles smaller than 2 mm can pass out of the stomach into the duodenum in the fed state. The emptying of the stomach contents during the fed state appears to follow a first–order-emptying pattern controlled by the volume within the stomach.

During the fasting state, four primary phases of gastric motility can be observed. The first (phase I), a period referred to as quiescence, is characterized by no significant contractile activity within the stomach. During the next phase (phase II), there are an irregular number of intermittent contractions. Phase III is denoted by a relatively short period of very intense contractions. It is during this phase that much of the remaining particulate matter within the stomach is forced into the duodenum. Phase IV is a relatively transient phase that represents the transition between phase III behavior and that of phase I. The contractile activity that begins within the stomach traverses down the gastrointestinal tract by the segmental contraction of portions of the small intestine. This contractile activity aids in the propulsion of intestinal contents along the length of the small and large intestine. In the fasted state, the cycle of phasic contractile activity repeats itself on the order of every 2 h. In the fed state, however, there is no movement of large, indigestible particles out of the stomach until a fasted state motility pattern takes place.

1. *Oral Suspensions*

Oral suspensions contain the drug in particulate form, suspended by dispersing agents present in the vehicle. This dosage form is frequently selected for development because the drug, or a more stable precursor, is poorly soluble in acceptable drug vehicles, or because a soluble form of the drug formulated as a syrup may not mask the taste of a drug as well as a suspension dosage form. In addition, sometimes a liquid dosage form is desirable because of the difficulty the very young and the very old have in swallowing tablets or capsules. Oral suspensions vary widely in composition. The vehicle can be an oil, water, or consist of an emulsion base (discussed later in more detail); it can vary in viscosity, pH, and buffer capacity. The drug particle size can range from micron-sized to nearly granule-sized. In addition, wetting agents, preservatives, flavoring agents, and coloring agents are also present in solution. Even though the dosage form is widely accepted, there are disadvantages to its use. Because of the physical instability of suspensions, they must be shaken vigorously before dispensing, or an inaccurate dose will result. The finished suspension can be flocculated or deflocculated. In fact, the formation of agglomerates in the suspension can sometimes reduce the bioavailability of the suspension to less than that of a tablet formulation [95].

The aqueous suspension is often used as a reference formulation to which all other formulations of the same drug are compared in bioavailability studies. For poorly soluble drugs, the oral suspension is considered the preferred dosage form because of safety. The oral suspension is often chosen in human studies over intravenous administration to avoid the risk of toxicity that exists with most drugs when they are given parenterally.

When the oral suspension is chosen as the reference formulation, a relative bioavailability determination can be made using Eq. (22). This equation has an advantage over the use of Eq. (18) in that, if the resulting fraction is less than 1, the formulation, and not biological differences is most likely responsible for the decrease. Although Eq. (18) accurately expresses the fraction of the dose reaching systemic circulation, whenever $F < 1$, the decrease in absorption cannot only be due to inadequate release from the dosage form, but also hepatic metabolism, or a slow or negligible rate of permeability across the gastrointestinal barrier. In Eq. (22) the AUC measurements in both the numerator and denominator represent identical oral routes of administration, whereas the same measurements in Eq. (18) represent oral and intravenous routes of administration.

Physicochemical properties of the drug and vehicle determine the physical properties of an oral suspension. These properties have been extensively studied relative to sedimentation rate and physicochemical stability. However, human studies that carefully and systematically evaluate each property for bioavailability are lacking. The effect of viscosity of suspending agents has been studied in human subjects. There is difficulty, however, in accurately assessing the effect of viscosity, partly because a variety of suspending agents are often studied concurrently, and partly, because once the dose is mixed with the stomach fluids, the physical properties of the mixture are unknown.

Recently, Sirois et al., [96] have reported on the effect of viscosity, particle size, and particle density on the gastric emptying of nondigestible solids. Using various grades of methylcellulose to adjust the viscosity of a large volume multiparticulate suspension, significant differences in the emptying rates of various sizes and densities were observed. At low viscosity (normal saline ~ 1 cP) very few particles emptied from the stomach with the fluid fraction. As the viscosity increased (3,300 and 30,000 cP), greater amounts of all particles emptied with the fluid fraction. In addition, more of the smaller particles (1.6 mm) emptied with the fluid fraction than did the larger particles (4 mm). In general, drug particles that are small, the densities of which are near that of the gastric contents, will empty more rapidly. Therefore, depending on the site of optimal absorption, selecting appropriate drug particle sizes, particle densities, and to a more limited extent, vehicle viscosities can be used to optimize the bioavailability of oral suspensions.

Soci and Parrott [97] measured the excretion of 200 mg of nitrofurantoin after administering the drug suspended in five different viscous, suspending agents. An increase in viscosity delayed absorption, resulting in the extension of clinically effective concentrations for a longer time. Complexation between nitrofurantoin and methycellulose or carbomer was demonstrated by dialysis; however, the extent of absorption was not affected by the interaction.

In another study, the bioavailability of sulfathiazole was studied as a function of the viscosity of various suspending agents [98]. As the viscosity of the suspending agent increased, the extent of absorption increased. When the drug was suspended in water, the rate and extent of absorption significantly decreased. The investigators concluded that the suspending agent imparted improved wetting and particle deaggregation to yield increased effective surface area, prolonged gastrointestinal transit time, and greater dispersibility, all of which contributed to the improved bioavailability of the products.

Oral suspensions intended for pediatric use, particularly commercial preparations of penicillin derivatives, have been studied for differences in bioavailability [99,100]. In these studies, the bioavailability of the dosage form followed the order of the solubility of the salts they contained. Solutions, tablets, or capsules of potassium salts, for example, generally yielded higher peak concentrations of the penicillin derivative than suspensions of slightly soluble calcium or benzathine salts. The authors noted that the poor bioavailability of the slightly soluble penicillin salts was probably responsible for the loose stools that practicing physicians had observed with these products, since a larger proportion of unabsorbed antibiotic in the large intestine would be expected to induce changes in the bowel flora.

In anticipation of substituting a suspension of carbamazepine for tablets in pediatric use, Wada et al. [101] measured plasma levels of the drug following administration of 200 mg of suspension or tablet dosage forms in nine adult male volunteers. The suspension yielded a more rapid rate of absorption, producing peak concentrations one-third higher than plasma levels from the tablet. In a similar study, Bloomer et al. [102] also found that a suspension formulation of carbamazepine resulted in higher C_{max} and shorter t_{max} values than found with commercial carbamazepine tablets, yet the extent of absorption for each dosage form was similar. Nearly identical results were obtained with phenytoin when a suspension dosage form was compared with commercial tablets or capsules. For the suspension study, the commercial preparations were purchased in Finland [103], whereas, in the tablet study the products were obtained in Australia [104].

Aqueous suspensions of griseofulvin and phenytoin have been studied in animals to determine whether a change in formulation could improve the erratic and incomplete absorption profile of these drugs when administered orally in tablet or capsule form. Several investigators demonstrated that griseofulvin absorption could be enhanced if administered with meals high in fat content [105–107]. Shinkuma and colleagues [108] conducted a very thorough study comparing the absorption of phenytoin from sesame oil or oleic acid (a principal fatty acid in sesame oil) suspensions. The C_{max} for the oleic acid suspension was about one-half that found with sesame oil, and the t_{max} was somewhat longer. However, the AUC for the oleic acid suspension was significantly higher than the sesame oil suspension. The differences in C_{max} and t_{max} were attributed to a delay in gastric emptying in the presence of oleic acid that did not occur with sesame oil. Oleic acid suspensions administered intraduodenally, instead of orally, resulted in plasma levels greater than those from the sesame oil suspension. This can most easily be explained by the difference in solubility and distribution coefficient for phenytoin in the two oils. The solubility of phenytoin in sesame oil was reported to be 332.7 mg/ml and in oleic acid was 745.2 mg/ml. As long as excess phenytoin was present, the higher concentration of phenytoin in solution in oleic acid resulted in a greater driving force for drug absorption across the intestinal membrane.

Al-Hammanu and Richards [109] tested the effect of similar physiological and physicochemical mechanisms on the absorption of a sodium salicylate, the salt of a water-soluble weak acid, suspended in fractionated coconut oil. This formulation's bioavailability was compared with that from an aqueous solution. Rabbits were given equal oral doses by gastric lavage, and salicylate blood levels were measured over time. The plasma AUC indicated that the oil suspension was responsible for a 1.32-fold increase in the extent of absorption. The peak time and peak concentration obtained for these two dosage forms showed a decrease in the rate of absorption for the coconut oil suspension; however, only differences in peak time were statistically significant. The investigators suggested that the increase in extent of absorption occurred because of the increased residence time of the drug in the stomach owing to the presence of the oil. A delay was observed for the peak time, partly because the oil acted as a reservoir to control the release of drug, and partly because of the potentially slower rate of absorption of drug from the stomach compared with the small intestine with its greater surface area.

Methoxsalen, an antipsoriatic agent, is a drug with poor aqueous solubility. Consequently, it is a candidate for enhanced absorption from an oily vehicle. In a bioavailability study by Steiner et al. [110] in nine volunteers, peak plasma levels ranged from 0.15 to 4.58 mg/ml. The peak time also varied considerably. In light of these results, Kreuter and Higuchi [111] compared peanut oil solutions and aqueous suspensions of methoxsalen with a capsule dosage form of methoxsalen in both the rat and dog. The peanut oil solution considerably enhanced the absorption rate and the maximal blood levels in the rat and dog when compared with the aqueous suspension. An identical dose was also given intravenously. For methoxsalen, the intravenous dose yielded plasma AUCs that were about one-fourth the AUC observed for the oral formulations. The authors [111] proposed two reasons for the lower bioavailability of the intravenous dose. Either methoxalen did not follow a linear relation between dose and plasma concentration, or the drug precipitated after intravenous administration and only very slowly redissolved to produce plasma levels below the detection level of the assay.

Similar results were observed for the oral preparations of a lipophilic steroid formulated in a sesame oil solution and in an aqueous suspension [112]. Both formulations were administered to rats orally in a 0.4-ml volume. The suspension contained 0.5% methylcellulose and 0.4% polysorbate 80, and the drug was micronized. The mean plasma AUC was greater for the sesame oil solution than for the aqueous suspension. Additional studies indicated that, as the drug exceeded its equilibrium solubility in sesame oil, the extent of absorption was no longer proportional to the administered dose, but showed a decrease.

With a fasted beagle dog as an animal model, the bioavailability of prednisolone was determined following an oral dose of a tablet, a triturated tablet suspended in 50 ml water, and an aqueous solution of prednisolone sodium phosphate [113]. All dosage forms were administered through a stomach tube. Although prednisolone sodium phosphate is rapidly converted to prednisolone in vivo by ester hydrolysis, the plasma AUC for the solution was about 75% of that obtained for the suspension. This was attributed to the fact that a considerable portion of the prednisolone sodium phosphate was in the ionized form in the stomach; therefore, it was not readily absorbed. The results also showed that about twice as much prednisolone was absorbed from the suspension as from the tablet dosage form. Tablet disintegration characteristics were assumed responsible for the results.

Bioavailability studies of oral suspensions have been conducted in various animal models and with water-soluble or poorly soluble drugs formulated as suspensions, solutions, or solid dosage forms. Although a solution can be considered more bioavailable than a suspension, tablet, or capsule dosage form, enough exceptions can be cited to lead one to be cautious in selecting a suspension over a tablet or capsule as the next most bioavailable dosage form. If doubt exists about which dosage form is the most bioavailable, animal studies should be conducted to answer the question. Once these studies are completed, human studies can be conducted to choose the optimal formulation.

Quite often pediatric or geriatric patients cannot swallow a solid dosage form without undue difficulty. As a result, the solid dosage form is crushed, or for a capsule, the contents emptied into a suitable vehicle for easy administration by the patient. Milk, fruit juices, applesauce, or other food that the patient will take becomes the vehicle by which the drug is administered. In one study, ketoconazole was tested for absorption efficacy using commercially available tablets that were thoroughly crushed and suspended in either water or applesauce [114]. The plasma AUC associated with the oral administration of granules from a crushed tablet suspended in applesauce was approximately twofold greater than the AUC from a suspension of the crushed tablet in water. Previous studies had shown that ketoconazole absorption was unaffected by the presence of food in the gastrointestinal tract [114].

2. Oral Emulsions

For emulsions, the drug can be suspended or dissolved in either the oily or the aqueous phase. In most studies, the details on the physical characteristics of the emulsion are lacking. The factors that affect the stability and release of drug from an emulsion, such as droplet size and emulsifier type, have not been well studied with regard to bioavailability. Even so, once the emulsion mixes with the contents of the gastrointestinal tract, its physical form would not be expected to remain intact for very long. Consequently, the effect of formulation variables may not be detectable from the evaluation of plasma AUCs. Yet, enough examples of increased bioavailabilities from emulsion systems exist to warrant further investigation.

Carrigan and Bates [115,116] studied the absorption characteristics of micronized griseofulvin from an O/W emulsion dosage form, an oil suspension, and an aqueous suspension in the rat. These investigators observed that there was no significant difference between the fraction of the oral dose of griseofulvin absorbed from the aqueous and oil suspension. However, a statistically significant 1.6- and 2.5-fold increase was observed for the emulsion dosage form when compared with the aqueous and oil suspension dosage forms, respectively. A follow-up study on the effect of absorption of micronized griseofulvin from corn oil–water emulsion and aqueous suspension dosage forms was conducted by Bates and Sequeira [117] after completion of their rat studies. Figure 9 shows the mean results of the excretion rate of 6-desmethylgriseofulvin, the metabolite through which nearly all of the dose is eliminated. Two commercial tablets, a corn oil–water (30 g) emulsion and an aqueous suspension (30 g) were carefully administered to five subjects at different times. The results showed that the emulsion dosage form was responsible for a three- to fourfold greater cumulative amount excreted than

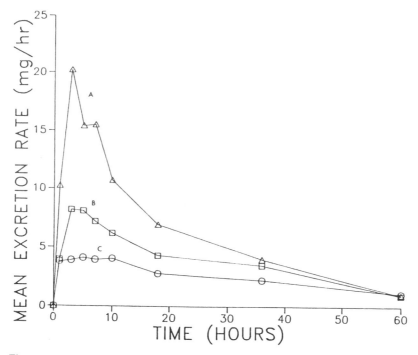

Fig. 9 Excretion rate of 6-desmethylgriseofulvin observed over time following the oral administration of 500 mg micronized griseofulvin to human subjects ($n = 5$) of a corn oil–water emulsion (A), and two tablet formulations (B and C).

the tablet or the aqueous suspension. Because the drug was absorbed over about 30 h, the assumption was made that absorption occurred throughout the gastrointestinal tract. One individual was given propantheline (30 mg) just before taking the aqueous suspension to retard stomach emptying. In this case, both the rate and extent of absorption of griseofulvin were identical from either the emulsion or the aqueous suspension. Therefore, absorption from the stomach was considered significant. In the same individual 6 g of lipid enhanced drug absorption.

Chakrabarti and Belpaire [118] studied the absorption profile of micronized phenytoin after its oral administration to rats as an aqueous suspension, a corn oil suspension, or a corn oil emulsion. Figure 10 shows their results. The corn oil suspension as well as the corn oil emulsion were statistically better than the aqueous suspension reference standard in both rate and extent of absorption.

Several investigators have attempted to increase the bioavailability of cyclosporine, a lipophilic, cyclic peptide compound used as an immunosuppressant. Johnston and colleagues [119] compared the bioavailability of an oily solution and the same oily solution dispersed in orange juice, or in regular or chocolate-flavored milk. They found no difference between the bioavailabilities of the four liquid formulations. There was significant variability in the absorption of cyclosporine from each of the dosage forms, and this variability may have masked any differences caused by the vehicles themselves. Ritschel and co-workers [120] also found no significant differences between the bioavailabilities of an oily solution; a capsule containing Gelucire (glycerides and polyglycide fatty esters), Pluronic F 68, and sodium taurocholate; and a capsule containing

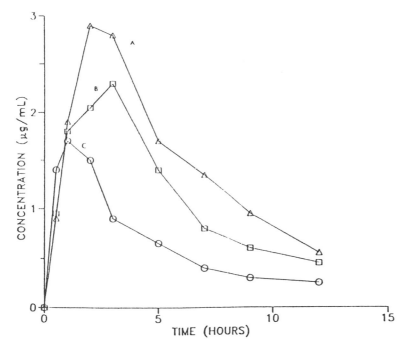

Fig. 10 Serum concentration of phenytoin observed over time following oral administration of 20 mg/kg to rats of a corn oil emulsion (A), corn oil suspension (B), and an aqueous suspension (C).

a suspension of cycloporine in a water–oil microemulsion vehicle gelled with silicon dioxide. In comparison, a fast-releasing oil–water microemulsion and a solid micellar solution of cyclosporine with fast in vitro release both increased the bioavailability of the peptide compared with the marketed soft gelatin capsule dosage form [121]. A slow-releasing microemulsion dosage form, containing components identical to the fast-releasing form, showed no difference in bioavailability from that of the soft gel capsule. The investigators [121] attributed much of the increased bioavailability to the release of cyclosporine in the upper small intestine, the region of the gastrointestinal tract where cyclosporine is most readily absorbed or to changes in intestinal physiology in the distal GI tract that provide a less-than-optimal environment for complete cyclosporine absorption.

The mechanisms responsible for the improvement in absorption of these poorly soluble drugs suspended in an O/W emulsion vehicle is not entirely clear, but has been explained by both physiological and physicochemical properties. Biliary secretions may have contributed to an increase in the dissolution rate which, in turn, permitted a faster rate of absorption to occur and also contributed to a greater extent of absorption. Alternatively, Bates and Sequeira [117] proposed that the bile components, through emulsification, increased the digestion rate of the lipids in the emulsion vehicle. This latter process is required to stimulate the fat-sensitive receptors in the duodenum, which would be responsible for the inhibition of gastric emptying. Therefore, it is conceivable that an emulsion vehicle results in a delay of gastric emptying, with an accompanying increase in bile secretion. The resulting increase in residence time would then permit a greater amount of the ingested dose to be absorbed.

3. Oral Gels

Liversidge and co-workers [123] investigated the bioavailability and ulcerogenicity of indomethacin from an oral suspension and an oral gel. Although the degree of gastric irritation is frequently high following exposure to oral doses of indomethacin, severe ulceration is also observed following intravenous administration. These investigators found that administration of indomethacin in an amphoteric gel significantly increased its bioavailability compared with the oral suspension, and no gastric irritation was observed. The gel was composed of oleic acid, egg phosphatide, arginine, and water. The final concentration of indomethacin in the gel was 0.1%, however, the gel was reported to have an indomethacin capacity of approximately 200 mg/g which would permit the administration of significantly greater amounts of the drug than those studied. The indomethacin exists in the gel as a dilute molecular dispersion. It was observed that the gel spontaneously formed a dispersion when it came into contact with gastric contents, and it is believed that the phospholipids present in the gel spontaneously form liposomes on dilution. The specific mechanisms by which the gel increases indomethacin bioavailability and decreases ulcerogenicity are still unclear, however. The indomethacin oral suspension, in comparison, resulted in a bioavailability of 68%, almost one-half that of the gel formulation and was severely irritating to the gastric mucosa.

4. Macroparticulate Drug Carriers

Very small particulates, <1 μm, have been observed to be absorbed through the tissues of both the small and large intestine [124]. Dosage forms containing drugs entrapped in microparticulates (liposomes, nanocapsules, or similar systems) have gained increasing attention as oral delivery systems for drugs that are not well absorbed or are subject to luminal degradation in the GI tract. Polystyrene nanoparticles are taken up by the Peyer's patches (lymphoidal tissues dispersed throughout the intestine) and are subsequently transported from the mesenteric lymph to the venous circulation [124]. Approximately one-third of the mass of 50-nm latex particles was taken up over a 10-day–dosing period. In comparison, only 7% of 1-μm particles was absorbed. There was no evidence of the systemic absorption of 3-μm particles [125]. The bulk of the particulates transported through the intestinal tissues lodge in the organs of the reticuloendothelial system (liver, spleen, bone marrow). The entrapment of drug within biodegradable nanocapsules, or nanocapsules that are permeable to the drug, would allow the systemic distribution of the drug, regardless of the distribution pattern of the particulate carriers. Aprahamian et al. [126] reported that nanocapsules beween 100 and 200 nm in diameter within which Lipiodol, an iodized oil, was entrapped, could be traced being transported from the intestinal villi through the intercellular spaces to the mesenteric venous circulation. Although these studies were conducted using an intestinal loop system, their results indicate that the use of nanoparticles can open up secondary routes of transport to the systemic circulation for poorly bioavailable drugs.

Fukui et al. [127] studied the effect of a mixed micellar solution of oleic acid–polyoxyethylene hydrogenated castor oil (HCO60) on the absorption of several different colloidal particles within various regions of the lower GI tract. The particles selected were Rotring ink (100–800 nm), platinum ink (2.4–10 nm), and colloidal gold (5, 20, or 40 nm). The Rotring ink particles were not absorbed from any region of the lower GI tract, with or without the addition of the mixed micelles. Platinum ink, in comparison, appeared in the thoracic lymph when administered in the mixed micellar solution, yet no plasma levels of the ink were measurable. No colloidal gold particles, regardless of size, could be detected in either lymph or blood following administration to the large intestine. When formulated in the mixed micellar solution, however, all three size ranges of colloidal gold were found both in the lymph and blood, although the amounts of the 40-nm particles found were significantly less than for the 5- or 20-nm colloid. Finally, in a comparison of the ability of the mixed micellar formulation to enhance the absorption of colloidal particles in either the colon or rectum, the uptake of particles had greater enhancement in the rectum than in the colon. This suggests that there may be anatomical or physiological differences between these two regions that mediate the uptake of particulate matter into the systemic or lymphatic circulation.

The development of several different controlled-release dosage forms has involved the use of granule-sized (> 100 μm) particles treated in a way such that they cause prolonged plasma levels of the drug agent involved. Generally, this is accomplished by coating the particles with various polymers that dissolve at varying rates within the GI tract. Frequently, the controlled-release particles are contained within a traditional dosage form (capsule or tablet) that on disintegration in the GI tract, releases the particulate units. In an elegant study combining both radiolabeled and cold drug containing extended-release spheres (1.0–1.4 mm), Graffner and co-workers [128] showed that remoxipride, a neuroleptic agent, would be suitable for formulation in an extended-release, multiple-unit, capsule dosage form. They observed that the primary capsule containing the remoxipride units dissolved in the gastric fluids within 30 min, and the remoxipride microcapsules emptied from the stomach of the fasted subjects within the next 30 min. The microcapsules were then observed to disperse throughout the small intestine and, subsequently, disperse throughout the large intestine within the following 5 h, where they remained for up to 48 h. Complete remoxipride absorption was observed within 24 h following administration.

5. Microparticulate Carriers

a. Liposomes

There have been several reports of liposomes improving the oral absorption of certain drugs. Insulin was reported to be absorbed orally in diabetic rats, demonstrated by significant reductions in blood glucose levels [129,130]. These results have been difficult to produce in normal animals, even though insulin could be shown to be absorbed. Heparin, an anionic anticoagulant biopolymer, has shown some oral activity after entrapment in cationic liposomes [131]. Oral immunization may also be feasible with liposomally entrapped antigens. When tetanus toxoid-loaded liposomes were administered orally to cats, an antibody titer equivalent to that found after subcutaneous inoculation was obtained [132]. Similar results have been shown for oral immunization against snake venom [133]. Such oral absorption can be due to one of two effects: stabilization of the entrapped drug to GI enzymes and pH or enhancement of absorption by Peyer's patches or other lipid absorption mechanisms.

b. Nanocapsules

Andrieu et al. [134] investigated the feasibility of delivering indomethacin, an NSAID which can cause severe GI irritation, in a nanocapsule formulation to protect the GI mucosa from damage. Indomethacin-loaded polyisobutylcyanocrylate nanocapsules (200–300 nm) were infused either intravenously or intragastrically to rats over a 60-min interval. Interestingly, the bioavailability of the nanocapsules administered orally was 133%, as compared with those administered intravenously. The reason for this was not clear from the data presented. The investigators noted that several of the pharmacokinetic parameters for indomethacin were altered in the nanocapsule formulation, most notably the volume of distribution for the nanocapsules was nearly twice that of an indomethacin solution. The difference in disposition patterns of the indomethacin nanocapsules following either intravenous or gastrointestinal delivery was thought to influence the measurement of the bioavailability.

C. Rectal Bioavailability

1. *Rectal Suspensions (Enemas)*

Historically, the administration of drug solutions or suspensions by the rectum was accomplished with an enema system. Enemas are frequently large in volume (50–100 ml) and have limited patient acceptability. In particular disease states which directly affect the colon (e.g., ulcerative colitis), delivery of medicaments directly to the rectum and colon in a large volume can be useful. For example, Bondesen et al. [135] reported on the absorption and efficacy of a 5-aminosalicylic acid (5-ASA) enema in patients with ulcerative colitis. Two different enema formulations were investigated: the first consisted of a 1000-mg/dl solution of 5-ASA at pH 7.4; the second formulation was a 1000-mg/dl suspension of 5-ASA buffered at pH 4.8 with about 200 mg/dl in solution. Plasma concentrations of 5-ASA and its acetylated metabolite following administration of the solution enema (pH 7.4) indicated that 5-ASA was rapidly absorbed from the rectal tissues of patients with chronic ulcerative colitis and resulted in plasma concentrations two to three times greater than those observed in individuals receiving oral sulfasalazine therapy. In comparison, the buffered suspension (pH 4.8) resulted in plasma concentration profiles that resembled those following oral therapy. Seven of 16 patients, in a 10-day multiple-dose study of the 5-ASA suspension, achieved clinical remission during this time. However, there was no correlation between the plasma levels of 5-ASA and the remission status of the patients. This observation may indicate that plasma concentrations may not be the best measures of the local effectiveness of a rectal dosage form.

Graves and co-workers [136] have studied the absorption of carbamazepine from a microenema suspension as a possible replacement therapy for individuals unable to ingest the marketed oral tablets. A comparison of the bioavailability of conventional oral tablets or a suspension of carbamazepine in propylene glycol, sorbitol, and sucrose, administered orally or rectally revealed that the rate of absorption and bioavailability from the oral tablet and the rectal suspension were equivalent. The bioavailability from the oral suspension, however, exceeded that from either of the other two dosage forms. It is likely that slow dissolution of the hydrophobic carbamazepine from the rectal suspension and oral tablet limited their bioavailabilities. The oral suspension, in comparison, may have had sufficient particle surface area for good dissolution in the gastric fluids in the presence of the cosolvents present in the formulation.

2. *Rectal Suppositories*

The absorption of drugs from rectal suppositories is a complex process of suppository melting or dissolution, drug release from the suppository base, drug dissolution in the rectal fluids, and drug permeation across the rectal membranes. In general, there are three primary types of suppository bases: fatty, oleaginous bases (Witepsol, cocoa butter, and such); water-soluble bases (PEGs); and emulsifying bases. The fatty bases melt at body temperature and are immiscible with the fluids in the rectum. Drugs incorporated into these bases partition between the oily base and the rectal fluids or tissues. The water-soluble bases dissolve rapidly in the rectal fluids, and the emulsifying bases, although not miscible with water, form in situ emulsions as water from the rectal fluids is incorporated into the suppository. Often drug release is more rapid and more complete from fatty base suppositories owing to the rapid melting of the base following insertion. One drawback of cocoa butter or fatty bases is that oil-soluble drugs depress the melting point of suppositories prepared from such materials. Chloral hydrate, menthol, camphor, and phenol are examples of such drugs. This problem can be ameliorated by the addition of white wax or other higher-melting waxy materials that raise the melting point of the base.

Minkov et al. [137] compared the bioavailability of phenobarbital and sodium phenobarbital from four different suppository bases. They observed that the C_{max} and relative bioavailability (compared with Witepsol H-15 base) in each of the suppository bases was independent of the salt or acidic form of the incorporated drug. The plasma levels of phenobarbital following administration in Witepsol H-15, Witepsol H-15 with 2% Tween 80, or Novosup (a mixture of polyethylene glycol esters with free fatty acids of sunflower oil and lard, Tween 20 and 80, Mirj 45, and Brij 58) were not statistically different from those measured following the administration of a phenobarbital aqueous suspension or a sodium phenobarbital aqueous solution. These results indicated that drug release from the suppository base was not rate-limiting, rather drug permeability across the rectal tissues was controlling the bioavailability of phenobarbital (Fig. 11).

In a similar study, Ghazy and colleagues [138] studied the in vitro release of ethosuximide from four different suppository bases: Witepsol W-35, Witepsol E-76, PEG 400:4000, and PEG 400:6000. The bioavailabilities of the two PEG suppositories were nearly equal (89 vs. 82%, respectively). The bioavailability of the Witepsol E-76 suppository was 59%, and that of the Witepsol W-35 suppository was 47%. These bioavailability values parallel the results of the drug release from the suppositories into normal saline at 37°C. It appears that, in the case of ethosuximide, a very water-soluble compound, drug release from the suppository base affects its bioavailability and that the rapidly dissolving water-soluble bases result in higher bioavailabilities than do the fatty bases.

Similar results were obtained by Vromans et al. [139] while investigating the absorption of metronidazole from an aqueous rectal suspension (containing 0.5% methylcellulose), a triglyceride base suppository (Elysol), and three PEG bases: PEG 1000, PEG 6000, and a 1:1 mixture of PEG 1000 + 6000. The bioavailabilities from the PEG suppositories were greater than those from the fatty base suppository, but the bioavailabilities of each of the PEG bases were not statistically different from each other or from the rectal suspension. These results seem to confirm previous in vitro studies of Schoonen et al. [140], who found that the rate-limiting step in drug release from a fatty base suppository was the transport of the metronidazole away from the lipid–water interface.

Cole and Kunka [141] have studied the bioavailability of theophylline from an oral elixir, a rectal enema, and a rectal suppository. The rate and extent of theophylline absorption was identical following administration by the oral elixir or the rectal solution. The rate of absorption for the suppository was much slower than for the other two dosage forms, but the extent of absorption was identical. Since theophylline is relatively water-insoluble and the suppository base is highly lipophilic, it is likely that release of

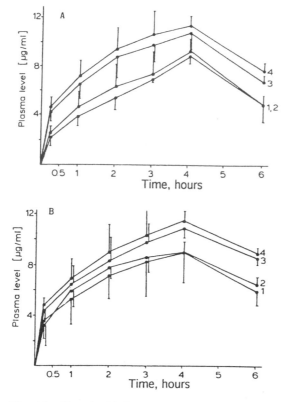

Fig. 11 Phenobarbital plasma levels after single-dose rectal or oral administration of 20 mg/kg phenobarbital (A) or 22 mg/kg sodium phenobarbital (B) in rabbits; 1, Witepsol H 15; 2, aqueous oral suspension (phenobarbital) or aqueous oral solution (sodium phenobarbital); 3, Novosup; 4, Witepsol H 15 with 2% Tween 80.

the drug from the dosage form significantly reduced the rate of absorption into the systemic circulation.

Itoh et al. [142] have attempted to develop a new type of suppository base by combining a fatty base (Pharmasol B115), a water-soluble base (PEG 4000), and an emulsifying base (Unilube) to produce a suppository of aminopyrine, with desirable release characteristics, that remains a solid at room temperature. Although the combination of the fatty base with the water-soluble base seemed to yield a suppository with excellent bioavailability, the addition of the emulsifying base to the system reduced the bioavailability, most probably owing to its slower dissolution than PEG.

3. Rectal Foams

Currently available rectal foams contain corticosteroids for use in inflammatory conditions in the lower bowel. Various investigators have studied the systemic absorption of these steroids following delivery by foam dosage forms [143]. Although there is disagreement over whether all of the steroids are absorbed following rectal foam administration, there is convincing evidence that these dosage forms are as efficacious as retention enemas. Because of the lower volume needed of the foam, it is also more acceptable to patients. In a rather detailed letter, Rodrigues et al. [144] describe both rectal tissue concentrations and plasma concentrations in patients receiving prednisolone metasulfobenzoate rectal foam (20 mg/20ml). At 6 h after administration, the rectal tissue levels averaged 4874 ng/ml, whereas the corresponding plasma level was only 107 ng/ml. The rectal tissue levels were also higher than those measured following rectal administration of a 0.2 mg/ml enema, but were similar to those following a 0.6 mg/ml enema.

D. Dermal Bioavailability

In general, topical application of drugs to the skin is intended for local effects either on or within the skin. Flynn [145], in a detailed discussion of drug absorption of dermatologicals, classified five distinct targets, beginning with the surface of the skin and progressing through the various layers of the skin to the sweat glands, with systemic absorption representing the least accessible target. Unfortunately, measuring drug bioavailability in each of these skin regions is limited, in part, by assay sensitivity and, in part, by the inability to adequately sample these various regions. Attempts to directly measure local drug concentrations at specific depths within the skin by carefully sectioning excised skin samples, homogenizing, and assaying for drug content have been reported [146]. In addition, the improvement in microdialysis techniques and instrumentation will likely result in improved capabilities to measure drug concentrations within the skin directly.

1. *Skin-Directed Bioavailability*

Bioavailability measurements of skin penetration were initially conducted with the corticosteroids because of their easily measured and graded blanching response. Stoughton [147] compared the results of the blanching assay with in vitro penetration of five corticosteroids across excised hairless mouse and human skin (Table 1). The steroids were applied to the skin of either species in 0.02 ml of 95% alcoholic solutions so that drug release was not a significant factor. From these studies, an important distinction was made between pharmacological activity and skin penetration. Although either factor can predominate in contribution to an increase in steroid effectiveness, Stoughton concluded that pharmacological activity was a greater contributor to overall effectiveness than

Table 1 Comparison of Vasoconstrictor Bioassay and In Vitro Penetration of Glucocorticosteroids

Steroid	In vitro penetration[a]		Vasoconstrictor bioassay[a]
	Human skin	Hairless mouse skin	Human skin in vivo
Fluocinolone	1.0	1.0	1
Betamethasone	1.6	2.2	1
Betamethasone valerate	1.7	2.1	125
Fluocinolone acetonide acetate	9.1	13.0	625
Fluocinolone acetonide	14.0	23.0	125

[a]Scores are relative to fluocinolone.
Source: From Ref. 147.

penetration. For example, betamethasone valerate was 625 times more effective in blanching than betamethasone alcohol, yet Table 1 indicates their skin permeability is equal and slightly higher in mouse skin, compared with human skin [147].

Place [148] used the blanching test to relate chemical structure of corticosteroids to vasoconstriction following the application of alcoholic solutions of drug to human skin. The contribution of skin penetration was not separated from the overall blanching effect. Nevertheless, the results, which were obtained from over 32,000 sites on the arms of 642 volunteers, clearly identified the overall effectiveness of various steroids. Each site was graded as having responded or not. The final results were tabulated as a percentage of sites responding and expressed as median effective dose responding (ED_{50}).

The ED_{50} values from this study, as well as a similarly conducted study [149], are summarized in Table 2 for several topically active corticosteroids. The results show that marked enhancement of topical activity of a particular steroid could be achieved, although not in a consistent manner, with various substitutions to the relatively unsubstituted steroid structure. For example, triamcinolone is only slightly more active than a placebo. The addition of another fluorine to the 6-α position of triamcinolone produces some enhancement of activity. However, a dramatic increase in activity occurs when the 16- and 17-α-hydroxy positions are joined through the acetonide functionality. The addition of an acetate to the 21 position of paramethasone produced a significant increase in activity. Likewise, fluocinolide, the 21-acetate of fluocinolone acetonide, had a fivefold increase in potency over fluocinolone acetonide. However, the addition of a 21-acetate to hydrocortisone did not alter the activity of the parent molecule. These results seem to indicate that no single functionality that produces an increase in activity in one steroid structure can be expected to produce a similar increase in another.

There are a large number of semisolids for use as topical vehicles for steroids and an equally large list of ingredients used as adjuvants in these semisolids. Consequently, the possible combinations of drugs and semisolids, to say nothing of the different skin diseases and possible infected sites, presents an enormous set of permutations to study.

Table 2 Log Concentration of the Dose Required to Produce Vasoconstriction in 50% of the Sites (ED_{50})

Steroid	ED_{50}^{a}
Fluocinolone acetonide	−5.11
Hydrocortisone	−0.25
6α,9α-Difluoro-16α-hydroxy prednisolone	−2.11
Triamcinolone acetonide	−5.41
9α-11β-Dichloro-6α-fluoro-16α,17α,21-trihydroxy-pregna-1,4-diene-3,20-dione-16,17-acetonide	−5.59
21-Acetate of above	−5.58
Paramethasone	−1.00
Paramethasone acetate	−5.16
Betamethasone acetate	−4.23
Betamethasone 17-valerate	−5.66
Fluocinolide	−6.27

[a]log (% w/v).
Source: From Refs. 148 and 149.

In an effort to reduce the confusion, Barry [150] and Flynn [144] provided guidelines for optimal release of drug from a particular semisolid. They stated that a drug must be soluble in the vehicle, since diffusion through the bulk phase determines its release. However, if the drug is very soluble in the vehicle, it will tend to remain there and not partition into the outer skin layer. Optimal release occurs when the drug is at or near its upper limit of solubility. At saturation solubility, the escaping tendency (i.e., activity) of the drug is at its maximum. Consequently, for optimal release, the vehicle and adjuvants should be chosen so that the drug is nearly saturated in the final formulation [150].

Barry [150] further modified the blanching test by creating a range of response observations from 0 to 4 with half point ratings from 6 to 96 h after application. The range was sufficient so that the kinetics of the blanching response could be studied for each preparation applied to the skin. A pharmacokinetic approach of this type permitted the identification of the input rate, which was controlled by the physicochemical properties of the vehicle or the permeability coefficient of drug into the skin [150,151]. Figure 12 gives the kinetic profiles for occluded applications of betamethasone 17-benzoate in foam, ointment, cream, and gel formulations. The results were expressed as a relative bioavailability relationship shown below:

$$\text{Bioavailability} = \frac{\text{score achieved by product}}{\text{score achieved by most active formulation}} \tag{30}$$

In Fig. 12 the foam would be considered the most active formulation to which all other formulations would be compared.

Although the blanching test may not directly correlate with anti-inflammatory activity or to the concentrations of drug in the skin, the effect of dosage form variation can be measured and expressed in relative bioavailability terms.

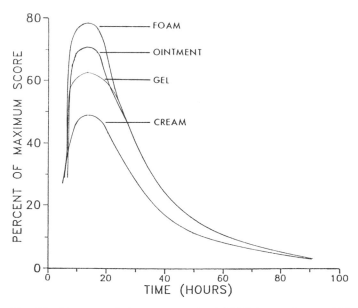

Fig. 12 Vasoconstriction response for 0.025% betamethasone 17-benzoate applied to occluded human skin as foam, ointment, gel, and cream formulations.

An additional concept important to drug release from various topical vehicles is that of thermodynamic activity. Higuchi [75] indicated that drug diffusional flux should be proportional to its activity in the vehicle, assuming other parameters remain constant. The maximal activity occurs when excess drug is present in the vehicle (i.e., a suspension) because the activity of dissolved drug and suspended drug are equal. Since the activity of a solid is taken as 1, the drug in solution also has an activity of 1. Changes in the vehicle that alter drug solubility should not alter drug release rates, as long as excess suspended drug is present. For subsaturated drug concentrations, there would be a decrease in activity proportional to concentration and activity coefficient. This concept of activity, being important to skin permeation, has been evaluated in a series of papers by Barry and co-workers [152–155]. Vapor-phase permeation of benzyl alcohol through human skin from various solvents is shown in Fig.13 [152,154]. As expected, the flux was proportional to the thermodynamic activity, as measured by equilibrium vapor pressures of benzyl alcohol in the various vehicles. When the vehicle with dissolved benzyl alcohol was in direct contact with the skin, higher diffusional fluxes were obtained than from the vapor phase [153,154]. Such results suggest the presence of interfacial barriers that contribute to overall permeation rates from the vapor phase that are not present or are greatly reduced in liquid-phase studies. A similar rationale can be deduced from work on the percutaneous penetration of diflorasone diacetate as a function of solubilizers [156]. Proportional, but opposite, effects of propylene glycol and polyoxypropylene-15-stearyl ether on solubility and partition coefficient were observed in mineral oil. These opposing factors led to penetration fluxes as a function of the weight fraction of solubilizer, which could be predicted reasonably well on the basis of activity considerations (i.e., a product of solubility and partition coefficients).

Finally, it is important to recognize that both activity and diffusional considerations must be included in any comprehensive consideration of topical drug delivery. To rationalize vehicle modification effects on skin penetration, thermodynamic activity considerations are important. On the other hand, to accurately represent the time course of

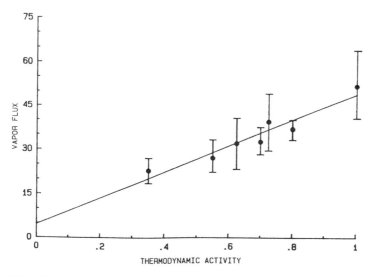

Fig. 13 Benzyl alcohol vapor flux through human skin from neat benzyl alcohol (activity = 1) and from 0.5-mol fraction binary mixtures (.35 ≤ activity ≤ .8).

drug release or of skin permeation, diffusional considerations must be included. Thus, one must decide whether rank-order correlations with formulation factors are satisfactory, or whether more detailed time course analysis is required to optimize or rationalize drug release from dermatological delivery systems.

In addition to the aformentioned physicochemical factors that affect skin permeability, skin penetration enhancers have been used to promote drug permeation for local and systemic effects [157]. Penetration enhancers increase skin permeability by reducing the diffusional resistance of stratum corneum by inducing reversible or irreversible changes in the protein structure, hydration level, or lipid content. The efficacy of proposed permeability enhancers must be viewed cautiously in light of their potential to cause permanent alterations in the skin and their ability to promote penetration of formulation excipients as well as therapeutic agents.

The more classic penetration enhancers have been dimethyl sulfoxide [158] and liquid amides, such as dimethylformamide and dimethylacetamide [159,160]. Even though they increase skin penetration for a wide variety of drugs, enthusiasm for their use has been dampened by irritancy, toxicity, and odor. An alkyl sulfoxide, decylmethyl sulfoxide, which is similar to dimethyl sulfoxide enhances the efficacy of topical tetracycline in the treatment of acne [161]. It is currently a component of a marketed formulation for acne (Topicycline) and is apparently effective at a level of only 0.125%. Other, longer-chain length *n*-alkanoic *N,N*-dimethylamides also have enhancing effects on dermal penetration [162]. *N,N*-Dimethyloctanamide and *N,N*-dimethyldecanamide were highly effective in the enhancement of ibuprofen and naproxen penetration across isolated rat skin. The dimethylamides showed good enhancement of both ibuprofen and naproxen in suspension vehicles composed of 50% propylene glycol. However, none were more effective than the control when the drugs were formulated in a liquid petroleum vehicle. These observations again demonstrate the importance of the drug partition coefficient between the formulation and the skin in determining permeability.

Pyrrolidones, which are cyclic amides, also promote skin penetration and increase drug uptake into the stratum corneum [163]. Azone (1-dodecylazocycloheptan-2-one), which is a cyclic amide, has produced skin penetration enhancements of 100-fold for polar drugs, which normally do not penetrate skin at significant rates [164,165]. Azone also appears to be an effective enhancer for some nonpolar drug agents. In a study investigating the enhancement of triamcinolone acetonide absorption in the presence of 1.6% Azone, Wiechers et al. found that the absorption of this steroidal agent was significantly greater than for triamcinolone alone [166]. In addition, they showed that Azone did not enhance triamcinolone depot formation in the stratum corneum, as had been previously observed for dimethyl sulfoxide [158], *N*-methyl-2-pyrrolidone [163], and dimethylformamide [159]. Hou and Flynn [167] studied the absorption of a similar steroid, hydrocortisone, in the presence of various concentrations of Azone (0.1–10%) in an oil–water emulsion system. They found that, although Azone consistently enhanced the permeability of hydrocortisone through excised skin segments, the permeability values were inversely proportional to the Azone concentration. The authors explain this observation based on the activity of hydrocortisone in the oil–water emulsion system. Azone itself is present in the oil phase of the emulsion, and the Azone/water partition coefficient of hydrocortisone was 331. Therefore, increasing Azone concentrations lowered the thermodynamic activity of hydrocortisone within the water phase of the emulsion, which correspondingly lowered the concentration gradient of hydrocortisone across the skin. Banerjee and Ritschel [168] reported on Azone's ability to enhance the permeability of vasopressin, a peptide drug compound, across the skin. Species differences were observed between the permeation enhancement across mouse (70 × enhancement) and rat (15 × enhancement) skin. When applied in vivo, vasopressin in the presence of Azone exerted its pharmacological effect in rats by significantly reducing urine volume and increasing urine osmolality. Other N-alkyl caprolactams similar to Azone have been studied for their ability to promote skin permeation [169]. Permeability enhancement with these N-alkyl caprolactams (methyl, propyl, hexyl, and dodecyl) was a function of donor vehicle polarity, permeant polarity, and enhancer concentration. More polar permeants appear to show the largest increases in permeation rates when formulated with these caprolactams.

Another group of investigators has recently reported on the effectiveness of cyclic monoterpenes as percutaneous absorption enhancers [170–172]. Although the effects of cyclic terpene gel formulations appear to be a result of a combination of effects owing to the presence of both a high concentration of alcohol in the formulation along with the enhancer, the inclusion of either d-limonene or l-menthol resulted in higher bioavailabilities of indomethacin and diclofenac sodium, respectively, than did Azone.

The use of fatty acids as topical absorption enhancers has also received considerable attention. Kurosaki and co-workers investigated the effectiveness of lipid dispersions of phosphatidylcholine or glycosylceramide in the enhancement of flufenamic acid permeation [173]. In an elegant series of experiments using rat abdominal skin, stratum corneum from hamster cheek pouch, and Silastic membrane, they demonstrated that dispersions containing either 20 μmol/ml of phosphatidylcholine or 18 μmol/ml of phosphatidylcholine with 2 μmol/ml of glycosylceramide enhanced the permeation of flufenamic acid in both rat skin and hamster stratum corneum. Dispersions containing either 40 μmol/ml or 60 μmol/ml did not enhance permeation, however. Interestingly, the permeation of flufenamic acid was not enhanced through Silastic membrane in the presence of the lipid dispersion at any concentration. This strongly suggests that the lipids in the formulation intereact with the lipids within the skin, thereby increasing the permeability of drug substances through this phase. Similar results were reported by Ogiso and Shintani [174] in their investigation of the enhancement capabilities of a series of fatty acids on propranolol permeability. In this case, the authors propose that a propranolol–fatty acid complex is formed that enhances propranolol's permeability through the lipids of the stratum corneum. They postulate that this complex must dissociate before propranolol can effectively traverse the tissues of the epidermis and dermis.

More traditional additives, such as ethanol, propylene glycol, and surfactants, have been employed to promote skin penetration. Frequently, ethanol and propylene glycol act as cosolvents in a formulation. Ethanol also acts directly on the skin by altering the conformation of the keratin fibrils within the stratum corneum, disrupting the crystalline lipid structure in the intercellular spaces, and by directly extracting lipids from the stratum corneum [175,176]. Propylene glycol may also act by disrupting the packing of the keratin fibrils [177]. It is rather clear that surfactants, particularly anionic surfactants, do penetrate the skin [178]. Anionic surfactants bind to skin proteins and promote swelling of the stratum corneum [179]. Cationic and nonionic surfactants exhibit less dramatic effects on stratum corneum and skin permeability. Regardless of their direct effects on the skin, however, the presence of surfactants in a topical formulation alters the thermodynamic activity of the drug. The resulting permeability through the skin is frequently a combination of an increased permeability owing to the direct effects on the stratum corneum and a decrease in activity gradient because of the solubilizing capability of the surfactant within the formulation [180].

2. *Systemic Bioavailability*

With a transdermal dosage form, the drug is intended to directly enter the systemic blood circulation. A reservoir of drug is applied to the skin, such that the input rate is slow and continuous, resulting in blood levels that eliminate the wide differences in maxima and minima experienced with oral administration. Drugs with short half-lives can be given by the transdermal route without frequent administration. Another advantage applies to drugs with high hepatic extraction ratios that can be given transdermally without a large loss of drug by first-pass metabolic effect. Consequently, the variable extent of absorption inherent with these types of drugs is minimized. Nevertheless, the transdermal route is not suitable for drugs that irritate or sensitize the skin, or for drugs that are not very potent or require a relatively large permeability rate that could not be attained across the skin barrier [181]. Flynn and Stewart [182] have described a relatively simple method to identify drug compounds that may show reasonable bioavailability from the transdermal route. By using a knowledge of the drug solubility and an estimate of its permeability through the skin from a measured octanol/water partition coefficient, the maximum amount of drug that could penetrate across the skin per day can be estimated. Comparing this amount with the known daily dose of the drug can be useful for rapidly identifying good candidate drug compounds for further investigation as transdermal drug products.

Nitroglycerin was one of the first drugs tested for transdermal delivery, primarily because its biopharmaceutic properties necessitate a nonoral route of delivery. It is potent, undergoes extensive first-pass metabolism, has a very short half-life of less than 20 min, and readily penetrates the skin [183,184]. A 2% nitroglycerin ointment has been available for over 30 years for angina pectoris. The topical administration of 2% ointment to the rhesus monkey indicated that the absolute bioavailability of nitroglycerin could be increased to 60% from the observed 2% for oral tablets and 30% for sublingual tablets [184]. The ointment dosage form provides therapeutic blood levels for approximately 8 h and is recommended for prophylactic protection from anginal attacks [185]. Fifteen milligrams of nitroglycerin, suspended in 1 in. of petrolatum ointment, is applied to various sites on the skin so that skin irritation and sensitization can be avoided. Because of its slow onset, however, the ointment dosage form is not recommended for acute anginal attacks.

The topical bioavailability of 2% nitroglycerin ointment has been questioned by various investigators [185–187]. When a 1-in. ribbon of ointment is spread over different areas, a potential difference in bioavailability can occur, even though 16 mg of drug is applied in each case. Sved et al. [185], using a simple crossover design, applied 16 mg (2% nitroglycerin) to three volunteers over 25 or 100 cm^2 of surface area. An additional volunteer was administered two different doses, each spread over 100 cm^2. Table 3 gives the results for plasma concentrations of nitroglycerin measured at 30–90 min for each application. Even though the applied dose was identical, plasma levels increased about twofold for the larger area of application. When the dose was doubled, but the surface area was held constant, the AUC between 30–90 min increased by 76%. These results, although conducted on only a few subjects, illustrate the importance of the relationship between area of application and the concentration of drug applied.

Table 3 Effect of Dose and Surface Area on the Bioavailability of Nitroglycerin Ointment in Volunteers (n = 4)

Treatment[a]	AUC (0–90 min; ng mL^{-1} min)
A	<0.2[b]
B	0.40
C	0.72

[a]A = 16 mg of nitroglycerin ointment (2%) spread over 25 cm^2; B = 16 mg of nitroglycerin ointment (2%) spread over 100 cm^2; C = 32 mg of nitroglycerin ointment (2%) spread over 100 cm^2.
[b]90-minute sample was below assay sensitivity, making calculations inaccurate.
Source: From Ref. 185.

In a more extensive study in which ten normal volunteers were used, plasma levels of nitroglycerin, heart rate, and blood pressure were evaluated as a function of area of application and dose [187]. Each subject received either a 1/2- or 1-in. ribbon of 2% nitroglycerin ointment applied over an area of 25 or 50 cm^2 of the chest. Ten plasma samples were assayed for drug over 360 min following application. Although inter- and intrasubject variation was large, statistical differences in plasma levels were observed for each dose when surface area was held constant. However, as shown in Table 4, and in opposition to the conclusion obtained from the Sved study [185], a change in surface area had no effect on AUC, time to peak, or peak concentration. Differences in application of the ointment were not well controlled. As a result, minor differences in thicknesses of the ointment spread over the skin, along with the relatively small doses that were applied over large and small areas, were considered the reason surface area had no effect on bioavailability.

Table 4 Comparison of Bioavailability Parameters Following Different Treatments of Nitroglycerin Ointment to Volunteers (n = 10)

Treatment[a]	AUC[b] (ng · mL^{-1} min)	C_{max}[c] (ng/mL)	t_{max}[d] (min)
A	552.5 (357.6)[b]	3.7 (1.4)	231.0 (125.0)
B	743.6 (545.5)	5.4 (4.6)	204.0 (121.7)
C	1729.7 (1250.8)	11.2 (9.4)	243.0 (132.2)
D	2276.7 (1942.7)	13.6 (8.8)	229.5 (112.7)

[a]A = ½ inch of nitroglycerin ointment spread over a 1¾ × 2¼ inch area (3.94 in.^{2}); B = ½ inch of nitroglycerin ointment spread over a 3½ × 2¼ inch area (7.88 in.^{2}); C = 1 inch of nitroglycerin ointment spread over a 1¾ × 2¼ inch area (3.94 in.^{2}); D = 1 inch of nitroglycerin ointment spread over a 3½ × 2¼ inch area (7.88 in.^{2}).
[b]Standard deviation.
[c]A versus C and B versus D are statistically different; whereas, A versus B and C versus D are statistically insignificant.
[d]A versus C, B versus D, A versus D, and C versus D are all statistically insignificant.
Source: From Ref. 187.

In an elegant series of experiments, Chiang and colleagues have characterized the permeation of minoxidil through excised sections of human cadaver skin from several different topical formulations [188–190]. Initially, minoxidil transport from a water–oil cream, an oil–water cream, and an ointment were studied in vitro using a finite dose technique and analysis scheme. The resulting data are shown in Fig. 14. Minoxidil was present in excess of its solubility in each of the formulations. The permeation from the water–oil cream was far superior to those from either of the other two formulations. The authors suggest that, since the differences in permeabilities are greatest at high minoxidil concentrations (increasing amounts of excess solid), that dissolution into the vehicle may play a role in minoxidil permeation. In a follow-up report, the permeation of minoxidil across human cadaver skin was studied from a suspension of minoxidil in an ointment dosage form and from a propylene glycol/ethanol/water minoxidil solution. Steady-state transport of minoxidil from the ointment was achieved after a relatively long time interval (6–8 h), whereas the flux of minoxidil from the solution increased monotonically throughout the duration of the experiment. The authors attribute this behavior to the evaporation of the solution vehicle resulting in a changing thermodynamic activity of the minoxidil over time. At short times (i.e., immediately following alcohol evaporation), it is likely that the minoxidil solution is supersaturated, providing a significantly larger driving force for permeation than that present within the initial solution or within the ointment. Further investigation of the effect of vehicle evaporation on minoxidil flux revealed that the precipitation of excess drug from solution with evaporation significantly reduced the flux across human cadaver skin. The flux increased systematically from 1, 2, and 3% solutions in the mixed propylene glycol/ethanol/water vehicle, yet as 5% minoxidil, the flux was significantly reduced. Careful examination of the solutions revealed that both the ethanol and water phases were subject to evaporation, and minoxidil at high concentration rapidly precipitated from the vehicle once evaporation was initiated. Again, the precipitation of minoxidil reduced the thermodynamic activity in the vehicle, thereby reducing the flux compared with the systems in which supersaturated conditions were likely to occur.

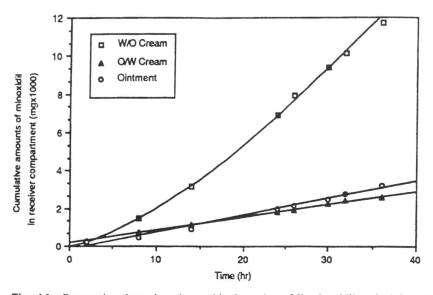

Fig. 14 Permeation through cadaver skin from three 2% minoxidil topical formulations.

Other investigators have also attempted to capitalize on the in situ formation of supersaturated systems to increase the bioavailability of several different drugs by formulating them as water-free microemulsions that imbibe water to form microemulsions on application to the skin [191–193]. The solubility of the drugs was observed to be lower in the water-containing microemulsion; therefore, transiently supersaturated systems were frequently created in situ. These microemulsion systems increased the pharmacological activity of the drugs compared with that observed following release from a transdermal matrix system. Although the direct effects of the components on drug penetration were uncharacterized, the use of self-emulsifying systems shows the potential for increasing the bioavailability of topically applied agents.

Many variables exist that can affect the bioavailability of ointments intended for transdermal delivery, such as surface area and thickness of the application, as well as the physicochemical parameters of the ointment. Given the multitude of parameters involved, most of which are difficult to control in a clinical setting, it is not surprising that systemic drug delivery through the intact skin has been developed more extensively with the use of polymer-controlled, drug delivery devices instead of delivery from an ointment [194–196].

3. *Liposomal Formulations*

The ability of fatty acids and phospholipids to act as absorption promoters indicates that liposomal delivery systems may be effective in the improvement of topical and systemic bioavailability from formulations applied to the skin. Although it is unlikely, because of their size, that liposomes would be absorbed intact across the skin, they may remain intact within the epidermis, resulting in a localized depot of active drug. One of the first reports by Mezei and Gulasekharam [197] indicated that the levels of triamcinolone acetonide in the dermis and epidermis were four- to fivefold higher when applied to the skin in a liposomal formulation, compared with control ointment. Also, systemic uptake was two- to threefold lower, which gives rise to fewer side effects. Similarly, liposomal cortisone penetrates 10- to 15-fold more efficiently than from an ointment [198]. Therapeutically, herpes lesions have been more effectively treated with liposomal interferon in hairless guinea pigs, when compared with either an aqueous solution or an emulsion [199]. A similar enhancement of activity has been seen in the therapeutic treatment of burn wounds with liposomal aminoglycosides [200]. The mechanism by which liposomes promote the penetration of drugs into the skin is not completely resolved, but it is clear that they are efficient, assisting the penetration of both hydrophobic and hydrophilic drugs into various strata of the skin.

4. *In Vitro–In Vivo Correlations*

Because of the ready availability of excised skin samples, either animal or human, much of the information on the performance of topical formulations has been gathered from in vitro diffusion experiments. As with any other in vitro system, the extrapolation of permeability data as an estimator of bioavailability is tenuous without further in vivo validation. This is of particular significance for skin-directed bioavailability where the ability of the drug to permeate through all of the layers of the skin is frequently inversely proportional to the activity of the drug within the skin itself. The use of in vitro systems to predict systemic bioavailability is often quite successful, however. Bronaugh and Franz [201] compared the permeability of benzoic acid, caffeine, and testosterone in each of three different vehicles (petrolatum, ethylene glycol/Carbopol 940 gel, and water/

Carbopol 940 gel) through excised human skin sections to the bioavailability measured in human volunteers. Because of experimental constraints, the data from the in vitro experiments were often not optimized for greatest in vitro performance, but rather, were selected to permit the most straightforward in vitro–in vivo comparisons. In vitro, the best predictor of permeability through the skin was the partition coefficient of the drug between the vehicle and the skin. When the percentage of each of the compounds transported through the skin sample was compared with the percentage excreted in the urine following topical application, good correlations were observed. In general, the in vitro permeabilities were slightly less than those observed in vivo, yet rank order correlations between in vitro and in vivo performance were quite good.

Another group of investigators [202] did not observe the same degree of in vitro–in vivo correlation when they compared the in vitro release of verapamil from a Carbopol 934 gel with the plasma levels of verapamil in rats following topical application of the gel. Surprisingly, the gel formulation that showed the most rapid verapamil release through a cellulose membrane into a phosphate buffer solution resulted in the lowest bioavailability in the rats. The in vitro performance of other gel formulations containing various solvents and putative absorption enhancers was also not easy to correlate with their in vivo performance. These results indicate that the experimental conditions required for the most optimal in vitro–in vivo correlations involve those that most closely mimic the in vivo case. The use of synthetic membranes in vitro limits the ability to detect changes induced in the stratum corneum that will affect drug permeation. In addition, since the skin is a multilaminate membrane, the use of a single membrane to predict in vivo performance often results in rather poor correlation with the actual in vivo response. Finally, even if more biologically relevant membranes, such as excised animal (rat, mouse, or other) skin, are used in the in vitro systems, they may or may not serve as good predictors of in vivo human performance.

E. Ophthalmic Bioavailability

Ophthalmologists prefer topical application to the eye as a method of treating eye disease, since systemic involvement is usually, but not always, minimal. For some drugs, such as anticholinesterase inhibitors and most cholinergic drugs, treatment of the eye by systemic routes would be impossible because of their toxicity. On the other hand, certain antibiotics, such as the cephalosporins and other synthetic penicillin derivatives, do not appreciably penetrate the eye; therefore, internal eye tissues can be treated only by the systemic route.

Although the proximity of eye tissues clearly favors topical instillation, absorption across the cornea is severely limited by anatomical and physiological constraints. The narrow pH range of the eye, rapid drainage and facilitated elimination by blinking, induced tearing from chemical or mechanical stimulation, and the small surface area available for absorption, all contribute to relatively poor ocular bioavailability (i.e., 2–10% of the applied dose) [203].

The albino rabbit has been used over the years to determine whether significant corneal penetration has occurred for a particular drug and also to determine whether formulations differ in bioavailability. The rabbit has been chosen over other species for the testing of ophthalmic products because it is sensitive to changes in physicochemical and formulation differences and because historically, it has been an adequate model for ocular toxicology.

Although the rabbit eye is anatomically different from the human eye relative to tear fluid dynamics, the blinking rate, and the presence of a nictitating membrane [204], the net effect of these differences on ocular pharmacokinetics has not been very significant. This is reasoned from the results of a study by Leibowitz et al. [205], in which 0.05 ml of 1% prednisolone acetate was administered to both rabbit and human eyes. Aqueous humor was obtained from human eyes of patients undergoing ocular surgery and assayed for drug. Drug was instilled at various times before surgery so that enough time intervals could be represented in the total patient population. Figure 15 shows a comparison of drug levels obtained from each species with time. With the exception that the extent of absorption appears greater for the rabbit than for humans, the aqueous humor–time curves for the rabbit and human eye show similar rates of absorption and elimination based on a similar upslope, t_{max}, and downslope for each curve.

Although ocular penetration studies have been reported for anesthetics, antibiotics, antibacterials, anti-inflammatory agents, antivirals, and autonomic drugs [206], these preparations were made in laboratory batches. In addition, they usually differed from commercial preparations in either pH, tonicity, buffering capacity, or in the specific adjuvants that were added. Commercial preparations were not often compared from production batches because radioactive tracer methodology was required to analyze the aqueous humor samples, which necessitated special preparation of a laboratory batch.

1. *Ophthalmic Suspensions*

Aqueous suspensions of lipophilic steroids were developed for the eye primarily because water-soluble analogues would not adequately penetrate the cornea to reach therapeutic levels within the eye. The bioavailability of ophthalmic suspensions is influenced primarily by the viscosity of the vehicle and the particle size of the suspended drug particles. Polymers, such as cellulosic derivatives, polyvinyl alcohol, and polyvinylpyrrolidone, have been used as vehicles to impart adequate viscosity to retard settling of particles and also to provide comfort. After many years of commercial use, investigators also learned that polymers retard the drainage rate of the instilled drop from the eye and, therefore, promote a longer retention time of the drug on the cornea.

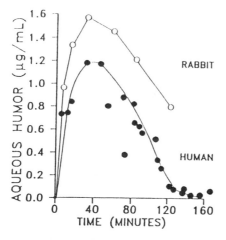

Fig. 15 A comparison of tritiated prednisolone acetate concentration in the aqueous humor of eyes over time following instillation of 50 µl of a 1% suspension.

The particle size of suspended drugs is usually below 10 μm to ensure that no abrasion of the cornea occurs. Particle size is also important because of its relation to the dissolution rate as well as retention within the conjunctival sac. Particles either dissolve or are expelled out of the eye at the lid margin or at the inner canthus. The time required for dissolution and corneal absorption must be less than the residence time of the drug in the conjunctival sac to take advantage of the retained particles. The saturated solution of a suspension likely provides the initial response, whereas the retained particles maintain the response as particles dissolve and drug is absorbed.

Sieg and Robinson [207] studied the bioavailability of fluometholone as a 0.1% aqueous suspension and ointment in the rabbit eye and compared the aqueous humor levels of drug representing the suspension with an aqueous humor–time curve generated from a saturated solution of the same drug. The aqueous humor–time AUC for the saturated solution was approximately 22% of the AUC determined from the suspension that contained the same concentration of steroid in solution. Although 78% of the AUC presumably comes from dissolution and subsequent absorption of the retained particles, only 2.4% of the fluometholone present in the saturated solution was responsible for 22% of the total AUC. However, the dissolution rate of the particles in relation to their residence time has the most significant effect on the rate and extent of ocular absorption. Hui and Robinson [208] studied the absorption of a 0.4% suspension of fluometholone, in addition to the 0.05 and 0.1% concentrations previously studied by Sieg and Robinson. Although no statistically significant differences in aqueous humor drug levels were found for the 0.05 and 0.1% suspensions, the 0.4% suspension resulted in aqueous humor levels in excess of either of the other two suspensions. This is initially somewhat surprising, since the free-drug concentration in solution is the same, regardless of the suspension concentration. The increased bioavailability of the 0.4% suspension is best explained by the realization that because of the higher particulate content of this suspension, a greater mass of drug remains in the cul-de-sac following drainage of the applied volume. These remaining particles then dissolve in the tear fluids and provide an additional driving force for fluometholone transport across the cornea into the aqueous humor. Even though the final suspension concentration would be limited by drug cost, formulation considerations, and the onset of side effects from the systemic absorption of the excess drug, it seems practical to attempt to administer a suspension with as high a concentration of drug as possible, rather than to administer a suspension for which the concentration is not much greater than that of a saturated solution. As expected, the bioavailability of a fluometholone suspension was increased as the particle size of the suspension was decreased. The authors also developed a pharmacokinetic model capable of predicting aqueous humor drug levels following fluometholone suspension administration. With this model, 2–6 μm was determined to be a reasonable size for these drug particles for optimal bioavailability using conventional particle size reduction techniques.

In a study of Schoenwald and Stewart [209], three suspensions of 0.1% [^{3}H]dexamethasone were prepared, with mean particle sizes of 5.75, 11.5, and 22.0 μm. After instilling each preparation into the right eye of rabbits, their aqueous humor and corneal levels were measured over 5 h. The results showed a statistically significant rank-order correlation between increasing blood levels and decreasing particle size. The particle size must be small enough to prevent corneal abrasion. However, even mild irritation can induce lacrimation and facilitate drug removal. If the particle size is too small, then the possibility exists that they may be swept away by drainage.

This latter phenomenon was studied by Sieg and Triplett [210] by instilling 3% suspensions of radiolabeled tracer microspheres to rabbit eyes. Figure 16 gives the results and shows the excellent retention of either 25- or 50-μl doses containing 25-μm particles. For a smaller particle size of 3 μm, retention was greater for the 25-μl than the 50-μl dose. For the two dosing volumes of 25 and 50 μl there was a proportional relation with the percentage retained, which was 30 and 70% for each dosing volume, respectively. The 25-μm particles were well retained in the conjunctival sac, but when the 3-μm–particle size was tested, retention was dependent on the volume instilled.

Lack of therapeutic efficacy when using a suspension may occur simply because the patient has not followed instructions and shaken the bottle thoroughly. Apt et al. [211] reported that, in a study of 100 patients who were instructed to shake a steroid suspension just before instilling, 63 patients completely ignored the instructions. However, it was more surprising to learn that after shaking the bottle as many as 40 times, one product dispensed 90% of the labeled amount, but three other products yielded only 82, 71, and 22% of label. The authors concluded that manufacturers should state on the label the number of times the bottle must be shaken to fully resuspend the particles.

2. Ophthalmic Ointments

Ophthalmic ointments are, in general, somewhat softer than dermatological ointments. At the temperature of the eye, ophthalmic ointments do not liquefy, but readily soften and, with blinking action or eyeball movement, continuously spread throughout the conjunctival sac. This action promotes mixing and uptake by the tears so that absorption into the cornea can occur. In contrast, rigid petrolatum ointment might be ineffective, since the shearing action from blinking would not create a new surface from which drug could readily partition into tears. The factors that determine the bioavailability of ophthalmic drugs from ointment vehicles are ocular contact time, diffusion through the

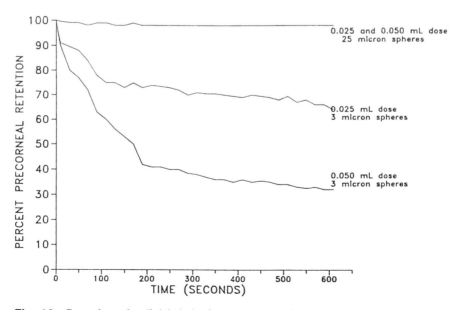

Fig. 16 Retention of radiolabeled microspheres applied to the conjunctival sac of rabbit eyes as a function of particle size and dose.

bulk of the ointment, effective concentration of drug at the cornea, and shear-facilitated release.

With any ophthalmic preparation, contact time is of primary importance. If the drug is not well retained in the conjunctival sac, significant drug absorption cannot take place. In general, 50% of an ointment instilled in the eye is retained for 30 min, whereas the same percentage of a viscous solution is retained for only 1–2 min. Although ointments provide a stable and nonirritating environment for ophthalmic drugs, their ability to increase contact time relative to viscous solutions prompted development of the ophthalmic ointment form for nighttime use when around-the-clock treatment was important.

Hanna and co-workers [212,213] compared the ocular bioavailability of commercial chloramphenicol solutions and ointments in both rabbit and human eyes. Chloramphenicol, a lipophilic compound that penetrates the cornea at relatively high rates, was assayed in various eye tissues by gas–liquid chromatography (GLC), using a nitrogen detector. Figure 17 shows the aqueous humor profiles following application of 50 μl of 1% chloramphenicol ointment in the rabbit eye. The peak concentrations range from 26 to 38 μg/ml at 2 h; however, the AUCs are nearly identical for ointment products A–C [212]. Hanna et al. [213] compared drop versus ointment therapy for 1% chloramphenicol in patients awaiting cataract surgery. They found that the ointment prolonged the drug concentration in aqueous humor above the minimum effective concentration for 2–4 h. In opposition to these results, the solution had to be instilled every 15 min for a total of 13 doses to attain comparable drug levels, which rapidly fell when the instillations were discontinued.

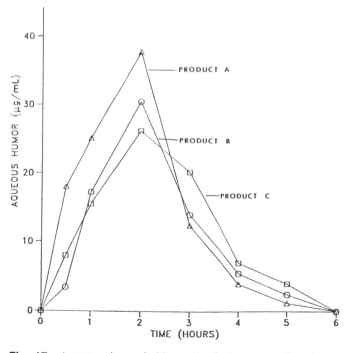

Fig. 17 A comparison of chloramphenicol concentrations in aqueous humor of the rabbit eye following application of 1% commercial ointments.

In a series of reports, Robinson and co-workers [214–216] studied the release of pilocarpine from water–oil emulsion systems and a suspension system in an attempt to identify those variables responsible for improved bioavailability. Table 5 expresses their AUC results between 0 and 30 min. Although the AUCs do not represent a complete profile, by 30 min most of the drug had been absorbed, and the differences are great enough to identify formulation variables that can influence bioavailability. The aqueous solution showed the poorest bioavailability. Although the aqueous solution readily mixes with tears, it is drained away from the eye too quickly for sufficient drug to be absorbed. For the water–oil emulsion ointments, the emulsifying efficiency inversely correlated with increased bioavailability. In Table 5, where a reduced level of water was used in the composition of the emulsion, the bioavailability increased because the effective concentration of pilocarpine increased. When a surfactant was added to stabilize the emulsion, the force of blinking or of eyeball movement had a reduced effect on rupturing the emulsion and releasing the drug. As a consequence, bioavailability was reduced compared with the same preparation without the emulsifying agent.

The ointment containing suspended particles of pilocarpine without the presence of water was less bioavailable than two of the emulsion systems. For the suspended system, the diffusional flux through the bulk gel was essentially zero because of the insolubility of pilocarpine in petrolatum. Nevertheless, one might expect that the effective concentration of surface particles, coupled with the high aqueous solubility of the drug in tears, would be sufficient to generate the highest aqueous humor levels. The authors concluded that the particles are coated with a film of petrolatum such that partitioning into tear fluids is neither rapid nor extensive.

In a study using 0.1% fluorometholone [207] in a suspension or an ointment, the ointment consisted of suspended particles, which, in contrast with pilocarpine, were partially soluble in the petrolatum vehicle. With this formulation, both bulk diffusion and shear-facilitated release contributed to the amount of fluorometholone available for corneal penetration.

Shrewsbury et al. [217] and Lee et al. [218] both reported on the disposition of cromolyn sodium (sodium cromoglicate) from various vehicles. Lee et al. studied a 2% aqueous solution or 4% cromolyn sodium in a hypoallergenic, acetylated lanolin base; a semisolid, oleaginous base (polyethylene and mineral oil); and a water-soluble, polyvinyl alcohol base. The water-soluble base was not as effective in prolonging ocular retention as were the two oil-based formulations. Shrewsbury and colleagues compared

Table 5 Effect of Ointment Formulation Variables on Aqueous Humor Levels of Pilocarpine (10^{-2}M) Following Instillation of 25 mg or 25 μl

Treatment	AUC (μg mL^{-1} min; 0–90 min)
1. Solution	22.5
2. Absorption base/liquid pet./25% H$_2$O	27.9
3. Absorption base/liquid pet./5% H$_2$O	40.5
4. Petrolatum base	53.3
5. Petrolatum base/surfactant/5% H$_2$O	61.5
6. Petrolatum base/5% H$_2$O	81.3

Source: From Ref. 216.

Lee's acetylated lanolin formulation to two oily suspensions composed of either 2 or 4% cromolyn sodium in Plastibase 5W (polyethylene and mineral oil). The levels of cromolyn sodium in tears, cornea, conjunctiva, aqueous humor, and iris–ciliary body were greatest at all time points following the administration of the acetylated lanolin base. The authors suggest that this is due to rapid release of the drug from the base in the eye and the limited clearance of the dosage form from the corneal surface. The oily suspensions, on the other hand, did not allow rapid release of the drug and, although slower than the aqueous solution, were rapidly cleared from the eye.

Mosteller and co-workers [219] have also reported the success of 10% cyclosporine incorporated in a lanolin petrolatum vehicle in producing elevated corneal cyclosporine levels with negligible aqueous humor and serum levels. This type of disposition is necessary for the successful ocular use of cyclosporin in corneal transplants and in intraocular inflammation unresponsive to corticosteroid treatment. Cyclosporine, a hydrophobic peptide, partitions readily out of the base and appears to concentrate in the corneal epithelium owing to its inability to traverse the hydrophilic stromal layer.

Robinson and co-workers [220] studied viscosity, independently of other parameters, and concluded that when either methylcellulose or polyvinyl alcohol was used as a vehicle at equal viscosities, there was no difference in the improvement of pilocarpine nitrate bioavailability in the rabbit eye. The increase in viscosity because of the presence of the polymer retards drainage and promotes contact time with the cornea. Hydrophilic drugs show slightly greater improvement in ocular bioavailability than lipophilic drugs when contact time of the drug with the cornea is increased. This occurs because the epithelial layer imparts a greater diffusional resistance to absorption for hydrophilic drugs. Robinson [220] showed that, when methylcellulose was used to increase viscosity from 1 to 15 cP, the rate of drainage from the eye was reduced by a factor of three. By increasing the viscosity from 15 to 100 cP another threefold reduction in drainage occurs; however, the drops become sticky and uncomfortable to use. Also, filter sterilization and mixing are made more difficult in the manufacture of the product.

3. *Liposomes*

Liposomal suspensions of several hydrophilic and hydrophobic drugs have been investigated for their ability to increase the ocular tissue drug concentrations. Since it is unlikely that liposomes are absorbed intact across the cornea, a liposomal formulation likely serves as a reservoir for drug at the corneal surface. This type of behavior was observed by Taniguchi et al. [221] in their investigation of ocular corticosteroid bioavailability from liposomal formulations. When using liposomes prepared from egg yolk lecithin, the investigators found that dexamethasone and dexamethasone palmitate liposomal formulations were less bioavailable than their equivalent aqueous suspensions. Dexamethasone valerate, in contrast, showed a much greater bioavailability (measured as dexamethasone plus dexamethasone valerate) following its administration in a liposomal vehicle. Previous in vitro-release studies had shown that no measurable levels of free dexamethasone palmitate were present in the liposomal formulation, nor was any entrapped dexamethasone palmitate released from the liposomes. It is not surprising, therefore, that dexamethasone palmitate in a lipsomal formulation shows little promise as an ocular delivery system. Similarly, the free dexamethasone concentration in the liposomal vehicle is far below the drug's saturated solubility; thus, it is not unexpected that a suspension formulation outperforms the liposomal formulation. With dexamethasone valerate, however, although more than 99% of the drug is incorporated into the liposomes, drug release from the liposomes is also rapid. Once the liposomal formulation is instilled into the eye, equilibration with the tear fluids takes place, resulting in a dexamethasone valerate concentration near that of the free-drug concentration in the formulation. As the dexamethasone valerate diffuses into the cornea and is hydrolyzed to dexamethasone, more dexamethasone valerate is released from the liposomes to reestablish the concentration equilibrium. As long as the liposomes remain at the corneal surface, this depot of drug allows greater concentrations of dexamethasone to build up in the ocular tissues.

4. *Nanoparticles*

Wood et al. [222] studied the disposition of radiolabeled polyhexyl-2-cyanoacrylate nanoparticles following ocular administration. They found that the nanoparticles were rapidly cleared from the eye, and approximately 1% of the instilled dose adhered to the corneal or conjunctival surfaces. The nanoparticles also biodegraded rapidly in the tear fluids. Since some of the nanoparticles adhered to the corneal surface, a further study was carried out by Li et al. [223] to investigate the bioavailability of progesterone associated with polybutylcyanoacrylate nanoparticles administered ophthalmically. When compared with a control aqueous progesterone solution, the bioavailability of nanoparticulate progesterone was less in the cornea, conjunctiva, and aqueous humor. These results indicate that the rapid clearance of the nanoparticles from the eye caused this dosage form to behave in a manner similar to a simple ophthalmic suspension. In addition, to this formulation's disadvantage, progesterone is highly associated with the nanoparticles; consequently, the free-drug concentration in the tear fluids is quite low and likely to be significantly less than a concentrated aqueous solution of the drug. Therefore, the low bioavailability can be explained by both a low free-drug concentration and a short retention time. These results indicate that it is necessary to increase the retention time of a nanoparticle ophthalmic formulation for it to enhance the bioavailability of any drug substance.

REFERENCES

1. A. S. Noyes and W. R. Whitney, *J. Am. Chem. Soc.*, 19:930 (1897).
2. A. S. Noyes and W. R. Whitney, *Z. Phys. Chem.*, 23:689 (1897).
3. W. Nernst, *Z. Physik. Chem. (Leipzig)*, 47:52 (1904).
4. W. Hixson and J. H. Crowell, *Ind. Eng. Chem.*, 23:93 (1931).
5. E. L. Parrott, D. E. Wurster, and T. Higuchi, *J. Am. Pharm. Assoc. Sci. Ed.*, 44:269 (1955).
6. P. J. Niebergall and J. E. Goyan, *J. Pharm. Sci.*, 52:29 (1963).
7. P. J. Niebergall and J. E. Goyan, *J. Pharm. Sci.*, 52:236 (1963).
8. W. L. Higuchi and E. N. Hiestand, *J. Pharm. Sci.*, 52:67 (1963).
9. W. L. Higuchi, E. L. Rowe, and E. N. Hiestand, *J. Pharm. Sci.*, 52:162 (1963).
10. J. G. Wagner, *Biopharmaceutics and Relevant Pharmacokinetics*, Drug Intell. Pub., Hamilton, IL, 1971, pp. 107–108.
11. P. Potishiri and J. T. Carstensen, *J. Pharm. Sci.*, 52:1468 (1973).
12. J. W. Mauger and S. A. Howard, *J. Pharm. Sci.*, 65:1042 (1976).
13. J. W. Mauger, S. A. Howard, and K. Amin, *J. Pharm. Sci.*, 72:190 (1983).
14. A. E. Nielsen, *J. Phys. Chem.* 65:46 (1961).
15. J. T. Carstensen and M. N. Musa, *J. Pharm. Sci.*, 61:223 (1972).
16. L. Z. Benet, in *Dissolution Technology* (L. J. Leeson and J. T. Carstensen, eds.), American Pharmaceutical Association, Washington, DC, 1974, pp. 47–50.

17. D. Brooke, *J. Pharm. Sci.*, 62:795 (1973).
18. P. Veng-Pedersen, and K. F. Brown, *J. Pharm. Sci.*, 64:1192 (1975).
19. P. Veng-Pedersen and K. F. Brown, *J. Pharm. Sci.*, 65:1437 (1976).
20. P. Veng-Pedersen and K. F. Brown, *J. Pharm. Sci.*, 64:1442 (1976).
21. P. Veng-Pedersen, *J. Pharm. Sci.*, 66:761 (1977).
22. P. Veng-Pedersen and K. F. Brown, *J. Pharm. Sci.*, 66:1436 (1977).
23. P. Veng-Pedersen and K. F. Brown, *J. Pharm. Sci.*, 64:1981 (1975).
24. I. Matsuura, *Yakugaku Zasshi*, 102:264 (1982).
25. I. Matsuura, *Yakugaku Zasshi*, 102:678 (1982).
26. D. E. Wurster and P. W. Taylor, *J. Pharm. Sci.*, 54:169 (1965).
27. D. E. Wurster and P. W. Taylor, *J. Pharm. Sci.*, 54:170 (1965).
28. D. E. Wurster and P. W. Taylor, *J. Pharm. Sci.*, 54:1654 (1965).
29. D. E. Wurster and D. O. Kildsig, *J. Pharm. Sci.*, 54:1491 (1965).
30. J. Piccolo and R. Tawashi, *J. Pharm. Sci.*, 59:56 (1970).
31. J. Piccolo and R. Tawashi, *J. Pharm. Sci.*, 60:59 (1971).
32. J. Piccolo and R. Tawashi, *J. Pharm. Sci.*, 60:1818 (1971).
33. W. I. Higuchi, S. Prakongpan, and F.-D. Young, *J. Pharm. Sci.*, 62:945 (1973).
34. S. L. Gupta, W. I. Higuchi, and N. F. H. Ho, *J. Pharm. Sci.*, 74:1172 (1985).
35. S. L. Gupta, W. I. Higuchi, and N. F. H. Ho, *J. Pharm. Sci.*, 74:1178 (1985).
36. W.-H. Wong, Ph.D. thesis, University of Iowa, Iowa City, IA 1982
37. A. P. Lötter, D. R. Flanagan, N. R. Palepu, and J. K. Guillory, *Pharm. Technol.*, 7:56 (1983).
38. T. Bates, H. Rosenberg, and A. Tembo, *J. Pharm. Sci.*, 62:2057 (1973).
39. S. A. Howard, J. W. Mauger, and L. Phusanti, *J. Pharm. Sci.*, 66:557 (1977).
40. J. W. Mauger, S. A. Howard, and K. Amin, *J. Pharm. Sci.*, 72:190 (1983).
41. A. C. Shah, C. B. Peot, and J. F. Ochs, *J. Pharm. Sci.*, 62:671 (1973).
42. W. I. Higuchi, and T. Higuchi, *J. Am. Pharm. Assoc. Sci. Ed.*, 49:589 (1960).
43. A. H. Goldberg, W. I. Higuchi, N. F. H. Ho, and G. Zografi, *J. Pharm. Sci.*, 56:1432 (1967).
44. A.-H. Ghanem, W. I. Higuchi, and A. P. Simonelli, *J. Pharm. Sci.*, 58:165 (1969).
45. G. Levy, and J. A. Procknal, *J. Pharm. Sci.*, 53:656 (1964).
46. J. R. Rapin, Y. Pourcelot, and P. Lespinasse, in *Topics in Pharmaceutical Sciences* (D. D. Breimer, and P. Speiser, eds.), Elsevier/North-Holland Biomedical Press, Amsterdam, 1981, pp. 217–229.
47. B. E. Cabana, in *Towards Better Safety of Drugs and Pharmaceutical Products* (D. D. Breimer, ed.), Elsevier/North Holland Biomedical Press, Amsterdam, 1977, pp. 153–168.
48. B. E. Cabana, in *Controlled Drug Bioavailability*, Vol. 2 (V. F. Smolen and L. A. Ball, eds.), Wiley-Interscience, New York, 1985, pp. 91–111.
49. U. S. Food and Drug Administration, Bioavailability/bioequivalence regulations, *Fed. Reg.*, 45(5):1634 (1977).
50. T. R. Bates, D. A. Lambert, and W. H. Johns, *J. Pharm. Sci.*, 58:1468 (1969).
51. A. Pilbrant, P. O. Glenne, A. Sundwall, J. Vessman, and M. Wretlind, *Acta Pharmacol. Toxicol.* [Suppl.], 40:7 (1977).
52. J. D. Strum, J. L. Colaizzi, T. J. Goehl, J. M. Jaffe, W. H. Pitlick, V. P. Shah, and R. I. Poust, *J. Pharm. Sci.*, 67:1399 (1978).
53. L. K. Mathur, J. M. Jaffee, R. I. Poust, H. Barry, III, T. J. Goehl, V. P. Shah, and J. L. Colaizzi, *J. Pharm. Sci.*, 68:699 (1979).
54. M. E. Dowty and J. R. Robinson, in *Drug Delivery to the Oral Mucosa* (J. G. Hardy, S. S. Davis,
55. M. Gibaldi and D. Perrier, *Pharmacokinetics*, 2nd ed., Marcel Dekker, New York, 1982, pp. 145–198.
56. K. K. H. Chan, and M. Gibaldi, *J. Pharm. Sci.*, 74:388 (1985).

57. H. G. Boxenbaum, S. Riegelman, and Elashoff, R. M. J. Pharmacokinet. Biopharm., 2, 123 (1974).
58. J. G. Wagner, *J. Pharm. Sci.*, 72:838 (1983).
59. D. W. Osborne, *Pharm. Manuf.* 3:41 (1986).
60. Y. W. Chien, *Novel Drug Delivery Systems*, Marcel Dekker, New York, 1982, pp. 149–217.
61. B. W. Barry, *Dermatological Formulations*, Marcel Dekker, New York, 1983, pp. 49–126.
62. G. L. Flynn, in *Modern Pharmaceutics*, Vol. 7 (G. S. Banker, and C. T. Rhodes, eds.), Marcel Dekker, New York, 1979, pp. 263–327.
63. G. L. Flynn, in *Percutaneous Absorption: Mechanisms—Methodology—Drug Delivery* (R. L. Bronaugh and H. I. Maibach, eds.), Marcel Dekker, New York, 1985, pp. 17–42.
64. G. P. Kushla and J. L. Zatz, *Int. J. Pharm.*, 71:167 (1991).
65. D. E. Wurster and S. F. Kramer, *J. Pharm. Sci.*, 50:288 (1961).
66. D. E. Wurster and R. Munies, *J. Pharm. Sci.*, 54:554 (1965).
67. M. Amin, Ph.D. thesis, University of Wisconsin, Madison, WI, 1967.
68. J. A. Ostrenga, Ph.D. thesis, University of Wisconsin, Madison, WI, 1967.
69. C. R. Behl, et al., *J. Invest. Dermatol.*, 75:346 (1980).
70. C. R. Behl and M. Barrett, *J. Pharm. Sci.*, 70:1212 (1981).
71. C. R. Behl, A. A. El-Sayed, and G. L. Flynn, *J. Pharm. Sci.*, 72:79 (1983).
72. I. H. Blank, in *Percutaneous Absorption: Mechanisms—Methodology—Drug Delivery* (R. L. Bronaugh and H. I. Maibach, eds.), Marcel Dekker, New York, 1985, pp. 97–106.
73. R. C. Wester, and H. I. Maibach, in *Percutaneous Absorption: Mechanisms—Methodology—Drug Delivery* (R. L. Bronaugh and H. I. Maibach, eds.), Marcel Dekker, New York, 1985, pp. 231–242.
74. D. E. Wurster, Curr. Prob. Dermatol., 7:156 (1978).
75. T. Higuchi, *J. Soc. Cosmet. Chem.*, 11:85 (1960).
76. T. Higuchi, *J. Pharm. Sci.*, 50:874 (1961).
77. W. I. Higuchi, *J. Pharm. Sci.*, 51:802 (1962).
78. B. J. Poulsen and G. L. Flynn, in *Percutaneous Absorption: Mechanisms—Methodology—Drug Delivery* (R. L. Bronaugh and H. I. Maibach, eds.), Marcel Dekker, New York, 1985, pp. 431–459.
79. J. Ostrenga, J. Halblian, B. Poulsen, B. Ferrell, N. Mueller, and S. Shastri, *J. Invest. Dermatol.*, 56:392 (1971).
80. B. J. Poulsen, *Br. J. Dermatol.*, 82:49 (Suppl. 6) (1970).
81. M. F. Coldman, B. J. Poulsen, and T. Higuchi, *J. Pharm. Sci.*, 58:1098 (1969).
82. J. Ostrenga, C. Steinmetz, and B. Poulson, *J. Pharm. Sci.*, 60:1175 (1971).
83. K. S. E. Su, J. F. Quay, K. M. Campanale, and J. F. Stucky, *J. Pharmacol. Exp. Ther.*, 147:376 (1965).
84. V. H. Guerrini, P. B. English, L. J. Filippich, J. Schneider, and D. W. A. Bourne, *Am. J. Vet. Res.*, 47:2057 (1986).
85. P. L. Toutain, M. Alvinerie, P. Fayolle, and Y. Ruckebusch, *J. Pharmacol. Exp. Ther.*, 236:794 (1985).
86. S. Benita, D. Friedman, and M. Weinstock, *J. Pharm. Pharmacol.*, 38:653 (1986).
87. W. J. Martone, W. W. Williams, M. L. Mortensen, R. P. Gaynes, J. W. White, V. Lorch, M. D. Murphy, S. N. Sinha, D. J. Frank, N. Kismetatos, C. J. Bodenstein, and R. J. Roberts, *Pediatrics*, 78:591 (1986).
88. J. L. Pedraz, B. Calvo, A. Bortolotti, A. Celardo, and M. Bonati, *J. Pharm. Pharmacol.*, 41:415 (1988).
89. M. Bonati, *Dev. Pharmacol. Ther.*, 16:13 (1991).
90. R. Perez-Soler, G. Lopez-Berestein, M. Jahns, K. Wright, and L. P. Kasi, *Int. J. Nucl. Med. Biol.*, 12, 261 (1985).
91. M. P. Osborne, V. J. Richardson, K. Jeyasingh, and B. E. Ryman, *Int. J. Nucl. Med. Biol.*, 6:75 (1979).

92. H. Sasaki, T. Kakutani, M. Hashida, and H. Sezaki, *J. Pharm. Pharmacol.*, 37:461 (1984).

93. R. W. Stevenson, H. M. Patel, J. A. Parsons, and B. E. Ryman, *Diabetologia*, 19:317 (1980).

94. R. W. Stevenson, H. M. Patel, J. A. Parsons, and B. E. Ryman, Diabetes, 31:506 (1982).

95. V. Rovei, M. Mitchard, M. S. Benedetti, and M. J. Kendall, *Int. J. Clin. Pharmacol. Ther. Toxicol.*, 22:56 (1984).

96. P. J. Sirois, G. L. Amidon, J. H. Meyer, J. Doty, and J. B. Dressman, *Am. J. Physiol.*, 258:G65 (1990).

97. M. M. Soci and E. L. Parrott, *J. Pharm. Sci.*, 69:403 (1980).

98. H. O. Alpar, and J. A. Hersey, *Il Farmaco*, 34:532 (1978).

99. H. Rollag, Jr., T. Midtvedt, and S. Wetterhus, *Acta Paediatr. Scand.*, 64:421 (1975).

100. T. Bergan, B. P. Berdal, and V. Halm, *Acta Pharmacol. Toxicol.*, 38:308 (1976).

101. J. A. Wada, A. S. Troupin, P. Friel, R. Remick, K. Leal, and J. Pearlman, *Epilepsia*, 19:251 (1978).

102. D. Bloomer, L. L. Dupuis, D. MacGregor, and S. J. Soldin, *Clin Pharm.*, 6:646 (1987).

103. P. J. Pentikainer, P. J. Neuvonen, and S. M. Elfving, *Eur. J. Clin. Pharmacol.*, 9:213 (1975).

104. L. Sansom, W. J. O'Reilly, C. W. Wiseman, L. M. Stern, and J. Derham, *Med. J. Aust.*, 2:593 (1975).

105. G. A. Greco, E. L. Moss, Jr., and E. J. Foley, *Antibiot. Ann.*, 7:553 (1959–1960).

106. M. Kraml, J. Dubuc, and D. Beall, *Can J. Biochem. Physiol.*, 40:1449 (1962).

107. P. Kabasakalian, M. Katz, B. Rosenkrantz, and E. Tounley, *J. Pharm. Sci.*, 59:595 (1970).

108. D. Shinkuma, Hamaguchi, Y. Yamanaka, N. Mizuno, and N. Yata, *Chem. Pharm. Bull.*, 33:4989.

109. O. M. O. Al-Hammanu, and J. H. Richards, *J. Acta Helv.*, 58:237 (1983).

110. I. Steiner, T. Prey, F. Gschnait, J. Washuttl, and Greiter, *Dermatol. Res.*, 259:299 (1977).

111. J. Kreuter, and T. Higuchi, *J. Pharm. Sci.*, 68:451 (1979).

112. L. S. Abrams, H. S. Weintraub, J. E. Patrick, and J. L. McGuire, *J. Pharm. Sci.*, 67:1287 (1978).

113. F. L. S. Tse, and P. G. Welling, *J. Pharm. Sci.*, 66:1751 (1977).

114. C. M. Ginsburg, G. H. McCracken, Jr., and K. Olsen, *Antimicrob. Agents Chemother.*, 23:787 (1983).

115. P. J. Carrigan, and T. R. Bates, *J. Pharm. Sci.*, 62:1476 (1973).

116. P. J. Carrigan, Ph.D. thesis, University of Connecticut, Storrs, CT, 1974.

117. T. R. Bates, and J. A. Sequeira, *J. Pharm. Sci.*, 64:793 (1975).

118. S. Chakrabarti, and F. M. Belpaire, *J. Pharm. Sci.*, 30:330 (1978).

119. A. Johnston, J. T. Marsden, K. K. Hla, J. A. Henry, and D. W. Holt, *Br. J. Clin. Pharmacol.*, 21:331 (1986).

120. W. A. Ritschel, G. B. Ritschel, A. Sabouni, D. Wolochuk, and T. Schroeder, *Methods Find. Exp. Clin. Pharmacol.*, 11:281 (1989).

121. J. Drewe, R. Meier, J. Vonderscher, D. Kiss, U. Posanski, T. Kissel, and K. Gyr, *Br. J. Clin. Pharmacol.*, 34:60 (1992).

122. R. Wassef, Z. Cohen, and B. Langer, *Dis. Colon Rectum*, 28:908 (1985).

123. G. G. Liversidge, J. Dent, and W. M. Eickhoff, *Pharm. Res.*, 6:44 (1989).

124. P. Jani, G. W. Halbert, J. Langridge, and A. T. Florence, *J. Pharm. Pharmacol.*, 41:809 (1989).

125. P. Jani, G. W. Halbert, J. Langridge, and A. T. Florence, *J. Pharm Pharmacol.*, 42:821 (1990).

126. M. Aprahamian, C. Michel, W. Humbert, J.-P. Devissaguet, and C. Damge, *Biol. Cell*, 61:69 (1987).

127. H. Fukui, M. Murakami, H. Yoshikawa, and S. Muranishi, *J. Pharmacobiodyn.*, 10:236 (1987).

128. C. Graffner, Z. Wagner, M.-I. Nilsson, and E. Widerlov, *Pharm. Res.*, 7:54 (1990).

129. G. Dapergolas, and G. Gregoriadis, *Lancet* 2:824 (1976).

130. H. M. Patel, and B. E. Ryman, *FEBS Lett.*, 62:60 (1976).

131. M. Ueno, in *Liposomes as Drug Carriers* (G. Gregoriadis, ed.), J. W. Wiley, New York, 1988, pp. 609–619.

132. C. Hirage, F. Ishii, and Y. Ichikawa, *J. Jpn. Assoc. Infect. Dis.*, 63:1308 (1989).

133. R. R. C. New, R. D. G. Theakston, D. Zumbuehl, D. Iddon, and J. Friend, *N. Engl. J. Med.*, 311:56 (1984).

134. V. Andrieu, H. Fessi, M. Dubrasquet, J.-P. Devissaguet, F. Puisieux, and S. Benita, *Drug Design Delivery*, 4:295 (1989).

135. S. Bondesen, O. H. Nielsen, O. Jacobsen, S. N. Rasmussen, S. H. Hansen, S. Halskov, V. Binder, and E. F. Hvidberg, *Scand. J. Gastroenterol.*, 19:677 (1984).

136. N. M. Graves, R. L. Kriel, C. Jones-Saete, and J. C. Cloyd, *Epilepsia*, 26:429 (1985).

137. E. Minkov, N. Lambov, D. Kirchev, I. Bantutova, and J. Tencheva, *Pharmazie*, 40:257 (1985).

138. F. S. Ghazy, M. S. Mohamed, A. A. Kassem, and B. M. Elhoseiny, *Pharmazie*, 43:484 (1988).

139. H. Vromans, F. Moolenaar, J. Visser, and D. K. F. Meijer, *Pharm. Weekbld Sci. Ed.*, 6:18 (1984).

140. A. J. M. Schoonen, F. Moolenaar, and T. Huizinga, *Pharm. Weekbl.*, 30:585 (1976).

141. M. L. Cole, and R. L. Kunka, *Biopharm. Drug Dispos.*, 5:229 (1984).

142. S. Itoh, N. Morishita, M. Yamazaki, A. Suginaka, K. Tanabe, and M. Sawanoi, *J. Pharmacobiodyn*, 10:173 (1987).

143. G. Neumann, Y. Niv, L. Bat, D. Abramowich, and E. Shemesh, *Isr. J. Med. Sci.*, 25:189 (1989).

144. C. Rodrigues, J. E. Lennard-Jones, J. English, and D. G. Parsons, *Lancet, 1:* 1497 (1987).

145. G. L. Flynn, in *Modern Pharmaceutics*, Vol. 7 (G. S. Banker, and C. T. Rhodes, eds.), Marcel Dekker, New York, 1979, pp. 263–327.

146. D. B. Guzek, A. H. Kennedy, S. C. McNeill, E. Wakshull, and R. O. Potts, *Pharm. Res.*, 6:33 (1989).

147. R. B. Stoughton, *Arch. Derm.*, 99:753 (1969).

148. V. A. Place, J. G. Velazquez, and K. H. Burdeck, *Arch. Dermatol.*, 101:531 (1970).

149. R. Woodford and B. W. Barry, *Curr. Ther. Res.*, 16:338 (1974).

150. B. W. Barry, *Dermatologica*, 152:47 (1976).

151. B. W. Barry, A. R. Brace, A. C. Norris, and R. Woodford, *J. Pharm. Pharmacol.*, 27:75P (1976).

152. S. M. Harrison, B. W. Barry, and P. H. Dugard, *J. Pharm. Pharmacol.*, 34 (Suppl.): 36P (1982).

153. S. M. Harrison, B. W. Barry, and P. H. Dugard, *J. Pharm. Pharmacol.*, 35(Suppl.): 32P (1983).

154. B. W. Barry, S. M. Harrison, and P. H. Dugart, *J. Pharm. Pharmacol.*, 37:84 (1985).

155. B. W. Barry, S. M. Harrison, and P. H. Dugard, *J. Pharm. Pharmacol.*, 37:226 (1985).

156. J. S. Turi, D. Danielson, and J. W. Woltresom, *J. Pharm. Sci.*, 68:275 (1979).

157. J. Hadgraft, *Pharm. Int.*, 5:252 (1984).

158. S. W. Jacob, and R. Herschler, (eds.), *Biological Actions of Dimethyl Sulfoxide*, Ann. N. Y. Acad. Sci., 243 (1975).

159. D. D. Munro, and R. B. Stoughton, *Arch. Dermatol.*, 92:585 (1965).

160. L. E. Matheson, D. E. Wurster, and J. Ostrenga, *J. Pharm. Sci.*, 68:1410 (1979).

161. H. L. Wechsler, J. Kirk, and J. Slowe, *Int. J. Dermatol.*, 17:237 (1978).

162. W. J. Irwin, F. D. Sanderson, and L. W. Po, *Int. J. Pharm.*, 66:(1990).

163. B. W. Barry, D. Southwell, R. Woodford, *J. Invest. Dermatol.*, 82:49 (1984).

164. R. B. Stoughton, *Arch. Dermatol.*, 118:474 (1982).

165. R. B. Stoughton, and W. McClure, *Drug Dev. Ind. Pharm.*, 9:725 (1983).

166. J. W. Wiechers, B. F. H. Drenth, J. H. G. Jonkman, and R. A. De Zeeuw, *Int. J. Pharm.*, 66:53 (1990).
167. S. Y. E., Hou and G. L. Flynn, *Int. J. Pharm.*, 66:79 (1990).
168. P. S. Banerjee, and W. A. Ritschel, *Int. J. Pharm.*, 49:199 (1989).
169. J. C. Kristof, Ph.D. thesis, University of Iowa, Iowa City, IA, 1985.
170. H. Okabe, K. Takayama, A. Ogura, and T. Nagai, *Drug Design Deliv.*, 4:313 (1989).
171. H. Okabe, Y. Obata, K. Takayama, and T. Nagai, *Drug Design Deliv.* 6:229 (1990).
172. Y. Obata, K. Takayama, H. Okabe, and T. Nagai, *Drug Design Deliv.*, 6:319 (1990).
173. Y. Kurosaki, N. Nagahara, T. Tanizawa, H. Nishimura, T. Nakayama, and T. Kimura, *Int. J. Pharm.*, 67:1 (1991).
174. T. Ogiso, and M. Shintani, *J. Pharm. Sci.*, 79:1065 (1990).
175. D. Bommannum, R. O. Potts, and R. H. Guy, *J. Controlled Release*, 16:299 (1991).
176. T. Kurihara-Bergstrom, K. Knutson, L. J. De Noble, and C. Y. Goates, *Pharm. Res.*, 7:762 (1990).
177. B. W. Barry, *J. Controlled Release*, 6:85 (1987).
178. R. J. Scheuplein, in *The Physiology and Pathophysiology of the Skin*, Vol. 5 (A. Jarrett, ed.), Academic Press, New York, 1978, pp. 1669–1730.
179. G. J. Putterman, N. F. Wolejska, M. A. Wolfram, and K. Laden, *J. Soc. Cosmet. Chem.*, 28:521 (1977).
180. G. Di Colo, C. Giannessi, E. Nannipieri, M. F. Serafini, and D. Vitale, *Int. J. Pharm.*, 50:27 (1989).
181. E. F. McNiff, A. Yacobi, F. M. Young-Chang, L. H. Golden, A. Goldfarb, and H. L. Fung, *J. Pharm. Sci.*, 70:1054 (1981).
182. G. L. Flynn, and B. Stewart, *Drug Dev. Res.*, 13:169 (1988).
183. A. Karim, *Angiology*, 34:11 (1983).
184. R. C. Wester, P. K. Noonan, S. Smeach, and L. Kasolad, *J. Pharm. Sci.*, 72:745 (1983).
185. S. Sved, W. M. McLean, and I. J. McGilveray, *J. Pharm. Sci.*, 70:1368 (1981).
186. P. K. Noonan and R. C. Wester, *J. Pharm. Sci.*, 69:365 (1980).
187. R. P. Iafrate, R. L. Yost, S. H. Curry, V. P. Gotz, and G. J. Caranasos, *Pharmacotherapy*, 3: 118 (1983).
188. C.-M. Chiang, G. L. Flynn, N. D. Weiner, W. J. Addicks, and G. J. Szpunar, *Int. J. Pharm.*, 49:109 (1989).
189. C.-M. Chiang, G. L. Flynn, N. D. Weiner, and G. J. Szpunar, *Int. J. Pharm.*, 50:21 (1989).
190. C.-M. Chiang, G. L. Flynn, N. D. Weiner, and G. J. Szpunar, *Int. J. Pharm.*, 55:229 (1989).
191. J. Kemken, A. Ziegler, and B. W. Muller, *J. Pharm. Pharmacol.*, 43:679 (1991).
192. J. Kemken, A. Ziegler, and B. W. Muller, *Pharm. Res.*, 9:554 (1992).
193. J. Kemken, A. Ziegler, and B. W. Muller, *Methods Find. Exp. Clin. Pharmacol.*, 13:361 (1991).
194. V. A. Place, in *Controlled Drug Bioavailability*, Vol. 3 (V. F. Smolen, and L. A. Ball, eds.), Wiley-Interscience, 1985, pp. 65–107.
195. Y. W. Chien, *Novel Drug Delivery Systems*, Marcel Dekker, New York, 1982, pp. 149–218.
196. G. W. Cleary, in *Medical Applications of Controlled Release*, Vol. 1 (R. S. Langer, and D. L. Wise, eds.), CRC Press, Boca Raton, FL, 1984, pp. 203–251.
197. M. Mezei and G. Gulasekharam, *Abstracts of the 39th Congress of Pharmaceutical Sciences*, FIP, Brighton, England, 1979, p. 134.
198. J. Lasch, and W. Wohlrab, *Biomed. Bichim. Acta,* 10:1295 (1986).
199. N. Weiner, N. Williams, G. Birch, C. Ramachandran, C. Shipman, Jr., and G. Flynn, *Antimicrob. Agents Chemother.*, 33:1217 (1989).
200. C. I. Price, J. W. Horton, and C. R. Baxter, *Gynecol. Obstet.*, 174:414 (1992).

201. R. L. Bronaugh, and T. J. Franz, *Br. J. Dermatol.*, 115:1 (1986).
202. T. Sekine, Y. Machida, and T. Nagai, *Drug Design Deliv.*, 1:245 (1987).
203. S. P. Erikson, in *Ophthalmic Drug Delivery Systems* (J. R. Robinson, ed.) A.Ph.A. Academy of Pharmaceutical Sciences, Washington, DC, 1980, pp. 55–70.
204. K. M. DeSantis, and R. D. Schoenwald, *J. Pharm. Sci.*, 67:1189 (1978).
205. H. M. Leibowitz, A. R. Berrospi, A. Kupfurman, G. V. Restropo, V. Galvis, and J. A. Alvarez, *Am. J. Ophthalmol.*, 83:402 (1977).
206. H. Benson, *Arch. Ophthalmol.*, 91:313 (1974).
207. J. W. Sieg, and J. R. Robinson, *J. Pharm. Sci.*, 64:931 (1975).
208. H.-W. Hui, and J. R. Robinson, *J. Pharm. Sci.*, 75:280 (1986).
209. R. D. Schoenwald, and P. Stewart, *J. Pharm. Sci.*, 60:39 (1980).
210. J. W. Sieg, and J. W. Triplett, *J. Pharm. Sci.*, 69:863 (1980).
211. L. Apt, A. Henrick, and L. M. Silverman, *Am. J. Ophthalmol.*, 87:210 (1977).
212. F. J. George and C. Hanna, *Arch. Ophthalmol.*, 95:879 (1977).
213. C. Hanna, J. Y. Massey, R. O. Hendrickson, J. Williamson, E. M. Jones, and P. Wilson, *Arch. Ophthalmol.*, 96:1258 (1978).
214. T. F. Patton and J. R. Robinson, *J. Pharm. Sci.*, 64:1312 (1975).
215. J. W. Sieg and J. R. Robinson, *J. Pharm. Sci.*, 66:1222 (1977).
216. J. W. Sieg and J. R. Robinson, *J. Pharm. Sci.*, 68:724 (1979).
217. R. P. Shrewsbury, J. Swarbrick, K. S. Newton, and L. C. Riggs, *J. Pharm. Pharmacol.*, 37:614 (1985).
218. V. H. L. Lee, J. Swarbrick, R. E. Stratford, and K. W. Morimoto, *J. Pharm. Pharmacol.*, 35:445 (1983).
219. M. W. Mosteller, B. M. Gebhardt, A. M. Hamilton, and H. E. Kaufman, *Arch. Ophthalmol.* 103:101 (1985).
220. S. S. Chrai, and J. R. Robinson, *J. Pharm. Sci.*, 63:1218 (1974).
221. K. Taniguchi, K. Itakura, N. Yamazawa, K. Morisaki, S. Hayashi, and Y. Yamada, *J. Pharmacobiodyn.*, 11:39 (1988).
222. R. W. Wood, V. H. Li, J. Kreuter, and J. R. Robinson, *Int. J. Pharm.*, 23:175 (1985).
223. V. H. K. Li, R. W. Wood, J. Kreuter, T. Harmia, and J. R. Robinson, *J. Microencapsul.*, 3:213 (1986).

9

Preservation of Dispersed Systems

Claude B. Anger, David Rupp, and Priscilla Lo

Allergan, Inc., Irvine, California

Harun Takruri

IOLAB Corporation, Claremont, California

I. OVERVIEW

Dispersed pharmaceutical systems require safeguards from microbial contamination that can affect the product and infect the consumer. This is accomplished by the addition of antimicrobial agents to destroy or inhibit the growth of those organisms that may contaminate the product during manufacture or use.

Both sterile and nonsterile multidose products can become contaminated with microbes through consumer use, misuse, or abuse. Thus, it is necessary to preserve all multiple-dose pharmaceutical products to protect (a) the product formulation and active ingredients from microbial degradation and (b) the consumer from infection that could be acquired through product use.

The preservation of nonsterile pharmaceutical products became a concern during the late 1950s and 1960s when many reports concerning the microbial contamination of such products were published [1,2]. Consequently, it became necessary to consider recognized standards for acceptable amounts and types of bacterial content in nonsterile pharmaceuticals. Much of the pioneering work in this area has been done by cosmetics manufacturers, whose products are generally more at risk from contamination than are pharmaceuticals. Little information was published on the preservation of cosmetics and pharmaceuticals during the pioneering era of preservative development. Manufacturers considered information generated as proprietary, thus restricting publications [3]. The association of the use of contaminated products with the development of clinical infection [4–7], increased regulatory control, and increased public awareness of product ingredients through consumer groups, has stimulated the generation of published research in the area of preservatives and microbiological product safety.

The challenge for the formulator is to find a balance between effective preservative and consumer safety. This can be considered as the balance between concentrations of preservative that are toxic to microbes and those that are toxic to people.

There is a very wide spectrum of compounds that efficiently kill microbes, even when toxic ones are eliminated from consideration. However, the requirements of solubility, stability, and compatibility with formulation ingredients or packaging components restrict this spectrum to a relative few. Figure 1 is a simple scheme showing some of the relationships between product ingredients, preservatives, and microbes. These interlocking relationships demonstrate the necessity for a well-planned preservation system that is integrated with the formulation. Preservation should never be an afterthought.

A preservative should never be chosen solely on a theoretical basis; therefore, it is essential to design a system for testing the efficacy of a preservative *in the formulation and in the intended container*. Design of the test program should also include testing the preservative efficacy and chemical stability of a product formulation over a given time period and under varying conditions (temperature, humidity). Manufactured product formulation should also be assessed for preservative efficacy and chemical stability to ensure that the manufacturing process did not alter the preservative system of the product formulation. In instances when a product formulation is marginally preserved, it is an option to include an in-use study to evaluate preservative effectiveness after consumer use in a controlled clinical situation.

In addition to a formulation-integrated preservative system and a testing program, the use of Good Manufacturing Practices (GMPs) is required to keep a product microbe-free [8]. These three methods for reducing microbial contamination are very closely related. Deficiencies in any one cannot be made up simply by adding more preservative "for insurance." The GMPs, although beyond the scope of this chapter, are a necessary precondition for successful preservation of pharmaceuticals. We will concern ourselves instead with the design of preservative systems and testing programs. This chapter will address:

The problem (microbial contamination and its effects)
The solution (commonly used preservatives)
The effects of formulation ingredients on preservative efficacy
The measurement of preservative efficacy
Future trends in this field

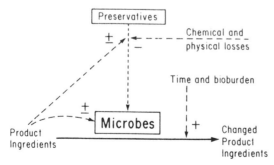

Fig. 1 Relationships among product ingredients, microbes, preservatives, and other factors. Microbes act on product ingredients (heavy arrow); this action is inhibited by preservatives (dashed arrow). Product ingredients can help or hinder ($\pm$) both the degradation process and the inhibition of egradation by preservatives. Chemical and physical losses of a preservative decrease its ability ot inihbit degradation of product ingredients by microbes. Microbial metabolism of product ingredients is increased with time and with greater numbers of microbes (bioburden).

II. GENERAL CHARACTERISTICS

A. Definition of Terms

During the process of developing recognized standards for the reduction of microbial contamination, many terms required definition, and many new terms were introduced. Sterilization, disinfection, and preservation, all are terms for the same general process— that of killing, removing, or reducing microbial contamination from formulations or surfaces. However, the terms differ from one another in their spectrum of activity and speed of action. In fact, a single compound can function in each of these three ways under different conditions. For example, temperature is a sterilant at 125°C, a disinfectant at 55°C, and a preservative at 5°C. Glutaraldehyde is a sterilant at 4.0%, a disinfectant at 0.4%, and a preservative at 0.003%. More exact definitions of these three terms and others that are used in this chapter and in the relevant literature are as follows.

Sterilization is a process that kills or removes *all* microbial contaminants, including bacterial and fungal spores.

Disinfection is a process that kills or removes all vegetative microbial contaminants (i.e., it does not destroy bacterial or fungal spores). Disinfection generally is quick, requiring only about 10–15 min contact with the appropriate agent. This term is not applied to pharmaceuticals and is reserved for surfaces that can come into contact with living tissue. Antiseptics are similar to distinfectants, but are applied directly onto living tissue. Antiseptics, therefore, are less toxic than disinfectants.

Preservation of pharmaceutical products is not so easily defined. In the pharmaceutical sense, a preservative prevents or inhibits microbial growth in the formulation to which it is added. However, there is little agreement on the quantitation of this process in terms of what number of organisms should be killed per which unit of time. Most criteria call for a 99.9% reduction of bacteria (0.1% survival or a 3-log reduction) in a specified time, which can range from 6 h to 14 days. There is also disagreement over the requirements for antifungal activity. One of the most stringent definitions of preservative action was offered by Kohn and associates, who stated that an ophthalmic formula having a self-sterilizing time of greater than 1 h, under their test conditions, was inadequately preserved [9]. For the purposes of this chapter, the word preservation will be used in the general sense of antimicrobial activity, without implying specific test criteria. We will discuss these criteria further in Section V.

Self-sterilization is a term used, historically, to mean the ability of a product to kill microbial contaminants. A product that is self-sterilizing can be said to be adequately preserved (i.e., no microbes can be recovered after a deliberate contamination, or challenge. However, the use of the word "sterilization" in this context is misleading, since preservatives kill vegetable cells, but do not destroy bacterial spores. Thus, even though a product is self-sterilizing and adequately preserved, it is not necessarily sterile. In practice, the definition of self-sterilization is based on some specified test procedure. Some procedures, however, cannot detect as many as 50–200 viable cells per milliliter or gram of product.

Neutralization is the elimination of a preservative's antimicrobial activity by the action of an added chemical agent (neutralizer), by filtration, or by dilution of the test sample. Exposure of microbes to dispersed products containing preservatives creates a population of surviving cells that exhibit different degrees of stress (i.e., sublethal injury from the lack of nutrients and the chemical–cellular interaction of preservative agents). For chemically induced cell injury, the effects observed are dependent on the chemical molecule/cell number ratio and removal of this stress can only be achieved by neutralization of the agent [10]. Neutralizers are now used in tests of preservative efficacy: aliquots of a formulation that has been challenged with microbes are taken, and the number of survivors are determined. Since preservatives are carried over in such a procedure, neutralizers are used in the recovery medium. They must act on the preservative without being toxic to the stressed microbial cells and without causing losses of viable cells by other means (e.g., precipitation). An example is polysorbate 80, which neutralizes quaternary ammonium compounds by trapping them in micelles. Before about 1975, neutralizers were not commonly used in tests of preservative efficacy. Therefore, caution should be exercised when interpreting the results of earlier preservative efficacy tests.

A *bactericidal* agent is one that kills vegetable bacterial cells. It may also have activity against fungi (fungicidal) and spores (sporicidal). A *bacteriostatic* agent is one that prevents the growth and replication of vegetative bacterial cells, but does not kill them. It may have activity against fungi (fungistatic). A compound with -static activity may have -cidal activity and vice versa, depending on the organism and the concentration of the preservative.

Bioburden refers to the microbial load or insult presented to a sample, formulation, or other potential home for microbes. Bioburden is expressed in terms of viable *organisms* per volume or weight [i.e., colony forming units (CFU) per milliliter or gram].

The microbial limits test is a comprehensive test developed by the United States Pharmacopeial Convention and published in the *United States Pharmacopeia* (*USP*) to assess nonsterile pharmaceutical products for the presence of bacteria and fungal bioburden [11]. It is not a test of preservative efficacy. This test requires the absence of *Staphylococcus aureus, Pseudomonas aeruginosa, Escherichia coli*, and *Salmonella* sp.; the time necessary for any product to kill these bacteria is not specified. Other microbes can be present up to a total of 10^3 CFU/g. Variations in procedures for testing the preservative efficacy or microbial limits of dispersed products (such as suspensions, emulsions, gels, ointments, and solid stick-type products) must be validated to ensure that these test procedures still recover small numbers of challenge bacteria. The microbial limits test is not applicable to multiple-dose otic, ophthalmic, nasal, or injectable products, which must be sterile and must pass preservative efficacy criteria.

The *minimal inhibitory concentration* (MIC) is that concentration of a preservative that prevents cells from growing under established conditions. However, the conditions and microbes used can vary from laboratory to laboratory, making comparisons of MICs problematic. The MIC is best considered a rough estimate of a preservative's ability to kill microbes.

The foregoing terms—preservation, bioburden, microbial limits test, and MIC—refer to aerobic bacterial and fungal (yeasts and molds) contamination only and do not consider viral, anaerobic, mycobacterial, actinomycete, or protozoal types of microbial contaminants.

B. Risks to Consumers

In the context of preservation, the risks to the consumer are preservative toxicity and microbial contamination (i.e., too much or too little preservative). It is important to consider the intended use of a multiple-dose pharmaceutical when estimating these risks, as this will determine the tolerable levels of both microbial contamination and preservative concentration. No contamination is allowed for sterile, multidose pharmaceuticals, such as injectables and ophthalmic products. Acceptable levels of contamination differ widely among nonsterile, multidose oral products, topical products for skin, and topical products for mucous membranes. In addition, the use of products on injured or diseased tissue further restricts both the acceptable degree of contamination and the concentration of preservative. This is of special concern for nonsterile topical creams and lotions that are often used to treat pain, inflammation, and dry skin. Such products are excellent environments for bacterial growth, and the compromised integument of a consumer in need of these products allows entry of pathogenic organisms to the body. Infections acquired in a hospital (nosocomial) have been traced to contaminated bottles of hand lotion [1,2]. In these studies the "infections caused by *S. [Serratia] marcescens* highly suggest transmission by contaminated hands. . . ." Sites of infection included burns, wounds, and catheters. Septicemia caused by *Klebsiella pneumoniae*, *P. aeruginosa*, *E. coli*, or *S. aureus* infections were also reported in the same studies.

In addition to causing direct infections, microbial contaminants can be harmful owing to their effects on the product. Fungi can metabolize complex carbohydrates, surfactants, and even steroids. This can change the physical properties of the formulation and can also deprive the consumer of the benefits of the product. Bacterial metabolism, even without the destruction of active ingredients, can damage a formulation by the formation of acidic end products that lower the pH of the product. This, in turn, can result in the growth of molds and fungi and the inactivation of the preservative. Some microbes can slowly metabolize emulsifiers, dispersing agents, and surfactants, which can cause separation of the dispersed phases (e.g., cracking of the emulsion).

The agents used to decrease the risks of bacterial contamination can themselves be harmful. Extreme care must be taken in the choice of compounds used in formulations that come in contact with sensitive tissues. Toxicity and irritation are dependent on the concentration of the compound in question. Thus, the appropriate concentration of a preservative is always the minimum amount that will do the job of preservation.

C. The Ideal Preservative

Several workers have devised lists of properties of the ideal preservative [12,13], which usually include the following:

Effective at low concentration against a wide spectrum of microbes
Soluble in the formulation at the required concentration
Nontoxic and nonsensitizing at in-use concentration
Compatible with formulation components and packaging
No effect on color, odor, or rheological properties of the formulation
Stable over wide ranges of pH and temperature
Relatively inexpensive

As with most ideals, this one is probably unattainable, and a balance must be struck among these requirements.

D. Special Considerations of Dispersed Systems

In principle, the preservation of dispersed pharmaceuticals is no different from the preservation of solution dosage forms. The complexity of such systems, however, necessitates special care in the selection and use of a preservative.

Lotions and creams are especially favorable environments for microbes. Such formulations contain more than enough carbon, nitrogen, and water for the metabolic needs of microbes. In addition, the complexity of a dispersed dosage form tends to work against the preservative—the more compounds there are in a formulation, the greater the chance that one or more will somehow inactivate it. (Only rarely will such an interation increase a preservative's efficacy.) These interactions will be discussed in Section V.

As an example of the problems associated with dispersed formulations, consider the partitioning of preservatives between the two or more phases of an emulsion. Partitioning can reduce the concentration of a preservative in the aqueous phase, where it must be present for antimicrobial activity, to the point that it is no longer effective. Another complexity is pH, which affects the efficacy of many preservatives. The nature of dispersed systems makes the meaning and measurement of pH problematic. Since microbes live on a microscale, often living within water droplets or on the interfaces between phases, they experience only the local pH. The formulator can either measure only the pH of the aqueous phase or an overall, "apparent," pH. This latter measurement is subject to large errors resulting from the presence of organic phases and particles. An additional difficulty is that particles are not always neutral and can add or take up hydrogen ions. This results in local pH gradients that can affect microbial growth and preservative efficacy and stability.

Another problem associated with preservation of dispersed systems is the effect of processing on a preservative's efficacy in a formulation. The manufacturing processes for dispersed systems are especially complex and can cause the inactivation, volatilization, degradation, or localization of the preservative. A compound might meet the requirements of an ideal preservative for a specific formulation, yet will not be useful because of the problems associated with the required manufacturing processes.

The complexity of dispersed systems leads to the special considerations decreased in the foregoing. The selection and use of preservatives, as detailed in the remainder of this chapter, are constrained by the interactions that can occur in these systems.

III. MICROBIAL CONTAMINATION

Reseachers at the U. S. Food and Drug Administration (FDA) reported 1550 isolations of gram-negative bacteria from raw materials and finished products between 1968 and 1971 [14]. This is hardly surprising given that microbes "are absent only in those places where a sterilizing influence prevails or in the interior tissues of healthy animals and plants" [13]. Microbes flourish whenever the balance between advantageous and hostile factors tips in their favor.

Bacteria are considered the most serious contamination, as they usually grow much faster than yeasts or molds. This is emphasized in the *USP* criteria for the microbial limits test for nonsterile pharmaceuticals. These requirements call for the absence of certain bacteria, namely *P. aeruginosa*, *S. aureus*, *E. coli*, and *Salmonella* spp., but do not recognize a concern for yeasts and filamentous fungi (molds). A list of objectionable microbial genera is presented in Table 1.

A. Sources of Microbial Contamination

1. *Air and Water*

Common airborne microbes are the gram-positive bacteria, *Staphyloccus,* Micrococcus, and Corynebacterium spp., and the spore-forming *Bacillus* and *Clostridium* spp.; the yeast *Rhodotorula* spp., and the molds *Aspergillus*, *Cladosporium*, and Penicillium spp.

Table 1 Microbial
Genera Considered
Objectional for
Dispersed Products

Gram-negative bacteria
Acinetobacter
Escherichia
Enterobacter
Klebsiella
Proteus
Pseudomonas
Salmonella
Serratia
Gram-positive bacteria
Clostridium
Staphylococcus
Molds
Aspergillus
Dermatophytes
Yeast
Candida

Source: Refs. 15 and 16.

The microbial flora of city water usually includes gram-negative nonfermentative bacilli, including *Pseudomonas, Alicaligenes, Acinetobacter, Flavobacterium*, and *Achromobacter* spp. Other soil and sewage bacteria, such as *Bacillus* spp.; the gram-negative fermenters *Serratia, Klebsiella, Proteus*, and *Enterobacter* spp.; and *E. coli*, can be found in tap water used for manufacturing. Thus, all but two of the objectionable genera listed in Table 1 are likely to be found in air and water.

Deionized water is often used in pharmaceutical formulations and is made by passing city main water through ion-exchange resin beds. These resin beds can become havens for bacterial contamination (usually *Pseudomonas* spp.), especially if the resin is not frequently regenerated. As a result, deionized water may be more heavily contaminated than tap water. By contrast, freshly distilled water is sterile. However, microbial contamination of distilled water frequently results from faulty cooling, storage, or distribution systems. Distilled water for pharmaceutical products is sometimes ozonized or maintained at 80°C in a holding loop to maintain its sterility.

2. *Raw Materials*

Pharmaceuticals are often derived from plant or animal sources; thus, they carry a natural microbial flora [17]. Plant materials can contain the microbes mentioned in the last section: the airborne molds, plus yeasts (*Saccharomyes* and *Rhodotorula* spp.) and other molds (*Mucor, Alternaria, Fusarium*, and *Auriobastidiums* spp.). Plant materials, including various natural gums, usually contain from 1000 to 100,000 microorganisms per gram. Synthetic ingredients generally have lower bioburdens than natural materials [16]. Raw materials of animal origin usually contain only bacteria, rarely yeasts or molds, but this flora may contain pathogens (e.g., *Pasteurella, Shigella*, and *Salmonella* spp.).

Consequently, many of these raw materials are treated with heat, irradiation, or alcohol to greatly reduce or eliminate their bioburden before use.

3. *Equipment*

Contamination from this source can be kept to a minimum by simple good-housekeeping measures. Cleanliness is greatly abetted by designing ease of maintenance into the machinery. This includes accessibility to all parts, elimination of crevices and dead ends where fluids might accumulate, and the use of smooth, easily cleaned parts wherever possible. Equipment for aseptic filling of sterile dispersed products must always be thoroughly cleaned, disinfected, and rinsed between uses.

4. *Personnel*

Manufacturing personnel often transfer microbes from their skin and respiratory passages to nonsterile pharmaceutical products. The skin flora is difficult to predict, as personal hygiene plays a large role in defining the transient population of gram-negative coliform bacteria. However, the staphylococci and diphtheroids are normally present, along with yeasts from the genera *Candida* and *Pityrosporum (Malassezia)*. The primary concern is transfer of *S. aureus* or coliforms from personnel to the product during manufacture. Coughing or sneezing in the bulk-manufacturing and filling areas can produce aerosols of bacteria such as staphylococci (including *S. aureus*), steptococci (viridans group), and occasionally *Haemophilus*, Klebsiella, or *Neisseria* spp. The use of protective garments by machinery operators is advised, as is training of personnel. Everyone who can come into contact with batch materials should understand that they are an important source of microbes and should be trained to avoid contaminating the product.

5. *Consumers*

Bacterial contamination of products through consumer use often results in a mixed microbial flora being present in the product [18]. This bacterial flora often is made up of gram-positive cocci and rods, with a few gram-negative rods. Since this source of contamination can introduce pathogens [18], it is essential that the preservative system be able to handle the bioburden that the consumer can be expected to add. It is almost impossible to prove that product contamination occurred after it left the factory. Thus, for both ethical and financial reasons, the manufacturer must be sure of the preservation of the product.

B. Survival and Growth of Microbial Flora: Factors Other Than Preservatives

1. *Water*

Water is the single most important requirement for microbial growth. In a multiphase system, microbes will grow in only the aqueous phase (although they can collect at interfaces). Anhydrous pharmaceuticals will rarely support microbial survival unless extraneous water has entered the product container.

Water activity, A_w, is a measurement of the water that is not bound by some interaction to components in a formulation. In other words, A_w quantitates the water available for microbial use. The higher the solute concentration, the lower the A_w. Water activity is temperature-dependent and is equal to the vapor pressure of the formulation divided by the vapor pressure of pure water at the same temperature. Most bacteria require high A_w values for growth, about 0.92 and above [20]. Gram-positive cocci can tolerate lower water activity (e.g., *S. aureus* can grow at an A_w of 0.86). Fungi prefer an A_w of about 0.90, although osmophilic yeasts can withstand an A_w as low as 0.62. The ability of microbes to thrive at a given A_w is greatly influenced by temperature and pH.

High concentrations of sugars increase osmotic pressure and decrease A_w to levels incompatible with most microbial life. However, osmophilic yeasts have grown, albeit slowly, in very high concentrations of sugars. Syrup BP, for example, is 66% surcrose with an A_w of 0.86 and is occasionally contaminated with osmophilic yeasts. Water activity can be estimated from the following equation:

$$A_w = \frac{\text{vapor pressure of the product}}{\text{vapor pressure of water}} \quad \text{(at the same temperature)} \qquad [21].$$

Formulators also have the option to use sodium chloride (100 ppm), added as a concentrate in a "little bit" of water, to lower the A_w of their "anhydrous" ointments after removal of preservatives. The addition of sodium chloride in this manner serves to increase the antimicrobial safety of those products that are currently required by compendia to be only "microbiostatic," but we believe ointments should at least significantly kill vegetative bacteria. Also, water films can develop on products through misuse, humidity, and daily temperature cycling, creating a localized area of lower sugar concentration. Such a film is a foothold for further microbial attack because of its increased A_w (and reduced osmotic pressure). Semisolid products are especially susceptible to this sort of attack, which is made possible by a localized area of reduced preservative concentration that does not mix with the rest of the product.

2. Nutrition

Nearly all microorganisms require certain basic nutrients to survive and grow in a pharmaceutical product. Many of these nutrients are found in dispersed dosage forms. These include carbohydrates, proteins, lipids (waxes, fatty acids, or fatty alcohols), organic acids, inorganic salts, and vitamins. Molds and yeasts are saprophytes (i.e., they obtain energy from the metabolism of dead organic matter). They are common to the bioburden of natural raw materials such as gums, pectins, starch, vegetable oils, and plant extracts. These organisms require water, air, a source of carbon, such as fats or carbohydrates (sugars or cellulose), very little protein, and a temperature of 18–25°C. Table 2 is a list of nutritional sources for microbes that are commonly found in contaminated dispersed pharmaceutical products.

Some bacteria possess the ability to adapt to extremely low nutritional levels, especially members of the genus *Pseudomonas*. *Pseudomonas cepacia* can survive in distilled water with only trace quantities of nutrients [22]. Likewise, *P. aeruginosa* can grow in distilled water in hospital mist therapy units [23,24]. The bacteria isolated from the therapy units were more resistant to antimicrobial agents when they were grown in distilled water than when they were subcultured on simple media. In the last decade, *Pseudomonas* species have become the contamination plague of the pharmaceutical industry.

Table 2 Sources of Microbial Nutrition in Dispersed
Pharmaceuticals

Emulsifiers	Anionic, cationic, nonionic, and amphoteric surfactants
Thickeners	Polyethylene glycols
Humectants	Sorbitol, mannitol, glycerol
Flavorings	Peppermint water, syrups
Natural products	Gums, proteins, starches
Fats and oils	
Steroids	

3. pH

The pH can have a limiting effect on the survival and growth of microorganisms. Unfortunately, this occurs only at the pH extremes of 3.5 or below and 10 or above. Few if any formulations are that acidic or basic; most fall in the pH range of 3.5–9.0. Bacteria are tolerant of pH and are able to thrive in the pH range of 5.5–8.5. Yeasts and filamentous fungi prefer more acidic conditions of pH 4–6. Microbial growth in formulations usually alters the pH, and changes in pH often greatly affect preservative activity. This problem will be addressed in more detail in Section V.

The pH of an acidic formulation can be increased by the metabolic activity of fungi—this change then allows bacteria to grow. Bacterial metabolism of sugars and fats produces acidic end products, which make the environment more favorable for molds and yeasts. The process of microbes creating conditions for their own death and for the growth of others is termed autogenic succession. A preservative, therefore, must be able to kill the first contaminants (the "pioneers") that create the conditions for spoilage. There is little point to a preservative that is effective against only the microbes found in a spoiled product–it must be able to kill the entire range of possible contaminants.

4. Temperature

Storage temperature can greatly affect the survival and growth of microbes in pharmaceutical products. Although molds and yeasts prefer temperatures of 18–25°C, bacteria prefer 30–37°C.Many molds and bacteria are inhibited and even destroyed by temperatures of 42–50°C. Storage of finished products at 23°C encourages molds and yeasts to grow and germinate. This temperature also tends to keep bacteria static, but alive, and able to respond to future changes in temperature. Temperatures of 4–15°C tend to hold microbial contaminants in a state of dormancy. However, the antimicrobial activity of preservatives is severely hampered by lower temperatures. Conversely, even though higher temperatures increase the rate of microbial growth, they also increase the efficacy of a preservative, by 2–50 times for a 10°C increase [25].

5. Interfaces and Attachment Substrates

Suspended particles can adsorb microbes; this affords greater protection and, thereby, greater survival for them. Dispersed liquid antacid preparations are often found contaminated with gram-negative bacteria, including *Pseudomonas, Klebsiella, Serratia,* and *Enterobacter* spp. [26,27]. Adhesion of *E. coli* to magnesium trisilicate was demonstrated by Beveridge and Todd [28]. These authors suggest that the bacterial attachment has some analogy to Langmuir adsorption, which implies an evenly dispersed monolayer of cells on the surface of the particles. Electrostatic attraction was ruled out as the mechanism of binding, since both the bacteria and the magnesium trisilicate particles have slight negative charges. Binding, therefore, was ascribed to van der Waals forces. In addition to the problem of protecting microbes, nutrients present in low concentration in a formulation may be concentrated at particle surfaces and thus be available for attached microbes.

6. *Bioburden*

The number of microorganisms introduced into a formulation greatly affects the potential for product deterioration. Very low contamination levels, fewer than 10 microbes per gram, require a rather long lag period before growth or product degradation can be expected (in an inadequately preserved formulation). In contrast, a very large inoculum may overwhelm a preservative system in short order. Also, the greater the number of cells contaminating a formulation, the greater the chance that cells resistant to the preservative may develop. A weakness of most microbiological testing programs is the failure to detect low levels of contamination, which, after a 3-month storage period, may grow into thousands of organisms per milliliter.

7. *Product Ingredients as Preservatives*

In a few cases, a product is self-sterilizing without an additional preservative (i.e., it is self-preserving). Alcohol is bactericidal at concentrations over 20%. This limits its use in many dispersed systems—the high concentration strongly affects the physical properties of the product. Another example is lauricidin (glyceryl monolaurate), a useful nonionic surfactant that also has bactericidal activity [29].

C. Effects of Contamination on Products

"Living organisms propagate at the expense of their environment and in considering any spoilage problem created by the presence of microorganisms, the variety of chemical reactions they can carry out and the rate at which these occur should be taken into account" [13]. The environment, here the product itself, must be protected from the changes microbes might make, for reasons of safety and efficacy.

Dispersed products are nutritional havens for microbes. Thickeners and emulsifiers are good carbon sources for fungi; creams, lotions, and gels are very susceptible to fungal attack. Bacterial metabolism of ester- and ester-based surfactants has been demonstrated [30,31] and can contribute to changes in the rheological properties of a formulation.

Products usually have shelf lives of about 2–3 years, during which time the concentration of active ingredients must remain within about 10–20% of the nominal concentration. Microbial metabolism of active ingredients, although rare, can accelerate degradation and reduce shelf life.

Carbohydrates are usually metabolized to acids, a process that may be accompanied by gas formation. These metabolites can cause products to develop odors, change color, shift pH, and cause phase separation. If thickeners are metabolized by microbes, the product will become considerably less thick, and the product's rheological properties will change accordingly.

A change of pH can greatly affect surfactants and other components that maintain the dispersion of phases in a product. Loss of some of these components through metabolism or loss of their efficacy through a change in pH can result in a separation of phases.

Even minor changes in physical properties are noticeable and can be disconcerting for the consumer. Since consumers cannot assay the active ingredients, they depend on their senses to tell them the quality of the product. Changes in a product's gross physical properties are likely to be interpreted as a loss of efficacy of the product.

It is desirable that dispersed parenteral formations, whether preserved or not, be free of pyrogens (substances that produce fever in humans and animals). The vast majority of pyrogens are bacterial endotoxins. The endotoxins are composed of lipopolysaccharides (LPSs) and are part of the outer membrane layer of gram-negative bacteria. The LPSs consist of a heteropolysaccharide, small amounts of protein, and covalently bound lipid A, which is responsible for the pyrogenicity of the LPSs.

Even when parenteral suspensions are sterile, they may contain LPSs shed from dead bacteria. However, it requires 1×10^5 organisms per gram to make enough endotoxin to be detected. Thus, these dispersed pharmaceutical products should be prepared endotoxin-free by dry heat depyrogenation of glass containers [32] and by filtration of the suspending medium through alumina or other adsorbents [33].

D. Risks to Consumer

The indirect risks of microbial contamination have already been mentioned (i.e., physical and chemical changes in the dispersed dosage form, resulting in an unacceptable or ineffective product). The direct risk of microbial contamination is infection. *Pseudomonas* spp. are particularly virulent, and special care must be taken with ophthalmic preparations. Some species are known to cause permanent damage to the eye in less than 24 h [34].

Viral contamination is not generally a concern; there have been no reports of viral infections that are due to pharmaceutical preparations. It is possible for viruses to enter a product; however, pathogenic viruses cannot multiply in formulations.

IV. PRESERVATIVES

In this section we will present brief descriptions of the commonly used preservatives. These descriptions are meant to be brief outlines of the use of these compounds, rather than monographs of all the data that may be needed by a pharmacist. For more information on particular agents, the interested reader is referred to various texts [35,36]. The compounds listed here are a narrower spectrum of preservatives than that available for use in cosmetics, owing to the nature of the typical applications of dispersed pharmaceuticals. The great majority of preserved pharmaceuticals use the compounds listed here [37]. Other preservatives, useful in their time, but now banned or simply disused, are not included in this section. Indeed, with on-going research and changes in safety and efficacy criteria, some of the preservatives in our list may be out of favor in a few years, and new ones may take their places. We recommend a cautious approach to new preservatives until they have been thoroughly tested.

It is important that antibiotics for the therapeutic treatment of disease states are never to be employed as preservative agents in pharmaceutical dosage forms. This includes the following classes of compounds: β-lactams (penicillins and cephalosporins); aminoglycosides (amikacin, gentamicin, and tobramicin); tetracyclines (minocycline, oxycycline, and such); sulfonamides and trimethoprim; macrolides, quinolones, and the peptide antibiotics, such as polymyxins or colistins. This edict is essential to medical treatment of infectious disease, because the indiscriminant use of antibiotics as preservatives would create a world of antibiotic-resistant microorganisms, with little to no treatment available for systemic infection. Antibiotics are those antimicrobial agents that elicit a high therapeutic index at which their toxic concentration to microbes is far (orders of magnitude) below their toxic concentration to human beings, which allows them to be administered through the bloodstream to reach infected organs. For instance, the quinolones usually kill bacteria in the 0.025- to 8.0-μg/ml range and are toxic to humans at 10,000 μg/ml. In contrast, preservative and disinfectant agents are usually toxic to humans when taken internally at use concentrations or only slightly above the ineffective range, but are safe for topical use and, sometimes, for digestive tract use. There is already a problem in this area from the use of antibiotics in animal feed. Anecdotally, a company was developing a line of contact lens care products that were preserved with trimethoprim. However, when the drug branch of the FDA found out that the device branch was considering approving these products, they put an immediate halt to the process. The development company lost a few million dollars in product development costs they could have saved by consulting with a knowledgable microbiologist.

A. Alcohols

1. *Alcohol* CH$_3$CH$_2$OH

Synonyms: Ethyl alcohol, ethanol. M.W. 46.07. Clear, colorless liquid, b. 78.5°C. Miscible with water. Forms binary azeotrope with 5% water, b. 78.15°C. The term "alcohol USP" refers to this mixture, 95/5 (v/v) alcohol and water. Typical concentration for preservation > 20%. The antimicrobial activity of alcohols is due to their ability to disorganize lipid membranes by penetrating into the hydrocarbon microbial membrane region. In general, short-chain alcohols produce greater changes in membrane disorganization than the higher homologues. Alcohols also exert antimicrobial activity by denaturing proteins. The activity of alcohols has also been recognized to increase with branching (primary < secondary < tertiary).

In dispersed systems, alcohol is used as a preservative in dermatological, parenteral, and oral products. It is most useful as a preservative when it is also useful as a solvent. However, the nature of dispersed systems places an upper limit to the concentration of alcohol that can be used. Too high a concentration of alcohol is incompatible with many emulsions and suspensions.

2. *Propylene Glycol* $H_2C-\underset{\underset{H}{|}}{\overset{\overset{OH}{|}}{C}}-CH_3$ (with OH on the first two carbons)

Synonyms: 1,2-Propanediol, 1,2-dihydroxypropane, methyl glycol. M.W. 76.09. Clear, colorless, viscous, hygroscropic liquid with a slightly acrid taste, b. 188°C. Miscible with water, alcohol, glycerin; immiscible with mineral oil and fixed oils. Dissolves in some essential oils. Typical concentrations for preservation: 15–30%.

Propylene glycol shares the antimicrobial and solvent properties of alcohol. It is a humectant and most of its activity is based on its ability to reduce water activity. At concentrations greater than 20%, it is often used as the sole preservative in a product. Propylene glycol has been shown to enhance the bactericidal activity of parabens when used at concentrations of 2–5% [38]. Like alcohol, propylene glycol causes burning and stinging on application. Its advantages over alcohol are greatly reduced volatility and better physical compatibility with suspensions and emulsions.

3. *Benzyl Alcohol*

Synonyms: Phenylmethanol, phenylcarbinol, M.W. 108.14. Colorless, oily liquid having a faint aromatic odor, b. 203–207°C. Solubility: 4% in water, miscible with alcohol and fixed and volatile oils. Typical concentrations for preservation (dermal products): 0.5–3%.

Benzyl alcohol is an excellent cosolvent for many pharamceutical formulations. It has moderate antimicrobial activity, especially at neutral to acidic pH. Formulations containing benzyl alcohol as preservative or cosolvent must be studied carefully because of interactions with plastics, especially polyethylene and polystyrene. The use of benzyl alcohol as a preservative has been discontinued in parenteral formulations for pediatric use because of safety concerns. Benzyl alcohol is rarely used in ophthalmic products because its antimicrobial activity is slow and it may cause ocular irritation if not properly formulated. It has been shown by Russel et al. [39] to penetrate closures. Magnesium trisilicate and polysorbate 80 reduce the bactericidal activities of benzyl alcohol [40].

4. *Chlorobutanol*

Synonyms: 1,1,1-Trichloro-2-methyl-2-propanol, chlorbutol.M.W. 177.46 (anhyd.). Colorless to white crystals, volatile at room temperature. One gram dissolves in 130 ml water, 1 ml alcohol, 10 ml glycerin. Very soluble in propylene glycol, soluble in vegetable and mineral oils. Typical concentration for preservation: 0.5%.

Chlorobutanol has lost much of its popularity in recent years owing to its lack of stability in many formulations. It is unstable at pH greater than 6 (Table 3). It is partially inactivated by polysorbate 80 and polyvinyl pyrrolidone [40,41], and can be absorbed by rubber closures. Magnesium trisilicate reduces the bactericidal activities of chlorobutanol [40]. Chlorobutanol is unstable in polyethylene containers [42]. It is volatile and can be lost through the headspace or plastic of the container [43,44]. Also, it has the odor and taste of camphor, which excludes it from oral use. Despite all this, chlorobutanol is still useful in certain preparations, such as ophthalmic ointments, where, owing to its solubility in petrolatum, the likelihood of loss through the headspace or the container is minimized.

5. *Phenylethyl Alcohol*

Synonyms: 2-Phenylethanol, phenethyl alcohol, β-phenylethyl alcohol. M. W. 122.17. Colorless liquid with roselike odor and sharp, burning taste. One milliliter dissolves in

Table 3 The Effect of
pH on the Stability of
Chlorobutanol

pH	$t_{1/2}$ (yr)
3.0	90
5.0	40.3
5.5	23.2
6.0	9
6.5	2.4
7.0	0.61
7.5	0.23

Source: Ref. 45.

60 ml water. Very soluble in alcohol, glyercin, propylene glycol, and fixed oils; slightly soluble in mineral oil. Typical concentrations for preservation: 0.25–0.5%.

Phenylethyl alcohol by itself is not a particularly effective preservative. It is weakly microbicidal against certain fungi and *Pseudomonas* spp. and can be considreed a bacteriostatic agent. Phenyethyl alcohol (1%, 20-min contact time) has been reported by Staal and Rowe [46] to inactivate mycoplasmas. However, the same authors reported that enveloped viruses were resistant when tested under the same conditions. It is useful in enhancing the activity of other preservatives [benzalkonium chloride (BAK), phenylmercuric nitrate, chlorhexidine, chlorobutanol], especially quaternary, amines and organic mercurials. Enhancement has been attributed to an effect on the cell envelope such that higher concentrations of other preservatives may enter the cell [47].

6. *Bronopol* $HOCH_2-\underset{\underset{NO_2}{|}}{\overset{\overset{Br}{|}}{C}}-CH_2OH$

Synonym: 2-Bromo-2-nitropropane-1,3-diol. M.W. 200.0. Off-white, odorless, slightly hygroscopic crystalline powder, m. 121°C. One gram dissolves in 4 ml water, 2 ml alcohol, 7 ml propylene glycol, and 100 ml glycerin. Bronopol is only slightly soluble in oils (less than 0.5%). Typical concentrations for preservation: 0.01–0.1%.

Bronopol possesses many of the properties of an ideal preservative: it is colorless, odorless, highly water-soluble, and nontoxic at typical concentrations. Bronopol partitions into the aqueous phase in most aqueous–organic solvent combinations, where it can come into contact with contaminating microorganisms. Bronopol is unaffected by the presence of surfactants [48–51] and works synergistically with certain nonionic surfactants [51]. Cysteine hydrochloride, dimercaprol, cystine hydrochloride, sodium thiosulfate, sodium metabisulfite, and sulfhydryl compounds have been reported to decrease bronopol's activity [48,52]. Bronopol is incompatible with some metals (iron, aluminum) limiting its use with certain packaging. It discolors solutions brown or yellow when exposed to light, especially under alkaline conditions at higher temperatures [55] and degrades in solution when exposed to gamma irradiation in clear glass ampules [56]. The use of bronopol is limited by its instability at alkaline pH. Formaldehyde release from bronopol has been reported at neutral and alkaline pHs [53,54]. The decomposition of bronopol yields nitrite, which can react with amines to form carcinogenic *N*-nitrosamines. The formation of *N*-nitrosamines can be prevented by the addition of antioxidants [57]. Besides nitrite and formaldehyde, other bronopol decomposition products include bromide, 2-bromo-2-nitroethanol, and 2-hydroxymethyl-2-nitropropane-1,3-diol. Decomposition of 2-hydroxymethyl-2-nitropropane-1,3-diol can lead to further release of formaldehyde. The Cosmetic Ingredient Review group concurred in 1984 that bronopol is safe to use up to 0.1% [58]. However, the group did mention possible sensitization to subjects with sensitive damaged skin.

7. *2,4-Dichlorobenzyl Alcohol*

Synonym: Myacide SP. M.W. 177. White to slightly yellow crystals, nonhygroscopic. Typical concentration for preservation: 0.04%–0.15%.

2,4-Dichlorobenzyl alcohol is especially effective against fungi and is compatible with cationic systems. In the presence of nonionics or anionics, some reduction in activity may result. In aqueous solutions, 2,4-dichlorobenzyl alcohol may oxidize to the corresponding acid and aldehyde. Solutions prepared in alcohol and glycols are stable. 2,4-Dichlorobenzyl alcohol can be combined with other preservatives, such as bronopol.

B. Dimethylol Dimethylhydantoin

Synonym: 1,3-Dimethylol-5,5-dimethylhydantoin, DMDMH, M.W. 188.19. White crystals, m. 102–104. Available as a 55% aqueous solution (Glydant). Clear solution with a mild odor and a specific gravity (25°C) of 1.16; miscible with water and alcohol. Typical concentrations for preservation: 0.15–0.4%.

DMDMH is a formaldehyde-releasing agent, with a broad antimicrobial spectrum. It is stable at a temperature of 80°C. Heating at 80°C will reduce the concentration of free formaldehyde, without changing the concentration of combined formaldehyde [59]. It is effective against *Pseudomonas* spp. but has weaker activity against fungi. DMDMH is compatible with surfactants and proteins, is stable over wide ranges of pH and temperature, and is nonirritating and nontoxic. Monomethylol dimethylhydantoin has similar properties (including antimicrobial activity) but has MIC values about double that of DMDMH [61]. The Cosmetic Ingredient Review group concluded that DMDMH was safe when used at concentrations up to 1.0% [60].

C. Sodium Hydroxymethylglycinate

Synonym: Suttocide A. M.W. 127.10 $C_3H_6NO_3 \cdot Na$. A 50% solution in water is marketed as Suttocide A. The solution is colorless to pale yellow with a mild odor. Typical concentration for preservation: 0.1–1.0%.

Sodium hydroxymethylglycinate is broad-spectrum agent against gram-negative and gram-positive bacteria, yeast, and molds. In combination with other preservatives, such as Kathon CG or parabens, sodium hydroxymethylglycinate can be used at lower concentrations. The combination of sodium hydroxymethylglycinate and Kathon CG is reported to be synergistic and is patented [62].

D. Quaternary Amines

1. *Quaternium 15*

Synonyms: *N*-(2-Chloroallyl)hexaminium chloride, Dowicil 200. M.W. 251.17. Cream-colored hygroscopic odorless powder. Solubility: 127 g dissolves in 100 ml water. Concentrated solutions in propylene glycol contain 18.7%, in glycerol 12.6%; in ethanol 1.85%; in isopropanol 0.25%; in paraffin oil 0.1%; in glycerine 12.6%; and in mineral oil 0.1%. Typical concentrations for preservation: 0.02–0.3%.

Quaternium 15 has a broad antimicrobial range and is effective against yeasts, molds, fungi, and gram-positive and gram-negative bacteria, including *P. aeruginosa*. Quaternium 15 is compatible with anionic, cationic, and nonionic surfactants as well as protein and other preservatives. It is unstable below pH 4 and above pH 10 and at temperatures above 60°C. Formaldehyde will volatilize from solutions warmed to temperatures above 60°C [63]. Paraformaldehyde deposits may form if warmed solutions are cooled below 15°C. Quaternium 15 may discolor acidic formulations yellow. Discoloration may be prevented by adding small quantities of sodium borate or sodium sulfite (0.05–0.1%). The Cosmetic Ingredient Review group concluded that quaternium 15 was safe when used at concentrations up to 1.0% [64].

2. *Benzalkonium Chloride*

Synonym: Alkylbenzyldimethylammonium chloride. Yellowish-white amorphous gel or gelatinous flakes with aromatic odor and bitter taste. Very soluble in water and alcohol. Typical concentrations for preservation: 0.004–0.02%.

Benzalkonium chloride (BAK) is a mixture of alkyldimethylbenzylammonium chlorides (mostly C_{12}, C_{14}, and C_{16}), as indicated in the foregoing structure. It is a cationic surfactant and has a broad spectrum of antimicrobial activity. The *USP* has a broad specification for BAK, which can adversely affect the efficacy of products that are formulated with different sources of BAK raw material. The *USP* specification for the C_{12} and C_{14} homologue components is that the $C_{12}H_{25}$ homologue represents no less than 40%, the $C_{14}H_{29}$ homologue represents no less than 20%, and that the two homologues togther must constitute no less than 70% of the total alkyldimethylbenzylammonium chloride content. Superior activity has been reported to be displayed by the C_{14} homolog [65–69], indicating that its content may indicate the efficacy of products formulated with different sources of BAK. BAK is active over a wide pH range and is very stable at room temperature. Its activity, however is enhanced at neutral to alkaline pHs at which the cell wall of microorganisms are usually negatively charged, thereby facilitating a cationic interaction with BAK [70,71]. BAK is subject to neutralization by many anionic compounds (especially anionic surfactants and soaps), which greatly limits its usefulness. It also binds to nonionic surfactants and can be precipitated by nitrate and other anions. Inactivation by nonionic surfactants (polysorbate 80) has been reported to be due to micelle formation [72]. BAK has also been reported to undergo self-micellization [73]. Bismuth carbonate, talc, calamine, calcium carbonate, kaolin, magnesium trisilicate, magnesium oxide, titanium oxide and starch absorb BAK in solution [40,74,75].

Benzalkonium chloride is used in most ophthalmic, nasal, and otic pharmaceuticals. Its efficacy (and that of other quarterny compounds) is enhanced by the presence of edetate disodium (EDTA) at concentrations of 0.01–0.1% [71,76]. Its activity is also enhanced by benzyl alcohol, phenyl propanol, and phenylethyl alcohol [77,78]. It is also used for the preservation of small-volume parenteral products.

For best results with this compound, the homologue distribution should be controlled to avoid unpredictable loss of activity. This is generally attributed to the loss of the C_{16} and C_{18} homologues, which are more susceptible to precipitation by counterions and adsorption into plastic surfaces than are the lower homologues.

3. *Cetrimide*
$$H_3C - \overset{\overset{\textstyle CH_3}{|}}{\underset{\underset{\textstyle CH_3}{|}}{N^+}} - C_nH_{2n+1} \quad Br^-$$

(n = 12,14 or 16)

Synonyms: Alkyltrimethylammonium bromide, cetrimonium bromide. M.W. 364.48. White to creamy white powder, m. 237–243°C. Soluble in water up to 10%, freely soluble in alcohol. Typical concentrations for preservation: 0.005–0.01%

Cetrimide is composed of a mixture of three alkyltrimethylammonium bromide compounds, differing only in alkyl chain length (C_{12}, C_{14}, C_{16}). The C_{14} compound was shown by Al-Taae et al. [79] to possess the greatest amount of activity. It shares many characteristics of benzalkonium chloride, especially incompatibility with anionic and nonionic surfactants.

In connection with cetrimide, it should be remembered that differential bacteriology methods employ "cetrimide agar" as a utilizable substrate for the identification of *P. aeruginosa*, which is able to grow in the presence of cetrimide. For this medium, the *Difco Manual* says: "cetrimide is added to inhibit bacteria other than *Pseudomonas aeruginosa*." Consequently, it is not wise to employ cetrimide as a preservative in dispersed pharmaceuticals. An example of the potential end result is noted in the reference of Spooner and Davison (1993) where their "antibiotic cream T" preserved with 0.2% cetrimide plus 100 ppm benzalkonium chloride was overwhelmingly contaminated with *P. aeruginosa* (46,000 CFU/ml) after consumer use.

E. Imidazolidinyl Urea Compounds

1. *Imidazolidinyl Urea*

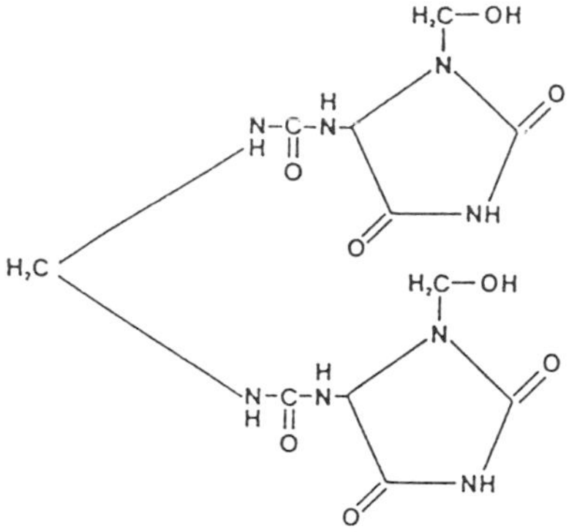

Synonyms: Germall 115; imidurea, NF; Biopure 100; Euxyl K200. M.W. 406.33, $C_{11}H_{16}N_8O_8 \cdot H_2O$. Tasteless, very hygroscopic powder, decomposes at 160°C. Typical concentration for preservation: 0.2%–0.6%.

Imidazolidinyl urea is very water-soluble, stable, and is effective against most microbes. The antimicrobial weakness of this preservative is fungi, but this can be surmounted by the addition of parabens and other antifungal agents. It can be combined with other preservatives, such as methylparaben and propylparaben, to provide broad-spectrum activity. Imidazolidinyl urea works synergistically with parabens [80–85]. and with sorbic acid, dehydroacetic acid, quaternaries, and Triclosan [86]. The concentration of imidazolidinyl urea may have to be increased when formulating with imidazolidinyl urea and parabens if known paraben inactivators, such as nonionic emulsifiers, proteins, or others, are present. Imidazolidinyl urea is compatible with all common formulation ingredients, such as surfactants or proteins. It is not inactivated in the presence of polyoxyethylene nonionic emulsifiers or lecithin [87].

2. *Diazolidinyl Urea*

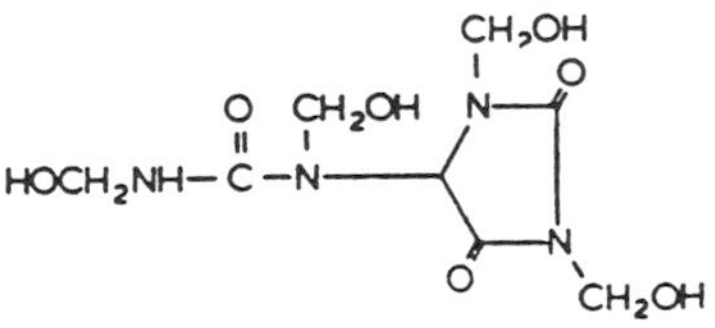

Synonym: Germall II. M.W. 278.23 $C_8H_{14}N_4O_7 \cdot H_2O$. White, hygroscopic powder. Typical concentration for preservation: 0.1–0.5%.

Diazolidinyl urea is a broad-spectrum agent against gram-negative and gram-positive bacteria, but has slight activity against fungi. In combination with other preservatives, such as methylparaben and propylparaben, it provides broad-spectrum activity against both bacteria and fungi.

The combination of 30% Germall II, 11% methylparaben, 3% propylparaben, and 56% propylene glycol is marketed as Germaben II. A combination of 20% Germall II, 10% methylparaben, 10% propylparaben, and 60% propylene glycol is marketed as Germaben II-E.

F. Acids

1. *Sorbic Acid*   H₃C–C=C–C=C–COOH (with H atoms shown)

Synonyms: 2,4-Hexadienoic acid, 2-propenylacrylic acid. M.W. 112.13. Crystalline needles with faint characteristic odor, m. 135°C. pK_a: 4.76. Solubility: 0.25% in water (30°C), 0.29% in 20% alcohol, 0.5–1.0% in oils. Typical concentrations for preservation: 0.05–0.2%.

Sorbic acid has a long history of effective preservation in the food industry. Historically, it has been used as an antifungal preservative, even though there have been reports of molds that have displayed resistance to sorbic acid; some even capable of metabolizing it [88,89]. It is one of the least toxic preservatives and is metabolized by mammalian cells by beta and omega oxidation, as are long-chain fatty acids [90]. Its use in pharmaceuticals is limited, however, because the antimicrobial activity is primarily due to the un-ionized form. The undissociated molecule exhibits greater activity than does the dissociated molecule [91–94]. Thus, sorbic acid is not recommended for use in alkaline formulations, although it is effective at acidic pH (optimum pH 5.5–6.5). Formulators should be aware that "sorbic acid" is not stable at the pH of optimum antimicrobial activity. Sorbic acid has few incompatibilities with typical formulation ingredients. It works synergistically with Germall 115 [86] and dehydroacetic acid [95]. There are, however, stability concerns when formulating with sorbic acid. Sorbic acid is sensitive to oxidation [96] and will discolor. It is unstable at temperatures above 38°C and is unstable in brown glass bottle containers, polyvinyl chloride containers, and polypropylene containers [97,98]. It degrades in solution when exposed to gamma irradiation in clear glass ampules [56].

2. *Benzoic Acid*   (benzene ring)–COOH

Synonym: Benzenecarboxylic acid. M.W. 122.12. White powder, m. 122°C. pK_a: 4.19. Solubility: 0.29% in water (20°C), 1 g in 3 ml alcohol (25°C). Typical concentrations for preservation: 0.1–0.5%.

Benzoic acid is effective only in the un-ionized form and, therefore, is useful only in acidic formulations [91,100]. It has optimal antimicrobial activity at a pH below 4.5. Loss of activity has been displayed in the presence of proteins and glycerol [86]. Benzoic acid is incompatible with nonionics, quaternary compounds, and gelatin [86], and with ferric, calcium, and heavy metal salts. Garret [101] found that pH effects the partioning of benzoic acid in certain oil–water systems, in that more benzoic acid was present in the aqueous phase as the pH was increased. It has moderate activity against gram-positive bacteria, mold, and yeast, but is less effective against gram-negative bacteria. Benzoic acid has been used as an antiseptic at concentrations up to 5% in combination with 3% salicyclic acid for fungistatic activity.

3. *Dehydroacetic Acid*

Synonyms: 3-Acetyl-6-methyl-2*H*-pyran-2,4(3*H*)-dione; 2-acetyl-5-hydroxy-3-oxo-4 hexenoic acid δ lactone. M.W. 168.15.White to cream crystalline powder, m. 109–111°C. Solubility: <0.1% in water, 3% in alcohol, <0.1% in olive oil, and <1% in glycerol. Typical concentrations for preservation: 0.02–0.2%.

Dehydroacetic acid is similar to the aforementioned acids in that it is effective as a preservative only in acidic formulations [92,102]. However it is a better antimicrobial at higher pH levels than are sorbic and benzoic acids [91]. Dehydroacetic acid is neutralized by nonionic surfactants [103] and discolors in the presence of iron [104]. Dehydroacetic acid is unstable in brown glass bottle containers, polyvinyl chloride containers, and polyethylene containers [97]. It has been reported to work synergistically with Germall 115 [86].

G. Parabens $R = CH_3$ to C_4H_9

The properties of the parabens and the typical concentrations at which they are used for preservation are listed in Table 4.

Parabens, esters of *p*-hydroxybenzoic acid, have been used as preservatives of cosmetics for over 60 years. The methyl and propylparabens are the most commonly used preservatives for cosmetics, and they are widely used for pharmaceuticals as well. As has been demonstrated over their long history, the parabens are very safe. They can, however, sensitize the skin and cause contact dermatitis, although the incidence of this is low.

The parabens are effective against mold, yeast, and gram-positive bacteria. Some molds are resistant, however. For example there is a report in the literature of a case

Table 4   Properties of the Parabens

Property	Methyl	Ethyl	Propyl	Butyl
Molecular weight	152.14	166.17	180.20	194.23
Melting point (°C)	125–127	116–118	96–98	69–71
Solubility (g/100 g)				
Water, 10°	0.20	0.07	0.025	0.005
25°	0.25	0.17	0.05	0.02
80°	2	0.86	0.30	0.15
Alcohol, 25°	52	70	95	210
Propylene glycol, 25°	22	25	26	110
Glycerin, 25°	1.7	~0.5	0.4	~0.3
Peanut oil, 25°	0.5	1	1.4	5
Mineral oil, USP, 25°	0.01	0.025	0.03	0.1

Source: Ref. 99.

in which methylparaben was hydrolyzed by *Cladosporium resinae* [105]. The parabens can be considered only bacteriostatic against *Pseudomonas* spp. and, as such, are not adequate by themselves to preserve ophthalmic products. Combining parabens with bactericidal agents is a common means of ensuring complete microbicidal activity of a formulation. In addition, combinations of parabens are used if two different phases are present. For example, methylparaben will protect the aqueous phase, in which it is more soluble, and propylparaben and butylparaben will provide protection in the oil phase, in which they dissolve more freely. Some marketed combinations are Phenonip, a blend of methyl-, ethyl, propyl-, isobutyl-, and *n*-butylparabens in phenylethyl alcohol, and Germaben II has already been described.

The usefulness of parabens is often limited by their low water solubility. They are readily extracted into organic solvents and oils and can also be lost from a product by absorption into rubber closures. The presence of propylene glycol increases the activities of the parabens by increasing their solubilities [106]. Parabens are subject to neutralization by nonionic surfactants: they bind or become trapped into micelles [107–109]. These properties all serve to reduce the concentration of preservative in the aqueous phase, where it is needed. Patel and Kostenbauder [110] reported that 78% of the total methylparaben and 95.5% of the total propylparaben were bound to polysorbate 80 when polysorbate 80 was present at a concentration of 5%. Studies performed by Pisano [111] confirm that the antimicrobial activity of paraben–polysorbate systems is a function of unbound paraben. Parabens have also been reported to bind to nylon and to be inactivated in the presence of nonionic macromolecules, such as polysorbate 80 (polyoxyethylene sorbitan mono-oleate) [40,112], Myrj 52 (polyoxyethylene sorbitan mono0leate), polyethylene glycol 4000 and 6000, and Pluronic F-68 (polyethylene propylene glycol) [112]. Magnesium trisilicate inactivates the activity of methyl paraben [40,113]. Paraben esters were not inactivated by kaolin [113], methylcellulose [114], polyvinylpyrrolidone, or gelatin [115]. Increasing the length of the alkyl group generally increases antimicrobial activity, but decreases water solubility [116] limiting their use in certain formulations [117]. Activity has also been decreased with branching [116]. The pentyl and higher esters are too insoluble for practical use. Methyl- and propylparabens are often combined to increase efficacy: antimicrobial activity is the sum of the concentrations, whereas the solubilities of the two compounds are independent.

Parabens are stable and effective in the pH range of 4–8 [118]. However, the pK_a of the hydroxyl group is about 8.5. At pH 8.5, 50% of the compound is ionized; thus, at the higher end of the effective pH range, the parabens ionize. The charged species cannot cross the microbial membrane; hence, the efficacy of the preservative is reduced. In addition, the parabens are subject to base-catalyzed hydrolysis following ionization [119] and, therefore, are not used in strongly basic formulations.

H. Phenols

1. *Phenol*

Synonyms: Carbolic acid, hydroxybenzene. M.W. 94.11. Colorless crystals with characteristic odor, m. 41°C. Solubility: 1 g dissolves in 15 ml water or 12 ml benzene. Very soluble in alcohol, glycerin, and oils.

Phenol is one of the oldest preservatives and is still the standard against which others are compared. Phenol is now used mainly as a disinfectant, rather than a preservative.

It is toxic, irritating, and has an unpleasant odor. In addition, it is neutralized by non-ionic surfactants and by reaction with proteins.

2. *4-Chloro-3,5-xylenol*

Synonyms: *p*-Chloro-*m*-xylenol, PCMX. M.W. 156.61. Crystalline powder with phenolic odor, m. 116°C. Solubility: 1 g dissolves in 3 L water. Typical concentration for preservation: 0.5%

At typical concentrations, chloroxylenol is much less toxic and irritating than phenol, but is considerably more potent as an antimicrobial. EDTA enhances the activity of chloroxylenol against chloroxylenol-resistant strains of *P. aeruginosa* [120]. Chloroxylenol does, however, share some disadvantages with phenol. It has an unpleasant odor and is neutralized by nonionic and cationic surfactants. For example, Judis [121] determined that polysorbate 80 would protect *E. coli* from chloroxylenol, while also preventing cell leakage.

3. *Chlorocresol*

Synonyms: Parachlorometacresol, 4-chloro-3-methylphenol, PCMC. M.W. 142.58. Dimorphous crystals, m. 64–66°C. Solubility 1 g dissolves in 260 ml water (20°C), freely soluble in alcohols, glycerine, and oils, pK_a: 9.2. Typical concentrations for preservation: 0.1–0.2%.

Cholorcresol has good antimicrobial activity against both gram-negative and gram-positive bacteria, including *P. aeruginosa,* and it is active against molds and yeasts. Its antimicrobial activity decreases with increasing pH, and it has no activity above pH 9. Chlorocresol is absorbed by rubber and, therefore, is lost through rubber closures [123]. It is unstable in polyethylene and polypropylene containers [92]. Cetomacrogol 1000 (Ceteth-20) complexes with chlorocresol [122] and also adsorbs to bismuth carbonate, calamine, calcium carbonate, kaolin, magnesium carbonate, magnesium trisilicate, magnesium oxide, titanium oxide, talc, and starch in solution [74]. Furthermore, oils, fats, and nonionic surfactants inactivate chlorocresol [40], and iron salts will discolor it in solution. Aqueous solutions of chlorocresol can turn yellow in light or in contact with air. Chlorocresol is commonly used for injectables.

4. *Triclosan*

Synonyms: 2,4,4'-Trichloro-2'-hydroxydiphenylether; Irgasan DP 300. M.W. 289.5. White crystalline powder, faint aromatic odor, m. 60–61°C. Solubility: 0.001% in water, about 100% in 70% alcohol, 60–90% in vegetable oils. Typical concentrations for preservation: 0.1–0.3%.

Triclosan is nonirritating, nonsensitizing, has a broad antimicrobial spectrum, and is especially effective against dermal microbial flora. It is, therefore, very common in cosmetic products, particularly deodorants and deodorant soaps. Triclosan is neutralized by nonionic surfactants (especially polysorbates) and lecithin. It works synergistically with Germall 115 [86].

I. Miscellaneous Preservatives

1. *Zinc Pyrithione*

Synonyms: Zinc bis-(2-pyridinethiol-1-oxide); bis-(2-pyridylthio)zinc-1,1'-dioxide; zinc omadine. M.W. 317.7. White to yellowish crystalline powder, mild odor. Solubility: 15 ppm in water, 100 ppm in alcohol, 2000 ppm in PEG 400. Typical concentrations for preservation: 0.025–0.1%.

Zinc pyrithione has broad antimicrobial activity and is effective against bacteria and fungi. However, *Pseudomonas* spp. are somewhat resistant to it. It is partially neutralized by nonionic surfactants and emulsifiers in MIC tests. Zinc can be chelated away from the pyrithione complex. Thus, the preservative is not compatible with EDTA or other chelating agents. Zinc pyrithione can transchelate (i.e., exchange its metal ion for another one). Transchelation can be prevented by adding zinc ions in the form of a salt [124]. Zinc pyrithione will degrade when exposed to light [125]. Photoprotectants can be incorporated into formulations or into containers to overcome this problem.

The sodium salt of pyrithione also has antimicrobial properties. In general, it is less potent than the zinc salt. Sodium pyrithione is compatible with many of the common preservatives and shows, with two exceptions, neither synergism nor antagonism. The exceptions are bronopol and lauricidin, which are antagonistic to the action of sodium pyrithione [126]. Both zinc and sodium pyrithione are used in dermal products and shampoos.

2. *Chlorhexidine*

Synonym: Bis(*p*-chlorophenyldiguanido)hexane. M.W. 505.5. Odorless, white crystalline powder, m. 132–134°C. Solubility of salts in water: digluconate, >70%; diacetate, 1.8%; dihydrochloride, 0.06%. Typical concentrations for preservatoin: 0.01–0.05%.

Chlorhexidine is used in various different dispersed systems: dusting powders, creams, aerosols, and medicated dressings. It is a broad-spectrum antimicrobial at in-use concentrations, but sensitivity to the preservative varies widely. Gram-positive bacteria are more sensitive than gram-negative, and *Pseudomonas* spp. can be resistant. Chlorhexidine is less potent, although active, against fungi and yeasts. It has very low toxicity in humans, and the incidence of skin sensitization is very low. The recommended concentration for use with mucous surfaces of 0.05%; irritation to the eye occurs with concentrations above 0.1%. Chlorhexidine is used as a disinfectant at concentrations of 0.5–1%.

Chlorhexidine has a relatively narrow effective pH range of 5–7. Its activity increases with increase in pH. However, it may precipitate out of solution at a pH greater than 8. Its activity also increases with a decrease in inoculum [127]. Chlorohexidine is inactivated by magnesium trisilicate and polysorbate 80 [40, 128] and adsorbs to bismuth carbonate, calamine, calcium carbonate, kaolin, magnesium carbonate, magnesium trisilicate, magnesium oxide, titanium oxide, talc, and starch in solution [74]. High concentrations of nonionic or cationic surfactants can cause inactivation of chlorhexidine, possibly by trapping into micelles [35].

3. *Thimerosal*

Synonyms: Sodium ethylmercurithiosalicylate, mercurothiolate, thiomersal. M.W. 404.84. Cream-colored crystalline powder, discolors in light. pK_a: 3.05. Solubility: 1 g is soluble in 1 ml of water or 8 ml alcohol. Typical concentrations for preservation: 0.002–0.02%.

Thimerosal is used in ophthalmic products because of its rapid antibacterial activity. It is especially effective against *P. aeruginosa*, a virulent pathogen of the eye. It is still one of the few valuable preservatives that can be used in a wide range of ophthalmic products.

Thimerosal is incompatible with other mercuric compounds, nonionic surfactants, and rubber closures. It has a complex stability profile: its sensitivity to heat and light depends on pH and the presence of certain metals. In general, thimerosal is most stable at pH 6–8 in the absence of light; the presence of Cu, Fe, and Zn ions accelerates its degradation. The stability of thimerosal in a formulation must be carefully evaluated because of its sensitivity to minor changes in the formulation, the packaging, and even the storage of the product.

Other organic mercurials, especially the acetate, borate, and nitrate salts of phenylmercuric acid, can be used as substitutes for thimerosal to meet special formulation requirements. The final pH of a formulation, the other constituents in the product, and the container in which the finished product is dispensed must be taken into consideration when deciding on which organic mercurial to use. Wallhauser cautions that phenylmercuric nitrate is active only above pH 6 [129]. In addition, organic mercurial compounds can be inactivated by organic material [130] and by nonionic surfactants [131] and they have been reported to adsorb to plastic, rubber, and polyethylene [132–134].

4. *Lauricidin*

Synonym: Glyceryl monolaurate. M.W. 274.4. Off-white solid powder or pastelike solid, m. 56°C. Solubility at 25°C: <0.1% in water, 80% in alcohol, 4.5% in propylene glycol, 0.2% in mineral oil. 250% in methanol, 60% in isopropyl alcohol, and 0.2% glycerin. Typical concentration for preservation: 0.5%.

Lauricidin is particularly effective against molds, yeasts, and gram-positive bacteria because it acts by affecting their membranes. It is not very effective against gram-negative bacteria owing to their protection by a more complex cell wall. Lauricidin does display antimicrobial activity against the gram-negative bacterium *Vibrio parahaem-olyticus* [135]. The inclusion of acidulants has been reported to increase its activity against other gram-negative bacteria [136]. In combination with edetate, it can be effective against gram-negative bacteria, especially *P. aeruginosa* [137,138]. Lauricidin has also been reported to work synergistically with sorbic acid [139]. Therefore, it should be considered as part of a "preservative system." Interestingly, it has strong antiviral activity [139].

The toxicity of lauricidin is extremely low. It is used as a preservative in cosmetics, but has not been used extensively otherwise.

5. *5-Chloro-2-methyl-4-isothiazolin-3-one and 2-Methyl-4-isothiazolin-3-one*

Synonyms: Methyl chloro isothiazolinone and methyl isothiazolinone; Kathon CG. M.W. 149.5 and 115. C_4H_4ClNOS and C_4H_5NOS. Clear amber liquid. Typical concentration for preservation: max. 0.1%. Kathon CG is a combination of 1.15% 5-chloro-2-methyl-4-isothiazolin-3-one and 0.35% 2-methyl-4-isothiazolin-3-one in an aqueous solution containing inert salts (magnesium chloride and magnesium nitrate).

Kathon CG exhibits broad-spectrum activity against gram-negative and gram-positive bacteria, as well as fungi. The combination of Kathon CG and Suttocide A is reported to be synergistic and was patented in 1990. Kathon CG is unstable at temperatures higher than 50°C. The presence of amine impurities in raw materials or some reducing agents, such as sulfite or bisulfites, has a deleterious effect on the stability of Kathon CG. Stearic acid can react with Mg^{2+} in formulatoins with Kathon CG and form insoluble magnesium stearate. Since the presence of calcium and magnesium ions has a signifciant positive effect on Kathon CG stability, it can be formulated with hard water.

Kathon CG is recommended for use in washoff products, such as shampoos, hair conditioners, and bubble baths, as well as surfactants and raw materials for cosmetics. It is not recommended for use in products such as toothpastes, lip balms, or eye products that come into direct contact with mucous membranes.

Kathon CG is soluble in water, lower alcohols, and glycols, but has low solubility in hydrocarbons.

6. *1,3-Bis(hydroxymethyl)-5,5-dimethylhy-dantoin and 3-Iodo-2-propynyl butylcar-bamate*

Synonyms: DMDM hydantoin and iodopropynyl butylcarbamate, Glydant Plus. White powder. Typical concentration for preservation: 0.03%–0.3%.

Glydant Plus is a combination of 1,3-bis(hydroxymethyl)-5,5-dimethylhydantoin and 3-iodo-2-propynyl butylcarbamate. Glydant Plus exhibits broad-spectrum activity and is especially good against yeast and molds. It is compatible with cationics, anionics, and nonionics. It is stable up to 80°C and over a wide pH range (pH 3–9). 1,3-Bis(hydroxymethyl)-5,5-dimethylhydantoin is marketed separately as Glydant XL-1000. 3-Iodo-2-propynyl butyl carbamate is marketed separately as Glycacil liquid or solid.

$$NC-\underset{\underset{Br}{|}}{\overset{\overset{CH_2Br}{|}}{C}}-CH_2-CH_2-CN$$

7. *1,2-Dibromo-2,4-dicyanobutane and 2-Phenoxyethanol*

$$\langle\text{phenyl ring}\rangle - O-CH_2-CH_2-OH$$

Synonym: Methyl dibromoglutaronitrile and phenoxyethanol Euxyl-K400, Merguard. Clear liquid mixture. Typical concentration for preservation: 0.03–0.3%.

Merguard is a combination of 19–21% 1,2-dibromo-2,4-dicyanobutane and 2-phenoxyethanol. Merguard exhibits broad-spectrum activity against gram-negative and gram-positive bacteria, as well as fungi. It is unstable at temperatures higher than 60°C. The presence of amines, alkalies, or sulfites has a deleterious effect on the stability of Merguard. It is soluble in water up to 0.4%. Merguard is recommended for use in all cosmetics and personal care products.

J. Polymeric Antimicrobials

Polymeric antimicrobials are compounds the structural chains of which contain integral antimicrobial groups, such as quaternary amines or biguanides. There is only one polymeric biguanide compound available as a preservative and that is polyhexamethylene biguanide or PHMB, sometimes called polyaminopropyl biguanide. The basic structure of the compound is as follows:

$$\left[-(CH_2)_6-NH-\underset{\underset{NH}{\|}}{C}-NH-\underset{\underset{NH}{\|}}{C}-NH-\right]_n$$

PHMB is soluble in water, glycols, and aliphatic alcohols. The pharmaceutical preservative-use concentrations run from 15 ppm to 1.0%, and the compound is available as a 20% solution under three different trade names: Cosmocil CQ, Baquacil, and Vantocil 1B (all from ICI Americas, Inc.). The spectrum of antimicrobial activity of PHMB includes bacteria, yeasts, molds, and protozoans. The mammalian host toxicity of PHMB is very low, with 5% solutions not causing eye irritation in rabbits or skin irritation in rats [140].

Polymeric quaternary ammonium compounds are often referred to as "ionenes" and have the general chemical structure as follows:

$$
\left[
\begin{array}{ccc}
R^2 & R^3 \quad R^5 & R^6 \\
\diagdown \; \diagup & & \diagdown \; \diagup \\
-R^1-N-R^4-N- \\
| & & | \\
A & & A
\end{array}
\right]_x
$$

where A is the anion of an acid and x is the degree of polymerization. These compounds are highly water-soluble and, in fact, one is termed WSCP which stands for water-soluble cationic polymer, from Buckman Laboratories. The other available polymeric quat is called Onamer M (sometimes called polyquad), from Onyx Chemical. The concentration range for use as a preservative for dispersed products is approximately 20–600 ppm. These compounds are nontoxic to mammalian hosts [140].

It is pertinent at this time to consider shifts in the use of various preservatives (Table 5). Particularly noteworthy are increases in the use of formaldehyde releasers.

K. Chelating (Sequestering) Agents

The deficiencies of one preservative can be made up by adding another, thus forming a preservative "system." The use of a mixture of parabens has been mentioned already. This is an effective and widely used technique that makes up for the low solubility of the individual compounds. Table 6 shows the effect of this combination on the growth of the fungus *Aspergillus niger.*

The parabens are safe and effective antifungal agents but are only moderately effective against bacteria, especially the pathogenic *Pseudomonas* species. To cover this deficiency, an antibacterial agent can be used. For example, the mixture of methyl- and propylparabens plus phenylethyl alcohol (sold as Phenonip) is effective against the entire spectrum of microbes. This is referred to as an additive effect (i.e., the different preservatives do not interact), and the total efficacy is simply the sum of the individual efficacies.

Synergism (or potentiation) can occur when two preservatives act on the same microbe by different mechanisms; the efficacy of the combination is greater than the sum of the individual efficacies [159,160]. A classic example of this is the use of edetate disodium with quaternary amines. Edetate disodium by itself has only very weak preservative activity. By combining it with benzalkonium chloride, lower concentrations of each can be used to obtain the desired microbicidal effect.

Chelating agents function to bind divalent cations such as Mg^{2+} or Ca^{2+} to stabilize certain chemicals. Ethylenediaminetetraacetic acid (edetic acid; EDTA) is a chelating agent often used in pharmaceutical formulations that has been inaccurately termed a preservative in some circles. Chelating agents, such as EDTA, sodium hexametaphosphate, or 1,10-phenanthroline, often act as potentiators of the antimicrobial effect of preservation agents (especially against gram-negative bacteria) in pharmaceutical formulations. In gram-negative bacteria, the lipophilic outer membrane is attached (stabilized) onto the peptidoglycan cell wall by divalent cation bridges [154]. Chelating agents, such as EDTA, nonlethally disrupt the permeability of the gram-negative outer membrane by

Table 5 Frequency of Use of Some Preservatives in Cosmetics as Disclosed to the FDA

	Number of products reported		
Chemical name	1993	1990	1984
Methylparaben	6738	7754	7694
Propylparaben	5400	6343	6796
Propylene glycol	3922	–	–
Citric acid	2317	136	162
Imidazolidinyl urea	2312	2749	2315
Butylparaben	1669	1200	803
Butylated hydroxyanisole (BHA)	1669	601	704
Butylated hydroxytoluene (BHT)	1610	551	375
Ethylparaben	1213	810	365
5-Chloro-2-methyl-4-isothiazolin-3-one-(methylchloroisothiazolinone)	1042	711	222
Phenoxyethanol	929	375	72
DMDM hydantoin	747	550	195
Quaternium 15	639	705	1126
Diazolidinyl urea	466	280	53
Triclosan	359	181	102
Sodium borate	358	29	25
Sorbic acid	251	178	396
Benzyl alcohol	237	64	49
2-Bromo-2-nitropropane-1,3-diol	223	321	429
Formaldehyde	185	441	711
Sodium benzoate	142	68	98
Benzoic acid	123	132	132
Potassium sorbate	112	78	94
Benzylparaben	106	26	39
Isobutylparaben	89	38	5
Benzalkonium chloride	86	161	34
Dehydroacetic acid	81	161	124
Chloroacetamide	75	82	23
5-Bromo-5-nitro-1,3-dioxane	60	58	17
Chloroxylenol	49	55	65
Paraformaldehyde	43	22	23
Sodium methylparaben	33	21	15
Chlorhexidine gluconate	27	18	8
Zinc pyrithione	25	28	32
Phenyl mercuric acetate	20	35	131
Dichlorobenzyl alcohol	11	12	2
Thimerosal	11	21	42

Source: Preservative frequency of use, *Cosmet. Toiletries*, 108 (Oct. 1993); 102 (Dec. 1984).

removal of these cation bridges. This allows the release of an important protein–lipo-polysaccharide complex, creating a greater influx of certain antimicrobial agents into the cells to cause more rapid killing action [155,156]. The bacteria most sensitive to this chelator action are in the genus *Pseudomonas* and, in fact, the minimal bacteriolytic activity is limited to *P. aeruginosa* and *P. alcaligenese*. Organic buffers, such as Tris, cysteine, and citric acid, also elicit chelating properties and can be employed to enhance

Table 6 Effect of Parabens on the Growth
of *Aspergillus niger*

% Methyl paraben	5 Propyl paraben	Growth
0.05	–	0
0.025	–	+ + +
–	0.015	0
–	0.01	+
–	0.005	+ + +
0.05	0.005	0
0.025	0.01	0
0.025	0.005	+

Source: Ref. 99.

the preservative efficacy of a formulation. A couple of excellent reviews on chelators
and EDTA are available to interested readers [157,158].

L. Combination Preservatives

Two new preservative systems introduced recently rely on a slow release of silver ions.
Both are described as follows:

1. *JM ActiCare*:

Synonyms: Johnson Matthey ActiCare; JMAC, an inorganic composite of silver chloride and titanium dioxide. White to cream pourable suspension. Typical concentration for preservation: 0.005–0.1%.

ActiCare is a silver chloride–titanium dioxide composite suspended and potentiated by a sulfosuccinate salt. The composite is a 10% suspension of 2% silver chloride and 8% titanium dioxide. The composite also contains 15% anionic surfactant composed of 10.5% sodium dioctylsulfosuccinate and 2.25% propane-1,2-diol. ActiCare is a broad-spectrum agent against gram-negative and gram-positive bacteria, as well as fungi. The antimicrobial activity is attributed to the inorganic composite, which allows a slow release of antimicrobial silver ions in an aqueous environment. ActiCare is not suitable for use in low-viscosity, single-phase liquid systems. The presence of cationic surfactants has a deleterious effect on the stability of ActiCare. ActiCare is soluble in water up to 0.4%. It is recommended for use in all products.

2. *Silver Borosilicate or Silver Aluminum Magnesium Phosphate*

Synonyms: Ion Pure type A; Ion Pure Type B; Ion Pure WA-29. White powder. Typical concentration for preservation: 0.25%–0.5%.

Silver borosilicate or Ion pure Type A is described as a water-dispersible silicate containing silver ion for broad-spectrum activity. Ion Pure Type A provides fast elution of silver ions. Silver aluminum magnesium phosphate or Ion Pure Type B provides slow release of silver ions when extended shelf life is needed. This preservative is broad-spectrum, nonmutagenic, and nonsensitizing.

Many suppliers of preservatives today offer proprietary mixtures of antimicrobial agents to add directly to your product formulation as the "preservative system." Examples are Germaben II from Sutton Laboratories, which combines parabens with diazolidinyl urea and propylene glycol; Midpol PHN from Tri-K Industries is a mixture of bronopol and phenoxyethanol; also from Tri-K a product called Midtect TF-60, which is a combination of 2,4-dichlorobenzyl alcohol and sodium dioctylsulfosuccinate; Paragon from McIntyre Group is a mixture of DMDM hydantoin(Glydant) and methylparaben in propylene glycol; and Glydant Pluspropylnyl from Lonza Inc., is a combination of DMDM hydantoin and iodopropylnyl butylcarbamate. Table 7 lists examples of marketed mixtures.

V. EFFECTS OF PRODUCT INGREDIENTS ON PRESERVATIVE ACTIVITY

The balance of many factors determines the success or failure of microbial growth in a complex environment such as a dispersed dosage form. The efficacy of a preservative is similarly determined by a balance of factors. This section is a guide to the likely interactions that affect (mostly adversely) the ability of a compound to keep a product well preserved. Of course not all such interactions are listed and, with the use of newer materials, new ones constantly come to light.

Given the complexity of dispersed pharamceuticals, it is apparent that a preservative system must be considered an integral part of the formulation from the outset of its design, not merely something thrown in to keep "bugs" away. The pharmacist can now make some very good guesses about how well a preservative will work. An adequate testing system is still essential, however.

A. pH

1. *Ionization*

For preservatives that are carboxylic acids, it is widely thought that only the un-ionized species is microbicidal. The pK_a of such preservatives, therefore, determines the effective pH range. The antimicrobial activity of benzoic acid, sorbic acid, and others, certainly decreases as pH increases past the pK_a.

However, the ionized species seems to have some degree of microbicidal activity, at least in the case of sorbic acid [141]. The activity of the sorbate ion was 10–600 times less than that of the un-ionized sorbic acid, depending on the organism tested. This result confirms our experience with sorbic acid as a preservative for simple solutions. Despite that the pH reduces the concentration of the un-ionized species to 2–3% of the total, such solutions are adequately preserved (Table 8). Sorbic acid at neutral pH can preserve a solution, but it takes more time for it to kill bacteria at the high end of its effective pH range. The length of time a preservative is allowed to contact the challenge microbes is clearly an important factor in the determination of preservative efficacy.

The pK_a of amines is generally higher than the pH of all but the most basic formulations. The antimicrobial activity of unchanged amine species has not, to our knowledge, been tested. However, the point appears to be moot as the higher pH required to form the un-ionized amines is lethal to microbes. Quaternary amines are charged at all pH values; their antimicrobial activity, therefore, is independent of pH.

Table 7 Combination Preservative Systems Available as Proprietary Mixtures

Actives	Recommended manufacturers use levels (%)	Trade names
Paraben combinations		
Methylparaben and propylbaraben	0.3–1.0	Combi-Steriline MP
Methylparaben, ethylparaben, and propylparaben	0.05–0.3	Nipasept
Isopropylparaben, isobutylparaben, and butyl paraben	Up to 0.5	LiquaPar
Methylparaben, ethylparaben, propylparaben, and butylparaben	0.05–0.3	Nipastat
Phenoxyethanol combinations		
Phenoxyethanol, methylparaben, ethylparaben, propylparaben, and butylparaben	0.6–1.4	Dekaben, Phenonip, Sepicide MB, Undebenzofene C, and Uniphen P-23
Phenoxyethanol and chloroxylenol	0.3–0.5	Emercide 1199
Phenoxyethanol and methyl dibromoglutaronitrile	0.03–0.3	Euxyl K400 and Merguard 1200
Phenoxyethanol and 2-bromo-2-nitropane-1,3-diol	0.04–.16	Midpol PHN
Phenoxyethanol, and 2,4-dichlorobenzyl alcohol	0.1–0.3	Midtect TPF
Phenoxyethanol, methylparaben, propyl paraben, and 2-bromo-2-nitropane-1,3-diol	0.25–0.5	Nipaguard BPX
Phenoxyethanol, triethylene glycol, and dichlorobenzyl alcohol	0.4–0.6	UniSupro S-25
Propylene glycol combinations		
Propylene glycol, sodium methylparaben, sodium dehydroacetate, sorbic acid, and tetrasodium EDTA	1–2	Fondix G Bis
Propylene glycol, diazolidinyl urea, methylparaben, and propylparaben	1	Germaben II
Propylene glycol, methylparaben, and propyl paraben	0.3–0.6	Nipaguard MPS
Propylene glycol, DMDM hydantoin, and methyl paraben	0.4–0.8	Paragon
Propylene glycol, DMDM hydantoin, methyl paraben, and propylparaben	0.4–0.8	Paragon II
Propylene glycol, methylparaben, ethylparaben propylparaben, and butylparaben		Paraoxiban
Butylene glycol combinations		
Butylene glycol, glycerin, and chlorphenesin	3.5 max.	Anti-MB
Butylene glycol, glycerin, chlorphenesin, and methyl paraben	3.5 max.	Killitol
Other combinations		
DMDM hydantoin, iodopropylnyl butylcarbamate	0.03–0.3	Glydant Plus
Methylchloroisothiazolinone and methylisothiazolinone	0.02–0.1	Kathon CG
Methyl dibromoglutaronitrile and dipropylene glycol	0.04–0.4	Merguard 1190
Polyaminopropyl biguanide and chloroxylenol	0.2	Mikrokill 2
Benzyl alcohol, methylchloroisothiazolinone and methylisothiazoline	0.03–0.15	Euxyl K100
Benzyl alcohol, methylparaben, and propylparaben	0.3–0.6	Nipaguard MPA

Table 8 Sorbic Acid Antimicrobial Activity Dependence on pH[a]

	pH			
	6.0	6.5	7.0	7.5
E. coli				
Day 0	0.0	0.0	0.0	0.0
Day 3	0.7	0.5	0.5	0.2
Day 7	6.0	2.0	0.5	0.8
Day 14	6.0	6.0	6.0	4.0
S. aureus	6.3	7.0		
Day 0	0.0	0.0		
Day 3	2.2	0.5		
Day 7	5.5	2.8		
Day 14	5.5	5.5		

[a]Log reduction of a 6-log microbial challenge of a saline solution preserved with 0.1% sorbic acid.

2. Stability

The chemical stability of some preservatives is strongly affected by pH. Bronopol is a good example of this [142]. At pH 4, the half-life of bronopol is over 5 years, whereas at pH 8 it has a half-life of 2 months. The stability of chlorobutanol as a function of pH has been discussed (see Table 3).

Sorbic acid, although less ionized at acidic pHs, is also unstable and is oxidized at pH less than 5. A balance between stability and efficacy, therefore, must be struck. This limits the useful pH range of sorbic acid to about 4–7.

B. Partitioning

Dispersed pharmaceuticals are, by definition, composed of more than one phase. Microbes inhabit only one phase, the aqueous. A preservative will be effective only when it is in contact with the microbes in the aqueous phase. Any process that reduces the concentration of the preservative in the aqueous phase reduces the preservative's efficacy. Most, although by no means all, preservatives favor the organic (or hydrophobic or oil) phase (Table 9). The concentration of preservatives in the aqueous phase is a function of the partition coefficient (K_w^o) and the organic/water volume ratio ($V_o/V_w = \varphi$; Fig. 2). The partition coefficient, in turn, is a function of temperature, pH, and the nature of the organic phase.

The obvious solution to the problem of a preservative's loss to the organic phase is to increase the total concentration of preservative in the formulation. This is often not a reasonable solution for two reasons. First, even if preservative efficacy is a function of concentration in the aqueous phase, preservative toxicity is a function of the total concentration in the formulation. Second, solubility is often limited for these compounds, in one phase or the other. For parabens, this can be obviated by using two different parabens, usually methyl- and propylparaben. Their solubilities are independent of each other and their efficacy is the total of both concentrations in the aqueous phase.

Surfactants, although necessary for most formulations, can be detrimental to preservative activity. The classic example of this is the interaction of nonionic surfactants,

Table 9 Partition Coefficients (K_w^o) for Common Preservatives

Preservative	$K_w^{o\,a}$	Oil
Benzyl alcohol	1.3	Peanut oil
	0.2	Liquid paraffin
Chlorhexidine	0.075	Liquid paraffin
	0.04	Arachis oil
Chloroscresol	1.53	Liquid paraffin
	117	Arachis oil
Phenethyl alcohol	21.5	Octanol
	0.58	Heptane
Methylparaben	0.03	Liquid paraffin
	7.0	Lanolin
	200	Diethyl adipate
Polyparaben	0.5	Liquid paraffin
	80.0	Arachis oil

[a] K_w^o = (concentration in oil)/(concentration in water) = C_o/C_w.
Source: From Ref. 35.

specifically polysorbate 80, with parabens [107]. The parabens become bound in micelles formed by the emulsifiers; this greatly reduces the concentration of preservatives in the aqueous phase. In simple systems this can be modeled, and good predictions of aqueous phase concentrations can be made [143–145]. Other preservatives are also susceptible to losses of efficacy from this type of interaction [146].

Certain surfactants are known to protect microbes from the action of a preservative. Polysorbate 80 seems to "plug up" the leaks in the bacterial membrane caused by

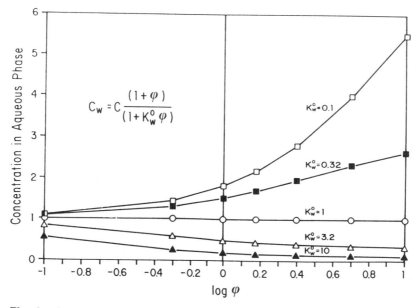

Fig. 2 Concentration in the aqueous phase (C_w) of preservatives with different partition coefficients (K_w^o) as a function of the ratio of volumes of the phases (ϕ). C is the total concentration of preservative.

phenol and related preservatives [147]. Although the mechanism is different here, the result is the same—the preservative is less effective in the presence of the surfactant.

Glycols have the opposite effect on preservative efficacy of the parabens and can reverse the neutralizing effects of steareth-20 [148].

Temperature does not affect solubilities equally in different phases. Generally, a higher temperature will cause preservatives to favor the organic phase. In other words, an increase in temperature effectively increases the partition coefficient, reducing the concentration of preservative in the aqueous phase.

The effect of temperature on partitioning can be illustrated by a topical cream. Consider, for example, a formulation consisting of mineral oil, cetyl alcohol, and stearic acid as the oil phase; sorbitan monooleate and polysorbate 80 as emulsifiers; benzyl alcohol and parabens as preservatives; and water. Assume that the oil and water phases are combined at 80°C with the preservatives added into either phase. At 80°C, cetyl alcohol, stearic acid, and sorbitan monoleate will melt and form a single liquid phase with the mineral oil. Benzyl alcohol and the parabens will have drastically different partition coefficients in this liquid than in mineral oil alone. The melted liquids acts as a seimpolar, rather than a nonpolar, solvent. As the emulsion cools and congeals, the preservatives will shuttle between the oil and water phases as the composition of the oil phase changes. As the solid components (cetyl alcohol, stearic acid, sorbitan monoleate) reach their congealing temperatures, the oil phase will take on the nonpolar properties of mineral oil and the partitioning of the preservatives will shift accordingly. In systems such as this, it is difficult to determine with certainty the concentration of each preservative in all phases of the complex dosage form.

C. Sorption

As with partitioning, sorption of the preservative reduces its concentration in the aqueous phase and thus its efficacy. Preservatives can bind to solid particles (e.g., talc, titanium dioxide) through a variety of mechanisms [149,150].

Plastics and rubbers can act as solid organic phases into which a preservative can partition [151]. Rubber stoppers are still used, especially for injectable formulations. Because rubber is itself a complex system, the effect of rubber products on a preservative system must be tested on a case-by-case basis.

Benzylkonium chloride and chlorhexidine gluconate can bind to polyethylene and polypropylene product containers [152]; thereby reducing their concentrations in formulations. This binding appears to be a surface adsorption process in that loss of the preservative quickly reaches a plateau. In the same set of experiments, the concentration of chlorobutanol and trimerosal decreased continuously over time to less than 10% of the stated content. This loss was shown to be due to sorption into polyethylene and polypropylene.

The degree of sorption into or through a plastic will also depend on the formulation. For example, a high alcohol content will prevent the loss of benzyl alcohol into plastic.

D. Processing

The manner in which the components of a dispersed system are added to each other strongly affects the properties of the final product. The order of addition of solvents can affect the partitioning of a preservative which, in turn, affects the preservative's efficacy. Although the final concentration of a preservative (or other component) in different phases is determined by the partition coefficient, the time necessary to reach that equilibrium can be affected by the order of addition.

Adequate control of pH and temperature during processing are also important here, especially in large batches of a formulation. Localized areas of high or low pH may cause precipitation or even destruction of a preservative (or other components). It may take considerable time for a precipitated preservative to redissolve. During that time, the formulation would be unprotected from microbial attack. For a volatile or heat-labile preservative, the longer cooling period of a large batch may cause its loss or destruction.

The manner of mixing is important when foams are produced. Foaming can cause surfactant preservatives (e.g., quaternary amines) to be trapped at the air–liquid interface. In this manner, the effective concentration of a preservative in a formulation can be reduced significantly.

Metal ions are known to enhance the destruction of many pharmaceutical ingredients, including preservatives. The less contact a formulation has with reactive metals, the less loss of preservative is likely to result. Edetate disodium is often added prophylactically to formulations to chelate metal ions and stabilize the product ingredients, including the preservative.

E. Packaging

Because the shelf life of dispersed pharmaceuticals is often from 2 to 5 years, the container–closure in which the product resides can have an important effect on preservative efficacy. Volatile peservatives can be lost from a formulation if the container is not tightly closed. Light can cause preservative degradation; thus, brown glass or opaque plastic is preferred for preservatives and product ingredients that are sensitive to visible or UV light.

Aluminum ions can bind to and inactivate bronopol [142]. Some preservatives can be extracted into rubber and plastics. These examples again point to the need for a testing program. A new formulation must be tested for antimicrobial activity in the *container-closure system in which it will be dispensed.*

F. Bioburden

In an adequately preserved product, the level of microbial contamination necessary to overpower the preservative is extremely high. However, if too many microbes are introduced into a poorly preserved formulation, they can overwhelm the preservative system. The most likely source of a bioburden that can overpower the preservative is the raw materials. Thus, the specifications for raw materials sometimes include passing a microbial limits test. Consumer contamination of products generally adds a much lower bioburden than the raw materials. The capacity test, described in Section IV, is a means of quantifying the bioburden that a preservative system can handle [153].

VI. EVALUATION OF PRESERVATIVE EFFICACY

A. Preservative Efficacy Test

The efficacy of a preservative must be evaluated in terms of the breadth and potency of the agent's antimicrobial activity. Usually, the manufacturer of a preservative has done the requiste efficacy testing of the pure preservative. This is done by using one or several of the many microbiological techniques that have been developed for this purpose. These include the following:

1. Determining the minimal inhibitory concentration (MIC) by incorporation of the preservative into agar or broth growth media
2. Determining the zone of growth inhibition around wells containing preservative solutions on agar plates
3. Measuring mold or bacterial spore swelling caused by preservatives in solution
4. Determining the rate of microbial death (survivor curves or D-values)

The criteria developed for assessing preservative activity dictate the methodologies to be used. The foregoing techniques all yield usable information and are convenient for comparing different preservatives. However, the process of preservation is complex and can be affected adversely, as described in the previous section. Thus the only valid way to determine the efficacy of a product's preservation is to challenge the agent(s) in a complete formulation.

In the United States, there are no compendial or regulatory tests or criteria specifically for dispersed dosage forms as separate from solution dosage forms. Therefore, we must look to the cosmetics industry for criteria, since that group of maufacturers pioneered the work in designing preservative challenge tests and efficacy criteria.

B. Preservative Challenge Test

A formulation cannot be considered adequately preserved until it has been tested for its ability to reduce a severe microbial challenge to zero viable cells. No matter how carefully the preservative system has been designed and how closely GMPs have been followed, the question must be asked: Can microbes survive in the formulation? The answer depends, to a great extent, on how the question is asked in practical, laboratory terms.

When a product sample is inoculated with challenge microorganisms, a population dynamics effect for microbial cell death begins. The challenge population contains a mixture of cells of which unknown portions are strongly, intermediate, or weakly resistant to the antimicrobial action of the formulation. The following process diagram depicts the dynamic changes in the population of challenge-cell types present in the test sample over the contact time period:

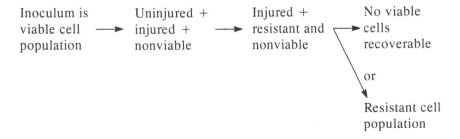

The time period to achieve each step in the foregoing process for decreasing challenge cell viability will be different for each product formula tested; some can complete the cycle in 1–7 days, some in 7–14 days, some in 14–28 days, and some may never complete the cycle, depending on the organism, the preservative system and the formulation constituents.

Rdzok and co-workers formalized the idea of a test system in 1955 [161]. Many variations on this theme have been reported since that time. All the described test systems were intended for use as research and development tools during the formulation and stability phases of product development. They were not meant to be product-release tests. Good reviews of preservative challenge test methods have been published [162–165]. From these reviews, plus the compendial tests in the *USP* and other pharmacopeias, one finds that there is no universally agreed-upon definition of adequate preservation of pharmaceutical products.

Even without clear criteria, a testing program must address the following to answer the larger question just posed:

Which organisms should be used to challenge the preservative?
How should the challenge organisms be prepared?
How many organisms should be used for a challenge?
Should the microbial challenges be single or mixed cultures?
How many challenges should be used?
At what times should aliquots be taken for the assay of survivors?
What neutralizer should be used in the recovery media?
What microbial assay method (e.g., pour plates, spread plates, or broth) should be used?

The rest of this section examines these questions.

1. *Test Organisms*

A preservative system must be effective against vegitative bacteria (both gram-positive and gram-negative), yeasts, and molds (spore-forming fungi). In addition, the preservative should be able to kill those organisms likely to get into the product from production or from consumer contamination. Consequently, the international compendial challenge organisms are:

Staphylococcus auereus, the most common gram-positive bacterial pathogen
Escherichia coli, the most common gram-negative fermentative enteric bacteria
Pseudomonas aeruginosa, the most common waterborne gram-negative nonfermentative bacteria
Candida albicans, the most common human skin yeast
Aspergillus niger, a very common air and soil fungus contaminant
Zygosaccharomyces rouxii, an osmophilic yeast

These six microorganisms are considered to be a reliable, representative sample, or bioindicators, of the microbial world. To make the data applicable to any product or laboratory in the world, controlled and cataloged strains of these organisms can be obtained from the American Type Culture Collection (ATCC) or the British National Collection of Type Cultures (NCTC). Preservative efficacy tests published by the *USP*, the British and European pharmacopeias, the Federal International Pharmaceutique, Cosmetic Toiletry and Fragrance Association, Society of Cosmetic Chemists, and the American Standard Test Methods, all recommend the use of the first five microorganisms above as challenges.

In addition, objectionable organisms (see Table 1) should be tested when there is reason to suspect they might contaminate a product, either from manufacturing processes or from consumer handling. These include

Pseudomonas multivorans	*Pseudomonas putida*
Klebsiella spp.	*Serratia marcescens*
Proteus mirabilis	*Penicillium* spp.
Candida parapsilosis	*Saccharomyces* spp.

The number of organisms recommended in published preservative challenge tests vary from the basic five to a comprehensive list of 25 organisms.

Additionally, it is recommended that organisms isolated from contaminated products be added to the challenge list. These "isochallenges" can be hardier than the laboratory strains and may even be strains that have developed resistance to certain preservatives [166,167].

2. Growth and Preparation of Inocula

The composition of the growth medium used to cultivate microorganisms can affect their resistance to preservatives. The addition or depletion of nutrients will influence the metabolic activity of microorganisms which, in turn, can affect their composition, function, and cell morphology. In nautral environments, microorganisms are starved and thus grow slower. Nutrient-deprived, slow-growing cells have been reported to be resistant to antimicrobial agents [168–170]. Peptidoglycan crosslinking varies with specific growth rate of gram-positive bacterial cells. Enhanced crosslinking increases cell wall stability by decreasing cell wall porosity, which may lead to resistance to antimicrobial agents. Gilbert and Brown [169] demonstrated that growth rate influenced the sensitivity of *Bacillus megaterium* to the actions of lysozyme, chlorhexidine, 2-phenoxyethanol, and certain antibiotics [170]. An increased growth rate increases the sensitivity of *P. aeruginosa* to polymyxin B in combination with EDTA [168] and to certain substituted phenols [169]. Sensitivity was related to changes in the lipopolysaccharide content of the outer membrane of *P. aeruginosa*. Richards et al. [67] demonstrated varying degrees of sensitivity of *E. coli* and *S. aureus* to BAK when grown to logarithmic phase, suggesting that the phase of growth will influence the suscepitibility of microorganisms to antimicrobial agents. Mayhall [171] found that *S. aureus* cells grown to log phase were more susceptible to antibiotics than were stationary-phase–grown cells.

Many studies have been performed demonstrating that the addition or depletion of nutrients in cultivation media can govern the outcome of results generated when studying the susceptibility of microorganisms to antimicrobial agents. In studying the correlation between lipid content and resistance to antimicrobial agents, Hugo et al. [172,173] demonstrated that *S. aureus*, grown in media containing 3% glycerol, grew cells that were "fat" in lipid content. These fattened cells were resistant to penicillins [172,173] and to alkyl phenols containing five or more carbon atoms in the alkyl chain [174]. Hugo et al. also demonstrated that *S. aureus* cells grown in media deficient in biotin grew lipid-deficient cells that were more susceptible to phenols and to cetrimonium bromide [174]. The presence of potassium has been shown by Nadir [175] to influence the adsorption of chlorhexidine to *B. megaterium*, thereby reducing this bacterium's susceptibility. Wilkinson reported increased resistance to EDTA when *P. aeruginosa* is grown in media deprived of magnesium [176]. Al Hiti and Gilbert [170,205] evaluated the depletion of carbon, nitrogen, and phosphate on the preservative efficacy of BAK, chlorhexidine, and thimerosal against the *USP* preservative panel of microorganisms. Their results indicate that BAK displayed the most variation to nutrient depletion and thimerosal the least. Ismail reported that resistance of *E. coli* to chlorhexidine increased when cells were grown in media depleted of carbon and that cells were more resistant to cetrimide and phenol when grown in media depleted of phosphate [177].

The pH of a medium and the temperature during incubation are two additional variables in growth conditions that may influence the susceptibility of an organism to an antimicrobial agent. The pH of a medium can fluctuate during incubation if a buffering system is not present. Organic acids produced during fermentation may be bactericidal, especially when the pH decreases [178]. Orth demonstrated that the pH of a medium decreases in the presence of glucose, thereby possibly increasing the sensitivity of microorganisms to the actions of preservatives [179]. Temperature influences the metabolic activity of both bacterial and fungal cells. The synthesis of cellular and extracellular molecules is favored under optimal temperature conditions. Increasing the production of certain molecules can directly or indirectly provide protection to organisms. The production of pigment by *S. marscescens* is enhanced when cells are grown at room temperature. The pigment produced has been reported to neutralize certain quaternary ammonium compounds.

Variation in the preservative and antimicrobial efficacy results reported in the literature may be attributed to differences in growth conditions employed by the laboratories performing the tests. Thus, challenge organisms must be cultured under standard conditions to ensure the reproducibility of the challenge test results. Bacteria are usually grown on trypticase soybean agar at 35°C for 18–24 h. Yeasts are grown on Sabouraud's dextrose agar at 25°C for 48 h (or 35°C for 24 h). Molds (filamentous fungi) are also grown on Sabouraud's dextrose agar at 25°C, but the incubation period is extended to 7 days.

Challenge organisms can be grown on an agar surface, as just described, or they may be grown in broth culture. There are differences of opinion on which is the best method for the purpose of a preservative challenge test. Orth et al. [179,180] studied the preservative efficacy of various preserved formulations against bacterial inocula prepared in broth and from an agar surface. The authors criticized the use of broth-prepared inocula in that they found that a decrease in rate of bacterial kill occurred. They attributed the decrease to carried-over broth that apparently inactivated the preservatives contained in the formulations or provided the bacteria with additional nutrients, enabling the bacteria to withstand the stress of the preservative systems. The authors confirmed their speculations by adding uninoculated broth to samples that were inoculated with agar-grown cells. Similar results were seen in that a decreased rate in kill was observed.

A valid criticism of preservative challenge tests is that standard, well-treated laboratory strains of organisms are not what the product will actually encounter. However, standardized microbial challenges do yield data that are reproducible from laboratory to laboratory. In addition, well-established strains do not require the complex media needed to grow more resistant or product-adapted cells. Other criticisms include the number of passages made before an organism is used. "The proposed revision to the *USP* stipulates that the organisms used for inoculation must be not more than five passages removed from the ATCC cultures, and mentioned that seed lot culture may be used" [181]. Other proposed revisions include phenol coefficient determinations, with required performance characteristics, before an organism can be used.

The preparation of the inoculum is as important to the results as the growth conditions. The harvest medium must be buffered and have the proper pH (about 6.8–7.4) and osmolarity so that it does not rupture or damage challenge cells. Surfactants (0.05% polysorbate 80) should be incorporated into the harvesting medium to facilitate single-cell dispersion. Orth and Brueggen [182] caution that "special care must be used to disperse cultures that are known to clump (i.e., *S. aureus* and some molds) before performing preservative efficacy tests." We believe that clumping could influence the rate of interaction between preservatives and microorganisms. It must also be emphasized that single-cell dispersion is a necessary prerequisite for accurate quantification.

Centrifugation is sometimes used in preparing challenge inocula. When used as a method of inoculum preparation, centrifugation enables microbiologists to wash cells free of growth medium and other potential contaminants. Improper control of centrifugation, however, can affect the results of tests evaluating the sensitivity of preservatives to microorganisms. Work performed by Gilbert et al. and by Rupp et al. [183–185] demonstrates how improperly controlled centrifugation can increase the susceptibility of microorganisms to antimicrobial agents. Gilbert et al. demonstrated that centrifugation at 10,000 g increased the susceptibility of *E. coli* to polyhexamethylene biguanide, while also affecting the adsorption of polyhexamethylene biguanide to the cell surface [183]. These authors attributed the increase in activity to loss of lipopolysaccharide from the cell envelope, which facilitated entry of the antimicrobial agent. Additional work performed by Gilbert et al. demonstrated that centrifugation (20,000 g) increased the susceptibility of *P. aeruginosa* to chlorhexidine and to cetrimide [184]. Work performed by Rupp et al. found that centrifugation (10,000 g) increased the susceptibility of *S. marcescens* to polyquad and to thimerosal/quaternium-16 [185].

3. *Amount of Challenge*

The volume of the microbial challenge should not exceed 1% of the volume of product (e.g., 0.1 ml inoculum into 10.0 ml of product). Creams, lotions, gels, and powder cakes usually have a sample size of 20 g, whereas 10-ml samples of aqueous suspensions are usually prepared. Once the inoculum is added to the product it is important that it be immediately mixed into the sample by a method that will yield uniform dispersion of the challenge cells. If uniform dispersion of the inoculum is not achieved, recoveries of viable cells from a fixed sample size can vary over a 5-logarithm (100,000-fold) range. This will tend to give erroneously low (or, less frequently, high) cell counts [i.e., apparently adequate (or inadequate) preservation].

The addition of an aqueous inoculum to an anhydrous product raises questions about the validity of such a challenge. The addition of water to the product may increase the odds of survival for the challenge microbes; therefore, the test might be a poor reflection of the survivability of typical contaminants. This can sometimes be circumvented by filtering the inoculum and adding the cell paste to the product.

A typical challenge is 10^6 cells per gram (or milliliter) of product. This level was chosen when neutralizers were not commonly used, and dilution of the challenged product (1:100) was used to negate the effect of preservative carryover. A second reason for this choice is that it is sufficient to observe the desired 3-logarithm (99.9%) reduction in viable cells.

The challenge should be performed on product that has been stored in the container–closure system in which the product will be used. This is essential, because preservatives can be lost through volatilization, adsorption, and other mechanisms, as was detailed in a previous section.

4. *Single Versus Mixed Challenges*

Most published tests recommend that each challenge organism be tested in separate aliquots of product (single challenge). Many times, however, it has been our experience that organisms that survive a mixed challenge (e.g., *P. aeruginosa, E. coli,* and *S. aureus)* would not have survived a single challenge. The presence of metabolites formed by the other microbes allowed these organisms to survive. Simultaneous inoculation of a sample with several different genera of microbes reduces the laboratory workload) while yielding information similar to, yet different from, that obtained from single challenges [161,165,186]. Mixed challenge should be reserved for circumstances under which the product's history of contamination supports the decision to use it. The value of data obtained from this method is questionable if the investigator does not identify the surviving organisms. If laboratory time is available, the use of both single and mixed challenges can be used to obtain a more complete picture of the preservative's efficacy in the formulation.

5. *Number of Challenges*

Multiple challenges of a product are performed to determine the antimicrobial capacity of the preservative system in the formula. A typical regimen is to repeat the original challenge at 14-day intervals a total of four times. This sort of "capacity test" yields very useful information about product safety in the hands of the consumer [153]. Multiple challenge tests should be reserved for testing final formulations. The FDA requires that all aqueous products for hydrophilic contact lens care (some of which are polydispersed systems) pass the *USP* preservative test with a rechallenge 14 days after the initial challenge. This is not required of other sterile ophthalmic eye drops or ointments. However, some manufacturers of nonsterile dispersed pharmaceuticals perform multiple challenges on their formulations to satisfy internal consumer safety standards.

6. *Assay Times*

The time intervals at which survivor assays are usually performed in our laboratories are immediately after mixing (zero time), and 1, 3, 7, 10, 14, and 28 days after the challenge. The addition of extra assay points during the first fortnight is useful for the rapid screening of preservative systems. Assays at 4 and 6 h following mixing are optional, but often yield data that adds to the understanding of the preservative's activity. For rapidly acting preservatives, the earlier time points are in indication of the margin of safety afforded the formulation. In addition to these advantages, the use of the listed time points allows evaluation of preservative efficacy in accordance with *all* compendial criteria.

7. *Use of Neutralizers*

Formulation constituents that are carried over to the growth medium in the survivor assay system can continue to inhibit microbial growth. Thus, the preservative's antimicrobial activity must be neutralized in some manner. Neutralizers are chemicals that inihbit the antimicrobial effects of preservatives. They are added to the dilution broth or the the agar plates [187]. The former is preferred because the preservative is neutralized immediately. We have found that neutralizers incorporated into the agar, but not into the broth, can decrease the ability of the medium to support the growth of stressed challenge cells, thereby yielding significantly lower plate counts of CFU per milliliter and causing the reporting of a marginal or inadequate preservative system as well preserved. Some useful neutralizing agents, and the preservatives against which they are effective, are presented in Table 10.

Some commercially available general-purpose preservative neutralization recovery media are Dey-Engly neutralizing medium (broth or agar) from Difco (0759-01-2), Letheen medium (agar or broth), and Clausen's medium from Oxoid. The efficacy of any of these media to neutralize the preservative system in a particular dispersed pharmaceutical must be validated in a specifically designed challenge test, as must its potential toxicity to the specific challenge organisms [188,189]. The Dey-Engly (D/E) medium has received the most use by industry. This is a very turbid complex medium that was formulated in 1970 to inhibit the activity of a wide variety of preservative agents in use at that time without being toxic to the five challenge organisms listed in the *USP* preservative efficacy test [63]. It contains bromcresol purple as a color indicator that turns yellow when the pH drops owing to acid production from bacterial growth. The formulations of D/E and Letheen (LM) media are as follows with figures being in grams per liter (g/L):

Constituent	D/E	LM
Lecithin	7.0	0.7
Polysorbate-80	5.0	5.0
Thiosulfate	6.0	0
Bisulfite	2.5	0
Thioglycollate	1.0	0

Test methods for assessing the efficacy and toxicity of a neutralizer recovery broth (NRB) are not readily available; hence, one is presented here. For the measurement of the efficacy of a NRB the growth pattern of each challenge organism must be the same in an inoculum serial dilution dose–response test of the NRB vs. NRB + product (at a

Table 10 Some Neutralizing Agents Employed in Recovery Broths or Solutions

Neutralizer	Preservatives
Polysorbate 80	Parabens, phenolics, quaternary amines, chlorhexidine, sorbic acid, alcohols
Sodium thiosulfate	Iodine, chlorine, hypochlorite, bronopol
Lecithin	Quaternary amines, phenolics, parabens, chlorhexidine
L-Cysteine, thioglycolate, and other sulfhydryls	Mercurials, bronopol
Neutralizing buffer[a]	Quaternary amines, chlorine

[a]Difco Laboratories, Detroit, Michigan. Contains monopotassium phosphate, sodium thiosulfate, aryl sulfonate complex, and sodium hydroxide, pH 7.2. Recommended as an adjunct to all neutralizing recovery media.

9-ml + 1-ml ratio, respectively). In the test, 1 ml of inoculum is added to tube 1, the tube vortexed and 1 ml is transferred to tube 2 and so on through tube 8 for each of the two media systems. The tubes are then incubated appropriately. The result is

Tube no.	1	2	3	4	5	6	7	8
CFU/ml	10^5	10^4	10^3	10^2	10	1	0.1	.01
CFU/tube	5 mil	500 K	50 K	5 K	500	50	5	.5
Growth	+	+	+	+	+	+	+	−

If growth does not occur in tubes 5–7 for NRB + product then the medium is not neutralizing properly and a new medium must be designed. If growth occurs in tubes 1–7 for both media systems then the NRB is validated for both neutralizer efficacy and lack of toxicity, as shown by growth of low numbers of challenge cells (50 or fewer per tube).

8. Assay of Surviving Microbes

To assay the survivors of the microbial challenge, an aliquot of the contaminated product is withdrawn and diluted, and survivors are allowed to grow on or in appropriate growth medium at an appropriate temperature. A proper control for this experiment is an identical challenge test on the same formulation minus the preservative(s). At assay times, 1 g or 1 ml of product is aseptically removed, added to 9 ml of dilution broth (containing the appropriate neutralizer), and mixed well. Two more sequential 1:10 dilutions of this suspension are made in dilution broth. The number of microbes per milliliter in each of the three dilutions is determined (in duplicate) by spreading 0.1 ml of the suspension on an agar plate.

The plates and the dilution broth suspensions are incubated at 35°C for 48–72 h (7 days for fungal spores). The number of colonies on the plates is counted, and the presence or absence of growth in the dilution broths is recorded. The number of colonies observed on a plate multiplied by the dilution factor of the plated suspension yeilds the number of microbes per gram or per milliliter of product. This calculation is valid only if the data from the three dilutions of an assay time point show the appropriate tenfold relationships, (e.g., 3 colonies for the 10^{-3} plate, 30 colonies for the 10^{-2} plate, and 300 colonies for the 10^{-1} plate).

Standard microbiological methods dictate that a count of fewer than 30 colonies per plate is not statistically valid. However, when there are only hundreds of microbes per gram, there will be fewer than ten colonies per plate for the first dilution (1:100) and no colonies for subsequent dilutions. Low numbers of colonies are reported and accepted as valid only when growth in the appropriate broth dilution supports the observation. The presence of growth in the broth dilutions with the absence of colonies on the plate for the first dilution is usually interpreted and reported as 10 CFU/g. In our laboratories, we use Table 11 to interpret the results from broth dilutions when there are very low levels of microbial survivors. If growth in the broth dilution tubes is not observed (i.e., only plate counts are used), the assay cannot validly detect fewer than 500 CFU/g.

Dispersed products can present problems with the assay phase of the preservative challenge test. Turbidity caused by particulates is difficult to distinguish from turbidity caused by microbial growth, especially for the first dilution broth tube (the 1:10 dilu-

Table 11 Interpretation of Results From
Recovery Broth Dilutions[a]

Product (CFU/ml)	Dilutions		
	10^{-1}	10^{-2}	10^{-3}
800	+	+	+
100	+	+	-/+
50	+	+	-
10	+	+/-	-
4	+	-	-

[a]Depending on the original concentration of microbes in the challenged product, and the dilution, microbial growth is (+) or is not (-) observed. Certain dilutions will sometimes show growth (+/-).

tion). The agar plate for this dilution may also contain particulates, which are difficult to distinguish from small microbial colonies. When this occurs, the sensitivity of the assay of microbial survivors is reduced, because only the higher dilutions of the challenged formulation will yield reliable results.

Some laboratories plate samples from the broth dilution tubes by the pour plate method. In this procedure, 22 ml of molten agar (at 50°C) is added to 1 ml of test sample and the mixture is swirled to disperse the cells. We do not recommend this method because many of the already-stressed challenge cells will die from the heat shock of going instantly from 22° to 50°C. This will yield erroneous data that may lead to a false sense of security about a preservative's efficacy.

The Cosmetic, Toiletry, and Fragrance Association (CTFA) in the United States has conducted a roundrobin collaborative study to validate an "efficacy of preservation" test proposed by the Association of Official Analytical Chemists (AOAC). This new test employs product challenges from four "selected pools of microorganisms," which are

1. Gram-positive cocci: *Staphylococcus aureus* plus *S. epidermidis*
2. Gram-negative fermentative bacilli: *Escherichia coli, Klebsiella pneumoniae,* plus *Enterobacter gergoviae*
3. Gram-negative nonfermentative bacilli: *Pseudomonas aeruginosa, P. cepacia,* plus *Acinetobacter calcoaceticus* var. *anitratus*
4. Yeast and mold: *Candida albicans* plus *Aspergillus niger*

The challenged products were sampled only three times (7, 14, and 28 days) and then rechallenged on day 28 and resampled as before. The criteria of acceptance are:

Bacteria: a 3-log (99.9%) reduction in 7 days contact and no increase thereafter
Fungi: a 1-log (90%) reduction in 7 days, followed by a 2-log (99%) kill in 14 days, and remain at or below that level for the next 14 days.

Microbiological data of this nature can vary significantly from sample to sample and the use of more sampling times tightens up this variance and provides added credibility to the data; accordingly, we would recommend that the foregoing test, whenever used, should include assay times at 1 day and 21 days to increase the accuracy and precision of the data generated.

C. Criteria for Adequate Product Preservation

Criteria for preservation efficacy are expressed as the percentage reduction in viable cells in a specific amount of time. To date, regulatory agencies, compendia, and industrial trade organizations throughout the world have not agreed on criteria for adequate product preservation. The established systems range in stringency from the *USP* to the *British Pharmacopeia*. To illustrate the diversity of preservation criteria, Table 12 summarizes and compares the compendial requirements for ophthalmic products. The product manufacturer and company microbiologist are left on their own to choose the appropriate criteria for their product. The nature of the product and the countries in which it will be marketed will influence this decision.

Criteria for preservation of oral products have been published by the *Federation International Pharmaceutique* and the *British Pharmacopoeia*, but not by the *USP*. The absence of such criteria in the United States may have contributed to problems with the preservation of oral antacid suspensions, as evidenced by the recall of 35 lots from six manufacturers in 1985 [27]. Two manufacturers' products, which accounted for most of the recalled lots, were presreved with parabens. The contaminants included *Pseudomonas, Klebsiella, Serratia*, and *Enterobacter* spp. A recent article clearly shows how aluminum hydroxide, simethicone, and polysorbate 80 inhibit the antimicrobial activity of parabens against gram-negative bacteria and, in particular, *P. aeurginosa* [191].

Some authors advocate the use of D-values (the average time required for a 1-log reduction of viable cells) as a screening procedure for developmental formulations [192, 193]. The D-value is determined by performing a preservative challenge test, assaying survivors several times in the first week, and plotting the logarithm of surviving microbes versus time. The slope of the resulting line is the first-order rate of death of the microbes, from which can be calcuated the average time for a 90% reduction of viable cells.

This concept has merit as a cost-reduction tool and certainly has a place in the armamentarium of the microbiologist. However, the technique lacks accuracy and precision in answering the basic question of preservative efficacy, especially in dispersed systems in which chemical and particulate interactions can affect kill rates. The D-value technique was developed for use with sterilizers and disinfectants, not with slower-acting preservatives. Reproducibility of D-values is often poor because the preservative-induced death of microbial challenge populations rarely follows first-order kinetics (i.e., the plot of logarithm of survivors versus time is not linear). Also, the method does not consider tailing effects and regrowth of the low-level survivors after a 3- or 4-week incubation [194].

Harmonization of compendial criteria for adequate preservative efficacy of pharmaceutical products worldwide has been going on from 1991 until 1994, with little compromise. The previous Table 12 shows the breadth of the harmonization chasm for preservative efficacy criteria. However, the following changes in criteria have been either adopted or proposed by the various compendia:

Table 12 A Comparison of Compendial Preservation Criteria for Pharmaceutical Products

Country: Pharmacopeia: Year:	United States USP XXI 1985	United Kingdom BP 80 1986 Addendum	Federal Republic of Germany DAB 9 1986	Italy Pharmacopeia 9th ed. 1985	Europe EP 1982
Contact times	7 d 14 d 21 d 28 d	6 h 24 h 7 d 14 d 28 d	24 h 7 d 14 d 28 d	6 h 24 h 7 d 14 d 28 d	24 h 7 d 28 d
Criteria for bacteria	*All products* Reduced by 99.9% (10^3) at 14 days; no increase thereafter	*Ophthalmics*[a] Reduced by 10^3 at 6 h; no recovery at 24 h and thereafter	*Sterile aqueous products* Reduced[b] by: 10^2 at 24 h 10^3 at 7 d 10^3 at 28 d	*Ophthalmics*[c] Reduced[b] by: 10^2 at 6 h, 10^3 at 24 h no recovery at 7 d (10^5 reduction); no increase at 28 d	*Ophthalmics* Reduced[b] by: 10^2 at 24 h 10^3 at 7 d 10^3 at 28 d
Criteria for yeasts and molds	No increase at 14 d and thereafter	Reduced by: 10^2 at 7 days; no increase thereafter	Reduced by: 10^1 at 14 d 10^1 at 28 d	No increase at 24 h; reduced by 10^2 at 7 d no increase at 14 d; no increase at 28 d	Reduced by: 10^1 at 14 d 10^1 at 14 d
Organism	*P. aeruginosa* ATCC902	Same	Same	Same	Same
	S. aureus ATCC 6538	Same	*S. aureus* ATCC 6538P	*S. aureus* ATCC 6538P	*S. aureus* ATCC 6538P
	E. coli	Same	Same	Same	Same
	C. albicans ATCC 10231	Same	Same	Same	Same
	A. niger ATCC 16404	Same	Same	Same	Same

[a]Desired criteria. Other considerations may be taken into account.
[b]*P. aeruginosa* and *S. aureus* only.
[c]Recommended criteria.

1. The British, German, French, and Italian pharmacopeias have decided to become one as the *European Pharmacopoeia*, with the following adopted final criteria presented as logarithms reduction in viable challenge cells at designated contact times.

Ophthalmics and parenterals	
Bacteria	*Target*: 2 logs/6 h, followed by 3 logs/24 h, followed by NR/7 days
	Minimum: 1 log/24 h, followed by 3 logs/7 days and NI thereafter
Yeast and mold	*Target*: 2 logs/7 days and NI thereafter
	Minimum: 1 log/14 days and NI thereafter
Topical (skin care)	
Bacteria	*Target*: 2 logs/2 days, followed by 3 logs/7 days and NI thereafter
	Minimum: 3 logs/14 days and NI thereafter
Yeast and mold	*Target*: 2 logs/14 day and NI thereafter
	Minimum: 1 log/14 days and NI thereafter
Oral (syrups and antacids)	
Bacteria	3 logs/14 day and NI thereafter
Yeast and mold	1 log/14 day and NI thereafter

NR, no recovery of viable cells; NI, no significant increase in CFU per milliliter.

2.   In contrast, the U. S. Pharmacopeial Convention have not changed their basic criteria for sterile multidose ophthalmics, parenterals, nasal, and otic products from those shown in Table 12. They have, however, proposed (a) criteria for topical products of a 2-log reduction of bacteria in 14 days, with no increase thereafter and stasis for the fungi; and (b) criteria for oral products of a 1-log reduction of bacteria in 14 days, with no increase thereafter and, again, stasis for fungi; plus, a special dispensation for oral antacids to be microbiostatic for all challenges for 28 days.

In addition, the *USP* is addressing the following issues that received a majority of support from industry representatives at a recent (1993) open conference on microbiological testing concerning preservative (antimicrobial) effectiveness:

1. Prefer a requirement for reduction in yeast plus mold counts, as opposed to stasis
2. Request a 24-h–assay point for ophthalmics and parenterals
3. Develop a panel of antimicrobials for testing organisms' resistance
4. Clarify the preparation of mold spore inocula and the interpretation of their data (spores do not reproduce by binary fision so they will not increase in viable numbers by growth: so, how do we judge a failure?)

A large chasm still exists in the acceptance criteria for the preservation of dispersed pharmaceutical products between the United States and Europe, with Japan leaning toward the European criteria. If one looks at the European criteria for ophthalmics and parenterals, with a focus on the 3-log reduction point, we see that the minimum time for this antibacterial kill is 7 days. Consequently, a possible attempt for United States harmonization would be to require a 3-log reduction in bacteria at 7 days, instead of 14 days, with no increase thereafter, and a 1-log reduction in the fungi over the 28 days of the test. This would at least go along with the European minimal criteria for ophthalmics and parenterals, which is probably at or below the internal standard employed by pharmaceutical companies.

VII. FUTURE TRENDS

The future of preservatives in dispersed pharmaceuticals is likely to involve changes based on developments in several areas. New avenues of research promise (a) new preservative agents, (b) new types of products, (c) new approaches to packaging, and (d) new or modified test methods.

A. New Preservative Agents

In the past 5 years, three mainstay preservative agents, thimerosal (and organic mercurials in general), benzyl alcohol, and benzalkonium chloride, have come under attack for safety reasons. Considerable effort is now directed to developing less-toxic and less-sensitizing agents. One approach being pursued is the development of polymerized forms of current preservatives (e.g., polymeric quaternary ammonium compounds) on the premise that polymeric compounds, in general, exhibit fewer undesirable biological effects. It remains to be seen whether such an approach leads to safer preservatives with appropriate microbiological profiles. As with present formulations, this can be determined only by thorough testing, especially in dispersed dosage forms.

A publication by Wallhäusser showed that over 90% of injectable, ophthalmic, and oral pharmaceuticals were preserved with only five different agents [37]. The most common preservatives for injectables were the parabens and alcohol; for ophthalmics, quaternary amines and organic mercurials; and for oral dosage forms, alcohol, benzoic acid, and the parabens. There are many more preservatives than these available. We would like to see a trend toward using the optimal preservative for a product, rather than the simple addition of the "tried and true" to a formulation. However, this is likely to occur very slowly, if at all, as economics and successful precedents both militate against the rapid adoption of newer preservatives.

As with pharmaceuticals themselves, the trend with new preservatives is toward "more powerful" ones (i.e., those that are effective at lower concentrations). Such agents have much higher therapeutic ratios and, therefore, can be used at lower concentrations. The lower the concentration of the preservative, the less chance it has of affecting bulk properties. However, the lower concentration means that a minor interaction with product ingredients or the container can cause a significant decrease in preservative efficacy.

To address the problem of microbial resistance to preservatives, new preservative compounds, new combinations of old agents, or a combination of new and old may be required. The genus *Pseudomonas*, and in particular the species *P. cepacia*, can be considered the plague of the 1980s for dispersed pharmaceuticals. Some of the conditions resulting in the development of antimicrobial resistance in *Pseudomonas* are discussed by Gilbert [195]. Borovian discusses the adaptation and growth of *P. cepacia* in the presence of two unrelated preservative systems: formaldehyde and benzoic acid [196]. Russell has reviewed the mechanisms of bacterial resistance to preservatives, disinfectants, and antiseptics [197].

B. Validity of Preservative Efficacy Test Criteria

Pharmaceutical product formulators and microbiologists are often asked if the preservative efficacy (PE) criteria applied to their products is a valid predictor of product safety (indicator of the frequency and amount of microbial contamination during consumer use) and, if the more stringent criteria applied in Europe have a valid rationale as a requirement to increase product safety over the criteria deemed adequate by U. S. Pharmacopeia.

Recently, a few authors have attempted to find a correlation of various products' abilities to pass different preservative efficacy criteria and their rate of contamination after consumer use (e.g., asking the questions: What is the validity of the various critieria for adequate preservative efficacy, and are more stringent criteria necessary?). This subject is of great interest because of the spectrum of requirements for adequate preservation of dispersed products around the world and the fact that neither the British nor the European pharamcopeias put forth a rational statement to substantiate their requirement for more stringent antimicrobial kill from pharmaceuticals, when in fact, no hazardous condition existed with consumer infections owing to inadequately preserved products over the 10–20 years of using the *USP* and corporate internal criteria for this safety test.

Brannan et al. [198] studied a unpreserved, marginally preserved, and well-preserved shampoo and lotion product with the CTFA mixed challenge PE test and then gave the products to 30 people to use. These investigators showed varying results in that the shampoo yielded contamination of 46% of the unpreserved, 21% of the marginal, and 0% of the well-preserved formulations, as compared with 90%, 0%, and 0% for the lotion, respectively. The authors concluded that how the product was used and the container design was more relevant than pass or fail PE challenge criteria when predicting consumer use contamination of a product. They stated, "if container design provides adequate protection, even poorly preserved products could withstand consumer use."

In 1991, Davison et al. [199] published the results of a pilot study to assess the validity of the *USP* versus the British pharamcopeial criteria for preservative efficacy. These authors assessed four products for their challenge test preservative efficacy profile and, then, let consumers use these products in three different settings, a ward (2 days), a clinic (0.5 days), and outpatient use (7 days). Two products were preserved with 50 ppm thimerosal (TMS, a saline and a dispersed steroid), a benoxinate solution with 100 ppm chlorhexidine (CX), and a steroid suspension with 100 ppm benzalkonium chloride (BAK). The results showed a 4.5–5.0% contamination rate for the TMS- and CX-preserved products and a 9.0% contamination of the best-preserved (100 ppm BAK) product—7/154, 9/221, 6/132, and 9/97, respectively. Although the CX-preserved product performed far superior to the two TMS-preserved products against *S. aureus* (total kill in 6 h at contact vs. a 4.5/6.8-log kill in 2 days of contact), their in-use contamination rates were identical. Since the contamination rate did not correlate with the PE test results, the authors decided to weight the data for used units showing greater than 1×10^3 CFU/ml (e.g., 800 CFU/ml = 1, and 1200 CFU/ml = 10) so that a distinction could be made between the "well-preserved" eye drops and the TMS-preserved products. The authors stated that "this study shows that the stringent criteria for multidose ophthalmic preparations in the BP efficacy of preservatives challenge test are realistic." However, we believe these investigators made an erroneous (and highly biased) conclusion, because the sample size variance (375 TMS-preserved vs. 229 CX- and BAK-preserved) created a circumstance for 150 more TMS-preserved units to show an increased level of contamination in a few units.

In 1993, Spooner and Davison [200] published a follow-up study (to their 1991 work) in which they assessed the contamination rate of 936 used cream (353/936), gel- (263/936), and injectable (320/936)-type products and performed PE challenge testing on 40 unopened products. These authors concluded that "For topical products the *British Pharmacopoeia* 1993 criteria and the proposed *European Pharmacopoeia* criteria–A for preservative efficacy are satisfactory, but the proposed *European Pharmacopoeia* criteria–B and the *U. S. Pharmacopeia* criteria may be potentially hazardous." We feel that these authors were erroneous in their conclusion because they misinterpreted the *USP* criteria in their Table 8 by saying that products that show growth of challenge bacteria (*P. aeruginosa*) between the day-7 and day-14 viable cell counts pass the *USP* criteria as long as the 14-day log reduction exceeds 3.0. This is completely wrong, because the *USP* states there can be no increase in bacterial challenge (CFU/ml) counts anywhere in the test data. It is interesting to see that the authors said nothing about the fact that the creams that passed the BP and EP–A criteria yielded between 12 and 35% contamination. Again, these authors stated that the less demanding European Pharmacopoeia criteria–B and the U. S. Pharmacopeia criteria would permit the use of products which could support the growth of adventitious contaminants and could therefore be potentially hazardous. This is a strong critical (and highly biased) statement that the data did not substantiate.

Interestingly, none of the three foregoing authors referenced the work of R. A. Cowen [202], published in 1974, in which he performed controlled consumer-use tests and PE tests on shampoos, bath additives, deodorants, and skin antiseptics. The correlation between in vitro laboratory test data and performance in practice was quite low for shampoos, deodorants, and skin antiseptics, but was fair for the bath additive products. Mr. Cowen said, *it is not known how resistance of various organisms actually on the skin differ in respect to individual antimicrobial agents or how this resistance matches that of the laboratory cultures (if tested). Such differences may well account for the discrepancy between the two sets of resultant data.* This information may well have influenced the foregoing authors' reports to include verbage saying that further work is necessary in the area of controlled in-use testing before correlations can be made between laboratory microbial challenge-testing data and actual consumer-use contamination rates. Also, they might have suggested a decent protocol for evaluating in-use contamination that discussed how the method of product use and the container designs influences the observed frequency and amount of in-use microbial contamination. Additionally, the performance of consumer-use testing on products used in clinical trials to identify a trend in the amount and type of microbial contamination was advocated by Lorenzetti in 1984 [203] as an adjunct to research and stability preservative challenge testing to fully assess a products safety in this area.

There are several literature articles describing the after-use contamination of dispersed pharmaceutical products; however, these reported product contaminations did not result in any clinically relevant hazardous situations to the users. Consequently, the assertion that stronger preserved products are safer products for the users is still an open issue for debate in the arena of pharmaceutical microbiology. Indeed, if the USP preservative efficacy criteria were as bad as Davidson and Spooner suggest than 25 years of its use in the United States should certainly have produced many user infections resulting in publicised consumer litigations. This is not true. We believe that the best preserved formula possible should be marketed for dispersed dosage forms. However, new chemical entities should not be kept from the marketplace if their formulations cannot be preserved as well as previous products, yet still do not deter from present safety afforded consumers of dispersed-type products.

C. New Packaging Approaches

One way to avoid the problems of sensitization and toxicity of preservatives is to eliminate the preservatives entirely. New packaging techniques allow this to be done in a safe manner. This is the idea behind the "unit dose" approach to packaging nonpreserved sterile pharmaceuticals. Unit-dosage is expensive for the consumer, who pays more for the packaging than the contents. However, clinical and regulatory concerns of safety, and the consumer movement in society calling for the elimination of preservatives from all products, are the forces behind the development of safe, nonpreserved, multidose pharmaceuticals which will require unique package, delivery system engineering.

D. New or Modified Test Methods

In considering new test methods, we have already seen that dispersed products often require alterations of compendial methods for testing ointments or suspensions. What lies ahead could be increased numbers and types of challenge microorganisms as well as multiple rechallenges. Also, with the poor laboratory reproducibility of preservative efficacy results seen over the past 15 years, the drive for better standardization will continue. For example, Al-Hiti and Gilbert recommend that microbiologists more closely scrutinize their inoculum preparation techniques [204]. Their earlier publication demonstrated that the ability of *P. aeruginosa* and *E. coli* to grow in the presence of chlorhexidine, thimerosal, or benzalkonium chloride varied markedly with various nutrient depletions of the inocula (as is likely to occur in nature) [205]. These are hints of new methods that may be used in the near future to improve the reliability and reproducibility of the preservative challenge test. A better understanding of the dynamics of testing methods will, one hopes, lead to standardization of methodologies and serve as an impetus to worldwide agreement on the definition of preservation for pharmaceutical products.

In the early 1990s, both the MCA in England and the *USP* in the United States have voiced concerns for standardizing the challenge microbial cell suspensions for PE testing. First, to avoid potential genetic changes that could effect test results, these agencies have recommended that no more than five passages (subcultures) of the test microorganisms be allowed between the primary culture (received from a known national culture repository) and the test product inoculum cell suspension. This request has been made even though no evidence has been presented that passage-10 cells are any different from passage-3 cells. This seems to be a very prudent scientific principle to include in preservative efficacy testing and is already carried out in many pharmaceutical company laboratories.

Also, there is a desire to measure and document the antimicrobial resistance of the challenge cell populations at the time of product testing. However, the problem here is exactly what to measure: the zones of inhibition to a battery of standard antibiotic disks (an antibiogram), or the kinetic kill rate of each organism to a standardized concentration of at least two different preservatives in some standard vehicle solution. Another problem with this proposed new test parameter is to establish the acceptable background variance, or the inherent experimental error, for the method chosen. Either method will undoubtedly produce day-to-day and technician-to-technician variability that must be considered in setting the standard performance expected from the cultures if the actual measurement of antimicrobial resistance can be done with repeated accuracy. This parameter in PE testing is finally being addressed, 20 years after R. A. Cowen's suggestion.

Additionally, the European and U. S. pharmacopeias are advocating that all PE testing on stability and clinical supplies of new products *be carried out in the final container*, as opposed to removing a measured aliquot of product from the final container (stored appropriately) and performing the challenge test in a closed test tube (plastic or glass). This proposal would require different inoculations for each different fill volume of the product, would reduce the uniform dispersion of the inoculum, and would create a tremendous increase in the storage space required for the PE test samples (product containers vs. test tube racks) to point out only a few problems. After input from industry, the pharmacopeias are reconsidering their proposal and will most likely allow both methods to be done, with a preference for some data generated in the final container.

A consideration of the foregoing proposed additions to the current PE tests performed around the world leads one to ask: What exactly is required in the submission of PE test data to a regulatory agency for approval of a product? The description of the PE test should include the following information:

1. The exact nomenclature of the organisms used and their source (strain numbers)
2. The exact procedures for preparation of the inocula (bacteria, yeast, and mold spores)
3. The manner of sample preparation, its exact amount, and the number of replicates
4. The level of CFU per millimeter challenge, proposed and observed, for each organism for each test
5. The incubation and storage conditions of the challenged test samples
6. The volume, number, and contact time periods at which samples are taken for CFU per milliliter counts
7. The exact method for determining the CFU per millimeter counts (spread vs. pour plates, or other)
8. The antimicrobial neutralization method employed and its validation testing for the recovery of low levels of each challenge organism and efficacy of inactivation.
9. The inoculum levels observed in the controls at time zero and the CFU per milliliter (or gram) of product at each assay point
10. A description of the trend in antimicrobial activity observed for all the PE tests performed on the product (includes both developmental and stability data)

One cannot simply say, "the *USP* or *EP* method was employed and all of the tests passed," one must describe the testing in great detail.

Finally, it is hoped that new preservation criteria reflect that different uses of products carry with them different risks. Products for oral, dermal, ocular, and injectable uses, therefore, should have different criteria for preservation, reflecting the differing potential hazards of the products if they are contaminated by microbes.

As long as product contamination is a risk to consumers, preservation of multidose pharmaceuticals will be a concern. A thorough understanding of the theory and practice of preservation must be applied by formulators and microbiologists early in the development process.

ACKNOWLEDGMENT

The authors gratefully acknowledge the assistance of Paul Laskar and Aaron Van Etten in the preparation of this chapter.

REFERENCES

1. L. J. Morse and L. E. Schonbeck, *N. Engl. J. Med.,* 278:376–378.
2. L. J. Morse, H. L. Williams, F .P. Grenn, E. E. Eldridge, and J. R. Rotta, *N. Engl. J. Med.,* 277:472–473 (1967).
3. M. J. Muscatiello and J. Penicnak, *Cosmet. Toiletries,* 101(12):47–50 (1986).
4. D. F. Spooner, Ellis Horwood, Chichester, 1988, pp. 15–34.
5. C. J. Holmes and M. C. Allwood, *J. Appl. Bacteriol.,* 46:247–267 (1979).
6. R. L. Berkelman, S. Lewin, J. R. Allen, R. L. Anderson, L. D. Budnick, S. Shapiro, S. M. Friedman, P. Nicholas, R. S. Holzman, and R. W. Haley, *Ann. Intern. Med.,* 95:32–36 (1981).
7. P. L. Parrott, P. M. Terry, E. W. Whiteworth, L. W. Frawley, R. S. Coble, I. K. Wachsmuth, and J. E. McGowan, *Lancet,* 2:683–685 (1982).
8. Code of Federal Regulations. Title 21. Office of the Federal Register, United States Government Printing Office. April 1, 1987:Sec. 211.
9. S. R. Kohn, L. Gershenfeld, and M. Barr, *J. Pharm. Sci.,* 52:967–974 (1963).
10. P. Gilbert, in *The Revival of Injured Microbes* (M. H. E. Andrew and A. D. Russell, eds.), Academic Press, London, 1984, pp. 175–191.
11. United States Pharmacopeial Convention. *The United States Pharmacopeia,* 22nd Rev. United States Pharmacopeial Convention, Rockville, Maryland, 1990, p. 1479.
12. B. Croshaw, *J. Soc. Cosmet. Chem.,* 28:3–16 (1977).
13. D. L. Wodderburn, *Adv. Pharm. Sci.,* 1:195–268 (1964).
14. J. R. Evans, Gilden, M. M., and Bruch, C. W., *J. Soc. Cosmet. Chem.,* 23:549–564 (1972).
15. C. W. Bruch, *Drug Cosmet. Ind.,* 109:26–30; 105–110 (1971).
16. C. W. Bruch, *Drug Cosmet. Ind.,* 110:32–37; 116–121 (1972).
17. G. Sykes, *J. Modern Pharm.,* 1–2(14):8–21 (1971).
18. L. A. Wilson, J. W. Kuehne, S. W. Hall, and D. G. Ahern, *Am. J. Ophthalmol.,* 71:1298–1302 (1971).
19. A. M. Duke, *J. Appl. Bacteriol.,* 44:Sxxxv-Sxlii (1978).
20. J. A. Troller, and J. H. Christian, *Water Activity and Food,* Academic Press, Orlando. 1978, pp. 86–102.
21. E. G. Beveridge, in *Pharmaceutical Microbiology* (W. B. Hugo, and A. D. Russell, eds.), Blackwell Scientific Publications, Cambridge, MA, 1992, Chap. 18.
22. S. M. Gelbart, G. F. Reinhardt, and H. B. Greenlee, *J. Clin. Microbiol.,* 3:62–66 (1976).
23. M. S. Favero, L. A. Carson, W. W. Bond, and N. J. Petersen, *Science,* 173:836–838 (1971).
24. L. A. Carson, M. S. Favero, W. W. Bond, and N. J. Petersen, *Appl. Microbiol.,* 23: 863–869 (1972).
25. A. D. Russell, in *Principles and Practice of Disinfection, Preservation, and Sterilization* (Russell, A. D., Hugo, W. B., and Ayliffe, G. A. J., eds.), Blackwell Scientific, Oxford, 1982, p. 115.
26. E. P. Robinson, *J. Pharm. Sci.,* 60:604–605 (1971).

27. M. S. Cooper, ed., *The Microbiological Update*. Microbiological Applications, Islamorada, FL, 1985.
28. E. G. Beveridge and K. Todd, *J. Pharm. Pharmacol.*, 25:741–744 (1973).
29. J. J. Kabara, *J. Soc. Cosmet. Chem.*, 29:733–741 (1978).
30. Y. Wachi, M. Yanagi, H. Katsura, and S. Ohta, *J. Soc. Cosmet. Chem.*, 31:67–84 (1980).
31. S. G. Hales, G. K. Watson, K. S. Dodgson, and G. F. White, *J. Gen. Microbiol.*, 132: 953–961 (1986).
32. M. J. Akers, K. M. Ketron, and B. R. Thompson, *J. Parent. Sci. Technol.*, 36:23–27 (1982).
33. C. Baggerman, J. A. Loos, and H. E. Junginger, *Int. J. Pharm.*, 27:17–27 (1985).
34. L. A. Wilson and D. G. Ahearn, *Am. J. Ophthalmol.*, 84:112–119 (1977).
35. American Pharmaceutical Association, *Handbook of Pharmaceutical Excipients*, Washington, DC, 1986.
36. Martindale, *The Extra Pharmacopoeia*, 28th Ed. (J. E. F. Reynolds, ed.), The Pharmaceutical Press, London, 1982.
37. K. H. Wallhäusser, *Pharm. Ind.*, 47:191–202 (1985).
38. P. S. Prickett, H. L. Murray, and H. N. Mercer, *J. Pharm. Sci.*, 50:316–320 (1961).
39. A. D. Russel, J. Jenkins, and I. H. Harrison, *Adv. Appl. Microbiol.*, 9:1–38 (1967).
40. R. T. Yousef, M. A. El-Nakeeb, and S. Salama, *Can. J. Pharm. Sci.*, 18:54–56 (1973).
41. C. K. Bahal and H. B. Kostenbauder, *J. Pharm. Sci.*, 53:1027–1029 (1964).
42. W. T. Friesen and M. Elmer, *Am. J. Pharm.* 28:507 (1974).
43. A. D. Nair and J. L. Lach, *J. Am. Pharm. Assoc.*, 48:390–395 (1959).
44. Lachman, *J. Pharm. Sci.*, 51:224–232 (1962).
45. A. D. Lair and J. L. Lach, *J. Am. Pharm. Assoc.*, (Sci. Ed.), 48:390–395 (1959).
46. S. P. Staal and W. P. Rowe, *J. Virol.*, 14:1620–1622 (1974).
47. R. M. E. Richards, and R. J. McBride, *J. Pharm. Pharmacol.*, 23:(Suppl.):141S–146S (1973).
48. B. Croshaw, M. J. Groves, and B. Lessel, *J. Pharm. Pharmacol.*, 16, (Suppl.):127T–130T (1964).
49. M. R. W. Brown, *J. Soc. Cosmet. Chem.*, 17:185–195 (1966).
50. Anonymous, *Cosmet. Toiletries*, 92:87–95 (1977).
51. M. C. Allwood, *Microbios*, 7:209–214 (1973).
52. R. J. Stretton, and T. W. Manson, *J. Appl. Bacteriol.*, 36:61–76 (1973).
53. R. L. Elder, Toxiology, 4: 47–61 (1980).
54. W. E. Rosen, and P. A. Berke, *J. Soc. Cosmet. Chem.*, 24:663–675 (1973).
55. D. M. Bryce and R. Smart, *J. Soc. Chem.*, 16:187–201 (1965).
56. T. J. McCarthy, *Pharm. Weekbl.*, 113:698–700 (1978).
57. P. C. Dunnett and G. M. Telling, *Int. J. Cosmet. Sci.*, 6:241–247 (1984).
58. Cosmetic Ingredient Review. *J. Am. Coll. Toxicol.*, 3:139–155 (1984).
59. H. Madea, N. Yamamota, T. Nagoya, K. Kurosawa, and F. Kobayashi, *Agric. Biol. Chem.*, 40:1705–1709 (1976).
60. Cosmetic Ingredient Review. *J. Am. Coll. Toxicol.*, 7:245–277 (1988).
61. P. A. Berke, D. C. Steinberg, and W. E. Rosen, *Cosmet. Toiletries*, 97(Nov):89–93 (1982).
62. P. A. Burke and W. Rosen, U. S. Patent 4,980,176, issued December 25, 1990.
63. T. J. McCarthy, in *Cosmetic and Drug Preservation* (J. J. Kabara, ed.), Marcel Dekker, New York, 1984, pp. 381.
64. Cosmetic Ingredient Review. *J. Am. Coll. Toxicol.*, 5:61–101 (1986).
65. R. A. Cutler, E. B. Cimijotti, T. J. Okolwich, and W. F. Wetterau, *CSMA Proceedings of the Annual Meeting*, 1966, pp. 102–113.
66. N. M. Daoud, N. A. Dickinson, P. Gilbert, *Microbios*, 37:73–85 (1983).
67. R. M. E. Richards and L. M. Mizrahi, *J. Pharm. Sci.*, 67:380–383 (1978).
68. E. J. Lien and S. M. Anderson, *J. Med. Chem.*, 11:430–441 (1968).

69. E. J. Lien, and J. H. Perrin, *J. Med. Chem.*, 19:849–850 (1976).
70. M. S. Karabit, O. T. Juneskans, and P. Lundgren, *Int. J. Pharm.*, 46:141–147 (1988).
71. D. C. Monkhouse and G. A. Groves, *Aust. J. Pharm.*, 48:S70–S75 (1967).
72. P. P. Deluca and H. B. Kostenbauder, *J. Am. Pharm. Assoc. (Sci. Ed.)*, 49:430–437 (1960).
73. J. A. Cella, et al., *J. Am. Chem. Soc.*, 74:2061–2062 (1952).
74. T. J. McCarthy, *J. Mondern Pharm.*, 4:321–329 (1969).
75. N. H. Batayilos and E. A. Brecht, *J. Am. Pharm. Assoc. (Sci. Ed.)* 46:524–531 (1957).
76. D. R. MacGregor and P. R. Elliker, *Can. J. Microbiol.*, 4:499–503 (1958).
77. R. M. E. Richards and R. J. McBride, *J. Pharm. Sci.*, 62:2035–2037 (1973).
78. R. M. E. Richards and R. J. McBride, *J. Pharm. Pharmacol.*, 23:141S–146S (1971).
79. A. A. N. Al-Taae, W. A. Dickinson, and P. Gilbert, Antimicrobial activity of some alkyl-trimethyl ammonium bromides, *J. Pharm. Pharmacol.*, 35(Suppl.):60P (1983).
80. W. R. Markland, Norda Briefs, No. 485 (1978).
81. W. E. Rosen and P. A. Berke, *Cosmet. Toiletries,* 92(Mar):88 (177).
82. W. E. Rosen and P. A. Berke, Are cosmetics emulsions adequately preserved against *Pseudomonas? J. Soc. Cosmet. Chem.*, 31:37–40 (1980).
83. W. E. Rosen, and P. A. Berke, Preservation of cosmetic lotions with imidazolidinyl urea plus parabens, *J. Soc. Cosmet. Chem.*, 28:83–87 (1977).
84. G. Jacobs, S. M. Henry, and V. R. Cotty, The influence of pH emulsifier, and accelerated aging upon preservative requirements of O/W emulsions, *J. Soc. Cosmet. Chem.*, 26: 105–117 (1975).
85. E. E. Boehm and D. N. Maddox, Preservative failures in cosmetics with special reference to combating contamination by *Pseudomonas* using binary and tertiary systems, *Am. Perfum. Cosmet.*, 85 (Mar): 31–34 (1970).
86. K. H. Wallhausser, Appendix B, in *Cosmetic and Drug Preservation*, (J. J. Kabara, ed.), Marcel Dekker, New York, 1984, pp. 605–745.
87. W. E. Rosen, and P. A. Berke, *Cosmet. Toiletries*, 94 (Dec): 47 (1979).
88. D. Melnick, F. H. Luckmann, and C. M. Gooding, *Food Res.*, 19:44–58 (1954).
89. J. A. Troller, *Can. J. Microbiol.*, 11:611–617 (1965).
90. H. J. Deuel, et al., *Food Res.*, 19:1–12 (1954).
91. F. J. Bandelin, *J. Am. Pharm. Assoc., (Sci. Ed.)*, 46:691–694 (1958).
92. B. Wickliffe and D. N. Entrekin, *J. Pharm. Sci.*, 53:769–773 (1964).
93. T. Ecklund, *J. Appl. Bacteriol.*, 54:383–389 (1983).
94. T. A. Bell, J. L. Etchells, and A. F. Borg, *J. Bacteriol.*, 77:573 (1959).
95. F. V. Wells and I. I. Lubowe, New York, Reinhold, pp. 1964, 586–598.
96. T. J. Mc Carthy and P. F. K. Eagles, *Cosmet. Toiletries,* 91 (June): 33–35 (1976).
97. T. J. Mc Carthy, *Cosmet. Perfum.*, 88 (Nov): 41–42 (1973).
98. T. J. Mc Carthy, *S. Afr. Pharm. J.*, 219:507–510 (1971).
99. T. R. Aalto, M. C. Firman, and N. E. Rigler, *J. Am. Pharm. Assoc (Sci. Ed.)*, 42:449–456 (1953).
100. O. Rahn and J. E. Conn, *Ind. Eng. Chem.*, 36:185–187 (1944).
101. E. R. Garrett, and O. R. Woods, *J. Am. Pharm. Assoc. (Sci. Ed.)*, 42:736–739 (1953).
102. T. J. McCarthy, *Cosmet. Perf.*, 89 (Dec.): 45–47 (1974).
103. D. L. Wedderburn, *J. Soc. Cosmet. Chem.*, 9:210–228 (1958).
104. S. M. Henry, and G. Jacobs, *Cosmet. Toiletries*, 96 (Mar.): 29–37 (1981).
105. W. T. Sokoski, C. G. Chidester, and G. E. Honeywell, *Dev. Ind. Microbiol.*, 3:179–187 (1962).
106. H. W. Hibbot, and J. Monks, *J. Soc. Cosmet. Chem.*, 12(2): 1–10 (1961).
107. M. M. Rieger, *Cosmet. Toiletries,* 96(May):39–43 (1981).
108. A. Aoki, A. Kameta, I. Yoshioka, and T. Matsuzaki, *J. Pharm. Soc. Jpn.*, 76:939–943 (1956).
109. W. Evans, *J. Pharm. Pharmacol.*, 16:323–331 (1964).

110. N. K. Patel, and H. B. Kostenbauder, *J. Am. Pharm. Assoc. (Sci. Ed.)*, 47:289–293 (1959).
111. F. D. Pisano and H. B. Kostenbauder, *J. Am. Pharm. Assoc.,(Sci. Ed.)*, 47:310–314 (1959).
112. S. M. Blaug, and S. S. Ahsan, *J. Pharm. Sci.*, 50:441–443 (1961).
113. M. C. Allwood, *Int. J. Pharm.*, 11:101–107 (1982).
114. W. Tillman and R. Kuramota, *J. Am. Pharm. Assoc.*, 46:211–214 (1957).
115. G. Miyawaki, N. Patel, and H. Kostenbauder, *J. Am. Phram. Assoc. (Sci. Ed.)*, 48:315 (1959).
116. M. Dymicky, and C. N. Huhtanen, 1979 15, 798–801.
117. W. B. Hugo and A. D. Russell, Types of antimicrobial agents. In *Principles and Practice of Disinfection, Preservation, and Sterilization* (A. D. Russell, W. B. Hugo, and G. A. Ayliffe, eds.), Blackwell Scientific Publications, Oxford, 1982, pp. 8–106.
118. I. R. Gucklhorn, 40:71–75 (1969).
119. S. M. Blaug and D. E. Grant, *J. Soc. Cosmet. Chem.*, 25:495–506 (1974).
120. A. D. Russell and J. R. Furr, *J. Appl. Bacteriol.*, 43:253–260 (1977).
121. J. Judis, *J. Pharm. Sci.*, 51:261 (1962).
122. T. J. McCarthy, *Pharm. Weekbl.*, 110:101–106 (1975).
123. O. Royce and G. Sykes, *J. Pharm. Pharmacol.*, 9, 914–822.
124. W. G. Gorman, U. S. Patent 4,161,562, Sterling Drug, Inc., July 17, 1979.
125. G. A. Hyde and M. M. Auerback, *Cosmet. Toiletries*, 94 (Apr.): 57–59 (1979).
126. G. A. Hyde and J. D. Nelson, in *Cosmetic and Drug Preservation* (J. J. Kabara, ed.), Marcel Dekker, New York, 1984, p. 124.
127. G. E. Davies, J. Francis, A. R. Martin, F. L. Rose, and G. Swain, *Br. J. Pharm. Chemother.*, 9:192–196 (1954).
128. D. D. Heard and R. W. Ashworth, *J. Pharm. Pharmacol.*, 20:505–512 (1968).
129. K. H. Wallhauser, *Pharm. Ind.*, 36:716–722 (1974).
130. G. Wilson, *Br. Med. J.*, 1:408–413 (1964).
131. W. A. Eckhardt, *Am. Perfumer Cosmet.*, 85:83–85 (1970).
132. K. Erikson, *Acta Pharm. Suec.*, 4:261 (1967).
133. D. Jaconia, Preservatives in pharmaceutical products. In *Quality Control in the Pharmaceutical Industry*, Vol. 1, Academic Press, New York, 1972.
134. L. Lachman, *Bull. Parenten. Drug Assoc.*, 22:127–144 (1968).
135. L. R. Beuchat, *Appl. Environ. Microbiol.*, 39:1178–1182 (1980).
136. N. Kato and I. Shibasaki, *J. Antibacterial Antifunal Agents Jpn.*, 4:254–261 (1966).
137. J. J. Kabara, *J. Soc. Cosmet. Chem.*, 31:1–10 (1980).
138. K. W. Nickerson, V. C. Kramer, and J. J. Kabara, *Soap Cosmet. Specialities*, (Feb.):50–58 (1982).
139. J. C. Hierholzer and J. J. Kabara, *J. Food Safety*, 4:1–12 (1982).
140. O. W. May, in *Disinfection, Sterilization, and Preservation*, 4th ed. (S. S. Block, ed.), Lea & Febiger, Philadelphia, 1991, pp. 322–333.
141. T. Eklund, *J. Appl. Bacteriol.*, 54:383–389 (1983).
142. B. Croshaw, and V. R. Holland, in *Cosmetic and Drug Preservation* (J. J. Kabara, ed.), Marcel Dekker, New York, 1984, pp. 31–62.
143. H. S. Bean, G. H. Konnig, and J. Thomas, *Am. Perf. Cosmet.*, 85(Mar): 61–65 (1970).
144. S. J. Kazmi and A. G. Mitchell, *J. Pharm. Sci.*, 67:1260–1266 (1978).
145. T. Shimamoto and H. Mima, *Chem. Pharm. Bull.*, 27:2743–2750 (1979).
146. J. Jacobs, *J. Soc. Cosmet. Chem.*, 26:105–117 (1975).
147. J. Judis, *J. Pharm. Sci.*, 51:261–265 (1962).
148. J. Poprzan and M. G. de Navarre, *J. Soc. Cosmet. Chem.*, 12:280–284 (1961).
149. T. J. McCarthy, J. A. Myburgh, and N. Butler, *Cosmet. Toiletries*, 92(Mar.):33–36 (1977).
150. T. Sakamoto, M. Yanagi, S. Fukushima, and T. Misui, *J. Soc. Cosmet. Chem.*, 38:83–98 (1987).
151. D. Coates, *Manuf. Chem. Aerosol News.* 19(Dec.):23 (1973).

152. N. E. Richardson, D. J. G. Davies, B. J. Meakin, and D. A. Norton, *J. Pharm. Pharmacol.*, 29:717–722 (1977).
153. M. Barnes and G. W. Denton, *Soap Perf. Cosmet.*, 42:729–733 (1969).
154. J. R. Hart, in *Cosmetic and Drug Preservation* (J. J. Kabara, ed.) Marcel Dekker, New York, 1983, Chap. 18.
155. L. Leive, *J. Biol. Chem.*, 243:2373–2380 (1968).
156. J. G. Voss, *J. Gen. Microbiol.*, 48:391–400 (1967).
157. W. B. Hugo and A. D. Russell, in *Principles and Practice of Disinfection, Preservation and Sterilization,* (A. D. Russell, W. B. Hugo, and G. A. J. Ayliffe, eds.) Blackwell Scientific Publications, London 192, pp. 55–57.
158. H. E. Morton and A. D. Russell, in *Disinfection, Preservation and Sterilization* (S. S. Block, ed.) Lea & Febiger, Philadelphia, 1983, pp. 410–411; 738–739.
159. S. P. Denyer, W. B. Hugo, and V. D. Harding, *Int. J. Pharm.*, 25:245–253 (1985).
160. P. G. Hugbo, *Cosmet. Toiletries*, 92(Mar.):52–56 (1977).
161. E. J. Rdzok, W. E. Grundy, F. J. Kirchmeyer, asnd J. C. Sylvester, *J. Am. Pharm. Assoc. (Sci. Ed.),* 44:613–616 (1955).
162. K. E. Moore, *J. Pharm. Pharmacol.*, 44:Sxliii–Sxlv (1978).
163. J. A. Ramp and R. J. Witkowski, *Dev. Ind. Microbiol.*, 16:48–56 (1975).
164. J. I. Yablonski, *Bull. Parenter. Drug Assoc.*, 26:220–227 (1972).
165. M. Leitz, *Bull. Parenter. Drug Assoc.*, 26:212–216 (1972).
166. J. Close and P. A. Nielsen, *Appl. Environ. Microbiol.*, 31:718–722 (1976).
167. B. T. Decicco, E. C. Lee, and J. V. Sorrentino, *J. Pharm. Sci.*, 71:1231–1234 (1982).
168. J. E. Finch and M. R. W. Brown, *J. Antimicrob. Chemother.*, 1:379–386 (1975).
169. P. Gilbert and M. R. W. Brown, *J. Bacteriol.*, 133:1066–1072 (1978).
170. P. Gilbert and M. R. W. Brown, *J. Appl. Bacteriol.*, 48:223–230 (1980).
171. C. G. Mayhall and E. Apollo, *Antimicrob. Agents* Chemother., 18:784–788 (1980).
172. W. B. Hugo and R. G. Stretton, *Nature*, 209:940–942 (1966).
173. W. B. Hugo and R. G. Stretton, *J. Gen Microbiol.*, 42:133–138 (1966).
174. W. B. Hugo and J. R. Davidson, *Microbios* 8:73–84 (1973).
175. M. T. Nadir and P. Gilbert, *Microbios* 26:51–63 (1980).
176. S. G. Wilkinson, in *Resistance of* Pseudomonas aeruginosa (M. R. W. Brown, ed.) John Wiley & Sons, London, 1975, pp. 145–183.
177. N. T. A. Ismail, R. M. E. Klemperer, and M. R. W. Brown, *J. Appl. Bacteriol.*, 43: xvi–xvii (1977).
178. E. Freese, C. W. Sheu, and E. Galliers, *Nature* 241:321–325 (1973).
179. D. S. Orth, C. M. Lutes, D. K. Smith, *J. Soc. Cosmet. Chem.*, 40(4):193–204 (1989).
180. D. S. Orth, 1979, J. Soc. Cosm. Chem., 30:321–332.
181. B. Mathews, *Regulatory Affairs J.*, (June):455–461 (1993).
182. D. S. Orth and L. R. Brueggen, *Cosmet. Toiletries,* 97 (May): 61–65 (1982).
183. P. Gilbert, D. Pemberton, and D. E. Wilkinson, *J. Appl. Bacteriol.*, 69:593–598 (1990).
184. P. Gilbert, F. Caplan, and M. R. W. Brown, *J. Antimicrob.* 27:550–551 (1991).
184. P. Gilbert, F. Caplan, and M. R. W. Brown, *J. Antimicrob.*, 27:550–551 (1991).
185. D. Rupp, M. Totaro, S. Kapadia, and C. Anger, American Society for Microbiology Meeting, May 26–30, 1992, Abstr. I–93.
186. G. Sykes, *J. Pharm. Pharmacol.*, 10:40T–46T (1958).
187. S. Singer, Cosmet. Toiletries, 102(Dec.):55–60 (1987).
188. S. W. Sutton, T. Wrzocek, and D. W. Proud, *J. Appl. Bacteriol.*, 70:351–354 (1991).
189. S. V. W. Sutton, *Int. Contact Lens Clinic.*, 19:167–173 (1992).
190. B. P. Dey and F. B. Engley, *Appl. Environ. Microbiol.*, 45:1533–1537 (1983).
191. S. Mizuba, and W. Sheikh, *J. Ind. Microbiol.*, 1:363–369 (1987).
192. D. S. Orth, *J. Soc. Cosmet. Chem.*, 31:165–172 (1980).
193. R. D. Houlsby, *J. Parenter. Drug Assoc.*, 34:272–276 (1980).

194. P. Gilbert, *Soc. Appl. Bacteriol. Symp. Ser.*, 12:175–197 (1984).
195. P. Gilbert, *Pharm. Int.*, (Aug.):209–212 (1985).
196. G. E. Borovian, *J. Soc. Cosmet. Chem.*, 34:197–203 (1983).
197. A. D. Russell, *Pharm. Int.*, (Dec.):300–308 (1986).
198. D. K. Brannan, J. C. Dille, and D. J. Kaufman, *Appl. Environ. Microbiol.*, 53:1827–1832 (1987).
199. A. L. Davidson, W. L. Hooper, D. F. Spooner, J. A. Farwell, and R. Baird, *Pharm. J.* 246:555–557 (1991).
200. D. F. Spooner and A. L. Davidson, *Pharm. J.*, 251:602–605 (1993).
201. S. M. Lindstrom and J. D. Hawthorn, *J. Soc. Cosmet. Chem.* 87:481–488 (1986).
202. R. A. Cowen, *J. Soc. Cosmet. Chem.*, 25:307–323 (1974).
203. O. J. Lorenzetti, in *Cosmetic and Drug Preservation* (J. J. Kabara, ed.) Marcel Dekker, New York, 1984, pp. 441–463.
204. M. M. A. Al-Hiti and P. Gilbert, *J. Appl. Bacteriol.*, 55:173–175 (1983).
205. M. M. A. Al-Hiti and P. Gilbert, *J. Appl. Bacteriol.*, 49:119–126 (1980).

10

Experimental Design, Modeling, and Optimization Strategies for Product and Process Development

Robert M. Franz and David C. Cooper

Glaxo-Wellcome Inc., Research Triangle Park, North Carolina

Jeffrey E. Browne

R. P. Scherer North America, St. Petersburg, Florida

Allen R. Lewis

The Upjohn Company, Kalamazoo, Michigan

I. INTRODUCTION

The efficient determination of a set of conditions that result in an optimally performing product or process is often the primary goal of the pharamceutical investigator. Although, ideally, this could be accomplished by the use of theoretical or mechanistic models, often pharmaceutical systems and processes are complex enough to require empirical models to describe product or process characteristics. Empirical modeling can generally be divided into two major categories. *Deterministic modeling* refers to model construction in which the input data are exactly known, whereas *stochastic modeling* employs probabilistic data.

This chapter will familiarize the reader with several experimental design, modeling, and optimization strategies that have proved useful in the pharmaceutical development process, as evidenced either through the literature or our own experiences. No attempt is made to cover specific fields in their entirety, and the reader is referred elsewhere for detailed information. Although there are numerous literature references to the use of these techniques for solid dosage form development [1–12], relatively little has been published concerning solution or disperse systems [13–16]. The techniques presented in this chapter are illustrated with examples relevant to disperse system development. Finally, these techniques not only allow the pharmaceutical investigator to develop an optimally performing product or process, but are also useful for determining rational limits for critical formulation or processing variables, outside of which unacceptable product would be produced.

II. DETERMINISTIC MODELING

A. Mathematical and Statistical Components

1. *Common Experimental Designs*

The "design" of an experiment can be simply defined as the plan that governs the performance of an experiment. The use of properly designed experiments helps reduce the procedural errors in the data collected. Randomization within the design helps average out the effects of extraneous variables that cause "noise" in the results. The effects of important variables, as well as the interrelation between these variables, can often be studied in a single well-designed experiment. Ultimately, the investigator wishes to obtain the maximum amount of reliable data at the least cost. Properly designed experiments help the investigator achieve this goal. The assumptions that must be made for valid conclusions to be drawn from the results of a statistically designed experiment are as follows: (a) the observations will be representative of the population about which conclusions are to be drawn; (b) the observations will be statistically independent, normally distributed, and of constant variance; and (c) outliers or missing values will not be observed in the design framework. The first assumption can be guaranteed by obtaining a random sample of the proper size from the appropriate population. Randomization will also ensure that the errors associated with measurment are independent. Parts of the second assumption can often be verified by simply examining the data or applying a specific test procedure. Various techniques for testing the hypothesis of homogeneous variances (e.g., Bartlett's test, Bartlett and Kendall's test, the Burr-Forster Q-test) [17,18], as well as data normality (e.g., W test, chi-square test) [17] are available. If the hypothesis of homogeneous variances or normal data is rejected, the data typically are "transformed" by using some mathematical function, such as the square root or logarithm, to ensure these properties. The assumption that missing or outlying data will not be observed is often difficult to predict. The necessary experiments can be repeated, or, if this is impossible owing to the constraints of the experiment, certain methods can be used to minimize the effects on the analysis [19,20].

The observations resulting from a designed experiment are often examined using analysis of variance (ANOVA) techniques in which the variance associated with a particular independent variable or interactions between independent variables (i.e., a treatment) is compared with the variance associated with the random error that occurs in the experiment [17, 20–22]. If there is a difference between the treatment and error variances, then the treatment being tested is considered to have a significant effect on the measured response. Comparisons between these variances are typically made using an F test or F distribution [21].

Many of the designs discussed in this chapter are "orthogonal" designs. Orthogonality can be thought of, in a geometric sense, as two perpendicular lines, neither having an effect on the direction of the other. For experimental design purposes, orthogonality is defined as follows [21,23]:

$$\sum_{u=1}^{N} x_{iu}x_{ju} = 0 \quad (i \neq j) \tag{1}$$

where independent variable levels are coded such that:

$$\sum_{u=1}^{N} x_{iu} = 0 \qquad \text{for} = 1, 2, \cdots, k \tag{2}$$

and

$$\sum_{u=1}^{N} x_{iu}^2 = N$$

In the foregoing equations, N is the number of experimental trials and x_{iu} and x_{ju} represent the uth level of variables i and j, respectively, for k variables. Typically, for factorial-type designs, the variable levels are fixed, equally spaced, and coded at -1 (low level), $+1$ (high level), and 0 (midpoint). The use of orthogonal designs not only simplifies the calculations used in the analysis but also guarantees that treatment effects on the measured response can be estimated independently. In other words, the effect of a selected treatment will have no projection on the effects of any of the other treatments in the experiment. From a statistical standpoint, this is highly desirable because independent tests of hypothesis (e.g., the F test mentioned previously) can be made on each treatment in the design.

Finally, the designs discussed in the following in no way represent the entirety of useful statistical designs. These designs are simply the ones that have been most frequently cited in the pharmaceutical literature, or that we have found to be useful for empirical modeling of pharmaceutical systems. For a complete and thorough analysis of statistical design methodology, the reader is referred elsewhere [17,20–23].

a. Full Factorials

Most of the designs discussed in this chapter are based on the full-factorial design. The full-factorial design is designated by the following nomenclature:

$$N = L^K \tag{3}$$

where
  K = number of variables
  L = number of variable levels
  N = number of experimental trials

Although 3^K designs are useful for obtaining curvature in a model, the most commonly used full factorial designs in the pharmaceutical literature are at two levels (i.e., 2^K) [24–27]. The 2^K designs will be discussed here. Only first-order regression models can be obtained from unaugmented 2^K designs. The major advantages of these designs are as follows:

1. A minimal number of trials per independent variable is required.
2. They form the basis for several other designs (Plackett-Burman, fractional factorial, composite, or other).
3. They can be used as building blocks to define a large response surface.
4. Both quantitative and qualitative variables can be examined.
5. The results of the design are easily interpreted.

For all practical purposes, in the pharmaceutical development area, full factorial designs are generally used when five or fewer variables are to be investigated, owing

Table 1a Design Matrix for a 2^3 Factorial Design: Suppository Example

Trial, i	Variables[a]			Drug release, y_i (% in 30 min)
	S	PS	CT	
1	−	−	−	60
2	+	−	−	85
3	−	+	−	50
4	+	+	−	55
5	−	−	+	75
6	+	−	+	100
7	−	+	+	65
8	+	+	+	70

[a]See Table 1b.

Table 1b Coded Units

Variable	Low level: −	High level: +
S, surfactant concentration	0.5%	5%
PS, bulk drug particle size (geometric mean diameter)	20 μm	80 μm
CT, cooling temperature of molten suppository	−5°C	25°C

to the exponentially increasing number of trials required. When large numbers of variables require investigation, other designs, which will be discussed later, are often used to minimize the experimental effort.

The design layout or "matrix" for a 2^3 factorial design presented in Table 1a can be used for determining the effects of two formulation variables (surfactant concentration and bulk drug particle size) and a processing variable (cooling temperature of molten suppository) on the release of drug from the dosage form (y_i). The levels of variables are coded at the low (−) and high (+) values for convention (see Table 1b). The geometric representation of the design and the results of the study are shown in Fig. 1.

The influence or "main effect" of surfactant concentration on the amount of drug released from the suppository can be calculated as the difference between the responses (y_i) at the high (+) and low (−) surfactant levels averaged over the four combinations of the remaining variables. The main effect of surfactant concentration (S) on the amount of drug released is calculated as follows:

$$S = \frac{(y_2 - y_1) + (y_4 - y_3) + (y_6 - y_5) + (y_8 - y_7)}{4}$$

$$= \frac{(85 - 60) + (55 - 50) + (100 - 75) + (70 - 65)}{4} \tag{4}$$

$$= 15$$

Similarly, the main effects of bulk drug particle size (PS) and suppository cooling temperature (CT) are calculated as follows:

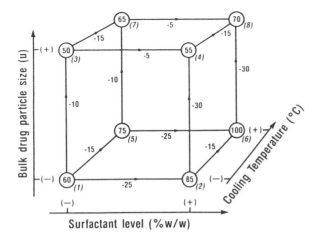

Fig. 1 Geometric representation of 2^3 factorial design, suppository example.

$$PS = \frac{(y_3 - y_1) + (y_4 - y_2) + (y_7 - y_5) + (y_8 - y_6)}{4}$$

$$= \frac{(50 - 60) + (55 - 85) + (65 - 75) + (70 - 100)}{4} \tag{5}$$

$$= -20$$

$$CT = \frac{(y_5 - y_1) + (y_6 - y_2) + (y_7 - y_3) + (y_8 - y_4)}{4}$$

$$= \frac{(75 - 60) + (100 - 85) + (65 - 50) + (70 - 55)}{4} \tag{6}$$

$$= 15$$

Careful examination of these calculations reveal that all the response data (y_i; drug release) are used to supply information on each of the main effects with the precision of four replications based on the differences between high and low levels. To obtain the same precision using "one factor at a time" experimental methodology, a total of 24 trials would be necessary. Four experiments at each variable level would have to be performed, while holding the remaining two variables constant at some predetermined, fixed value. It would have to be assumed that the effect of a variable would be the same at all levels of the remaining two variables (i.e., the main effects are additive). For this reason, one factor at a time methodology often does not detect "interaction" between variables. Interaction between two factors exists when a change in one variable produces a dissimilar magnitude of change in the response at different levels of the remaining variables. By employing a factorial design, interaction can easily be detected. For instance, in the suppository example, as the bulk drug particle size is increased at a high surfactant level, the amount of drug dissolved (averaged over both cooling temperatures) drops

30%, whereas at a low surfactant level, the drop is only 10%. This indicates that a significant interaction may exist between bulk drug particle size and surfactant concentration, as shown in Fig. 2a. One can exploit interaction effects to achieve a more robust product or process. For isntance, in this example the interaction between S and PS allows the selection of a formula having better dissolution properties than would normally be expected (i.e., low PS and high S in Fig. 2a). The example also indicates that the suppository-cooling temperature has the same magnitude of effect on drug release (averaged over both surfactant levels) at both bulk drug particle sizes. This indicates that significant interaction does not exist between bulk drug particle size and cooling temperature, as depicted in Fig. 2b. To calculate the $S \times PS$ interaction, the difference in average surfactant effect at high and low particle size is determined. By convention, half the difference is considered the interaction effect. The calculation is presented below (also see Fig. 1 and Table 1):

Particle size	Average surfactant effect	
High (+)	$= \dfrac{(y_4 - y_3) + (y_8 - y_7)}{2}$	(7)
	$= \dfrac{(55 - 50) + (70 - 65)}{2}$	
	$= 5$	

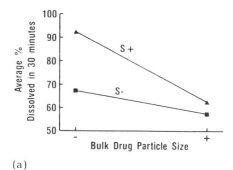

(a)

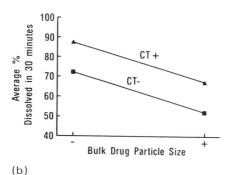

(b)

Fig. 2 An example of (a) interacting and (b) noninteracting variables in a factorial experiment; suppository example (S = surfactant level, CT = cooling temperature).

Low (–)
$$= \frac{(y_2 - y_1) + (y_6 - y_5)}{2} \tag{8}$$
$$= \frac{(85 - 60) + (100 - 75)}{2}$$
$$= 25$$

S × PS interaction
$$= \frac{1}{2} \text{ difference} = \frac{5 - 25}{2}$$
$$= -10$$

The effect of the particle size–cooling temperature interaction ($PS \times CT$) and the surfactant concentration–cooling temperature interaction ($S \times CT$) can be calculated similarly as follows:

Particle size	Average cooling rate effect

High (+)
$$= \frac{(y_8 - y_4) + (y_7 - y_3)}{2} \tag{9}$$
$$= \frac{(70 - 55) + (65 - 50)}{2}$$
$$= 15$$

Low (–)
$$= \frac{(y_6 - y_2) + (y_5 - y_1)}{2} \tag{10}$$
$$= \frac{(100 - 85) + (75 - 60)}{2}$$
$$= 15$$

PS × CT interaction
$$= \frac{1}{2} \text{ difference} = \frac{15 - 15}{2} = 0$$

Surfactant concentration	Average cooling rate effect

High (+)
$$= \frac{(y_6 - y_2) + (y_8 - y_4)}{2} \tag{11}$$
$$= \frac{(100 - 85) + (70 - 55)}{2}$$
$$= 15$$

Low (–)
$$= \frac{(y_5 - y_1) + (y_7 - y_3)}{2} \tag{12}$$
$$= \frac{(75 - 60) + (65 - 50)}{2}$$
$$= 15$$

$$\text{S} \times \text{CT interaction} \quad = \frac{1}{2} \text{ difference} = \frac{15 - 15}{2} = 0$$

Finally, the three-factor interaction effect ($S \times PS \times CT$) can be thought of as half the difference between the average surfactant concentration–particle size interaction ($S \times PS$) at each cooling temperature as described below:

Cooling temperature	Average $S \times PS$ interaction effect
High (+)	$= \dfrac{(y_8 - y_7) - (y_6 - y_5)}{2}$ $\qquad$ (13) $= \dfrac{(70 - 65) - (100 - 75)}{2}$ $= -10$
Low (−)	$= \dfrac{(y_4 - y_3) - (y_2 - y_1)}{2}$ $\qquad$ (14) $= \dfrac{(55 - 50) - (85 - 60)}{2}$ $= -10$

$$\text{S} \times \text{PS} \times \text{CT interaction} \quad = \frac{1}{2} \text{ difference} = \frac{-10 - (-10)}{2} = 0$$

Although the calculations shown here are for illustrative purposes, much faster methods, such as contrast tables or the Yates algorithm, are generally used to determine factor effects [17,20]. A summary of the analysis is presented in Table 2. The results indicate that increasing the suppository cooling rate between −5° and 25°C improves the percentage drug released in 30 min by 15%. The effects of surfactant concentration (S)

Table 2 Calculated Effects Using a 2^3 Factorial Design: Suppository Example

Effect	Estimate (% dissolved in 30 min)
Average	70
Main effects	
$\quad$ Surfactant concentration, S	15
$\quad$ Bulk drug particle size, PS	−20
$\quad$ Suppository cooling temperature, CT	15
Two-factor interactions	
$\quad S \times PS$	−10
$\quad S \times CT$	0
$\quad PS \times CT$	0
Three-factor interaction	
$\quad S \times PS \times CT$	0

and bulk drug particle size (*PS*) should be interpreted concurrently with the $S \times PS$ interaction, which is relatively large. Figure 2a shows that the $S \times PS$ interaction is due to a greater sensitivity of the small particle-sized bulk drug to surfactant level than the larger particle-sized material. Overall, the amount of active dissolved in 30 min is inversely proportional to the bulk drug particle size and directly proportional to the surfactant concentration of the suppository. The actual change in the amount of drug dissolved is dependent on both the main effects and the interaction term, as depicted in Figure 2a. The conclusions drawn pertain only to data within the independent variable levels tested (i.e., the design inference space). Extrapolation outside this region would require additional experimentation

In the foregoing example, no replicate trials were performed to obtain an estimate of the standard error (deviation) associated with the effects. Without this estimate, it is often difficult to determine whether a variable actually affects the measured response or whether the value obtained is simply due to experimental error. For a factorial design, the standard error of individual effects can be calculated using the following equation (assuming independent errors) [20]:

$$\text{s.e.} = \left(\frac{4}{N} s^2 \right)^{1/2} \tag{15}$$

where

$\quad$ s.e. = estimated standard error of an effect

$\quad N$ = total number of trials in a factorial or replicated factorial design

$\quad s^2$ = average of estimated sample variances (i.e., the pooled estimate of the population variance, σ^2)

The average estimated sample variance (s^2) can be obtained several ways, including replication of trials within the factorial design, and inclusion of several centerpoints if the variables are continuous (i.e., variables held at midpoint between low and high levels). The estimated standard error of an effect (s.e.) can also be determined by considering the influence of higher-order interaction terms negligible and using the obtained values as a measure of experimental error [20].

In summary, the use of 2^K factorial designs in experimental methodology allows both main effects and interaction terms to be calculated with a relatively small number of trials, as compared with one factor at a time techniques.

b. Plackett-Burman

The Plackett-Burman designs are described by the nomenclature K/N, where the fewest trials (N) that can be used is the smallest integer multiple of 4 greater than the number of variables (K) [28,29]. Designs of this type are especially useful in the early stages of experimentation for screening the high and low levels of a large number of unknown variables (i.e., ≥9) with a minimum of experimental trials. One hopes that this will allow the experimenter to reduce the number of variables for subsequent testing by eliminating any that demonstrate a lack of significance on the measured response. The assumption is made that interaction between variables is negligible compared with the main variable effects because, in the worse case ($N = K + 1$), most two-level interaction terms are confounded with the prime variables of interest. "Confounding" in a design simply implies that the effects of two or more treatments are inseparable and, therefore, the true source of any one effect cannot be determined. Even though Plackett-Burman designs are economical, they are also risky because improper conclusions may be drawn owing to confounding when the assumption of negligible interactions is violated. It is up to the experimenter to decide between economy and risk when using designs of this type. An example of the layout for an 11-variable, 12-trial Plackett-Burman design is presented in Table 3.

c. Fractional Factorials

Fractional factorials are simply a block of a full-factorial design. They take advantage of the fact that, when the number of variables is large, there is a hierarchy in the significance of the interaction terms. In other words, higher-order interactions tend to become negligible as the number of variables increases and, therefore, can be eliminated from the model. The major advantage of the fractional factorial is that a large number of variables can be examined at the main-effect and two-variable interaction level with a minimum of trials. However, the experimenter also loses degrees of freedom for testing purposes by performing a minimum number of experiments.

The designs are designated by the following nomenclature:

$$N = L_{R-F}^K = L_R^{K-F} \tag{16}$$

where

L = number of variable levels (typically 2)
R = resolution
K = number of variables
F = fraction of the full factorial (i.e., $F = 1$ then fraction is 1/2, $F = 2$ then fraction is 1/4, and so on, for a two-level design)
N = number of experimental trials

For example, a two-level, five-variable, half-fractional factorial would have 16 trials ($2^{5-1} = 2^4 = 16$). In this discussion, only two-level designs (i.e., $L = 2$) will be examined. This type of design has been extensively used in the pharmaceutical literature to investigate various product- and process-related variables [25,30–32].

Table 3 A 12-Trial, 11-Variable Plackett-Burman Design Matrix[a]

Trial	X_1	X_2	X_3	X_4	X_5	X_6	X_7	X_8	X_9	X_{10}	X_{11}
1	+	+	−	+	+	+	−	−	−	+	−
2	+	−	+	+	+	−	−	−	+	−	+
3	−	+	+	+	−	−	−	+	−	+	+
4	+	+	+	−	−	−	+	−	+	+	−
5	+	+	−	−	−	+	−	+	+	−	+
6	+	−	−	−	+	−	+	+	−	+	+
7	−	−	−	+	−	+	+	−	+	+	+
8	−	−	+	−	+	+	−	+	+	+	−
9	−	+	−	+	+	−	+	+	+	−	−
10	+	−	+	+	−	+	+	+	−	−	−
11	−	+	+	−	+	+	+	−	−	−	+
12	−	−	−	−	−	−	−	−	−	−	−

[a] +, high level of variable; −, low level of variable.

Table 4 Confounding Patterns According to the Resolution Code of a
Fractional Factorial Design

Resolution code	Worst-case confounding[a]
III	Main effects with two-level interactions
IV	Two-level interactions with two-level interactions
V	Two-level interactions with three-level interactions
VI	Three-level interactions with three-level interactions

[a]At least one.

The resolution (R) of a particular fractional factorial is reflective of the confounding pattern in the design, as described in Table 4 [20,28]. In general, as the resolution increases, fewer main effects and two-level interactions are confounded. Also, for designs with equal numbers of variables, the fractional factorial used (1/2, 1/4, 1/8,⋯.) is proportional to the design resolution R. Typically, fractional factorials have less confounding, given the same number of trials and variables, than the previously discussed Plackett-Burman designs.

Fractional designs and the confounding patterns are developed using a "defining relationship" or "design generator," which is simply an alias of another term in the linear model (i.e., terms are confounded) [17,20]. Efficient designs can be developed by careful selection of the defining relationship. For example, a design can be generated so that the interaction terms the experimenter feels are insignificant are confounded in such a way as to obtain maximum information on the speculated significant factors. Further discussion on fractional design generation is presented by Box et al. [20] and by Anderson and McLean [17,33].

Another advantage of a fractional factorial design is that a full factorial can be obtained in every set of $R - 1$ variables (R = resolution). This is especially useful when the experimenter has a large set of variables (i.e., in the screening stage), but suspects that only $R - 1$ of them may have a significant effect on the measured response. The use of a fractional factorial of resolution R would then give a complete factorial design, plus replicates, for the suspected significant variables. Geometric representation of the full factorials embedded in a 2_{III}^{3-1} fractional factorial is shown in Fig. 3.

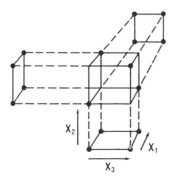

Fig. 3 A 2_{III}^{3-1} fractional factorial design showing projections into 2^2 full factorial designs.

Fractional factorials can also be augmented to help unravel confounded terms if the information is important to the experimenter. For example, two complementary half-fractional factorials can be performed as separate blocks and then combined to obtain a full-factorial design. The "block" effect, which is a result of incomplete randomization, can be confounded with a higher-order interaction, which, for all practical purposes, can be assumed to be negligible. Sequential use of fractional factorials is discussed in detail by Box et al. [20] and Daniel [22].

An extensive listing of various fractional factorial design layouts is presented by McLean and Anderson [33] and Bisgaard [34].

d. Central Composite

The central composite design is an extension of the two-level factorial or fractional factorial design. These designs have found wide acceptance for modeling pharmaceutical systems [25,35–40]. The basic second-order central composite design is used to estimate curvature in a continuous response (i.e., dependent variable) according to the following model:

$$y = \beta_0 + \beta_1 x_1 + \beta_2 x_2 + \cdots + \beta_K x_K + \beta_{12} x_{12} + \cdots + \beta_{(K-1)K} x_{K-1} x_K$$
$$+ \beta_{11} x_1^2 + \cdots + \beta_{KK} x_K^2 + \varepsilon \tag{17}$$

where

y = estimate of response (i.e., dependent variable)
x = independent variable
β_0 = overall mean response
β_i = regression model coefficients
K = number of independent variables
ε = random error

The design has three basic parts: (a) a two-level factorial or fractional factorial (2^{K-F}), (b) a centerpoint or centerpoints (C, thus the term "central" composite), and (c) additional points at the extremes of a single factor (α) and at the center of the remaining factors (i.e., starpoints, $2K$). The number of experimental trials (N) in a composite design is given by:

$$N = 2^{K-F} + 2K + C \tag{18}$$

where

K = number of variables
F = fraction of the full factorial
C = number of centerpoint replicates

The major advantage of designs of this type is the reduction in the number of experimental trials required to estimate the squared terms in the second-order model. Table 5 compares the number of experimental trials required for 3^K (or 3^{K-F}) designs and a typical composite design with a single centerpont ($2^{K-F} + 2K + 1$) for up to five independent variables. Disadvantages of the composite designs when compared with a three-level factorial design include (a) fewer degrees of freedom for estimation of the error term in the model; (b) inability to estimate certain interaction terms (i.e., linear by quadratic, quadratic by quadratic, and such); (c) unequal variances for certain main effect (i.e., squared terms) and interaction model coefficients; and (d) possibility, depending on the design, that the squared terms in the model will not be orthogonal to each other.

Table 5 Comparison of the Number of Experimental Trials Required for a Three-Level Factorial Design (3^{K-F}) Versus a Typical Composite Design ($2^{K-F} + 2K + 1$)

Number of independent variables, K	3^{K-F} factorial	$2^{K-F} + 2K + 1$ composite
2	9	9
3	27	15
4	81	25
5	243	43
5	81[a]	27[b]

[a]One-third fractional factorial three-level design (3^{5-1}).
[b]Half fractional factorial-based design (2^{5-1}).

These disadvantages are typically considered minor in comparison with the small number of experimental trials required to obtain a second-order model. The design layout and geometric representation for a general central composite design with three independent variables ($K = 3$) are presented in Table 6 and Fig. 4, respectively.

Although the starpoints can assume any location in the design and a simple nonorthogonal regression analysis can be performed to study variation in the data, several specific types of central composite designs have proved to be particularly advantageous.

Face-Centered Central Composite. This second-order design has starpoints spaced one unit from the centerpoint (i.e., $\alpha = 1$). With the exception of the two-variable case

Table 6 Design Layout for a General $2^{K-F} + 2K + C$ Design, Where $K = 3$ and $C = 1$

Trial[a]	Variable level[b]			
	X_1	X_2	X_3	
1	–	–	–	
2	+	–	–	
3	–	+	–	
4	+	+	–	
5	–	–	+	2^3 full factorial
6	+	–	+	
7	–	+	+	
8	+	+	+	
9	$-\alpha$	0	0	
10	$+\alpha$	0	0	
11	0	$-\alpha$	0	
12	0	$+\alpha$	0	Extreme or "starpoints"
13	0	0	$-\alpha$	
14	0	0	$+\alpha$	
15	0	0	0	Centerpoint

[a]Trial order is run randomly during actual experimentation.
[b]Symbols as follows: +, high levels; –, low level; 0, midpoint, α, Starpoint distance.

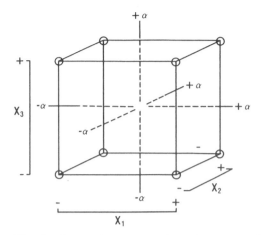

Fig. 4 Geometric representation of a general $2^{K-F} + 2K + C$ central composite design, where $K = 3$, $F = 0$, and $C = 1$.

($k = 2$), these designs are neither orthogonal nor rotatable (to be discussed later) outside the basic factorial design. Their major advantage lies in the ease of design construction, especially if the high and low levels of the basic factorial portion (which may be performed initially) are at the extremes of the desired inference space.

Orthogonal Central Composite.   Designs of this type have the advantage of having all terms (including squared terms) in the model orthogonal to each other and, therefore, all effects can be estimated independently (i.e., uncorrelated estimates of the model coefficients can be obtained). This is accomplished by locating the starpoints at a distance, α, from the centerpoint, as described by the following equation [17,23,41].

$$\alpha = \frac{[(F + T)^{1/2} - F^{1/2}]^2 F^{1/4}}{4n^2} \tag{19}$$

where
  F = number of treatment combinations in the factorial run (fractional or full)
  T = number of additional points multiplied by number of observations per treatment combination (n)

Rotatable Central Composite.   A design is considerable to be rotatable if the variance of the estimated response is a function of only the distance from the center of the design, not of the direction. Thus, for each of two points that are equidistant from the design center, the precision (or variance) of the estimates of the response is equivalent. Rotatable central composite designs have all points equally spaced from the centerpoint; therefore, rotation around this point does not change the variance of the response, hence, the name "rotatable." For a second-order rotatable design, the starpoint distance α is calculated by using the following equation [23,41].

$$\alpha = (F)^{1/4} \tag{20}$$

where F is the number of treatment combinations in the factorial run (fractional or full).

There are several types of second-order rotatable central composite designs. The *uniform precision* rotatable central composite design is based on the idea that the investigator desires uniform variance (or precision) in the estimates of the response within ± 1 coded unit of the centerpoint. A uniform precision design helps minimize bias in the regression coefficients caused by higher-order terms (i.e., third-order, and so on) in the true response surface [23]. The *orthogonal* rotatable central composite design is rotatable and orthogonal; therefore, uncorrelated effects of the model terms can be obtained (i.e., terms estimated independently). Both these designs are obtained by simply altering the number of centerpoint trials in the basic rotatable central composite design [23]. Table 7 compares the design parameters of the two types of rotatable central composite designs for up to eight variables.

In summary, for investigation of second-order models of the type described here, composite designs are generally recommended over three-level factorial designs (3^K) because of the major reduction in the number of experimental trials required. The composition of the second-order design is based on the starpoint distance to the design center, as well as the number of centerpoint trials conducted. Table 8 summarizes the starpoint distance α of the basic composite designs discussed here for up to eight variables. Several methods for comparing second-order composite designs have been developed that typically take into account the precision with which the model coefficients are estimated, the number of experimental trials required, and the bias of the model coefficients in the presence of higher-order terms in the true response surface [23,41]. When selecting a composite design, the investigator should take into account these factors, as well as the ease of applying the design to the overall experimental effort.

e. Mixture Designs

Mixture designs are specialized designs, particularly useful for formulation development [16,42–44] in which the measured response is a function of only the proportions of the components in the product. The ultimate objective of a mixture design is to obtain a response surface that can be optimized relative to the ingredient proportionalities. Process variables can also be included in mixture experiments by combining mixture and factorial designs. Although there are several types of mixture designs, only the simplex lattice, extreme vertices, and mixture–process variable designs will be discussed here.

Simplex Lattice. If there are k components in a mixture and the proportion of the ith component in the mixture is X_i, then the mixture problem can be described as follows:

$$X_i \geq 0 \qquad (1 \leq i \leq k)$$

$$\sum_{i=1}^{k} X_i = 1 \tag{21}$$

Since the proportion of X_i could be unity, a "mixture" could theoretically be composed of a single component. Therefore, the design points can be thought to geometrically represent the vertices of a $(k-1)$-dimensional regular-sided figure, or a "simplex." The design vertices represent single-component "mixtures," whereas the interior of the simplex contains points representing combinations of all components. The designs are referred to as (k,m)-simplex lattices, where k is the number of mixture components and m is related to the spacing of points between the values of 0 and 1 for X_i. For example,

Table 7 Comparison of Uniform Precision and Orthogonal *Rotatable* Central Composite Designs[a]

Design parameter	k								
	2	3	4	5	5 1/2 rep	6	6 1/2 rep	7 1/2 rep	8 1/2 rep
F	4	8	16	32	16	64	32	64	128
SP	4	6	8	10	10	12	12	14	16
$C(up)$	5	6	7	10	6	15	9	14	20
$C(orth)$	8	9	12	17	10	24	15	22	33
$N(up)$	13	20	31	52	32	91	53	92	164
$N(orth)$	16	23	36	59	36	100	59	100	177
α	1.414	1.682	2.000	2.378	2.000	2.828	2.378	2.828	3.364

[a]Symbols as follows:

k = number of variables

F = number of treatment combinations in the factorial run

SP = number of starpoints

$C(up)$ = number of center points for a uniform precision design

$C(orth)$ = number of center points for an orthogonal design

$N(up)$ = total number of trials for a uniform precision design

$N(orth)$ = total number of trials for an orthogonal design

α = starpoint distance from design center

1/2 rep = half-replicate (half fractional factorial)

Source: Adapted from Ref. 23, p. 153.

Table 8 Comparison of Starpoint Distances α for Three Types of Composite Designs

k	Face-centered central composite	Orthogonal central composite[a]	Rotatable central composite
2	1.000	1.000	1.414
3	1.000	1.216	1.682
4	1.000	1.414	2.000
5	1.000	1.596	2.378
5[b]	1.000	1.547	2.000
6	1.000	1.761	2.828
6[b]	1.000	1.724	2.378
7[b]	1.000	1.885	2.828
8[b]	1.000	2.029	3.364

[a]Assumes a single centerpoint ($C = 1$).
[b]Basic design is a half-fractional factorial.

a (3,2)-simplex lattice would have three components in a mixture at $m + 1$ equally spaced points between 0 and 1 (i.e., $X_i = 0, 1/2, 1$) as shown in Fig. 5. The number of points or trials required (n) for a (k,m)-simplex lattice is given by [45]:

$$n = \frac{(m + k - 1)!}{m!(k - 1)!} \tag{22}$$

Specific polynomial equations, containing n terms, are associated with the selected simplex and are used to describe the response surface. The equations take the form of the following for a first- and second-order polynomial, respectively [45]:

First-order:

$$y = \sum_{i}^{k} V_i X_i \tag{23}$$

where $V_i = B_0 + B_i$ for $i = 1, 2, \cdots, k$

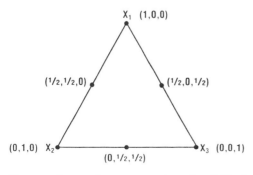

Fig. 5 Geometric representation of a (3,2) simplex-lattice design.

Second-order:

$$y = \sum_i^k V_i X_i + \sum_{i<j}^k \sum^k V_{ij} X_i X_j \qquad (24)$$

where

$$V_i = B_0 + B_i + B_{ii}$$
$$V_{ij} = B_{ij} - B_{ii} - B_{jj} \qquad \text{for } 1 \le i < j \le k$$

The special coefficients (V_i) in the foregoing equations are identified with the usual regression coefficients (B_i) because of the constraint that the sum of all component proportions (X_i) equals 1 [45].

Table 9 summarizes the number of trials (n), excluding replicates, for a first- and second-order simplex design for the listed number of components in the mixture. Further detailed information concerning simplex-lattice designs can be found elsewhere [17,45,46].

Extreme Vertices. In most mixture problems concerning pharmaceutical disperse systems, certain portions of all ingredients (viscosity imparting agents, surfactants, preservatives, or other) are required for the final product to perform satisfactorily. Often the investigator knows in advance the extremes of each component to be tested. The extreme vertices design is an extension of the simplex-lattice mixture design, which allows these constraints to be taken into account [17,47,48]. The constrained mixture problem can be described as follows [17]:

$$0 \le a_i \le X_i \le b_i \le 1 \ (1 \le i \le k)$$

and

$$\sum_{i=1}^k X_i = 1 \qquad (25)$$

where X_i is the ith of k components in the mixture, constrained between an upper (b_i) and a lower (a_i) limit. A technique was developed by McLean and Anderson for locating the vertices of a polyhedron that fall on the boundaries formed by the constraints of the mixture components within the original unconstrained simplex lattice [17]. Fig-

Table 9 Experimental Trials Required in a Simplex-Lattice Design (k,m)[a] for First- and Second-Order Simplex Polynomials

	Number of required trials	
Number of components	Linear, $m = 1$	Quadratic, $m = 2$
3	3	6
4	4	10
5	5	15
6	6	21

[a]k, number of mixture components; m, variable spacing.

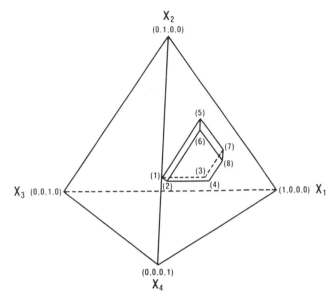

Fig. 6 Geometric representation of a four-component extreme vertices design (From Ref. 17.)

ure 6 geometrically depicts an example by McLean and Anderson of the extreme vertices polyhedron formed within the unconstrained simplex when the levels of the four mixture components were constrained within the following proportions [19]:

$$0.40 \leq X_1 \leq 0.60$$
$$0.10 \leq X_2 \leq 0.50$$
$$0.10 \leq X_3 \leq 0.50$$
$$0.03 \leq X_4 \leq 0.08$$

Typically, a second-order polynomial is fit to the data generated in the polyhedron and a response surface is generated. One potential problem with experiments of this type is that a nonuniformity of design points exist, resulting in poor precision of the response estimate in areas having minimal trials. A detailed discussion of extreme vertices can be found in the literature [17,47,48].

Mixture–Process Variable Designs.   Process variables can be included in mixture experiments by combining mixture designs (formulation variables) with factorial designs (process variables). Typically, lattice designs are used for the formulation variables and a factorial design, which covers the ranges of the process variables, is run at each point in the mixture design [49,50]. The design layout for a (3,2) simplex lattice in which three process variables are investigated in a full 2^3 factorial design ((3,2) simplex lattice $\times$ 2^3 design) is presented in Fig. 7. The design shown in Fig. 7 requires 48 experimental trials, illustrating the inefficiency of certain types of mixture–process variable designs. One way to improve the efficiency of mixture–process variable designs is the use fractional factorial designs [50]. If a 2^{3-1} fractional factorial was used to evaluate process variables instead of the full factorial shown in Fig. 7, then the number of experimental trials would be reduced to 24, half that of the original design. The number of experimental trials in the (3,2) simplex lattice $\times$ 2^{3-1} fractional factorial mixture–process

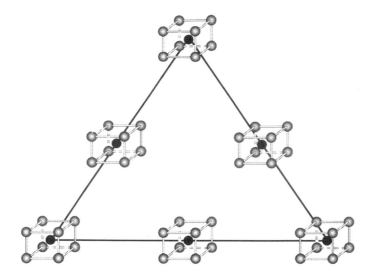

Fig. 7 Example of 3,2 simplex lattice × 2^3 factorial mixture/process variable design.

variable design approaches that of a highly efficient $2^{5-1} + 2(5) + 1$ five-factor central composite design encompassing 27 experimental trials (see Table 5).

The modeling and analysis of mixture–process variable designs is not as straightforward as those designs discussed previously. The model terms are a result of a cross product between the mixture terms and the process variable terms. A detailed description of the modeling and analysis of mixture–process variable designs is described in the literature [49–51].

f. D-Optimal Designs

There are some experimental situations in which the traditional designs mentioned so far are not applicable. These situations generally occur when practical considerations force the use of an irregularly shaped design region. For these situations, it can be helpful to create a computer-generated design that is customized for a particular situation. The most popular computer algorithms for generating such designs are called D-optimal algorithms. D-optimal designs have been used infrequently in pharmaceutical development [52,53].

For example, suppose that for a particular suspension milling problem, when the maximum mill speed is applied, the gap setting must exceed by 20% the minimum. This results in a nonrectangular design region as shown in Fig. 8a. Suppose further that suspension particle size is to be modeled throughout this experimental region using a quadratic equation. Traditional experimental designs, such as the central composites, do not cover this region very well; they will either be too small to cover the entire region of interest, or they will be too large and require some observations to be collected outside the feasible region.

To generate a custom design using a D-optimal algorithm, the following must be specified: (a) a set of candidate points (N) that cover the design region, (b) the desired statistical model, and (c) the number of points (n) to select from the candidate design points. The algorithm then searches for the best design; the set of n points selected from

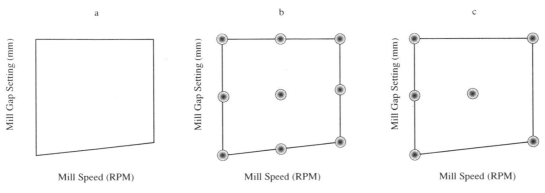

Fig. 8 Geometric representations of (a) design space, (b) N candidate points, and (c) algorithm selected points for a D-optimal design; suspension example.

N candidates that is "optimal" for fitting the desired model. The optimality criterion most often used is D-optimality, a criterion that ensures that the resulting design will estimate its parameters with low variance. The calculations and theory for variance minimization that support optimal designs are described in detail elsewhere [49,54].

For the D-optimal design problem just mentioned, a set of $N = 9$ candidate points will cover the design region, as shown in Fig. 8b. The quadratic model selected for mill speed (M) and gap setting (G) is provided in the following equation:

$$y_{\text{particle size}} = \beta_0 + \beta_1 M + \beta_2 G + \beta_{12} MG + \beta_{11} M^2 + \beta_{22} G^2 + \varepsilon \qquad (26)$$

In this example it is necessary to select the smallest design possible, since experimental materials are limited. The smallest design will have $n = 6$ points, since there must be at least as many points as there are parameters in the Eq. (26). Then, one of several D-optimal algorithms are used to search for the best 6-point design from the 9-point candidate set. The algorithm selects the points for the design shown in Fig. 8c. One could probably have intuitively selected an appropriate design for this problem with just two factors. However, with a larger number of factors, it becomes nearly impossible to intuitively select appropriate designs. D-optimal algorithms are necessary to select the appropriate experimental design in cases with larger sets of variables.

Another situation in which D-optimal designs can be very useful is for mixture experiments with constraints on the components (as described previously). Because of the constraints, the experimental region is usually an irregularly shaped polyhedron (see Fig. 6 for an example). In these situations, D-optimal algorithms can be used to select a design from a candidate set that includes the vertices, midedges, and midfaces of the polyhedron.

One should be aware that the designs generated by D-optimal algorithms are very sensitive to the statistical model on which the optimal design is based. Therefore, it is often advisable to specify a model that is slightly more complex than the model actually necessary. Additional design points will then be available if it is necessary to fit the more complex model, and the points will provide even coverage of the experimental region. For example, in the foregoing problem, it would be wise to specify a quadratic model (for the D-optimal algorithm), even if a linear interactions model (without squared terms) would suffice. In complex experimental situations, it is advisable to consult with a professional statistician when using D-optimal designs. For a more detailed introduction to D-optimal designs see Khuri [49] and Snee [54].

2. Modeling Using Regression Analysis

Simply stated, regression analysis is a technique to determine what meaningful relationships, if any, exist between experimental variables and a response variable. The specific relationship defined for a response variable (denoted Y) and the experimental or independent variables (denoted X) is known as the regression model. Most regression models are empirical and serve to approximate more complex theoretical models.

Although a given empirical model may represent an adequate approximation within the region or space defined by the experimental data, extrapolation of the model beyond this space can result in erroneous inferences. It is important for predictive purposes that the experimenter apply a regression model only to the experimental design inference space from which it was derived and realize the risks in applying it elsewhere.

In this section, only linear regression analysis (as opposed to nonlinear analysis) will be reviewed, since, in most experimental situations, a linear polynomial regression model can be used to approximate the relationship existing between the response variable and the independent variables. In the simplest case, a linear (referring to linearity in the β coefficients), first-order (referring to the highest power in X) polynomial of the following form is used:

$$Y = \beta_0 + \beta_1 X + \varepsilon \tag{27}$$

where Y and X_1, X_2, $\cdots$ denote the response and independent variables, respectively; β_0, β_1, $\cdots$ are the regression model coefficients that estimate the linear or main effects of the independent variables, and ε is the random error term, the standard deviation of which is zero. Sometimes more complicated polynomial functions are required to fit the experimental data. Consider, for example, the linear, second-order polynomial described by Eq. (17).

The selection of an appropriate experimental design "goes hand in hand" with regression analysis, since certain designs are better than others in estimating the regression coefficients for an assumed model. For example, an unaugmented two-level factorial design is well suited for making estimates of the β's in a linear first-order model [see Eq. (27)], but cannot be used to estimate a second-order model [see Eq. (17)]. Experimental designs for fitting a second-order polynomial must involve three levels for each variable so that the quadratic effects (β_{11}, β_{22}) can be estimated. In addition, if an experimental design is selected that incorporates evenly spaced levels of the independent variables X_i, the computational procedures for fitting a model to the experimental data are simplified through the use of orthogonal polynomials.

The following section on regression analysis should by no means be considered an exhaustive review of the subject. Rather, it is intended only to provide the reader with an appreciation of regression analysis as it relates to the models used for response surface exploration and optimization. A considerable amount of the ensuing discussion has been extracted from several excellent textbooks and papers on regression analysis. Some readers may want to refer to these for further information on a specific topic [23,55–59].

a. Least Squares Method

To determine how independent variables relate to a given response variable, a method of analysis known as the least squares method is typically employed to fit a mathematical

Table 10 Effect of NaCl Addition on Final
Product Viscosity

NaCl added (X) (% w/v)	Product viscosity (Y) (cP $\times$ 100)
0.0	21.0
0.1	27.5
0.2	37.5
0.2	33.5
0.2	44.5
0.2	39.5
0.3	50.0
0.4	61.5
0.5	79.0
0.5	80.0
0.5	76.5
0.6	92.0
0.7	122.5
0.8	127.5
0.9	147.5
1.4	220.0

equation or model to the data. For example consider the data given in Table 10 and plotted in Fig. 9, showing the effect of sodium chloride (NaCl) addition on the final viscosity of a shampoo product. Data of this type represent the simplest case, for which the dependence on one variable, viscosity, is proportional to another variable, NaCl addition. In this example, it is reasonable to initially assume that a linear, first-order regression model of the form

$$Y_i = \beta_0 + \beta_1 X_i + \varepsilon_i \qquad (28)$$

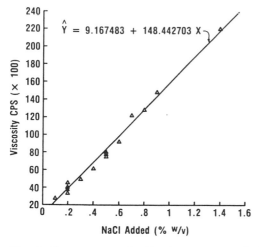

Fig. 9 Least-squares plot for shampoo example: Effect of percentage NaCl addition (% w/v) on final product viscosity (cP $\times$ 100).

adequately describes the population of data points representing the relationship between product viscosity (denoted Y) and sodium chloride addition (denoted X). It is assumed the data in Table 10 represent a random sample of observations from the population of interest. According to this model, for each X_i there is a corresponding value Y_i, which is a function of $\beta_0 + \beta_1 X_i$, plus a deviation or random error term ε_i. The unexplained variation in Y_i, namely ε_i, represents the amount by which any individual Y_i falls above or below the regression line.

The least squares method provides a procedure by which estimates of β_0 and β_1 (b_0 and b_1, respectively) in Eq. (28) can be obtained to minimize the deviations, ε_i. More precisely, estimates b_0 and b_1 are selected to minimize the sum of squares (SSE) of the ε_i's. The SSE is expressed mathematically as follows:

$$SSE = \sum_{i=1}^{n} \varepsilon_i^2 = \sum_{i=1}^{n} (Y_i - \beta_0 - \beta_1 X_i)^2 \tag{29}$$

where n is the number of experimental runs or trials (i.e., in the shampoo example, $n = 16$). By using algebra and calculus, the values of b_0 and b_1 that yield the smallest possible value of SSE in Eq. (28) can be calculated by the following equations:

$$b_1 = \frac{\Sigma X_i Y_i - [(\Sigma X_i)(\Sigma Y_i)]/n}{\Sigma X_i^2 - (\Sigma X_i)^2/n} = \frac{\Sigma(X_i - \bar{X})(Y_i - \bar{Y})}{\Sigma(X_i - \bar{X})^2} \tag{30}$$

and

$$b_0 = \bar{Y} - b_1\bar{X} \tag{31}$$

where

$$\bar{X} = \sum_{i=1}^{n} \frac{X_i}{n} \quad \text{and} \quad \bar{Y} = \sum_{i=1}^{n} \frac{Y_i}{n}$$

Thus, Eqs. (30) and (31) provide the prediction equation or model:

$$\hat{Y} = b_0 + b_1 X \tag{32}$$

where $\hat{Y}$ is the predicted value of Y at a given value of X. Applying these equations for b_1 and b_0 to the shampoo example, the prediction equation relating viscosity to salt added can readily be determined ($n = 16$):

$$\Sigma Y_i = 21.0 + 27.5 + \cdots + 220.0 = 1260.0$$

$$\bar{Y} = \frac{1260.0}{16} = 78.75$$

$$\Sigma X_i = 0.0 + 0.1 + \cdots + 1.4 = 7.5$$

$$\bar{X} = \frac{7.5}{16} = 0.46875$$

$$\Sigma X_i Y_i = (0.0)(21.0) + (0.1)(27.75) + \cdots + (1.4)(220.0) = 874.8$$

$$\Sigma X_i^2 = (0.0)^2 + (0.1)^2 + \cdots + (1.4)^2 = 5.43$$

$$b_1 = \frac{\Sigma X_i Y_i - [(\Sigma X_i)(\Sigma Y_i)]/n}{\Sigma X_i^2 - (\Sigma X_i)^2/n} = \frac{874.8 - (7.5)(1260.0)/16}{5.43 - (7.5)^2/16}$$

$$= \frac{284.175}{1.914375} = 148.442703$$

$$b_0 = \bar{Y} - b_1 \bar{X} = 78.75 - (148.442703)(0.46875) = 9.167483$$

$$\hat{Y} = 9.167483 + 148.442703X \quad \text{(see Fig. 9)}$$

Certain assumptions are inherent in using the least squares approach to fit regression models to experimental data. Specifically, the estimates of the regression coefficients (b_0 and b_1) and predicted values (Y) will be best, that is, unbiased and having the least variance, if the following holds true: (a) the X values are fixed and not random variables; (b) the deviations (ε_i) are independent, uncorrelated, and have a mean of zero; (c) the variance of the deviations (denoted σ^2) is constant; and (d) the deviations (ε_i) are normally distributed. The last assumption of normality is important in that it allows the investigator to find the distribution of estimates b_0, b_1, and Y, and to perform appropriate tests of significance (i.e., F tests and t statistics, which will be covered in a later section).

b. Residuals

The residual (denoted e_i) is defined as the difference in the observed Y value (Y_i) and the predicted Y value ($\hat{Y}_i$) that is calculated from the prediction equation. It can be thought of as the amount of the response value Y_i that the regression model does not explain, or as the observed errors associated with the experimental data if the model is correct. Residuals for the shampoo example are given in Table 11. Provided the residuals have a mean zero and constant variance, and are independent and follow a normal dis-

Table 11 Observed Values (Y_i), Predicted Values ($\hat{Y}_i$), and Residuals (e_i) for Shampoo Example

Y_i	$\hat{Y}_i$	e_i
21.0	9.17	11.83
27.5	24.01	3.49
37.5	38.86	-1.36
33.5	38.86	-5.36
44.5	38.86	0.54
39.5	38.86	0.64
50.0	53.70	-3.70
61.5	68.54	-7.04
79.0	83.39	-4.39
80.0	83.39	-3.39
76.5	83.39	-6.89
92.0	98.23	-6.23
122.5	113.08	9.42
127.5	127.92	-0.42
147.5	142.77	4.73
220.0	216.99	3.01

tribution, plots of the residuals associated with the experimental data should (a) appear as points randomly scattered about a horizontal line when e_i is plotted against X_i, and (b) be scattered randomly about a horizontal line when e_i is plotted against $\hat{Y}_i$.

Abnormalities in the scatter pattern may suggest that the variance is not constant or that the model is inadequate. Sometimes this situation can be rectified by transforming an independent or dependent variable, or by adding additional terms to the regression model. Examination of residual plots is beneficial when dealing with simple models, but may not be suitable for more complicated models. For the shampoo example, examination of the residual plots (Fig. 10) reveals a curved relationship between both e_i's and

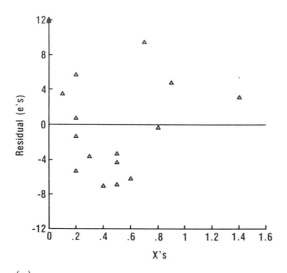

(a)

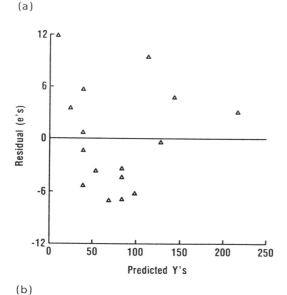

(b)

Fig. 10 Residual plots for shampoo example: (a) residuals (e's) against the independent variable, percentage NaCl added (X's); (b) residuals (e's) against the predicted dependent variable, final product viscosity ($\hat{Y}$'s).

X_i, and the e_i's and $\hat{Y}_i$. This suggests the regression equation should possibly contain a term(s) to account for quadratic effects.

c. The Coefficient of Determination, R^2

The residuals serve as a measure of how well the prediction equation fits the experimental data. Furthermore, that of the total variation in the observed values (Y_i's) about their mean, a portion can be explained by the predicted line, whereas the remainder is due to the random variation of the Y_i's about the line. More precisely,

$$\Sigma(Y_i - \overline{Y})^2 = \Sigma(Y_i - \hat{Y}_i)^2 + \Sigma(\hat{Y}_i - \overline{Y})^2 \tag{33}$$

Equation (33) states that the total sum of squares about the mean (*SST*) equals the sum of squares due to the regression equation (*SSR*) plus the sum of squares about the regression equation (*SSE*). This provides a method of assessing the strength of the regression equation; in other words, it is possible to determine how much of the variability in the experimental data is explained by the regression equation. By defining R^2, the coefficient of determination, as follows:

$$R^2 = \frac{SSR}{SST} \tag{34}$$

the amount of the total variation about the mean that is explained by the regression equation can be readily measured. The closer R^2 is to unity, the better the regression equation is at predicting the experimental data. This occurs when *SSE* approaches zero. For the shampoo example,

$$R^2 = \frac{SSR}{SST} = \frac{42183.7}{42699.5} = 0.988$$

d. The Analysis of Variance (ANOVA)

Equation (33) provides the basis for construction of the ANOVA table, a convenient representation of the components making up the variation associated with the dependent variable (Y_i). For the linear, first-order regression, model, $Y_i = b_0 + b_1X_i$, the analysis of variance is given in Table 12.

Using Table 12, the ANOVA for the shampoo example is shown below:

Source of variation	Degrees of freedom	Sum of squares	Mean square	Calculated *F* value
Total	15	42699.5		
Regression	1	42183.7	42183.7	1146.3
Residual	14	515.8	$s^2 = 36.8$	

e. The *F* Test

The ANOVA is useful in that it provides an *F* test for significance of the regression. In other words, when a regression model is fitted to experimental data, its adequacy can be tested with the *F* test. The test is essentially a comparison of two estimates of variance. The mean square for error (*MSE*) yields one unbiased estimate s^2 of the population variance σ^2. The mean square for the regression (*MSR*) provides a second unbiased estimate of the population variance σ^2, if the regression coefficients β_1, β_2, $\cdots$ are zero.

Table 12 ANOVA for a Linear, First-Order Regression Model of the Form $Y_i = b_0 + b_1X_i$

Source of variation	Degrees of freedom (d.f.)	Sum of squares (SS)	Mean square (MS)	Calculated F value
Total (about mean)	$n - 1$	$SST = \Sigma Y_i^2 - \dfrac{(\Sigma Y_i)^2}{n}$		
regression	1	$SSR = \dfrac{[\Sigma X_i Y_i - (\Sigma X_i)(\Sigma Y_i)/n]^2}{\Sigma X_i^2 - (\Sigma X_i)^2/n}$	$MSR = \dfrac{SSR}{d.f.}$	$F = \dfrac{MSR}{s^2}$
residual	$n - 2$	$SSE = SST - SSR$	$MSE = s^2 = \dfrac{SSE}{n - 2}$	

This becomes evident when one examines the expected values of *MSR* and s^2 [denoted $E(MSR)$ and $E(s^2)$, respectively] for the regression equation $\hat{Y} = b_0 + b_1 X$:

$$E(MSR) = \sigma^2 + \beta_1^2 \ \Sigma \ (X_i - \overline{X})^2 \qquad (35)$$

$$E(s^2) = \sigma^2$$

To test whether the regression coefficient b_1 differs significantly from zero, the *F* test ratio, $F = MSR/s^2$ is employed. For the first-order equation, $\hat{Y} = b_0 + b_1 X$, in testing b_1 for significance one is also testing the regression equation for significance.

A calculated *F* value greater than the tabulated critical $F (1, n - 2, 1 - \alpha)$ as illustrated in Fig. 11, indicates b_1 is nonzero and the regression is significant. *F* values less than the critical *F* suggest both *MSR* and s^2 provide reasonable unbiased estimates of σ^2, and the regression is nonsignificant.

f. Standard Error and Confidence Limits for the Regression Coefficients b_0 and b_1

The estimated standard error (s.e.) of b_1 is given by:

$$\text{s.e.}(b_1) = \frac{s}{\{\Sigma(X_i - \overline{X})^2\}^{1/2}} \qquad (36)$$

Assuming normality of the ε_i's, a confidence limit for b_1 of $100 (1 - \alpha)\%$ can be calculated using the *t* statistic:

$$b_1 \pm \frac{t(n - 2, 1 - \tfrac{1}{2}\alpha)s}{\{\Sigma(X_i - \overline{X})^2\}^{1/2}} \qquad (37)$$

where *t* is the $(1 - 1/2 \ \alpha)$ percentage point of a *t* distribution (Fig. 12) with $n - 2$ degrees of freedom.

The standard error and $100(1 - \alpha)\%$ confidence limits for the intercept b_0 can be calculated by using

$$\text{s.e.}(b_0) = \left\{ \frac{\Sigma X_i^2}{n\Sigma(X_i - \overline{X})^2} \right\}^{1/2} s \qquad (38)$$

$$b_0 \pm t(n - 2, 1 - \tfrac{1}{2}\alpha)\left\{ \frac{\Sigma X_i^2}{n\Sigma(X_i - \overline{X})^2} \right\}^{1/2} s \qquad (39)$$

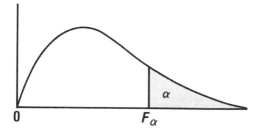

Fig. 11 Percentage points of the *F* distribution.

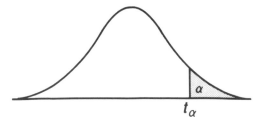

Fig. 12 Critical values of t.

Considering the shampoo example, the standard error and 95% confidence limit (95% C.L.) for b_1 and b_0 are as follows:

$$\text{s.e.}(b_1) = \frac{s}{\{\Sigma(X_i - \overline{X})^2\}^{1/2}}$$

$$= \frac{6.066}{1.91442} = 4.384$$

$$95\% \text{ C.L.} (b_1) = b_1 \pm \frac{t(n-2, 1 - \frac{1}{2}\alpha)s}{\{\Sigma(X_i - \overline{X})^2\}^{1/2}}$$

$$= 148.442703 \pm \frac{(2.145)(6.066)}{1.384} = 148.442703 \pm 9.401$$

$$139.041 \leq \beta_1 \leq 157.844$$

$$\text{s.e.}(b_0) = \left\{\frac{\Sigma X_i^2}{n\Sigma(X_i - \overline{X})^2}\right\}^{1/2} s$$

$$= \left[\frac{5.43}{16(1.91442)}\right]^{1/2} (6.066) = 2.554$$

$$95\% \text{ C.L.} (b_0) = b_0 \pm t(n-2, 1 - \frac{1}{2}\alpha)\left\{\frac{\Sigma X_i^2}{n\Sigma(X_i - \overline{X})^2}\right\}^{1/2} s$$

$$= 9.167483 \pm (2.145)\left[\frac{5.43}{16(1.91442)}\right]^{1/2} (6.066)$$

$$= 9.167483 \pm 5.478$$

$$3.689 \leq \beta_0 \leq 14.646$$

g. Standard Error and Confidence Limits for Predicted Values of $Y(\hat{Y}_k)$

As previously discussed (see least squares section), the predicted value of $Y(\hat{Y}_k)$ is equal to $\hat{Y}_k = b_0 + b_1 X_k$. The standard error of the predicted mean value of Y for a given X_k is:

$$\text{s.e.}(\hat{Y}_k) = s\left\{\frac{1}{n} + \frac{(X_k - \overline{X})^2}{\Sigma(X_i - \overline{X})^2}\right\}^{1/2} \tag{40}$$

From Eq. (40), it is obvious that the standard error is minimized as X_k approaches $\overline{X}$. In other words, the best predictions of Y_k for a given X_k occur close to the mean, $\overline{X}$. The confidence interval for the mean value of Y when $X = X_k$ is given by:

$$Y_k \pm t(n - 2, 1 - \tfrac{1}{2}\alpha) \, s\left\{\frac{1}{n} + \frac{(X_k - \overline{X})^2}{\Sigma(X_i - \overline{X})^2}\right\}^{1/2} \tag{41}$$

The predicted value of an individual value of Y is again $Y_k = b_0 + b_1 X_k$. However, here consideration must be given to the fact that an individual value of Y varies about a regression line with variance, σ^2. This leads to the following expression for confidence limits of an individual value of Y:

$$\hat{Y}_k \pm t(n - 2, 1 - \tfrac{1}{2}\alpha)\left\{1 + \frac{1}{n} + \frac{(X_k - \overline{X})^2}{\Sigma(X_i - \overline{X})^2}\right\}^{1/2} \tag{42}$$

By using the foregoing expressions the 95% confidence limits for the mean and individual values of Y are shown in Fig. 13 for the shampoo example.

h. Pure Error and Lack of Fit

As previously noted, the residuals and mean square for error (*MSE*) reflect the ways in which the selected regression model fails to explain the variation in Y. If the model is

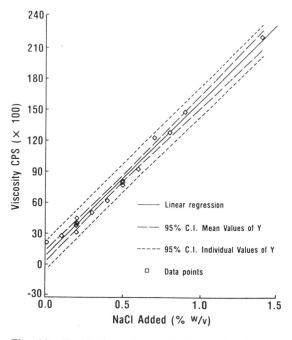

Fig. 13 The 95% confidence limits for the shampoo example.

less than optimal, *MSE* becomes larger, yet still provides an unbiased estimate of variance.

When a number of observations of Y are available at the same value of X, these repeated observations (or replicates) provide an estimate of the variance of Y. The mean square associated with the estimate is termed pure error, since it is an independent estimate of the variance of Y and is unaffected by the fitted regression model.

The mean square for pure error, denoted *MS(PE)* or s_e^2 is calculated using the following equation:

$$MS(PE) = s_e^2 = \left\{ \frac{\sum_{i=1}^{k}\sum_{u=1}^{n_i}(Y_{iu} - \bar{Y}_i)^2}{\sum_{i=1}^{k}n_i - k} \right\} \tag{43}$$

where subscript u refers to the number of replicates (n_i) at a given X_k. The calculation of the mean square for pure error in the shampoo example is as follows:

$$MS(PE) = s_e^2 = \frac{\begin{array}{c}(37.5 - 38.75)^2 + (33.5 - 38.75)^2 + (44.5 - 38.75)^2 \\ + (39.5 - 38.75)^2 + (79.0 - 78.5)^2 \\ + (80.0 - 78.5)^2 + (76.5 - 78.5)^2\end{array}}{7 - 2}$$

$$= \frac{69.25}{5} = 13.85$$

The pure error estimate for the variance σ^2 is readily incorporated into the ANOVA with the knowledge that the sum of squares for error (*SSE*) can be split into two components: the sum of squares owing to lack of fit, *SS(LOF)*, and the sum of squares from replicates, *SS(PE)*. Rewritten and rearranged in terms of the mean squares gives:

$$MS(LOF) = MSE - MS(PE) \tag{44}$$

The *F* ratio, $F = MS(LOF)/MS(PE)$, can then be used to test the adequacy of the regression model. If the calculated *F* value is larger than the tabulated critical *F* value for significance, the regression model has significant lack of fit and may be unacceptable. It should be noted that the critical *F* value is based on the degrees of freedom associated with each mean square. A nonsignificant *F*-test result indicates that the model is adequate and the value of *MSE* is a reasonable estimate of the variance that can be used for standard error and confidence interval limits. Incorporating lack of fit and pure error into the analysis of variance for the shampoo example yields:

Source	Degrees of freedom	Sum of squares	Mean square	Calculated *F* value
Total	15	42699.5		
Regression	1	42183.7	42183.7	1146.3
Residual	14	515.8	36.8	
Lack of fit	9	446.55	MS(LOF) = 49.6	3.58
Pure error	5	69.25	s_e^2 = 13.85	

The tabulated critical F value at $\alpha = 0.05$ with 9 degrees of freedom (d.f.) in the numerator and 5 d.f. in the denominator is:

$$F(9, 5, 0.95) = 4.77$$

Since the calculated F value of 3.58 is less than this value, the lack of fit is not signficant and the regression model $\hat{Y} = 9.167483 + 148.442703X$ is accepted.

i. Fitting More Complicated Regression Models to Experimental Data

Until this point, the least squares method and associated measures of precision have been applied to the simplest type of model, that is, a linear, first-order polynomial ($Y = \beta_0 + \beta_1 X + \varepsilon$) involving a single independent variable and response variable. In most real situations more complicated models having a greater number of variables or terms, and in many cases higher-order terms, are required to adequately fit the experimental data.

The same principles previously described for the least squares method can also be applied here provided that the coefficients β_1, β_2, $\cdot\cdot\cdot$ are linear. To do this, it is necessary to use matrix algebra. Although not reviewed here (see listed references), the matrix algebra approach can be used to accomplish the following: (a) obtain the least square estimates of the linear regression coefficients; (b) construct the analysis of variance [i.e., *SST, MSR, MSE, MS(LOF), MS(PE)*], thereby allowing one to determine the lack of fit, regression coefficient significance, and R^2; and (c) determine the variance, standard error, and confidence intervals for the regression model coefficients, the mean value of Y at X_k and an individual value of Y at X_k.

In summary, the principles of least squares analysis can be used to handle nearly all types of linear polynomial models through the matrix algebra approach. This approach to analysis has been facilitated by the use of computers for calculations involving more complicated regression models.

j. Selection of the "Optimum" Regression Model

When building a regression model, the experimenter must decide which variables should be included and which should not. To adequately explain the variability in the dependent variable (Y) and allow reliable values to be predicted, the model should include as many independent variables (X_k) as possible. However, because this often leads to complicated models that are difficult to understand, and the cost of running experiments with a large number of variables is high, a smaller model with fewer variables is desirable.

Several procedures have been frequently employed to determine which variables should be included in the regression equation. They include the all-possible regressions procedure, the backward elimination procedure, the forward selection procedure, and the stepwise procedure. For more details on these techniques the reader is referred to the listed references.

3. Mathematical Techniques for Locating an Optimum

After determining the mathematical relationship between the independent variables and the dependent or response variables(s), one of a number of techniques can be used to locate an optimal solution. For these techniques to produce a useful result, the mathematical model must be adequate in terms of predicting the response at any given value of the independent variables. Methods for assuring the adequacy of a regression model were described in the previous section.

The goals of optimization can be stated in terms of minimizing a function (called the objective function) of the response variables. By simply reversing the sign of the objective function, the problem can be changed to locate a maximum. Many applications of optimization have constraints or conditions imposed on the solutions. There can be both equality and inequality constraints on either the independent or response variables. For example, suspension viscosity (a secondary response variable) may have to be maintained within acceptable limits, while suspension potency (the primary response variable) is maximized. Likewise, the surfactant level in the suspension (an independent variable) might have to be maintained within practical limits. The introduction of constraints, although complicating the solution, increases the usefulness of the result. The basic optimization problem can be described mathematically as follows:

Select $x = (x_1, \cdots, x_n)$ to minimize the objective function A, where

$$A = f(x) \tag{45}$$

subject to m inequality constraints, $g(x)$:

$$g_k(x) \leq 0 \quad k = 1, \cdots, m$$

and l equality constraints, $c(x)$:

$$c_j(x) = 0 \qquad j = 1, \cdots, 1$$

As describe in the foregoing equations, optimization is simply finding the independent variable values that result in minimizing the objective function subject to constraints. Usually, convergence to a local minimum is partially dependent on the starting point. As seen in Fig. 14, a search beginning at either point A or point D will converge to a local minimum, whereas a search beginning at either B or C will find the global minimum or optima. Although there is no strategy that can guarantee global optimization, current practice calls for the use of multiple starting points to help protect against the local minimum phenomenon.

There are many optimization techniques available to the researcher; however, we will briefly describe only a few of the commonly used techniques. We will first describe some techniques for unconstrained optimization, followed by those for linear systems,

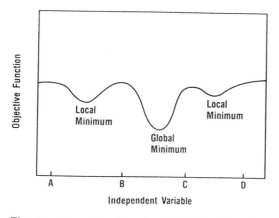

Fig. 14 Example of local and global minima in a known response surface.

and conclude with those for nonlinear systems. This list is not intended to be exhaustive. The interested reader is referred to the more detailed survey by Saguy et al. [60].

One of the simplest and earliest used unconstrained optimization techniques employs classic calculus to find the minimum of the objective function [61]. The first derivative of the objective function is set equal to zero and the resulting equation is solved for the independent variable value. This technique can be modified by the use of LaGrange multipliers to transform a system with equality constraints to an unconstrained problem. The addition of "slack variables" will likewise transform a system with inequality constraints. The application of this technique is limited to systems in which the objective function is differentiable, and the partial derivatives of the objective function, relative to the independent variables, must be continuous. As the number of variables or constraints increases or the complexity of the constraints increases, this technique becomes more unusable. An early example of the application of this technique to pharmaceutical systems was described by Fonner et al. [1].

Linear programming is one of the most widely used optimization techniques [62,63]. The principal advantage of linear programming is that it handles a large number of variables and constraints efficiently. Linear programming is applicable only to systems in which both the objective function and the constraints are linear and the model has no random error element. Thus, linear programming is not applicable to the type of response surface models described earlier [see Eq. (17)].

There are several techniques that can be used to find the unconstrained optima in the special case of only one independent variable. The most common of these are the grid search, the Fibonacci, and the quadratic techniques. The grid search and the Fibonacci technique involve observing the response values and computing the objective function at a series of specific intervals of the independent variable. The grid search uses equal interval spacing, while the Fibonacci search uses a series of progressively smaller intervals of which the width is based on the Fibonacci series. The optima is chosen from the setting that gives the minimum value of the objective function. The quadratic technique involves fitting a low-order polynomial (typically a quadratic) to the observed responses, much like interpolating to find the optima. The optimum can be determined by setting the first derivative to zero and solving for the value of the independent variable.

One of the more common techniques for unconstrained optimization with two or more independent variables is the simplex. The most basic form of the simplex, called a regular simplex, involves evaluating the objective function at $n + 1$ (where n is the number of independent variables) points equidistant about the starting point. A new point is added by reflecting from the vertex with the highest valued objective function to form a new simplex. This process is repeated, usually adjusting the span of the simplex to cover a narrower region, until the optima is located. Numerous variations have been developed to accelerate the convergence.

More computationally intensive methods are required to perform constrained optimization of systems of two or more independent variables. The most robust among these is the sequential unconstrained minimization technique (SUMT). This is an offshoot of the penalty function method [64]. The SUMT technique restricts the search to those points that satisfy the constraints, called the feasible points. This method can handle all types of constrained systems: linear and nonlinear, equality and inequality. The only requirement is that the objective function be computable.

B. Experimental Strategies for Response Surface Exploration and Optimization

This section deals with several *sequential experimentation* strategies for locating an optimal solution. Sequential experimentation allows the investigator to build on the knowledge gained at the completion of each part of the overall design strategy. If the entire experiment was designed and performed at the onset (i.e., *comprehensive experimentation*), the investigator would have to know (a) which variables were the most important, (b) the ranges of the variables to be studied, and (c) whether mathematical transformation of the data or responses was necessary. Early in the investigation, the experimenter is least able to answer questions of this type, but becomes more able to do so as the experimental strategy evolves.

Several of the algorithms used for determining the next set of experimental conditions in a sequential strategy are the same, or similar to, those used to search a mathematically defined response surface for an optimum (i.e., Fibonacci, simplex, as discussed earlier). During sequential experimentation, these algorithms are used to determine the conditions under which the next experiment or trial should be performed to further improve the measured response.

Finally, several sequential experimentation techniques, such as the univariate search and the sequential simplex, are not composed of randomly performed trials; therefore, some estimate of the experimental error is necessary to truly assess the results. Often this estimate can be obtained by randomly repeating selected trials near the optimal solution.

1. *Univariate Search*

Most researchers, at some time during experimentation, have used the "one variable at a time" method to obtain an "optimal" solution to a problem. Typically, this method involves changing one variable over a series of successive increments while holding the remaining variables constant. The direction in which the variable is moved is determined by whether improvement occurs in the measured response. When the best response is located, the adjusted variable is fixed at the appropriate level while another variable is successively incremented to determine further improvements in the measured response. The procedure continues until a tentative optimum is found for all variables. A second "cycle" is then initiated. Additional cycles are added until no further enhancement of the response takes place. At this point, an "optimum" is said to have been located. The size of the variable increment during the search can be fixed or randomly determined [60]. Other more efficient methodologies have also been developed for determining the increment size, including the Fibonacci technique and the golden section technique. These and other univariate techniques are discussed in detail elsewhere [17,25].

Interaction between variables may cause problems in locating the optimum when using univariate techniques. Figure 15 shows that interaction between variables, in the form of a rapidly rising or falling ridge, may lead to false conclusions about the location of the optimum. The univariate search initially conducted by varying X_1 (with X_2 fixed) along line AB indicates that point 0 is the optimum (see Fig. 15). By varying X_2 through point 0 (line CD), one falsely concludes that the optimum levels for X_1 and X_2 are found at point 0.

In summary, univariate techniques are often less efficient (i.e., more experimental trials are required) than other optimization strategies and, in the presence of significant variable interaction, may lead to false conclusions about the location of the optimum.

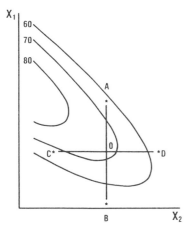

Fig. 15 Possibility of locating a false optimum (0) using the univariate technique on a rising ridge; asterisk indicates increment.

2. *Evolution Operations*

Evolutionary operation (EVOP) is a sequential optimization technique, first developed by Box and Draper [65], designed to be performed by process operators during full-scale manufacturing without endangering the final product. The procedure involves performing a simple experiment, typically a factorial design with a centerpoint, inside the range of operating conditions that will give acceptable product [66]. Changes in the processing variables are usually quite small, and often numerous trials are necessary to discern the effect of a variable from the experimental error. This is of little consequence, however, since a typical production operation is performed repetitively. When one set of data has been collected at all design points, a "cycle" is said to have been completed. Usually, a single cycle is not sufficient to detect any significant change in the response, so the experiment is repeated at the same design points (i.e., cycle 2). Additional cycles are performed until one or more processing variables, interactions, or the mean response proves to be significantly different from the experimental error. An estimate of the experimental error is obtained from the cycle data. After a significant effect has been detected, one "phase" is said to have been completed, and the processing variables are adjusted in a direction that improves the operation. The objective, as always, is to move in the direction of the optimum response. To facilitate EVOP procedures by production personnel, a simple form was developed for analysis of the data during the manufacturing operation [17,21,65]. Such forms have been adapted to the following example.

a. EVOP Example: Suspension Manufacturing

A large in-line rotor stator colloid mill with recirculating capabilities was adapted to a 5000-L tank for manufacture of a suspension. Because of active ingredient degradation, a 5% drug flush was added to the suspension to obtain a 24-month expiration dating. It was determined after production start-up that by reducing the heat generated during suspension homogenization, less active ingredients degraded and, therefore, a more stable product could be obtained. The improved stability would subsequently allow reduction of the drug flush, saving the company thousands of dollars, or an increased expiration dating, which was favorable from a marketing standpoint. Because product demand was great, the manufacturing operation could not be drastically disturbed for testing purposes. Evolutionary operation techniques were used to determine whether small changes in the rotor stator gap distances and total homogenization times could be made to minimize the final product temperature, without manufacturing material outside of company specifications.

A 2^2 factorial design, centered around the current operating conditions, was chosen for the study. The centerpont, taken at the currently used gap distance and homogenization time, allowed a check on possible changes in the mean suspension temperature that would indicate curvature in the response surface and the possibility that the current process was straddling a minimum (or maximum). Figure 16 shows the design setup and results of the first EVOP cycle in which each trial consisted of a separate production lot. The operating variable levels were coded at the upper ($+$), lower ($-$), and midpont (0) values, and the production lots were manufactured randomly. Table 13 is the first cycle worksheet results, tabulated by production personnel. The main effects and interaction term were calculated as described previously under common experimental designs. Unless a separate estimate of the experimental error is available, little information can be gleaned from the first cycle.

The second EVOP cycle was performed at the same operating levels. The results are presented in Table 14. Because none of the effects were greater than the error limits, which represent approximately a 95% confidence interval, any real effects could not be distinguished from experimental error. Some mathematical rationale behind the method of determining the standard deviation is presented elsewhere [21]. It is sufficient to say here that the standard deviation is based on the range and number of differences in the trial responses. The value $f_{k,n}$, where k is the number of design points (5) and n is the cycle number (2), is taken from a standard table [17].

A third cycle was performed under the same operating conditions and the worksheet results are presented in Table 15. In this cycle, the gap setting was shown to have a significant effect at the 95% confidence level. This ended the first EVOP phase and the results were presented to a special committee in the form shown in Fig. 17. After determining that the final suspensions were well within company specifications during phase 1 of the EVOP evaluation, a decision was made to reset the operating conditions at the high gap setting (0.016 in.) and, because it had no significant effect, a short homogeni-

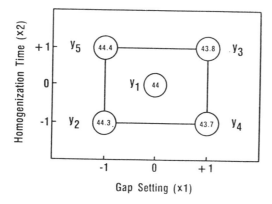

Fig. 16 Design setup and results for EVOP phase I, cycle 1: suspension example. The response y_i is product temperature (°C). Gap settings = 0.014 in. ($-$); 0.015 in. (0); 0.016 in. ($+$). Homogenization times = 55 min ($-$); 60 min (0); 65 min ($+$).

Table 13 EVOP Worksheet: First Cycle, Suspension Example

	5		3	Cycle: $n = 1$		Project: Suspension example
x_2		1		Response: Final product temperature		Phase: I
	2		x_1	4		Date: 9/9/85

	Calculation of averages					Calculation of standard deviation
Operating conditions:	1	2	3	4	5	
(i) Previous cycle sum						Previous sum $S =$
(ii) Previous cycle average						Previous average $S =$
(iii) New observations	44	44.3	43.8	43.7	44.4	Range of (iv) =
(iv) Differences [(ii) − (iii)]						New $S = $ range $\times f_{k,n} =$
(v) New sums [(i) + (iii)]	44	44.3	43.8	43.7	44.4	New sum $S =$
(vi) New averages Y_i [v/n]	44	44.4	43.8	43.7	44.4	New average $S = \dfrac{\text{new sum } S}{n - 1}$

Calculation of effects

Calculation of error limits

$x_1 = $ Gap setting effect $(G) = 1/2(Y_3 + Y_4 - Y_2 - Y_5) = -0.6$

$x_2 = $ Homogenization time effect $(H) = 1/2(Y_3 + Y_5 - Y_2 - Y_4) = 0.1$

$x_1 x_2 = G \times H$ interaction effect $= 1/2(Y_2 + Y_3 - Y_4 - Y_5) = 0$

Change in mean effect $1/5(Y_2 + Y_3 + Y_4 + Y_5 - 4Y_1) = 0.04$

For new average $= \dfrac{2S}{n^{1/2}} =$

For new effects $= \dfrac{2S}{n^{1/2}} =$

For change in mean $= \dfrac{1.78S}{n^{1/2}} =$

Table 14 EVOP Worksheet: Second Cycle, Suspension Example

	5	3
x_2	1	
	2	x_1 4

Cycle: $n = 2$
Response: Final product temperature

Project: Suspension example
Phase: I
Date: 9/19/85

Calculation of averages

Operating conditions:	1	2	3	4	5
(i) Previous cycle sum	44.0	44.3	43.8	43.7	44.4
(ii) Previous cycle average	44.0	44.3	43.8	43.7	44.4
(iii) New observations	43.6	43.0	43.9	44.0	43.2
(iv) Differences [(ii) − (iii)]	0.4	1.3	−0.1	−0.3	1.2
(v) New sums [(i) + (iii)]	87.6	87.3	87.7	87.7	87.6
(vi) New averages Y_i [v/n]	43.8	43.7	43.9	43.9	43.8

Calculation of standard deviation

Previous sum $S =$
Previous average $S =$
Range of (iv) = 1.6
New $S =$ range $\times f_{k,n} = 0.48$[a]
New sum $S = 0.48$

New average $S = \dfrac{\text{new sum } S}{n - 1} = 0.48$

Calculation of effects

$x_1 =$ Gap setting effect $(G) = 1/2(Y_3 + Y_4 - Y_2 - Y_5) = 0.15$

$x_2 =$ Homogenization time effect $(H) = 1/2(Y_3 + Y_5 - Y_2 - Y_4) = 0.05$

$x_1 x_2 = G \times H$ interaction effect $= 1/2(Y_2 + Y_3 - Y_4 - Y_5) = -0.05$

Change in mean effect $1/5(Y_2 + Y_3 + Y_4 + Y_5 - 4Y_1) = 0.02$

Calculation of error limits

For new average $= \dfrac{2S}{n^{1/2}} = 0.68$

For new effects $= \dfrac{2S}{n^{1/2}} = 0.68$

For change in mean $= \dfrac{1.78S}{n^{1/2}} = 0.60$

[a]$S =$ standard deviation, $f_{k,n} = f_{5,2} = 0.30$ where k is the number of design points and n is the cycle number.

Table 15 EVOP Worksheet: Third Cycle, Suspension Example

x_2 5   3
  1
  2   x_1 4

Cycle: $n = 3$
Response: Final product temperature

Project: Suspension example
Phase: I
Date: 9/29/85

Operating conditions:	\multicolumn{5}{c}{Calculation of averages}					Calculation of standard deviation
	1	2	3	4	5	
(i) Previous cycle sum	87.6	87.3	87.7	87.7	87.6	Previous sum $S = 0.48$
(ii) Previous cycle average	43.8	43.7	43.9	43.9	43.8	Previous average $S = 0.48$
(iii) New observations	44.2	46.2	41.2	41.0	46.0	Range of (iv) $= 5.4$
(iv) Differences [(ii) − (iii)]	−0.4	−2.5	2.7	2.9	−2.2	New S = range $\times f_{k,n} = 1.89^a$
(v) New sums [(i) + (iii)]	131.8	133.5	128.9	128.7	133.6	New sum $S = 2.37$
(vi) New averages Y_i [v/n]	43.9	44.5	43.0	42.9	44.5	New average $S = \dfrac{\text{new sum } S}{n-1} = 1.19$

Calculation of effects

x_1 = Gap setting effect $(G) = 1/2(Y_3 + Y_4 - Y_2 - Y_5) = -1.55^b$

x_2 = Homogenization time effect $(H) = 1/2(Y_3 + Y_5 - Y_2 - Y_4) = 0.05$

$x_1 x_2 = G \times H$ interaction effect $= 1/2(Y_2 + Y_3 - Y_4 - Y_5) = 0.05$

Change in mean effect $1/5(Y_2 + Y_3 + Y_4 + Y_5 - 4Y_1) = 0.14$

Calculation of error limits

For new average $= \dfrac{2S}{n^{1/2}} = 1.37$

For new effects $= \dfrac{2S}{n^{1/2}} = 1.37$

For change in mean $= \dfrac{1.78S}{n^{1/2}} = 1.22$

[a] S = standard deviation. $f_{k,n} = f_{5,3} = 0.35$, where k is the number of design points and n is the cycle number.
[b] Significant at 5% level.

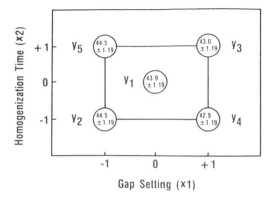

Fig. 17 EVOP phase I, cycle 3: Results for suspension example. The response (y_i) is average product temperature (°C $\pm$ standard deviation).

zation time (55 min). This resulted in a more stable product (i.e., longer shelf life), as well as a decrease in the overall production time.

Phase II of the project was then initiated around these new operating conditions (i.e., new design centerpoint), and EVOP was continued to further minimize the homogenized suspension temperature. This process was continued (i.e., phase III, phase IV) until no further decrease in temperature could be achieved without the possibility of jeopardizing the product integrity.

3. *Sequential Simplex*

The sequential simplex optimization technique was developed by Spendley et al. [67] and modified by Nelder and Mead [68]. Subsequent modifications of this technique have been made by others and are discussed elsewhere [60,69]. Geometrically, the simplex figures are similar to the mixture designs discussed previously (simplex lattice, extreme vertices) except that the sum of the levels of the factors does not have to add to 1. The simplex used in this technique is represented by $n + 1$ vertices of an n-dimensional figure, where n is the number of factors being examined. For example, to investigate two independent variables, the simplex design is a triangle. Typically, the independent variables are scaled to equivalent units. The results of previous experiments are used to define the variable levels for the next experiment in the search for an optimum. The simplex figure is then directed along the response surface following a set of rules that sequentially moves the response away from the poorest value. This technique does not require the generation of a mathematical model for response surface exploration. The methodology has been successfully applied in the pharmaceutical area to optimize a capsule formulation [70], obtain maximum solubility of caffeine in a mixed cosolvent system for parenteral administration [71], and the development of film coatings [72]. Chemical and analytical techniques have also been optimized using the sequential simplex technique [73].

The first step in the simplex procedure is to select the initial vertex, scale the independent variables to equivalent units, and generate the remaining vertices in the initial simplex. The experimental trials are then conducted at the initial simplex vertices and the responses are generated. Figure 18 shows an initial simplex (vertices $X_W X_S X_B$)

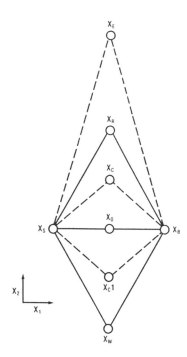

Fig. 18 Vertices of an initial two-dimensional simplex $(X_W X_S X_B)$ with operations to obtain the subsequent vertex: X_0 = centroid, X_W = vertex with worst response value; X_B = vertex with the best response value; X_S = vertex with the next best response value; X_R = new vertex obtained through reflection ($a = 1$), X_E = new vertex obtained through expansion ($b = 2$); X_C and X_C^1 = new vertices obtained through contraction ($c = 0.5$).

for a two-variable study. Three operations are then used to move the simplex along the response surface toward an optimum in the modified simplex technique:

Reflection. In Fig. 18, the worst response is found at vertex X_W, the best response at vertex X_B, and the second best response at X_S. By "reflecting" away from the vertex with the worst response (X_W) it is hoped that a value closer to the optimum will be located. Reflection away from X_W takes place through the centroid (X_0) of the remaining vertices (X_S and X_B; see Fig. 18), and the response at the new reflected vertex (X_R) is then evaluated. Mathematically, the reflected vertex is given by

$$X_R = (1 + a)X_0 - aX_W \tag{46}$$

where X_R is the reflected vertex, X_0 is the centroid of all the remaining vertices except for X_W, X_W is the vertex in the simplex having the worst response, and a is the reflection coefficient ($a > 0$), typically set at 1.0. The centroid X_0 can be calculated as follows:

$$X_0 = \frac{1}{n} \sum_{\substack{i=1 \\ i \neq W}}^{n+1} X_i \tag{47}$$

where n is the number of variables. If the response at vertex X_R lies between the responses at vertex X_S and X_B, then vertex X_R is retained and the new simplex ($X_S X_B X_R$; see Fig. 17) is evaluated.

Expansion. If the response during reflection at vertex X_R is better than the response at vertex X_B, then "expansion" of the simplex is attempted. The expansion operation is used in the modified sequential simplex technique to help the experimenter accelerate the process of locating an optimum. The point X_E in Fig. 18 represents a vertex found by expansion.

Mathematically, the expanded vertex X_E is given by:

$$X_E = bX_R + (1 - b)X_0 \tag{48}$$

where b is the expansion coefficient (>1), typically set at 2. If the response at vertex X_E is better than that at X_R, then X_R is replaced by X_E and the new simplex ($X_S X_B X_E$, see Fig. 18) is evaluated. If, on the other hand, the response at X_E is poorer than at X_R, the expansion process is considered unsuccessful. The vertex X_R is then retained and reflection begins again.

Contraction. If, during the reflection process, the response at X_R is worse than all the other responses in the simplex *except* for that at vertex X_W, we replace vertex X_W with vertex X_R and "contract" the new simplex $X_S X_B X_R$, see Fig. 18). Thus the new X_W will be X_R. The contraction operation not only accelerates the process of locating the optimum; but also allows the figure to better conform to the response surface, expecially if there are sharp ridges or valleys. Mathematically, the vertex generated by contraction X_C (see Fig. 18) is given by:

$$X_C = cX_W + (1 - c)X_0 \tag{49}$$

where c is the contraction coefficient ($0 \le c \le 1$), typically set at 0.5. If, during the reflection process, the response at vertex X_R is worse than all the other responses in the simplex, *including* vertex X_W, we retain X_W and locate the contracted vertex $X_C 1$ (see Fig. 18) using the same equation described earlier. If the contraction process produces a response at vertex X_C (or $X_C 1$) that is better than that at X_W, then the vertex X_W is replaced by vertex X_C (or $X_C 1$) and the reflection process proceeds. However, if the contracted vertex X_C (or $X_C 1$) produces a response that is worse than that at X_W, the contraction process is considered a failure and all X_i should be replaced by ($X_i + X_B$)/2 and the reflection process restarted.

The reflection, expansion, and contraction operations are performed until an optimum response is located, typically when several new vertices fail to produce a response better than a previous vertex. Other rules for sequential simplex optimization are found in the literature [74].

a. Modified Sequential Simplex Example: Emulsion Droplet Size Optimization

A pharmaceutical emulsion, after pilot plant scale-up, had become less stable owing to an increase in the average droplet size of the dispersed phase. During development, stable emulsions were fabricated having mean droplet sizes near 5 μm. After pilot scale-up, the droplet size of the product increased to 10 μm. The modified sequential simplex technique was used to determine if changing the levels of the two surfactants, Arlacel 80 and Tween 80, within their New Drug Application (NDA) limits would improve the stability of the emulsion by reducing the droplet size. The surfactant levels were scaled from 0 to 100% using the following equation:

$$F_S = \frac{F_i - F_{Lo}}{F_{Hi} - F_{Lo}} \times 100 \tag{50}$$

where F_S was the scaled surfactant level in percent, F_i was the actual surfactant level and F_{HI} and F_{LO} were the high and low limits for the surfactant level found in the NDA. The initial simplex was generated around the original formula having scaled values of 10% for both Arlacel 80 and Tween 80. The initial step for Arlacel 80 was chosen as 50% of the scaled values, and Tween 80 was set at 25%. The initial simplex and results of the experimental trials are shown in Table 16. Vertex 4 was generated by reflection away from vertex 1, which had the largest dispersed phase droplet size (i.e., 10 μm). The reflected point (X_R) and centroid (X_0) were calculated respectively using Eqs. (46) and (47) with a reflection coefficient (a) of 1 as shown below:

$$\text{Centroid} = \begin{pmatrix} \text{Tween level} \\ \text{Arlacel level} \end{pmatrix} = X_0 = \tfrac{1}{2} \times \begin{pmatrix} 35\% + 10\% \\ 10\% + 60\% \end{pmatrix} = \begin{pmatrix} 22.5\% \\ 35\% \end{pmatrix}$$

$$\text{Vertex 4} = \begin{pmatrix} \text{Tween level} \\ \text{Arlacel level} \end{pmatrix} = X_R = (1 + 1)\begin{pmatrix} 22.5\% \\ 35.0\% \end{pmatrix} - \begin{pmatrix} 10\% \\ 10\% \end{pmatrix} = \begin{pmatrix} 35\% \\ 60\% \end{pmatrix}$$

The experimental trial performed at this vertex (i.e., 35% Tween 80, 60% Arlacel 80) resulted in a dispersed phase droplet size of 6.8 μm (see Table 16). Since this response was better than any in the initial simplex, the next vertex was located in the direction

Table 16 Results of Modified Simplex Search: Emulsion Example

Vertex	Vertices retained[a]	Scaled factor level (%)		Dispersed phrase droplet size (mm)
		Tween 80	Arlacel 80	
1	–	10	10	10
2	–	35	10	7
3	–	10	60	9
4	2,3,R	35	60	6.8
5	2,3,E	47.5	85.0	5.4
6	2,5,R	72.5	35	8.0
7	2,5,C	56.9	41.3	6.0
8[b]	5,7,R	69.4	116.3	100[b]
8	5,7,C	43.6	36.6	6.5
9	5,7,R	60.8	89.7	5.8
10[b]	5,9,R	51.4	133.4	100[b]
10	5,9,C	55.5	64.3	4.0
11	5,10,R	42.2	59.6	5.5

[a]*R*, reflection; *E*, expansion; *C*; contraction.
[b]Boundary violation.

of the best response by using Eq. (48) and an expansion coefficient (*b*) of 2. The calculations were performed as follows:

$$\text{Vertex } 5 = \begin{pmatrix} \text{Tween level} \\ \text{Arlacel level} \end{pmatrix} = X_E = 2 \times \begin{pmatrix} 35\% \\ 60\% \end{pmatrix} + (1 - 2)\begin{pmatrix} 22.5\% \\ 35.0\% \end{pmatrix}$$

$$= \begin{pmatrix} 47.5 \\ 85.0 \end{pmatrix}$$

The experimental trial at this vertex again resulted in excellent improvement of the dispersed phase droplet size, which was determined to be 5.4 μm (see Table 16). This resulted in retention of vertex 5 and subsequent reflection away from vertex 3, which had the highest droplet size in the new simplex. The sequential simplex technique was continued, as shown in Table 16, until a minimum droplet size of 4 μm was obtained at a Tween 80 level of 55.5% and an Arlacel 80 level of 64.3%, resulting in an emulsion exhibiting acceptable stability properties. During the simplex procedure several boundary violations occurred in which the calculated scaled factor level exceeded 100% (see vertices 8 and 10, Table 16). Boundary violations are typically handled by arbitrarily assigning an unacceptable value to the response, in this example a 100-μm dispersed phase droplet size, and the simplex algorithm is then continued. The path of the simplex optimization is shown graphically in Fig. 19.

In summary, the simplex technique is a simple and often efficient method, useful for the development of pharmaceutical products or processes. The technique does not require the use of mathematical models, and experiments are performed iteratively to move in the direction of the optimum. Computer software can be used to greatly simplify the analysis [69]. Often, when an optimum is found, response surface models are generated to develop greater understanding of the area near the optimum point [70].

4. Response Surface Methodology

Response surface methodology (RSM), first developed by Box and Wilson [20], is composed of a particular set of mathematical and statistical techniques used to investigate

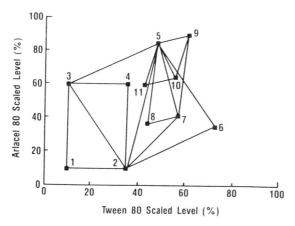

Fig. 19 Simplex path for emulsion optimization example. The numbers correspond to the vertices in Table 16.

the empirical relationship between one or more measured responses (i.e., dependent variables) and a number of independent variables, with the ultimate goal of obtaining an optimal problem solution. The basic components of this methodology include experimental design, regression analysis, and optimization algorithms, which were discussed in the preceding sections. The use of RSM not only allows the determination of an optimal set of experimental conditions that maximize (or minimize) a primary response, but it is also useful for examining changes in the response surface over a given range of independent variable levels. Response surface methodology can be broken down into three interrelated phases: the exploratory phase, the bounding phase, and the optimization phase.

In the *exploratory phase* the experimenter's objectives are to screen a large set (i.e., ≥ 9) of independent variables to determine whether they significantly affect the measured responses. Also, during this phase the direction toward the region most likely to include the optimal response is determined. In the *bounding phase*, the experimental region containing the optimum response is located and, in the *optimization phase*, levels of the independent variables that give the best response are determined. Typically, after location of the optimum, an experimenter may explore the area surrounding this point using several different analytical techniques. The RSM process is evolutionary and several experiments are usually performed to find a reliable optimal solution. In this discussion, an *experiment* is a set of related trials with the same variables and a common experimental region (i.e., the experimental design), whereas a *trial* is an experimental unit corresponding to a set combination of independent variable levels for which response values are measured.

Figure 20 is a flowchart showing how the three phases of RSM are interrelated. Notice that the exploratory or bounding phases often can be minimized or even eliminated if the investigator has a certain level of expertise or knowledge about the system

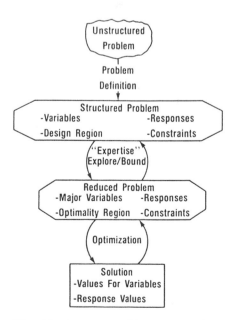

Fig. 20 Flowchart of interrelated phases used during response surface methodology.

and is relatively sure about the location of the optimum. By eliminating these phases, the investigator takes several risks, including (a) using an incorrect variable set, (b) choosing an experimental region that does not contain the optimum, and (c) choosing an experimental region that is too large to yield an accurate model using typical first- and second-order polynomial equations. In moving from the exploratory to the optimization phase of RSM, the number of independent variables is often reduced and the experimental region explored should become smaller.

a. Exploratory Phase

The exploratory phase is used to screen a large number of independent variables (i.e., ≥ 9) for significance as well as to determine the initial direction toward the experimental region containing the optimal response. Typically, minimal trial experimental designs, such as Plackett-Burman and fractional factorial designs, are used during this phase and, in most cases, the main effects are considered to dominate interaction terms. During this phase the investigator should determine a strategy for selecting experimental regions within the independent variable operating limits, design and conduct at least two experiments using this strategy and, finally, drop any variable that does not have a significant effect on the measured response(s) in at least one of the experiments. Two experiments are performed (with different independent variable intervals) to minimize the risk associated with improper interval width selection and with algebraic additivity of confounded effects. Figure 21 illustrates how selection of an improper independent variable interval width may lead to false conclusions about the area of optimal response. To help minimize errors of this type, a rule of thumb is to start in the middle of the operating limits and choose the interval width to be 20–25% of the operating range. A subsequent experiment is then performed in which the independent variable interval widths are adjusted, to move toward the region of optimal response.

b. Bounding Phase

The primary objective of the bounding phase is to locate the experimental region most likely to contain the optimal response. The experimental interval containing the optimum should be small enough to ensure that the first- and second-order polynomials frequently used in RSM will accurately estimate the true response surface. Also, if possible, the optimum should be located in the interior of the region (vs. boundary), to give the optimization algorithm the best chance of locating it. Typical experimental designs used during this stage include Plackett-Burman, fractional factorials, full factorials, and even central composite designs, if curvature estimation is required.

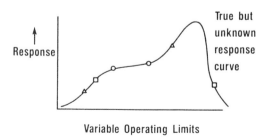

Fig. 21 The effect of the selected experimental independent variable interval width on the conclusions drawn about the measured response: circles, conclusion of no-effect (false); squares, conclusion of negative-effect (false); and triangles, conclusion of positive effect (true).

The basic strategy employed during the bounding phase is to keep moving the independent variable interval in a direction toward the optimum until no further improvement in the response is possible. Often, this will manifest itself in the form of a sign change (i.e., plus to minus) for the regression coefficient, as illustrated in Fig. 22. Figure 23 is a flowchart showing how a typical experimental strategy used during the exploratory and bounding phases can be applied in locating the optimal experimental region. Other strategies for moving toward the optimum experimental region include the steepest ascent technique [5,20], the method of parallel tangents [75], and the use of the sequential simplex, as discussed earlier.

c. Optimization Phase

When the optimal response is thought to be bounded, the optimization phase of RSM is implemented. The major objective of this phase is to find a set of independent variable values that optimize (i.e., maximize or minimize) a specific response. Typical experimental designs used in this phase include fractional and full factorials and various central composite designs if curvature in the response surface is apparent. Often, if the final design used in the bounding phase is suitable (i.e, fractional or full factorial with a design resolution of V or higher), it can be augmented with the appropriate starpoints and centerpoints to form a central composite design useful for determining a second-order polynomial model.

Once the model (or models, for multiple response systems) has been determined using regression techniques, an optimization algorithm is used to explore the primary response surface predicted by the derived equation and an optimal solution is located. For multiple response systems, the values of secondary responses are predicted at the independent variable levels giving the optimal primary response. Even though at certain times an investigator may be interested in maximizing (or minimizing) a primary response without considering the second responses (*unconstrained optimization*), most practical problems involve multiple response systems in which the secondary responses must fall within specified limits. The use of *constrained optimization* allows the investigator to find optimal levels of the independent variables to maximize (or minimize) a primary response while holding several secondary responses within an acceptable range.

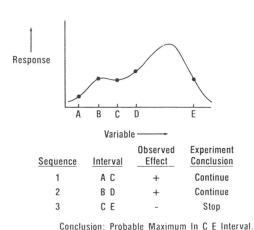

Sequence	Interval	Observed Effect	Experiment Conclusion
1	A C	+	Continue
2	B D	+	Continue
3	C E	−	Stop

Conclusion: Probable Maximum In C E Interval.

Fig. 22 Typical strategy used during the bounding phase of response surface methodology to locate the experimental region of optimal response (i.e., maximization).

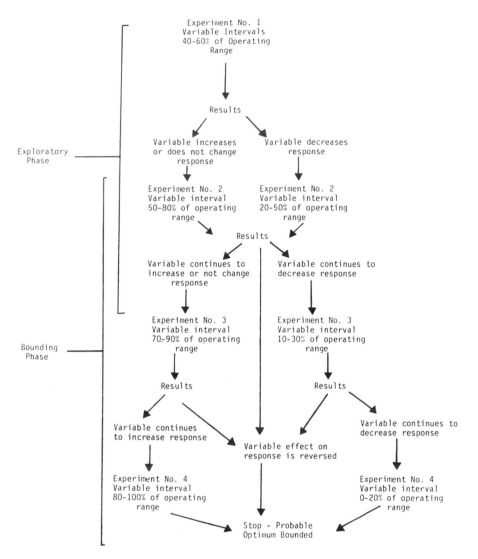

Fig. 23 Flowchart of experimental strategy used in the exploratory and bounding phases for a maximization problem.

Figure 24 graphically illustrates the difference between results obtained for an unconstrained optimization and those obtained when constraining a secondary response. After an optimal solution is determined, further evaluation of the results is usually undertaken.

   Model Verification. Assuming statistical analysis indicates that the model adequately represents the data, model verification is accomplished by performing an independent trial (or trials) using optimal levels of the variables and then comparing the measured response(s) with the results predicted by the empirical model(s). Ideally, model verification should include several trials over a range of the response surface to determine the model predictability at points remote from the optimum.

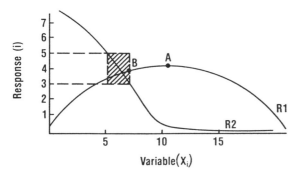

Fig. 24 Difference between the optimal primary response (R_1) for an unconstrained optimization and a constrained optimization where the secondary response (R_2) is constrained such that $3 \leq R_2 \leq 5$: A, optimal response; unconstrained optimization; B, optimal response, constrained optimization.

Graphic and Canonical Analysis. After locating an optimum, some form of graphic analysis is almost always performed in RSM. These techniques allow the experimenter to visually detect the true nature of the response surface generated by the empirical model; in particular, the magnitude of the relationship between the response and the independent variables. Figure 25 shows typical examples of contour plots fitted to a two-variable, second-order model having different values for the regression coefficients.

Canonical analysis consists of shifting the origin to a new point and rotating the axes through the new origin so they correspond to the contour axes. This methodology allows for easy interpretation of a second-order response function. Further details on canonical analysis are presented elsewhere [20,23].

Sensitivity Analysis. The object of sensitivity analysis is to allow the experimenter to determine how far the independent variables can vary without causing large changes in the optimal response. The usual goal of this type of analysis is to reduce the cost of the independent variables, while keeping the primary response at or near its optimum. For example, if the optimal point is at the top of a steep peak, small changes in the independent variables could cause drastic reductions in the primary response. If, on the other hand, an optimal solution is located on a stationary ridge (see Fig. 25), the independent variables often can be changed significantly while only minimally affecting the optimal response. Usually, the pharmaceutical investigator prefers the latter case as it gives flexibility in the independent variable levels without affecting final product quality. Sensitivity analysis can be performed graphically by simple examination of contour plots.

Another sensitivity analysis method frequently used is to constrain the *independent variable levels* to ranges close to their optimum level and search for a minimum (i.e., poorest response value) in the primary response. If the poorest primary response value in the constrained range of independent variables is acceptable (and the predicted secondary responses are also within limits), the constraints are iteratively broadened until an unacceptable minimum is located. This technique allows the experimenter to determine ranges of the independent variables that give satisfactory primary and secondary responses. Sensitivity analysis is an excellent technique for establishing rational limits

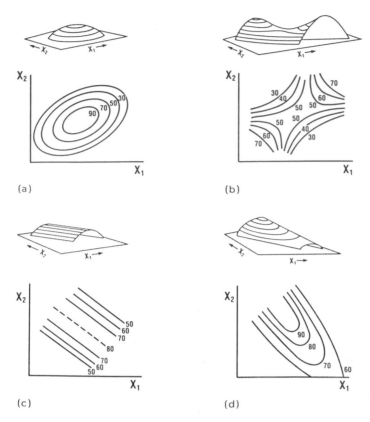

Fig. 25 Examples of response surface contour plots generated with the same second-order equation, $y = b_0 + b_1X_1 + b_2X_2 + b_{11}X_1^2\ b_{22}X_2^2 + b_{12}X_1X_2$, but with different coefficient values. (a) Peak or mound, (b) saddle point or minimax, (c) stationary ridge, and (d) rising ridge.

for formulation and process variables that are included in a New Drug Application.

Tradeoff Analysis. The major objective of tradeoff analysis is to find a set of independent variable levels that yields the best overall *set* of responses in a multiple response system. Typically, this type of analysis is performed by making successive optimization runs while varying the constraints on the *responses* assigned for tradeoff. The constraints are tightened during the successive trials until a set of acceptable solutions is located.

Figure 26 graphically illustrates a two-dependent-variable tradeoff problem and the resulting plot generated during the analysis. Many times tradeoff analysis results in several suitable solutions to a problem, and the "best" solution is often chosen subjectively by the experimenter. The use of *principal component analysis* allows identification of those responses that contribute the most information to the overall system being studied and, therefore, is useful for comparing multiple solutions or deciding which responses to constrain during tradeoff analysis [76,77].

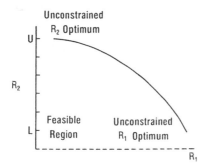

Fig. 26 Example of a two-response variable tradeoff plot where R_1 was maximized subject to the constraint $R_2 > K_I$, where K_I is an iteration between the upper (U) and lower (L) bounds of R_2 ($L \leq K_I \leq U$).

d. Response Surface Methdology: Suspension Example

During the development of a steroidal suspension, an investigator was interested in the effect of certain formulation and process variables on product stability. The independent variables, proposed operating limits, and the measured responses are presented in Table 17. Potency of the suspension was determined as the amount of drug remaining after 30 days storage at 75°C, and the viscosity (in centipoise; cP) was determined after exposure to the same accelerated conditions. The goal of the project was to maximize product potency after storage at 75°C for 30 days by determining the optimal levels of the independent variables. Suspension viscosity, a secondary response, had to be maintained within an acceptable range.

Two *exploratory* experiments were performed to determine which variables had a significant effect on the product potency as well as to determine the initial direction toward the optimal solution. The designs chosen for these first two experiments were 8/12 Plackett-Burman designs (i.e., 8-variables, 12 trials). The upper and lower levels

Table 17 Variables, Operating Limits, and Measured Responses: Suspension Example

Independent variable	Term	Operating limits
Temperature of H_2O for paraben dissolution (°C)	TEMP	60–100
Sodium carboxymethylcellulose (mg ml^{-1})	CMC	0–10
Number of passes through in-line homogenizer	PASS	1–6
Suspension pH	PH	3–7
Suspension buffer strength (% of hypothesized ideal)	BS	50–150%
Polysorbate 80NF (mg ml^{-1})	POLY	0–4
Methylparaben (mg ml^{-1})	MP	0–3
Propylparaben (mg ml^{-1})	PP	0–0.75

Responses

Potency, percent
Suspension viscosity, centipoise

of the independent variables were coded at +1 and –1, respectively. The experimental strategy used during the exploratory–bounding phase of this study was presented previously in Fig. 23. Any variable that did not significantly affect the product potency (i.e., regression coefficient confidence ≤75%) in *both* experiments was set at a fixed value for the remaining studies.

The trials were conducted and the data were entered into a statistical–mathematical computer program called POET (*P*rocess *O*ptimization through *E*xperimental *T*actics) frequently employed to solve problems using response surface methodology [28]. Basically, the POET package consists of a series of interactive programs that allow the experimenter to fit an empirical model to data from a designed experiment and to (optionally) optimize one of the responses with or without constraints on the independent or dependent variables. The optimization algorithm used by POET is the sequential unconstrained minimization technique (SUMT), which was discussed previously. Similar commercially available statistical computer programs for optimization studies are available [78], and many can even be used on a personal computer [79]. Software tools useful for experimental design and RSM are discussed later in this chapter. The results of the regression analysis for the primary response (potency) in both exploratory phase experiments are presented in Table 18.

Regression results were also generated for the secondary response, suspension viscosity, but are not presented here. The experimental variable interval widths (according to the strategy outlined in Fig. 23) and the interpretation of the regression results are presented in Table 19. The results of both experiments indicated that the number of passes through the in-line homogenizer (PASS), methylparaben level (MP), and propylparaben level (PP) did not significantly affect the product potency. These three variables were fixed at a level that would maximize product potency (as indicated by the regres-

Table 18 Summary of Regression Analysis on the Primary Response, Potency, for Two Experiments[a] Performed During the Exploratory Phase: Suspension Example

Term[b]	Experiment 1		Experiment 2	
	Regression coefficient	Confidence	Regression coefficient	Confidence
Intercept	68.413	100.00	73.7955	100.00
TEMP	0	0	1.6500	94.23
CMC	0.8665	99.26	0.9500	81.74
PASS	0	0	0.1500	19.72
PH	–0.6665	98.46	–1.5500	93.32
BS	1.8110	99.61	0.8205	76.75
POLY	–0.2940	88.54	–0.7990	75.78
MP	0.1335	60.90	0.5500	60.90
PP	–0.1335	60.90	–0.5500	60.90
Regression confidence	99.23		82.21	
R^2	0.9885		0.8977	
Estimated experimental error	0.4620		1.9055	

[a]Eight-variable, 12-trial Plackett-Burman design.
[b]For definitions, see Table 17.

Table 19 Summary of Exploratory Phase Experimental Strategy[a] and Results: Suspension Example

Variable	Experiment 1				Experiment 2			
	Variable interval[b]		Effect on potency[c]	Significant effect[d]	Variable interval[e]		Effect on potency[c]	Significant effect[d]
	−1	+1			−1	+1		
TEMP	76	84	0	No	80	92	+	Yes
CMC	4	6	+	Yes	5	8	+	Yes
PASS	3	4	0	No	4[f]	5	+	No
PH	4.6	5.4	−	Yes	3.8	5.0	−	Yes
BS	90	110	+	Yes	100	130	+	Yes
POLY	1.6	2.4	−	Yes	0.8	2.0	−	Yes
MP	1.2	1.8	+	No	1.5	2.4	+	No
PP	0.30	0.45	−	No	0.15	0.38[f]	−	No

[a]Eight-variable, 12-trial Plackett-Burman design.
[b]40–60% of operating range (see Table 18).
[c]+, increases potency; −, decreases potency; 0, remains the same.
[d]Confidence of regression coefficient ≥75%.
[e]50–80% of operating range if + or 0 effect on potency from experiment 1; 20–50% of operating range if − effect on potency from experiment 1.
[f]Rounded to nearest decimal.

sion coefficients) and a _bounding phase_ experiment was performed. The experimental design used during the bounding phase was a 2^{5-1} fractional factorial with a single centerpoint. The addition of a centerpoint allowed an estimate of the curvature present in the response surface [20,23]. At this stage in the experimental process, no reversal of effect (i.e., sign change of the regression coefficient) was observed for any of the variables, so the experimental strategy outlined in Fig. 23 was continued.

The results of the primary response (potency) regression analysis, including two-way interactions, are presented in Table 20 for the bounding experiment. The experimental variable interval widths and the interpretation of the regression results are shown in Table 21. The results indicated (a) that the variables did not significantly affect the potency within the range of tested values, indicating the existence of some kind of response surface plateau; and (b) that several variables (CMC, BS, and POLY) had a reverse effect on the suspension potency compared with the previous exploratory phase results, suggesting that the area of optimal response had been bounded. Table 22 summarizes the results from the three experiments performed in the exploratory–bounding phases and shows for each variable the experimental region that most likely contained the maximum potency.

Because the results of the bounding phase indicated significant curvature in the response surface, the _optimization phase_ was undertaken using a face-centered central

Table 20 Summary of Regression Analysis on the Primary Response Potency, During the Bounding Phase: Suspension Example[a]

Term	Regression coefficient	Confidence
Intercept	80.3450	98.26
TEMP	2.5500	53.71
CMC	−1.1870	30.68
PH	−1.147	29.79
BS	−1.580	38.73
POLY	0.0295	0.83
TEMP × CMC	0.9495	25.23
TEMP × PH	1.8135	42.92
TEMP × BS	0.8950	23.92
TEMP × POLY	0.5665	15.58
CMC × PH	−1.0455	27.49
CMC × BS	2.3675	51.35
CMC × POLY	−3.4405	62.88
PH × BS	2.2965	50.38
PH × POLY	0.7620	20.62
BS × POLY	−2.778	56.40
Regression confidence	22.80	
R^2	0.9052	
Estimated experimental error	9.0765	

[a] 2^{5-1} fractional factorial design with centerpoint.

Table 21 Summary of Bounding Phase Experimental Strategy and Results: Suspension Example[a]

Variable	Variable interval[b,c]		Effect on potency[d]	Significant effect[e]
	−1	+1		
TEMP	88	96	+	No
CMC	7	9	−	No
PASS	5[f]			
PH	3.4	4.2	−	No
BS	120	140	−	No
POLY	0.4	1.2	+	No
MP	2.4[f]			
PP	0.15[f]			

[a]2^{5-1} fractional factorial design.

[b]70–90% of operating range if coefficient from both previous exploratory experiments was + (or 0); 10–30% of range if −.

[c]The centerpoint for the experimental design was located at the midpoint of all ranges (0,0, 0,0,0).

[d]+, increases potency; −, decreases potency.

[e]Confidence of regression coefficient ≥75%

[f]Fixed from exploratory phase.

composite experimental design with three centerpoint replicates. The core of this design was a 2^{5-1} fractional factorial. The variable intervals, shown in Table 23, were widened slightly from those obtained during the bounding phase to obtain more information about the experimental region near the optimum. The experiments were performed and the data was input into the computer program. The regression results for potency and viscosity in the form typically generated by the POET computer package are shown in Tables 24 and 25, respectively.

Examination of the statistical output indicated that the models were acceptable and could be expected to accurately predict the responses within the inference space of the design. The regression results indicated that only the carboxymethylcellulose level (CMC), buffer strength (BS), and pH (PH) significantly affected the primary response, product potency, within the design limits. Curvature was evident by the significance of the squared terms (see Table 24). An unconstrained optimization was then performed, with the goal of maximizing suspension potency. An optimal predicted potency value of 93.210% was found at the independent variable levels shown in Table 26.

Because the predicted viscosity under these conditions was unacceptably low (i.e., 733.51 cP), the investigator decided to constrain this secondary response to greater than or equal to 800 cP to improve the suspension's rheological properties. The results are compared with those obtained during the unconstrained optimization in Table 26. An increase in product viscosity resulted in a suspension having poorer stability properties (i.e., potency: 86.882; see Table 26). Three-dimensional contour plots were constructed by varying the levels of two of the significant variables (i.e., CMC, BS, or PH), while holding the other variables constant at their optimal values and plotting the response. Figure 27 shows that when examining two variables at a time, the response surface was peaked or moundlike in appearance. The optimal potency was located at the top of the

Table 22 Summary of Exploratory–Bounding Phase Experiments and Probable Optimal Experimental Region for Significant Variables

Variable	Experiment 1		Experiment 2		Experiment 3		Probable location of maximum potency
	Variable interval	Regression coefficient sign	Variable interval	Regression coefficient sign	Variable interval	Regression coefficient sign	
TEMP	76–84	0	80–92	+	88–96	+	92–100
CMC	4–6	+	5–8	+	7–9	–	7–9
PH	4.6–5.4	–	3.8–5.0	–	3.4–4.2	–	3.4–3.8
BS	90–110	+	100–130	+	120–140	–	110–120
POLY	1.6–2.4	–	0.8–2.0	–	0.4–1.2	+	0.4–1.2

Table 23 Variables and Limits Included
in the Optimization Phase: Suspension
Example

Variable	Variable interval	
	−1	+1
TEMP	90	100
CMC	6	10
PH	3	4
BS	100	130
POLY	0.2	1.4

peak for the unconstrained optimization (see Fig. 27a–c), but was shifted down the side of the peak during the constrained optimization (see Fig. 27d–f). To obtain the best possible combination of suspension potency and viscosity, a tradeoff analysis was performed. The results, shown in Fig. 28, indicated that the product viscosity could be significantly increased to approximately 800 cP without a substantial reduction in suspension potency (i.e., ≥85%). At viscosities greater than 800 cP, suspension potency rapidly declined.

To verify the RSM study, the experimenter fabricated several trial suspension formulations at both the unconstrained and constrained optimal levels of the independent variables (see Table 26). Potency and viscosity were measured and good agreement existed between the predicted and actual results.

5. Robust Product and Process Design

a. Taguchi Methods

As part of product and process development, recent emphasis has been placed on designing products that are "robust" in nature. In the previous material, the primary criteria has been the optimization of a formulation or a manufacturing process to achieve the best possible product characteristics. Although this should always be a primary goal, it would also be advantageous from a cost and quality standpoint to design products that are insensitive to environmental, manufacturing, and component variation. Taguchi methods (TM), developed by Dr. Genichi Taguchi, have been successfully used to achieve this goal [80–82]. Although these techniques have not been extensively used in development of pharmaceutical products, they have been successfully used in other engineering applications [83] and are directly applicable to pharmaceutical formulation and process development.

The TM define product quality as the "loss a product causes society after being shipped, other than any losses caused by intrinsic functions" [80]. In TM, the product is said to lose quality as it deviates from a target value, even if it is within an acceptable specification range. Figure 29 graphically depicts the loss function, which, in its simplest form can be approximated by a quadratic equation. To minimize loss and, thereby, maximize product quality, a product should be manufactured at optimal levels of controllable variables, with minimum variation from target specifications caused by uncontrollable variables (noise). Controllable variables are those independent variables that can be specified or easily changed to control product characteristics. Noise variables

Table 24 Regression Results for Product Potency During Optimization Phase: Suspension Example

Term[a]	Coefficient	Confidence
INT	87.0637	100.00
POLY	-0.2062	20.32
CMC	-5.3728	99.99
BS	3.2383	99.69
TEMP	-0.4284	40.47
PH	-5.1626	99.96
POLY SQ	1.7874	64.80
CMC SQ	-9.7126	99.93
BS SQ	-7.2126	99.60
TEMP SQ	1.7874	64.80
PH SQ	-6.2126	99.11
POLY × CMC	0.5444	46.75
POLY × BS	0.5444	46.75
POLY × TEMP	0.2944	26.66
POLY × PH	-0.6295	46.91
CMC × BS	0.7944	63.09
CMC × TEMP	0.5444	46.75
CMC × PH	-0.8795	61.30
BS × TEMP	0.5444	46.75
BS × PH	0.3705	29.00
TEMP × PH	-0.8795	61.30

Source of variation	Sum of squares	Degrees of freedom	Mean square	Confidence
Regression SS	3467.4450	20	173.3722	99.99
Residual SS	64.0033	8	8.0004	
lack of fit	62.0033	6	10.3339	90.92
pure error	2.0000	2	1.000	
Total SS	3531.4483	28		

R^2 0.9819

Estimated experimental error 2.8285   Precision of model fit 15.9

Table 25 Regression Results for Product Viscosity During Optimization Phase: Suspension Example

Term	Coefficient	Confidence
INT	738.3705	100.00
POLY	−26.5079	99.99
CMC	51.8254	100.00
BS	−2.5635	46.62
TEMP	8.3810	93.38
PH	27.7630	99.97
POLY SQ	−18.3845	91.91
CMC SQ	−33.3845	99.33
BS SQ	19.1155	92.84
TEMP SQ	18.6155	92.22
PH SQ	−33.3845	99.33
POLY × CMC	−10.1786	95.65
POLY × BS	−10.5536	96.21
POLY × TEMP	4.8214	71.07
POLY × PH	9.7667	91.90
CMC × BS	−9.8036	95.01
CMC × TEMP	4.0714	63.40
CMC × PH	10.0167	92.51
BS × TEMP	3.6964	59.04
BS × PH	9.1417	90.13
TEMP × PH	−3.7333	53.26

Source of variation	Degrees of freedom	Sum of squares	Mean square	Confidence
Regression SS	20	104878.9180	5243.9459	100.00
Residual SS	8	1658.3923	207.2990	96.66
lack of fit	6	1639.7256	273.2876	
pure error	2	18.6667	9.3333	
Total SS	28	106537.3103		

R^2 0.9844

Estimated experimental error 14.3979   Precision of model fit 17.0

Table 26 Results of Unconstrained and Constrained Optimization: Suspension Example

	Optimal variable level	
Variable	Unconstrained	Constrained (viscosity > 800 cP)
POLY (mg ml^{-1})	0.2000	0.2000
CMC (mg ml^{-1})	7.3698	8.4235
BS (%)	116.87	126.79
TEMP (°C)	90	100
PH	3.366	3.4890
Predicted responses		
Potency (%)	93.210	86.882
Viscosity (cP)	733.51	800.00

are those that cannot be easily or cheaply controlled and can affect product characteristics over time. According to TM, there are three types of noise: (a) *outer noise*, caused by environmental factors such as temperature, humidity, or even operator variability; (b) *inner noise*, typically caused by deterioration in equipment or process variable control; and (c) *between product noise*, caused by unit-to-unit variation within a given batch or lot. As we reduce the effect of noise on product or process variability we improve the quality of a product. This is preferably done by reducing the sensitivity of the product to noise, rather than using higher cost components or new costly manufacturing technologies. In other words, we develop products to be robust against noise. The TM define the development of optimal formulation and process variables that are least sensitive to noise as the *parameter* design stage. It is this stage of product development at which the greatest improvement in quality is realized at the least cost.

The TM separately treat controllable and noise variables through the use of designed experiments having *inner* (controllable variables) and *outer* (noise variables) orthogonal arrays and the use of both response means and signal-to-noise ratios (S/N) during data analysis. Table 27 presents an example of a designed experimental layout using TM. Typically, the inner array is a type of fractional factorial design for the controllable variables. The outer array used for the noise variables is designed as a full or fractional factorial. Although noise variables cannot easily (or cost effectively) be controlled during actual operating conditions, significant effort (and cost) to control them during TM experimentation is undertaken. Data is collected on combinations of the controlled variables over the entire range of uncontrollable or noise variables. For extremely noisy systems, it may not be necessary to identify and control all the noise variables, but to simply perform several repetitions at each combination of controllable variable levels and analyze the data using S/N ratios. The S/N ratio is inversely proportional to the loss function (see Fig. 29). In other words, as the S/N ratio is maximized, loss is minimized, and quality is improved. The S/N ratio is based on the mean response at a given combination of controllable variable levels (signal) and the standard deviation caused by variation over the range of noise variables. Another way to view the S/N ratio is as a measure of dispersion of results around a target value. As the S/N ratio increases, the dispersion of results becomes narrower around the target value (i.e., the width of the

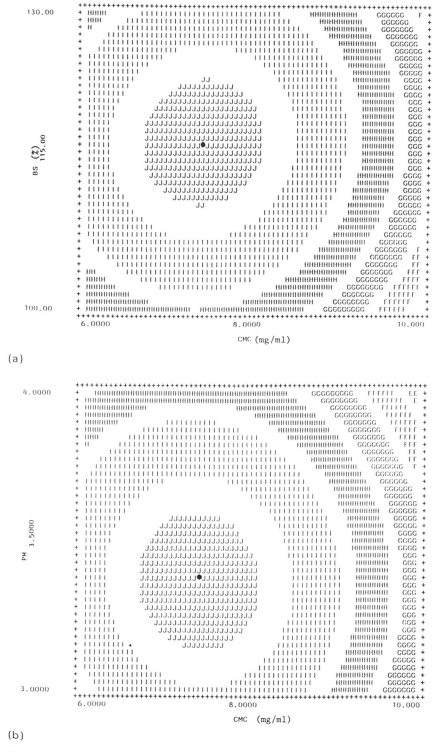

(a)

(b)

Fig. 27 Contour plots of product potency for (a–c) unconstrained and (d–f) constrained (i.e., viscosity ≥ 800 cP) optimization; suspension example. Two variables at a time were examined while the remaining variables were held at their optimal levels (solid circles indicates optimal potency). Key: Potency (%): E = 61.9–66.1; F = 67.9–72.1; G = 73.9–78.1; H = 79.9–84.1; I = 85.9–90.1; J = 91.9–96.1.

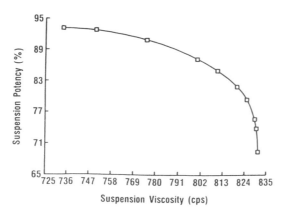

Fig. 28 Tradeoff analysis for product potency and viscosity: suspension sample.

distribution becomes narrower). The S/N ratio is calculated differently, depending on whether a target response is best, or if minimization or maximization of the response is best. The calculation differences allow a constant interpretation that the larger the S/N ratio, the better the product performance under "noisy" conditions. The calculations and theory behind S/N ratios are explained in detail in several references [80,84].

b. Taguchi Method: Suspension Example

A simple example of the use of TM to develop a robust suspension is presented in Table 27. The inner array of controllable formulation variables is based on a five-factor, resolution III, fractional factorial design. The noise variables in this example include shelf storage temperature, varied over the range expected to be found in the hands of the customer, and bulk drug particle size, which is costly to control from the supplier. The

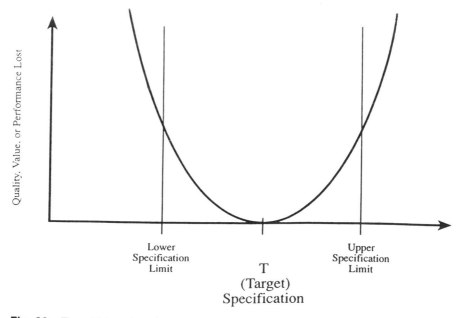

Fig. 29 Taguchi loss function.

Table 27 Experimental Design with Inner and Outer Arrays (Suspension Example with a Target Viscosity of 150 cps)[a]

| | Controllable Variables[b] | | | | | | | Noise Variables[c] | | | | | | | |
	A	B	C	D	E	F	G	0 / 0	- / -	+ / -	- / +	+ / +	Mean	Variance	S/N Ratio[d]
Trial	0	0	0	0	0	0	0	150	155	145	157	143	150	37.0	27.8
1	-	-	-	+	+			150	160	140	155	145	150	62.5	25.6
2	+	-	-	-	-			148	143	140	146	138	143	17.0	30.8
3	-	+	-	-	+			152	160	156	159	153	156	12.5	32.9
4	+	+	-	+	-			151	152	147	149	146	149	6.5	35.3
5	-	-	+	+	-			143	153	148	154	142	148	30.5	28.6
6	+	-	+	-	+			138	148	140	146	143	143	17.0	30.8
7	-	+	+	-	-			156	154	155	157	153	155	2.5	39.8
8	+	+	+	+	+			151	150	149	151	149	150	1.0	43.5

[a]Inner array (controllable variables)–2_{III}^{5-2} fractional factorial design. Outer array (noise variables)–2^2 factorial design.
[b]Suspension components: A, NaCl; B, sodium carboxymethylcellulose; C, surfactant 1; D, surfactant 2; E, surfactant 3
[c]F, shelf storage temperature; G, particle size of drug substance.
[d]S/N ratio for "target response is best" = $(S/N)_T = 10 \log_{10} (\bar{y}^2/s^2)$ where: $(S/N)_T$ = signal to noise ratio for target response is best
$\bar{y}$ = mean trial response averaged over the noise variables.
s^2 = variance of trial response averaged over the noise variables.

Table 28 Taguchi Method Comparison of Mean Responses and S/N Ratios for Suspension Example

Controllable Variable	Mean Response			S/N Ratio		
	+	–	Difference	+	–	Difference
A	146	152	–6	35.1	31.7	+3.4
B	153	146	+7	37.9	29.0	+8.9
C	149	150	–1	35.7	31.2	+4.5
D	149	149	0	33.3	33.6	–0.3
E	150	149	+1	33.2	33.6	–0.4

A, NaCl; B, sodium carboxymethylcellulose; C, surfactant 1; D, surfactant 2; E, surfactant 3.

product characteristic of importance is suspension viscosity. The objective is for the product to be as close to 150 cps viscosity as possible to minimize problems with delivery from a specialized device. The viscosity specification for the formulation is 145–155 cps when released under laboratory conditions. The current product formulation is represented by the values of controllable variables set at the midpoint (zeros) in the design, as shown in Table 27. It can be seen that this combination of controllable variables gives an optimal target viscosity of 150 cps. However, over the range of noise variables that could be experienced during production and in the field (bulk drug particle size and shelf temperature), the variation (variance = s^2 = 37.0 in Table 27) in viscosity associated with the current formulation could result in difficulties obtaining optimum delivery from the specialized device. Table 28 provides a simple TM comparison of the mean response and S/N ratios at low and high levels for each controllable variable. The results indicate the following: (a) Only controllable variables A (NaCl concentration) and B (sodium carboxymethylcellulose concentration; CMC) have a significant effect on the viscosity of the suspension. Viscosity is proportional to the sodium carboxymethylcellulose (CMC) concentration and inversely proportional to the NaCl concentration; (b) Variables A, B, and C (surfactant 1 concentration) can significantly effect the S/N ratio. The concentrations of these formulation variables are directly proportional to the S/N ratio. (c) The concentration of NaCl and CMC can be used to adjust the viscosity to the nominal value of 150 cps, whereas the levels of NaCl (factor A), CMC (factor B), and surfactant 1 (factor C) can be used to maximize the S/N ratio and thereby minimize variation in the product caused by the noise variables.

In the final analysis of the suspension example, the levels of NaCl and CMC were adjusted to the high end of the range tested to provide a suspension with a target viscosity of 150 cps. The upper limits of these controllable variables also resulted in a product that was most robust to the noise variables tested (i.e., maximum S/N ratio). The level of surfactant 1 was also adjusted to the upper end of the range tested to maximize the S/N ratio. Surfactants 2 and 3 had little effect on the target viscosity and S/N ratio and were relatively inexpensive; therefore, the levels of surfactants 2 and 3 were used at the high end of the range tested. These formula modifications (see trial 8 in Table 27) provided a product that met the target viscosity specification of 150 cps while greatly improving the robustness to variations in storage conditions and bulk drug particle size routinely experienced in the customer and manufacturing environments. Figure 30 compares the estimated normal distributions for product viscosity for the

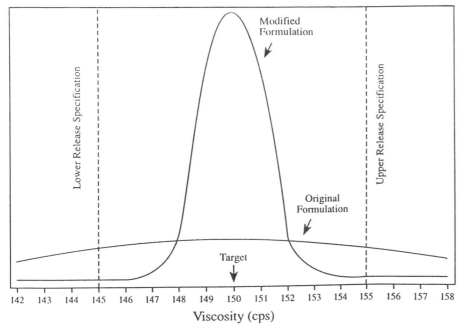

Fig. 30 Normal viscosity probability distributions under "noisy" conditions for the original suspension formulation ($s^2 = 37.0$) and the modified suspension formulation ($s^2 = 1.0$)

original formulation (see midpoint, Table 27) with that of the revised formulation (see trial 8, Table 27) when measured under "noisy" conditions.

c. Other Techniques for Robust Product and Process Design

Although the basic TM approach of improving product quality and robustness to environmental and component variation should be the goal of any pharmaceutical scientist, there are a number of criticisms of these technqiues in general. The major criticisms revolve around basic statistical assumptions and analysis promoted as part of the original TM techniques [85–87]. For example, noise factors may not vary independently as implied by the use of orthogonal outer arrays. In reality, correlation of noise factors may overestimate or underestimate the true variance of a response, thereby making it impossible to find the setting of control variables that minimizes noise [87]. Also, because of the correlation often seen between signal and noise, Box and Gunter suggest that response means and standard deviations be analyzed separately, rather than using the S/N ratios [85,87]. Taguchi methods also do not emphasize the determination and use of interactions between controllable variables as an effective means to improve product or process robustness [85,86]. There are a limited number of design types promoted by TM and many are relatively inefficient for derived information. In general, TM promotes the use of very large designs where the interactions are confounded with main effects. The results are then analyzed and a "best" set of controllable variables are "selected" from the experiments performed. Experiments of this type often involve numerous trials in regions that are nonoptimal. Determination of the effect of noise variables on controlled factor combinations that do not give acceptable product is inefficient use of experimental resources. A newer method called "robust product design" has been promoted that focuses only on evaluating control variable regions of interest relative to noise factors [88,89]. It has been recommended that sequential experimentation, regression analysis, response surface methodology, computer-generated graphics, and optimization algorithms (as previously described in the chapter) be substituted for the statistical techniques promoted by TM as a more efficient means of experimentation [85–89]. It has also been pointed out that noise due to long-term changes in processes or components may not be easily or well analyzed during short-term experimentation [88].

In conclusion, TM promotes the design of products and processes robust to "noisy" environments, which should be a key objective of any pharmaceutical scientist. By combining the goals of TM with the advanced statistical methodology promoted by Box [20,85] and others [86–88], advantages of each can be realized.

C. Software Tools

In the past 10 years there has been a great deal of interest in using software tools to automate the steps involved in experimental design and analysis. This interest includes both the use of computer-generated "algorithmic" designs (such as the D-optimal designs mentioned earlier) and the automated use of standard designs (such as factorials and response surface experiments). These tools have been very helpful in extending the use of statistically designed experiments beyond statisticians to engineers and scientists.

Some tools that are available seek to make statistical design easier for the non-statistician, and some tools seek to put a full range of mathematical tools into the hands of professional statisticians. Lack of clarity about the intended audience, unfortunately, can result in tools that try to do everything for everyone. These tools can be baffling to nonstatisticians.

The main problem with the design software of the past 10 years is that it simply has not been easy enough to use. Because of current rapid advances in software technology, this first generation of statistical design tools should soon be eclipsed by a second generation of tools based on graphic interfaces instead of character-based interfaces. We hope that this will result in statistical design products that are much easier to use, especially for nonstatisticians.

Because of the rapidly changing hardware and software environment, specific product recommendations will not be made. However, general guidelines for evaluating any software tool for statistical design follow:

1. It should help organize what is known about the variables—the number of variables and the range for each.
2. On the basis of how many variables are selected, it should provide some guidance for what designs are feasible (or even recommended) for the situation.
3. Once the feasible designs are selected, it should then generate the designs (using selected variable information), randomize the runs, and prepare a data collection form. This form should show the variables in their actual units, and the runs should be presented in random order.
4. After collection of the data, the software should guide you through a simple statistical analysis. Most current products simply provide a set of analysis tools, but it would be better if the software provided guidance for an analysis that was appropriate to the type of experiment conducted. For example, it should provide a graphic interpretation (i.e., normal probability plot), rather than a classic regression analysis, when the experiment is so small that few degrees of freedom exist for estimating error.
5. Unless the statistical software is to be used for other purposes, ease of use

should be the primary consideration in evaluating these products because they will probably be used only intermittently. Software that is too difficult to use will often get little use from the nonstatistician.

Some currently popular software packages for classic experimental designs (i.e., factorial) include Design Ease (Stat-Ease Inc., Minneapolis, MN), JASS (Joiner Associates, Inc., Madison, WI), X-STAT (Wiley Professional Software, New York, NY), and CADE (International Quality Technology, Ltd, Plymouth, MN). ECHIP (Expert in a Chip, Inc., Hockessin, DE) and RS/Discover (BBN Software Products Corp., Cambridge, MA) are useful software packages for classic, mixture, and optimal designs. For detailed information on specific software packages the reader is referred to an excellent review article by Nachtsheim [90].

III. STOCHASTIC MODELING

Stochastic or probabilistic modeling involves problems in which some or all the parameters are described by random variables, rather than the typical deterministic quantities. This type of modeling is often called "modeling under uncertainty," and one must resort to probability theory to describe the characteristics of a chance-dependent phenomenon. Although little has been published in the pharmaceutical literature on these techniques, stochastic modeling has been employed extensively in other industries [91–94]. Typical pharmaceutical applications have included comparison of tablet and capsule weight variation criteria using Monte Carlo simulation [95], cost evaluation of alternative pharmaceutical tableting processes using digital computer simulation [96–98] and evaluation of pharmaceutical process equipment and facility configurations [99–103]. While many methodologies exist for stochastic modeling, one of the most useful techniques for the investigator involved with the product and process development of disperse systems is digital computer simulation. In-depth descriptions of other techniques, such as stochastic linear and nonlinear programming and stochastic dynamic programming, can be found elsewhere [74,104,105]. No matter what methodology is employed, stochastic modeling involves the use of either discrete or continuous random variables. Discrete random variables, as the name implies, take only discrete values, whereas continuous random variables can take any value in a specified range. Both types of random variables can be described by a probability density function and a corresponding cumulative probability function, as depicted graphically in the examples shown in Figs. 31 and 32.

A. Digital Computer Simulation

Computer simulation can be broadly defined as the process of designing and developing a mathematical logical model of a system and performing experiments with this model on a computer [106,107]. A "system" in this case is a collection of interdependent elements that act together collectively to achieve some goal. Although data for a simulation can be determinisitic, there is generally a stochastic component involved in the model. Computer modeling and simulation are advantageous in that they permit the user to develop a thorough understanding of how a system behaves, as well as assisting in the evaluation of alternative conditions and strategies. This can be done without (a) building the system, if it is a proposed system; (b) disturbing the system, if it is an operating system that is costly or unsafe to experiment with; and (c) destroying the

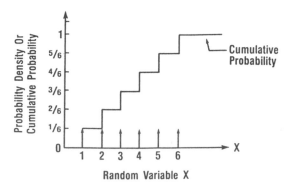

Fig. 31 Example of the probability density function and the corresponding cumulative probability function for a discrete random variable having a probability of 1/6.

system it the object of the experiment is to determine stress limits. Computer modeling and simulation also allow the user to maintain the same operating conditions for each replication or run of an experiment. This may be difficult to achieve using real systems. Obtaining a large sample size for an experiment may be difficult with some real systems owing to time and cost considerations. This can be overcome by using a simulated system.

Computer simulation should be considered when (a) a problem cannot be mathematically formulated, or when analytical techniques for solving the mathematical problem have not been developed; (b) mathematical techniques for problem solving are too complex or difficult to work with; (c) it is desired to view a simulated history of a process over a particular time span; (d) the only possibility of studying a phenomenon, owing to experimental difficulties, is to use simulation; and (e) the phenomenon being studied has an extremely long time span, and time compression would be useful [106,108]. The ideal simulation model, when complete, should be easily understood and goal oriented. Control and manipulation of the model should be simple, and updating or modifying it should require a minimum of effort. The simulation model should also be logical and

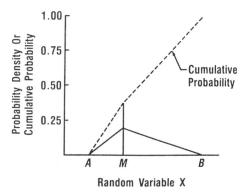

Fig. 32 Example of the probability density function (solid curve) and the corresponding cumulative probability function (dashed curve) for a continuous random variable in the form of a triangular distribution: (M = mode, A = minimum, B = maximum).

complete on issues involving the system, with the ability to be more complex if so desired.

Even though computer modeling and simulation seem to have numerous advantages over experimentation and analysis of real systems, there are certain disadvantages that the user of this type of analytical procedure should be aware of. These disadvantages may justify the use of an alternative analytical method or experimentation on the real system under investigation. For example, simulation models are artificial and can appear to represent the real system when, in actuality, they do not. A good simulation model often takes a great deal of time and money to develop, and lack of precision in the model often cannot be measured, which results in attributing a greater degree of validity than is justifiable to the simulation output [106,109,110].

Even though little has been published about the use of computer modeling and simulation in the pharmaceutical area, many other industries have used these techniques successfully. In the manufacturing environment, computer modeling and simulation can be useful in four major areas [111].

1. *Planning*—the effects of decisions on future production
2. *Scheduling*—the determination of policies that will increase production
3. *Logistics*—the coordination of system components to obtain desired objectives, such as new facility design
4. *Evaluation*—the determination of benefits derived from different manufacturing methods, increased levels of production, or different types of equipment.

The last area, evaluation, is the area most useful to the pharmaceutical investigator involved with the implementation of new manufacturing processes and equipment, whereas logistics modeling can be used for investigating material and product flow through a new facility and identifying bottlenecks caused by design restrictions.

The computer modeling and simulation process is composed of ten basic steps [106, 112–114]:

1. *Problem formulation.* This step requires defining the problem to be examined, as well as a statement of the problem-solving objective.
2. *Model building.* During this step, the actual or proposed system is reduced to a series of mathematically logical relationships, as defined by the problem formulation.
3. *Data acquisition.* This step involves identifying, specifying, and collecting the data needed for a specific example of the model.
4. *Model translation.* In this step, the model for computer processing is prepared.
5. *Verification.* In this step, it is established that the computer program is correct; that is, there are no "bugs" in the program.
6. *Validation.* This step requires the determination that the model represents the real system with a certain degree of accuracy.
7. *Experiment design.* In this step experimental conditions and factors that will help solve a given problem are chosen.
8. *Experimentation.* In this step the model is executed on a digital computer to obtain the desired experimental results.
9. *Analysis of results.* In this step, the model outputs are studied, to draw conclusions and make recommendations for problem resolution.
10. *Implementation and documentation.* This step involves the use of decisions

based on the simulation's results and documenting the model and its use.

Experimentation and analysis of a computer simulation can be undertaken using the experimental design [97] and response surface methodologies [115] described in the preceding sections.

Computer simulations can be grouped into two general categories: *Discrete simulation* models use time-advance mechanisms based on the occurrence of each significant event. "Events" used in this context mark the start and completion of an activity within the system. The dependent variables in this type of simulation model change discretely at specified points in simulated time. Discrete simulation is generally used in job shop, queueing, and batch-type simulations. *Continuous simulation* models use time-advance mechanisms based on fixed increments. The time in these models is updated at predetermined, fixed time intervals. Differential equations are often used to describe how a variable changes with time in simulations of this type. Continuous simulation is frequently used in biological and flow process modeling. In a *combined simulation* model, the dependent variable may change discretely or continuously.

Although a computer simulation can be programmed from the ground up using a language such as FORTRAN, there are several commercially available *simulation languages* that allow the user to interact with prewritten subroutines to greatly simplify the programming procedure. Table 29 gives a sample of some of the frequently used languages and appropriate references to each.

In recent years a new generation of computer simulation tools has been developed called *manufacturing simulators*. These tools are typically limited to discrete manufacturing models and incorporate higher level computer languages that allow the graphic assembly and subsequent animation of manufacturing system models. The manufacturing simulators are less flexible than simulation languages, but they have the advantage of being easy to learn and use, thereby allowing scientific and engineering staff not familiar with simulation programming to construct and analyze complex manufacturing systems on a personal computer [123]. Recently, a manufacturing simulator (WITNESS, AT&T Istel, Beachwood, Ohio) has been used to design and analyze a continuous process for solid dosage forms [124], a pharmaceutical packaging system [99], and a single-pot processing system for wet granulation [102]. Because of the large number of simulation languages and manufacturing simulators available, comparison of the advantages and disadvantages of each is beyond the scope of the discussion. The reader is referred elsewhere for this review [123].

Table 29 Some Widely Used Simulation Languages and References

Continuous model simulation languages	Discrete model simulation languages	Combination simulation language
MIMIC [116]	GPSS [113,117,118]	GASP IV [107]
DYNAMO [113,117]	SIMULA [117,118]	SIMAN [122]
	Simscript and Simscript II [113,117–120]	
	GASP II [113,121]	

The following discrete simulation example, patterned after a simple job shop problem [122], illustrates how computer modeling can be useful to the investigator involved with disperse system manufacturing equipment selection and process design.

1. *Computer Simulation: Cream Processing Example*

A manufacturer of semisolid products was interested in purchasing large-scale equipment for production of two different creams in a new facility. These products were high-volume pharmaceuticals and, although batch operations were used, the products were manufactured almost continuously. The initial capital investment included a large roller mill, necessary for dispersion purposes for cream A, and two large mixing vessels in which either cream A or cream B could be processed. Cream A was processed first on the roller mill and then in the mixing vessels, whereas cream B was processed using only the latter. Each lot of cream A was composed of five separate batches, and cream B was composed of eight batches per lot.

A first-in/first-out (FIFO) processing scheme was initially investigated because complete cleanup between each batch was necessary for proper equipment maintenance. This allowed FIFO scheduling of batches of two different products in the same equipment. Alternative scheduling procedures were later investigated using the simulated system. The maximum number of forecasted lots were 12 and 10 per month for creams A and B, respectively. The simulation was designed to move those numbers of lots through the modeled system before completion. The various processing and arrival times were estimated based on past experience with the product as well as historical tabulation of previous data. The data necessary to perform the simulation are presented in Table 30. The processing times shown in Table 30 include the preparation, processing, and cleaning times associated with each batch. A flow diagram of the modeled system and the events that take place during the simulation are shown in Fig. 33. Management was interested in determining the average in-process time for each lot of product in the production system. Equipment utilization and queue lengths were also of interest. The model was programmed using a commercially available simulation package and the simulation was performed.

Verification of the simulation was accomplished using data from another corporate division having a similar equipment setup for different products. The results of the simulation are presented in Table 31. The results indicated, on average, that lots of cream A spent a slightly longer in-process time in the system than did lots of cream B, as would be expected because of the processing differences. The average queue length for batches to be processed in the mixing vessel was larger than that for the roller mill, since both products were funneled into the mixing vessel queue.

Especially interesting was that the mixing vessel queue length reached 64 batches at some point during the simulation, even though the average mixing vessel utilization was only about 74% (i.e., 147.1%/200.00%; see Table 31). This would suggest that a change in scheduling procedure or equipment size or type might be advantageous. Changes such as these are easily made in a computer model. The simulation could then be rerun and the results compared. Finally, the total time necessary to process 10 lots of cream B and 12 lots of cream A was 182.3 hr (see Table 31). Under production conditions of 7-h shifts, one shift per day, it would take approximately 26 days to

Table 30 Data for Cream Processing Simulation

Cream	Maximum number of forecasted lots per month	Time between lot arrivals from central weighing areas (h)	Number of batches per lot	Roller mill processing time per batch (h)	Mixing tank processing time per batch (h)
A	12	14	5	3	Randomly selected from a uniform distribution between 1 and 2 h
B	10	Randomly selected from an exponential distribution having a mean of 3 h	8		Randomly selected from a uniform distribution between 2 and 3 h

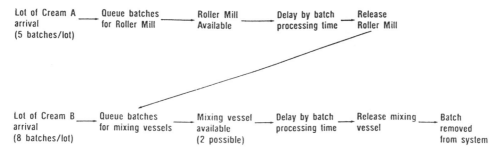

Fig. 33 Flow diagram of simulated system: cream example.

Table 31 Results of Computer Simulation: Cream Example

Output	Mean	Standard deviation	Minimum	Maximum
In-process lot time in system (h)				
Cream A	31.2	14.4	12.8	66.4
Cream B	26.5	14.7	1.3	50.2
Queue length (batches)				
Roller mill	3.8	1.9	0	8
Mixing vessel	15.6	20.6	0	64
Equipment utilization (%)[a]				
Roller mill	98.7	11.3	0	100%
Mixing vessel	147.1[b]	62.9	0	200%[b]
Total simulation time (h)	182.3			

[a]Equipment utilization = (time in use/total simulation time) × 100.
[b]Equipment utilization mixing vessel 1 plus equipment utilization mixing vessel 2.

manufacture all product lots. This manufacturing time would meet the predicted maximum marketing forecast for the products (i.e., 10 lots of cream B and 12 lots of cream A per month).

IV. CONCLUDING REMARKS

This chapter presents several experimental design, modeling, and optimization strategies that may prove useful to the pharmaceutical investigator involved with the product or process development of disperse systems. The choice of methodology resides with the investigator and is at least partially dependent on the type of problem to be solved. Each case should be judged according to time, money, labor, and effort involved. Improved reliability and performance of the final product or process is the ultimate goal of any optimization study when compared with trial-and-error development techniques.

While these techniques are well known, a recent survey of 68 pharmaceutical companies [125] indicated that only about 14% always use optimization techniques and 35% occasionally use them. Based on the recent emphasis of product and process justification during FDA pre-approval inspections, wider utilization of statistical design and optimization techniques should occur. Recent FDA-sponsored studies on the effects of formulation and process variables on physical and biopharmaceutical properties of immediate-release solid, oral dosage forms have emphasized the use of response surface techniques [126].

ACKNOWLEDGMENTS

The authors express their appreciation to Rodger Klassen and Vincent McCurdy for their helpful discussions on a variety of subjects. In addition, the authors especially thank Jan Sullivan, Melinda Young, and Linda Creech for their dedication in typing and preparing the manuscript. Special thanks to David Pearlswig for helpful discussion on computer simulation techniques and software.

REFERENCES

1. D. E. Fonner, Jr., J. R. Buck, and G. S. Banker, Mathematical optimization techniques in drug product design and process analysis. *J. Pharm. Sci.*, 59:1587 (1970).
2. M. R. Harris, J. B. Schwartz, and J. W. McGinity, Optimization of a slow-release tablet formulation containing sodium sulfathiazole and a montmorillonite clay, *Drug Dev. Ind. Pharm.*, 11:1089 (1985).
3. K. Takayama, H. Imaizumi, N. Nambu, and T. Nagai, Mathematical optimization of formulation of indomethacin/polyvinylpolypyrrolidone/methyl cellulose solid dispersions by the sequential unconstrained minimization technique, *Chem. Pharm. Bull.*, 33:292 (1985).
4. A. Devay, P. Fenkete, and I. Racz, Application of factorial design in the examination of Tofizopam microcapsules, *J. Microencapsulation*, 1:299 (1984).
5. S. Dincer and S. Ozdurmus, Mathematical model for enteric film coating of tablets, *J. Pharm. Sci.*, 66:1070 (1977).
6. R. M. Franz, J. A. Sytsma, B. P. Smith, and L. J. Lucisano, In vitro evaluation of a mixed polymeric sustained release matrix using response surface methodology, *J. Controlled Release* 5:159 (1987).
7. E. E. Hassan, R. C. Parish, and J. M. Gallo, Optimized formulation of magnetic chitosan microspheres containing the anticancer agent, oxantrazole, *Pharm. Res.*, 9:390 (1992).
8. K. Takayama and T. Nagai, Novel computer optimization methodology for pharmaceutical formulations investigated by using sustained-release granules of indomethacin, *Chem. Pharm. Bull.*, 37:160 (1989).
9. A. M. Falzone, G. E. Peck, and G. P. McCabe, Effects of changes in roller compactor parameters on granulation produced by compaction, *Drug Dev. Ind. Pharm.*, 18:469 (1992).
10. J. G. McGurk, D. W. Lendrem, C. J. Potter, Use of statistical experimental design in laboratory scale formulation optimization and progression to pilot plant, *Drug Dev. Ind. Pharm.*, 17:2341 (1991).
11. O. Shirakura, M. Yamada, M. Hashimoto, S. Ishimaru, K. Takayama, and T. Nagai, Particle size design using computer optimization technique, *Drug Dev. Ind. Pharm.*, 17:471 (1991).
12. M. J. Jozwiakowski, D. M. Jones, and R. M. Franz, Characterization of a hot-melt fluid bed coating process for fine granules, *Pharm. Res.*, 7:1119 (1990).
13. E. Senderak, H. Bonsignore, and D. Mungan, Response surface methodology as an approach to optimization of an oral solution, *Drug Dev. Ind. Pharm.*, 19:405 (1993).
14. D. E. Hagman, G. E. Peck, G. S. Banker, and J. R. Buck, An application of management science in pharmaceutical suspension design, School of Industrial Engineering Research Memorandum No. 73-1, Purdue University, West Lafayette, IN, April, 1973.

15. J. B. Schwartz, Optimization techniques in product formulation, *J. Soc. Cosmet. Chem.*, 32:287 (1981).
16. F. Pattarino, E. Marengo, M. R. Gasco, and R. Carpignano, Experimental design and partial least squares in the study of complex mixtures: Microemulsions as drug carriers, *Int. J. Pharm.*, 91:157 (1993).
17. V. L. Anderson and R. A. McLean, *Design of Experiments—A realistic Approach*. Marcel Dekker, New York, 1974.
18. I. W. Burr and L. A. Foster, A test for equality of variances. Department of Statistics Mimeo Series No. 282, Purdue University, West Lafayette, IN, 1972.
19. C. Yale and A. B. Forsythe, Winsorized regression, *Technometrics*, 18:291 (1976).
20. G. E. P. Box, W. G. Hunter, and J. S. Hunter, *Statistics for Experimenters*, John Wiley & Sons, New York, 1978.
21. C. R. Hicks, *Fundamental Concepts in the Design of Experiments*, Holt, Rinehart, & Winston, New York, 1973.
22. C. Daniel, *Applications of Statistics to Industrial Experimentation*. John Wiley & Sons, New York, 1976.
23. R. H. Myers, *Response Surface Methodology*, Virginia Polytechnic Institute and State University, Blacksburg, VA, Library of Congress Catalog Card. No. 71-125611, 1976.
24. J. Spitael and R. Kinget, Use of factorial design to evaluate the coating of powders in a fluidized bed, *Int. Conf. Powder Technol. Pharm.*, 7:1 (1978).
25. D. A. Doornbos, Optimization in pharmaceutical sciences, *Pharm. Weekbl. (Sci. Ed.)*, 3:33 (1981).
26. S. Bolton, J. Reinstein, and O. Alobe, Application of factorial designs in kinetic studies: Hydrolysis of benzylpenicillin solutions, *Int. J. Pharm. Technol. Prod. Manuf.*, 5:6 (1984).
27. S. Paschos, Y. Gonthier, and C. Jeannin, Evaluation of high temperature fluidized bed granulation parameters, *Int. J. Pharm. Technol. Prod. Manuf.*, 5:13 (1984).
28. "Process Optimization through Experimental Tactics—POET." Upjohn Technical Notes, Kalamazoo, MI, Feb. 2, 1984.
29. R. L. Plackett and J. P. Burman, The design of optimum mulifactorial experiments, *Biometrika*, 33:305 (1946).
30. V. I. Gorodnicher, H. M. El-Banna, and B. V. Andrew, The construction and uses of factorial designs in the preparation of solid dosage forms, *Pharmazie*, 36:270 (1981).
31. H. M. El-Banna, A. A. Ismail, and M. A. F. Gadalla, Factorial design of experiment for stability studies in the development of a tablet formulation, *Pharmazie*, 39:163 (1984).
32. V. A. Devay, B. Kovacs, J. Uderszky, and Z. Domotor, Multifactorial design optimization of film coating technique, *Pharm. Ind.*, 44:830 (1982).
33. R. A. McLean and V. L. Anderson, *Applied Factorial and Fractional Designs*, Marcel Dekker, New York, 1984.
34. S. Bisgaard, *A Practical Aid for Experimenters*, Starlight Press, Madison, WI, 1988.
35. K. Takayama, N. Nambu, and T. Nagai, Computer optimization of flufenamic acid/polyvinylpolypyrrolidone/methyl cellulose solid dispersion, *Chem. Pharm. Bull.*, 31:4496 (1983).
36. E. Fenyvesi, K. Takayama, J. Szejtli, and T. Nagai, Evaluation of cyclodextrin polymer as an additive for furosemide tablet, *Chem. Pharm. Bull.*, 32:670 (1984).
37. J. B. Schwartz, J. F. Flamholz, and R. H. Press, Computer optimization of pharmaceutical formulations. I: General procedure, *J. Pharm. Sci.*, 62:1165 (1973).
38. J. B. Schwartz, J. R. Flamholz, and R. H. Press, Computer optimization of pharmaceutical formulations. II. Application in troubleshooting, *J. Pharm. Sci.*, 62:1518 (1973).
39. N. Benkaddour, L. Bonnet, F. Rodriguez, and R. Rouffiac, Statistical optimization of paracetamol hydrophilic matrix formulations, *Lab. Pharma-Probl. Technol.*, 22:270 (1984).
40. J. B. Schwartz, Optimization techniques in pharmaceutical formulation and processing. In *Modern Pharmaceuticals* (G. S. Banker and C. T. Rhodes, eds.), Marcel Dekker, New York, 1979.

41. G. E. P. Box and N. B. Wilson, On the experimental attainment of optimum conditions, *J. R. Stat. Soc.*, 13:1 (1951).

42. M. Hirata, K. Takayama, T. Nagai, Formulation optimization of sustained-release tablet of chlorpheniramine maleate by means of extreme vertices design and simultaneous optimization technique, *Chem. Pharm. Bull.*, 40:741 (1992).

43. A. D. Johnson, V. L. Anderson, and G. E. Peck, A statistical approach for the development of an oral controlled-release matrix tablet, *Pharm. Res.*, 7:1092 (1990).

44. R. J. Belloto, Jr., A. M. Dean, M. A. Moustafa, A. M. Molokhia, M. W. Gouda, and T. D. Sokoloski, Statistical techniques applied to solubility predictions and pharmaceutical formulations: An approach to problem solving using mixture response surface methodology, *Int. J. Pharm.*, 23:195 (1985).

45. J. A. Cornell, Experiments with mixtures: A review, *Technometrics*, 15:437 (1973).

46. R. D. Snee, Techniques for the analysis of mixture data, *Technometrics,* 15:517 (1973).

47. R. A. McLean and V. L. Anderson, Extreme vertices design of mixture experiments, *Technometrics*, 8:447 (1966).

48. R. D. Snee and D. W. Marquardt, Extreme vertices designs for linear mixture models, *Technometrics,* 16:399 (1974).

49. A. I. Khuri and J. A. Cornell, *Response Surfaces—Designs and Analyses*, Marcel Dekker, New York, 1987.

50. J. A. Cornell and J. W. Gorman, Fractional design plans for process variables in mixture experiments, *J. Qual. Technol.,* 16:20 (1984).

51. J. W. Gorman and J. A. Cornell, A note on model reduction for experiments with both mixture components and process variables, *Technometrics*, 24:243 (1982).

52. M. Chariot, G. A. Lewis, D. Mathieu, R. Phan-Tan-Luu, and H. N. E. Stevens, Experimental design for pharmaceutical process characterization and optimization using an exchange algorithm, *Drug Dev. Ind. Pharm.,* 14:2535 (1988).

53. G. A. Lewis and M. Chariot, Nonclassical experimental designs in pharmaceutical formulation, *Drug Dev. Ind. Pharm.,* 17:1551 (1991).

54. R. D. Snee, Computer-aided design on experiments—some practical experience, *J. Qual. Technol.,* 17:222 (1985).

55. N. R. Draper and H. Smith, *Applied Regression Analysis,* John Wiley & Sons, New York, 1966.

56. R. J. Brook and G. C. Arnold, *Applied Regression Analysis and Experimental Design*, Marcel Dekker, New York, 1985.

57. W. Mendenhall, *Introduction to Probability and Statistics*, 4th ed., Suxbury Press, 1975.

58. G. J. Hohn, W. Q. Meeker, Jr., and P. I. Feder, The evaluation and comparison of experimental designs for fitting regression relationships, *J. Qual. Technol.,* 8:140 (1976).

59. G. E. P. Box, The exploration and exploitation of response surfaces: Some general considerations and examples, *Biometrics*, 10:16 (1954).

60. I. Saguy, M. A. Mishkin, and M. Karel, Optimization methods and available software, *CRC Crit. Rev. Food Sci.,* 20:275 (1984).

61. G. B. Thomas, *Calculus and Analytical Geometry,* Addison-Wesley, London, 1960.

62. S. I. Gass, *Linear Programming: Methods and Applications*, 3rd ed., McGraw-Hill, New York, 1969.

63. A. Charnes and W. W. Cooper, *Management Models and Industrial Applications of Linear Programming*, Vols. 1 and 2, John Wiley & Sons, New York, 1961.

64. A. V. Fiacco and G. P. McCormick, *Nonlinear Programming, Sequential Unconstrained Minimization Techniques,* John Wiley & Sons, New York, 1968.

65. G. E. P. Box and N. R. Draper, *Evolutionary Operation: A Statistical Method for Process Improvement*, John Wiley & Sons, New York.

66. M. H. Rubenstein, Evolutionary operations to optimize tablet manufacture, *Drug Cosmet. Ind.,* 4:44 (1975).

67. W. Spendley, G. R. Hext, and F. R. Himsworth, *Technometrics,* 4:441 (1962).
68. J. A. Nelder and R. Mead, A simplex method for function minimization, *Comput. J.,* 7:308 (1965).
69. L. J. Lucisano, Simplex-V vs. COPS: A comparative review of two simplex optimization programs, *Sci. Software.,* 4:166 (1988).
70. E. Shek, M. Ghani, and R. E. Jones, Simplex search in optimization of capsule formulation, *J. Pharm. Sci.,* 69:1135 (1980).
71. P. L. Gould, Optimisation methods for the development of dosage forms, *Int. J. Pharm. Technol. Prod. Manuf.,* 59:19 (1984).
72. C. J. Thoennes and V. E. McCurdy, Evaluation of a rapidly disintegrating, moisture resistant lacquer film coating, *Drug Dev. Ind. Pharm.,* 15:165 (1989).
73. D. E. Long, Simplex optimization of the response from chemical systems, *Anal. Chim. Acta,* 46:193 (1969).
74. S. S. Rao, *Optimization—Theory and Applications,* 2nd ed., Wiley Eastern, New Delhi, 1984.
75. R. J. Buehler, B. V. Shah, and O. KempThoren, Method of parallel tangents, *Chem. Eng. Prog. Symp. Ser.* 60 (1964).
76. N. R. Bohidar, F. A. Restaino, and J. B. Schwartz, Selecting key parameters in pharmaceutical formulations by principal component analysis, *J. Pharm. Sci.,* 64:966 (1975).
77. L. Benkerrour, D. Duchene, F. Poisieux, and J. Maccario, Granule and tablet formula study by principal component analysis, *Int. J. Pharm.,* 19:27 (1984).
78. COED: Computer optimized experimental design, User's guide CS-392, CompuServe Incorp, Columbus, OH, 1978.
79. J. S. Murray, *X-Stat-Statistical Experiment Design/Data Analysis/Nonlinear Optimization,* John Wiley & Sons, New York, 1984.
80. G. Taguchi, *Introduction to Quality Engineering—Designing Quality into Products and Processes,* Nordica International Limited, 1990.
81. G. Taguchi, Robust technology design, *Mech. Eng.,* 115:60 (1993).
82. D. M. Byrne and S. Taguchi, The Taguchi approach to parameter design, *Qual. Prog.,* 12:19 (1987).
83. J. C. Warner and J. O'Conner, Molding process is improved by using the Taguchi method, *Mod. Plast.,* 66:65 (1989).
84. G. Box, Signal-to-noise ratios, performance criteria, and transformations, *Technometrics,* 30:1 (1988).
85. G. Box, S. Bisgaard, and C. Fung, An explanation and critique of Taguchi's contributions to quality engineering, *Qual. Reliability Eng. Int.,* 4:123 (1988).
86. B. Gunter, A perspective on the Taguchi methods, *Qual. Prog.,* 20:44 (1987).
87. B. A. Jones, A robust approach to Taguchi methods, 12th Annual Rocky Mountain Quality Conference, Denver Colorado, June 8, 1988.
88. T. A. Donnelly, Robust product design, *Machine Design,* 59:77 (1987).
89. B. Wheeler, *ECHIP Course Text,* Expert In A Chip, Inc. (1987).
90. C. J. Nachtsheim, Tools for computer-aided design of experiments, *J. Qual. Technol.,* 19:132 (1987).
91. D. S. Surk and J. J. Talavage, A GASP IV model of steel ingot processing, *Simulation,* 29:49 (1977).
92. A. Levi and D. D. L. Cardillo, Simulation of a rotating track production line, *Simulation,* 31:155 (1978).
93. M. Cross and P. E. Wellstead, Some control and simulation aspects of the pelletizing of iron ore, *Simulation,* 33:181 (1979).
94. C. H. Falkner, Jointly optimal inventory and maintenance policies for stochastically failing equipment, *Oper. Res.,* 16:587 (1968).

95. M. E. Lacy, P. J. Davis, E. S. Johnson, and A. P. Koester, Comparison of tablet and capsule weight–variation criteria by Monte Carlo simulation, *Pharm. Technol.,* 9:98 (1985).

96. R. M. Franz, G. S. Banker, J. R. Buck, and G. E. Peck, Cost evaluation of alternative pharmaceutical tableting process by simulation, *J. Pharm. Sci.,* 69:621 (1980).

97. J. R. Buck, R. M. Franz, G. S. Banker, and G. E. Peck, Tableting production times, costs, and risks through simulation, *Drug Dev. Ind. Pharm.,* 6:237 (1980).

98. R. M. Franz, Tableting formulations and processes: Examination of the adsorptive properties of microcrystalline cellulose and the development of a comparative cost model and simulation for pharmaceutical tableting processes. [Ph.D. thesis] Purdue University, West Lafayette, IN, 1980.

99. L. R. Gibson and C. A. Winterberger, Simulation of a pharmaceutical packaging line, *Pharm. Eng.,* 12:24 (1992).

100. R. P. Poska, J. F. Glasscock, A. J. Badalamenti, D. B. Magerlein, and J. M. Magerlein, Evaluation of high-output tablet machines, *Pharm. Technol.,* 12:78 (1988).

101. D. Stapley, Pharmaceutical plant optimization and simulation, *Manufac. Chem.,* 59:47 (1988).

102. D. Pearlswig, P. Robin, and L. Lucisano, Simulation modeling applied to the development of a single pot process utilizing microwave vacuum drying, *Pharm. Technol.,* 18:44 (1994).

103. J. Branstrator and M. McCormick, Computer simulation justifies construction of Ciba-Geigy dyestuff production facility, *Ind. Eng.,* 21:17 (1989).

104. H. M. Wagner, *Principles of Operations Research,* Prentice-Hall, Englewood Cliffs, NJ, 1975.

105. H. M.Taylor and S. Karlin, *An Introduction to Stochastic Modeling,* Academic Press, Orlando, FL, 1984.

106. R. E. Shannon, *Systems Simulation—The Art and Science,* Prentice-Hall, Englewood Cliffs, NJ, 1975.

107. A. A. B. Pritsker, *The GASP IV Simulation Language,* John Wiley & Sons, New York, 1974.

108. F. F. Martin, *Computer Modeling and Simulation,* John Wiley & Sons, New York, 1968.

109. G. W. Evans, G. F. Wallace, and G. L. Sutherland, *Simulation Using Digital Computers,* Prentice-Hall, Englewood Cliffs, NJ, 1967.

110. R. S. Lehman, *Computer Simulation and Modeling,* Lawrence Erlbaum, Hillsdale, NJ, 1977.

111. D. Wortman, The potential role of statistical modeling for process evaluation. A report to the Management Conference for the Pharmaceutical Industry, Sept. 5–7, 1979, Purdue University, West Lafayette, IN.

112. D. N. Chorafas, *Systems and Simulation,* Academic Press, New York, 1965.

113. T. H. Naylor, J. L. Balintfy, D. S. Burdick, and K. Chu, *Computer Simulation Techniques,* John Wiley and Sons, New York, 1966.

114. J. M. Smith, *Mathematical Modeling and Digital Simulation for Engineers and Scientists,* John Wiley & Sons, New York, 1977.

115. D. C. Montgomery and D. M. Evans, Second-order response surface designs in computer simulation, *Simulation,* 25:169 (1975).

116. J. S. Rosko, *Digital Simulation of Physical Systems,* Addison-Wesley, Reading, MA, 1972.

117. J. E. Sammet, *Programming Languages: History and Fundamentals,* Prentice-Hall, Englewood Cliffs, NJ, 1969.

118. W. R. Franta, *The Process View of Simulation,* North-Holland, New York, 1977.

119. F. P. Wyman, *Simulation Modeling: A Guide to Using Simscript,* John Wiley & Sons, New York, 1970.

120. P. J. Kiviat, R. Villaneuva, and H. M. Markowitz, *The Simscript II Programming Language,* Prentice-Hall, Englewood Cliffs, NJ, 1969.

121. A. A. B. Pritsker and P. J. Kiviat, *Simulation with GASP II: A Fortran-Based Simulation Language,* Prentice-Hall Englewood Cliffs, NJ, 1969.

122. C. D. Pegden, *Introduction to Siman,* Systems Modeling Corp., Calder Square, PA, 1982.
123. A. H. Law and S. W. Haider, Selecting simulation software for manufacturing applications: Practical guidelines and software survey, *Ind. Eng.,* 21:33 (1989).
124. D. Pearlswig and J. Patton, Computer simulation techniques for process and facility design [Abstract], AAPS Arden House Conference, 1992.
125. R. F. Shangraw and D. A. Demarest, Jr., A survey of current industrial practices in the formulation and manufacture of tablets and capsules, *Pharm. Tech.,* 17:32 (1993).
126. L. J. Luciasano and R. M. Franz, FDA Proposed guidance for chemistry, manufacturing, and control changes for immediate-release solid doage forms: A review and industrial perspective, *Pharm. Technol.,* 19:30 (1995).

Index